Endocrine Pathophysiology

Eric I. Felner, MD, MSCR

Associate Professor of Pediatrics
Division of Pediatric Endocrinology
Director, Pediatric Endocrinology Fellowship Program
Director, Pediatric Clerkship
Emory University School of Medicine
Atlanta, Georgia

Adjunct Associate Professor of Chemical and Biomolecular Engineering
Georgia Institute of Technology
Atlanta, Georgia

Guillermo E. Umpierrez, MD, FACP, FACE

Professor of Medicine
Department of Medicine, Division of Endocrinology
Director, Diabetes and Endocrinology Section - Grady Health Care system
Emory University School of Medicine
Atlanta, Georgia

 Wolters Kluwer | Lippincott Williams & Wilkins
Health

Philadelphia · Baltimore · New York · London
Buenos Aires · Hong Kong · Sydney · Tokyo

Acquisitions Editor: Crystal Taylor
Product Manager: Lauren Pecarich
Production Project Manager: Priscilla Crater
Art Director: Doug Smock, Jennifer Clements
Designer: Joan Wendt
Production Service: Integra Software Services Pvt. Ltd.

Two Commerce Square
2001 Market Street
Philadelphia, PA 19103 USA
LWW.com

Printed in China

Library of Congress Cataloging-in-Publication Data
Endocrine pathophysiology (Felner)
  Endocrine pathophysiology / [edited by] Eric I. Felner, Guillermo E. Umpierrez.
    p. ; cm.
  Includes bibliographical references and index.
  ISBN 978-1-4511-7183-9 (paperback)
  I. Felner, Eric I., editor of compilation.   II. Umpierrez, Guillermo E., editor of compilation.   III. Title.
  [DNLM: 1. Endocrine Glands—physiopathology.   2. Endocrine System Diseases—physiopathology.
3. Endocrinology—methods. WK 100]
  RC649
  616.407—dc23

                                                                                        2013028725

Care has been taken to confirm the accuracy of the information presented and to describe generally accepted practices. However, the authors, editors, and publisher are not responsible for errors or omissions or for any consequences from application of the information in this book and make no warranty, expressed or implied, with respect to the currency, completeness, or accuracy of the contents of the publication. Application of the information in a particular situation remains the professional responsibility of the practitioner.

The authors, editors, and publisher have exerted every effort to ensure that drug selection and dosage set forth in this text are in accordance with current recommendations and practice at the time of publication. However, in view of ongoing research, changes in government regulations, and the constant flow of information relating to drug therapy and drug reactions, the reader is urged to check the package insert for each drug for any change in indications and dosage and for added warnings and precautions. This is particularly important when the recommended agent is a new or infrequently employed drug.

Some drugs and medical devices presented in the publication have Food and Drug Administration (FDA) clearance for limited use in restricted research settings. It is the responsibility of the health care provider to ascertain the FDA status of each drug or device planned for use in their clinical practice.

To purchase additional copies of this book, call our customer service department at (800) 638-3030 or fax orders to (301) 223-2320. International customers should call (301) 223-2300.

Visit Lippincott Williams & Wilkins on the Internet at: LWW.com. Lippincott Williams & Wilkins customer service representatives are available from 8:30 am to 6:00 pm, EST.

10   9   8   7   6   5   4   3   2   1

CCS1013

List of Contributors

STUDENT CONTRIBUTORS

Mark H. Adelman (MD 2011)

Sarah D. Turbow (MD 2012)

Bhavya S. Doshi (MD 2012)

Adva Eisenberg (MD 2013)

Kristina M. Cossen (MD 2012)

Steven A. Gay (MD 2013)

Robert S. Gerhard (MD 2013)

David L. Gutteridge (MD 2012)

Josh A. Hammel (MD 2011)

David Kappa (MD 2012)

Geoffrey S. Kelly (MD 2013)

Steven C. Kim (MD 2013)

Anna L. Lipowska (MD 2012)

Meredith MacNamara (MD 2013)

Stanislav Polioshenko (MD 2013)

Karen E. Schmitz (MD 2013)

Elicia D. Skelton (MD 2014)

Evan T. Tiderington (MD 2012)

Dane Todd (MD 2011)

Jason Zhu (MD 2013)

FACULTY CONTRIBUTORS

Milton R. Brown, PhD, MHA
Assistant Professor of Biochemistry
Division of Pediatric Endocrinology
Emory University School of Medicine

Mary S. Dolan, MD, MPH
Associate Professor of Gynecology/Obstetrics
Division Director, General Gynecology/Obstetrics
Department of Gynecology/Obstetrics
Emory University School of Medicine

Eric I. Felner, MD, MSCR
Associate Professor of Pediatrics
Division of Pediatric Endocrinology
Director, Pediatric Endocrinology Fellowship
   Program
Director, Pediatric Clerkship
Emory University School of Medicine

Raghuveer Halkar, MD
Associate Professor of Radiology
Division of Nuclear Medicine & Molecular
   Imaging
Emory University School of Medicine

Andrew B. Muir, MD
Bernard Marcus Professor of Pediatrics
Division Director, Pediatric Endocrinology
Emory University School of Medicine

Briana C. Patterson, MD, MSCR
Assistant Professor of Pediatrics
Division of Pediatric Endocrinology
Emory University School of Medicine

Jyotirmay Sharma, MD
Assistant Professor of Surgery
Emory University School of Medicine

Guillermo E. Umpierrez, MD, FACP, FACE
Professor of Medicine
Division of Endocrinology
Director, Diabetes and Endocrinology
   Section
Grady Health Care System
Emory University School of Medicine

All student contributors graduated or are on track to graduate from Emory University School of Medicine. All faculty contributors are on faculty at Emory University School of Medicine

Foreword

One of the best ways to learn is to teach. This is almost axiomatic for resident physicians and faculty; however, opportunities for medical students to teach are often limited. Moreover, the unavoidably large gap in knowledge between faculty members and those just starting their medical careers often leads to passive transfers of information, rather than active partnership in learning.

With this textbook of endocrine pathophysiology—the product of collaboration between 20 Emory medical students and 8 faculty members—Drs Felner and Umpierrez, together with their coauthors, have provided a shining example of how to involve medical students in educating themselves and others. The result is a textbook on a complex subject that perfectly addresses the needs of early phase learners including medical students and house staff. A consistent style is maintained throughout the book. Interest is maintained with clinical vignettes bracketing each chapter at the beginning and end; learning objectives are clearly outlined, and subsections are consistently organized. The learner can assess his or her progress with multiple-choice review questions accompanied by answers that are explained in detail. Reference lists consist mainly of appropriately selected review articles in widely available journals.

Many medical school pathophysiology courses are oriented strongly toward pathology as it occurs in adults. Yet children are not merely small adults and often are afflicted by distinct diseases. Moreover, they are far less likely than adults to have multiple medical problems or to suffer the long-term effects of poor lifestyle choices. Indeed, diseases in children often provide clearer insights into pathophysiology than can be gleaned by studying adults. This book strikes a particularly good balance between pediatric and adult pathophysiology by virtue of being edited by both a pediatric endocrinologist (Felner) and an adult endocrinologist (Umpierrez). Two additional specific chapters on pediatric endocrinology further ensure an appropriate balance between diseases of adults and children.

By integrating physiology, embryology, anatomy, and biochemistry with clinical endocrinology, this book is suitable for first- or second-year medical students taking an endocrinology core course, and for third- or fourth-year medical students on clinical rotations, as well as for residents who need a concise review of the subject to care for their patients. Medical students and residents have a lot that they need to learn, and Drs Felner and Umpierrez have greatly facilitated the acquisition of the basics of this complex and important field.

Perrin C White, MD
The Audry Newman Rapoport Distinguished Chair in Pediatric Endocrinology
University of Texas Southwestern Medical Center
Dallas, Texas

Preface

This book provides a comprehensive introduction to the pathophysiology of the endocrine system that is specifically geared toward medical students and house officers. Despite an abundance of endocrinology reference books, their content is primarily oriented to the description of their clinical presentation, diagnosis, and management of endocrine disorders, with limited information on pathophysiology. This can be overwhelming to a medical student who has yet to start his or her clinical years. This book aims to integrate physiology, embryology, anatomy, and biochemistry with the clinical patient encounters in the hospital and in the outpatient settings. It will assist medical students and trainees to better understand the physiologic and pathophysiologic conditions of the endocrine system. Emphasis is placed primarily on the basic physiology by which endocrine diseases develop, in order to facilitate understanding of both clinical diagnosis and therapy.

The motivation for writing this book was a perceived need by our first- and second-year medical students at Emory University School of Medicine. When our Medical School underwent a revision of its curriculum in 2007, with reduction of lecture time and greater emphasis on small group learning, students required a different approach to learning. This created an opportunity to develop a book that met the needs of our students in a new paradigm of learning. We realized that the best resource would be a pathophysiology textbook with major input from the students themselves. We believed that faculty guidance would further enhance each chapter and lend credence to the final product. By the time these young medical students entered the third and fourth years, they were capable of writing a cogent and easily readable chapter for their younger colleagues, with the help of an experienced faculty member.

This book is unique for a number of reasons. It is the first comprehensive endocrine pathophysiology text written by medical students and faculty. The goal for pairing a student with a faculty member was to focus on the needs of the student, while providing the expertise by the faculty. Since learning is enhanced by testing, every chapter concludes with a series of multiple-choice questions. Each question is annotated in detail, with the correct answer and each incorrect answer fully explained.

The first chapter is a basic introduction to endocrinology. The next 12 chapters follow a head-to-toe sequence as follows: hypothalamus and pituitary gland (Chapter 2), thyroid gland (Chapter 3), parathyroid gland (Chapters 4 and 5), pancreas (Chapters 6 to 8), obesity (Chapter 9), adrenal gland (Chapters 10 and 11), and reproduction (Chapters 12 and 13). The remaining chapters do not follow an anatomical format, but include important areas of endocrinology including pediatric endocrinology (Chapters 14 and 15), the autoimmune polyglandular syndromes (Chapter 16), multiple endocrine neoplasia (Chapter 17), endocrine biochemical testing (Chapter 18), stimulation and suppression testing (Chapter 19), radiologic and nuclear medicine approaches to endocrine diseases (Chapter 20), and surgical approaches to endocrine disorders (Chapter 21).

It has been a great opportunity for these 20 highly motivated medical students and a privilege for us to collaborate with them that spanned four graduation classes at Emory. Their enthusiasm, dedication, and attention to detail, while still involved in their medical school activities, have made this book a labor of love and created an easily readable and informative text for all of the students who will follow them. We are grateful to our faculty colleagues who coauthored each chapter for the time, effort, expertise, and commitment to this book.

Finally, a project of this magnitude that required more than 3 years to complete could not have occurred without the support and patience of our families—for whom we are both extremely grateful.

We hope that readers of this book will expand their understanding of the endocrine system, specifically the pathophysiology, and the specialty areas that few medical school textbooks have addressed. We also hope that this book provides a solid foundation for further learning and clinical care of your patients.

Eric I. Felner, MD, MSCR
Guillermo E. Umpierrez, MD, FACP, FACE

Contents

Basic Endocrinology and Function

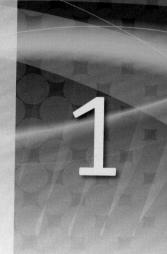

1

Eric I. Felner
Guillermo E. Umpierrez

CASE

You are called to see a 27-year-old previously healthy man who is in the local emergency center because he was involved in a motor vehicle accident 1 hour ago. He is conscious but not completely alert. He is afebrile and his blood pressure is 95/42 mmHg. He is able to move all of his extremities but complains of significant pain over his right thigh. He is wearing a medical identification bracelet, but the information has worn off. Due to concern for certain life-threatening conditions, a series of laboratory tests are ordered. After receiving intravenous fluids, his blood pressure improves to 125/75 mmHg, and he is now alert and oriented. A radiograph of his right leg shows a midfemur fracture. Prior to entering the operating room, he informs you that he wears the bracelet because he has a penicillin allergy. He receives pain medication, and, shortly prior to undergoing surgical reduction of his femur, the operating room nurse states that his electrolyte panel, blood count, liver function, and kidney function are normal. He does, however, have an elevated cortisol of 35 mcg/dL (normal = 8 to 22). Should the surgeon be concerned about operating on a man with an elevated cortisol level?

Knowledge of the anatomy and normal function of the endocrine glands is crucial to understanding and evaluating the diseases that affect the endocrine system. This chapter reviews the physiology of the endocrine system to help the learner recognize appropriate hormone responses to the above clinical scenario. We summarize the appropriate responses to a stressful event at the end of the chapter to give the learner a better understanding of endocrine physiology. The remaining chapters focus on pathophysiology.

CHAPTER OUTLINE

Endocrine System
  Endocrine Glands
  Hormone–Receptor Interactions
  Hormone Classification
    Peptides
    Steroid Hormones
    Amine Hormones
Endocrine Homeostasis and
Feedback Regulation
Hormone Excess, Deficiency, and
Resistance
Clinical Endocrinology

OBJECTIVES

1. Define endocrinology.

2. Recognize the components of the endocrine system.

3. Compare and contrast the two major classes of hormones.

4. List the hormones and the glands that produce them.

ENDOCRINE SYSTEM

The endocrine and nervous systems are the two major organ systems by which cells and tissues communicate. From a simple perspective, endocrinology can be defined as the study of glands, the hormones they produce, and the effects of the hormones. Hormones are secreted directly into circulation and exert their effects by binding to receptors in or on target cells. Hormones may act within the same cell (autocrine action), on neighboring cells (paracrine action), or on distal cells (endocrine action).

A more in-depth study of endocrinology encompasses the following: 1) regulation of hormone synthesis and secretion; 2) hormone–receptor interaction; 3) interaction between endocrine organs and target tissues; 4) hormone deficiency, excess, or resistance; and 5) regulation of energy metabolism, reproduction, and growth.

Endocrine Glands

The major glands that make up the endocrine system include the hypothalamus, pituitary, thyroid, parathyroid, pancreas, adrenal, ovary, testis, and placenta (Figure 1-1). Most of these glands produce hormones with a variety of effects. Under physiologic conditions, hormones are secreted from their glands, bind to a receptor, and initiate their action. In addition to these glands, nonendocrine organs (i.e., lungs and stomach) as well as a number of solid tumors can produce hormones.

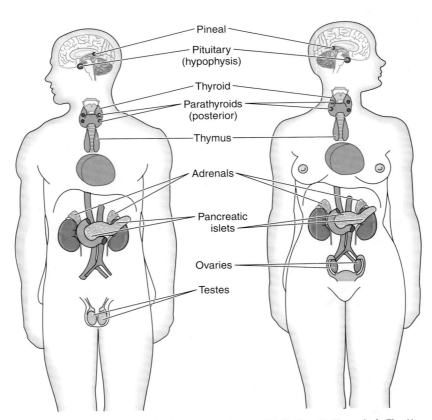

FIGURE 1-1. Location of the major endocrine glands. (Cohen BJ, Taylor JJ. Memmler's The Human Body in Health and Disease. 11th ed. Baltimore, MD: Wolters Kluwer Health; 2009.)

Hormone–Receptor Interactions

Hormone receptors are proteins that bind hormones with high affinity and specificity. Each receptor has a domain that recognizes a specific hormone and a domain that generates a signal once the hormone is bound (Figure 1-2).

Receptors in the cell membrane, known as **cell surface receptors**, are usually present in excess of the amount actually needed for maximum biologic response. Hormones are present in low concentration in the circulation so that the maximum biologic response of cell surface receptors is determined by hormone concentration.

Nuclear, or *intracellular*, **receptors**, on the other hand, are usually present in low concentration in the cell, and the number of receptors, rather than the hormone concentration, determines the extent of the biologic response.

Events at the postreceptor level are necessary for normal hormone action. Therefore, the cells must have a mechanism for release of bound hormone or the destruction of the hormone–receptor complex to turn off the action of the hormone.

Hormone Classification

Hormones are divided into three major classes: **peptides**, **steroids**, and **amines**. Peptide hormones include hormones secreted from the hypothalamus, pituitary gland, pancreas, and placenta (Table 1-1). Steroid hormones include hormones secreted from the adrenal cortex and gonad (Table 1-2). Amine hormones are synthesized from amino acids and are

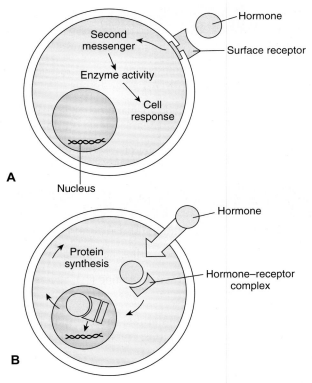

FIGURE 1-2. General mechanisms of hormone action for **(A)** peptide hormones and **(B)** steroid hormones. (Porth CM. Pathophysiology Concepts of Altered Health States. 7th ed. Philadelphia, PA: Lippincott Williams & Wilkins; 2005.)

TABLE 1-1.	Peptide Hormones
Location/Number of Hormones	**Names and Abbreviations**
Hypothalamus (4)	Corticotropin-releasing hormone (CRH), growth hormone–releasing hormone (GHRH), gonadotropin-releasing hormone (GnRH), thyrotropin-releasing hormone (TRH)
Anterior pituitary (6)	Adrenocorticotropic hormone (ACTH), follicle-stimulating hormone (FSH), luteinizing hormone (LH), growth hormone (GH), thyroid-stimulating hormone (TSH), prolactin (Prl)
Posterior pituitary (2)	Antidiuretic hormone (ADH), oxytocin
Pancreatic islets (3)	Glucagon, insulin, somatostatin
Calcium-regulating hormones (2)	Calcitonin, parathyroid hormone (PTH)
Placenta (2)	Human chorionic gonadotropin (hCG), human placental lactogen (hPL)
Gonad (1)	Inhibin
Liver (1)	Insulin-like growth factor-1 (IGF-1)

TABLE 1-2.	Steroid Hormones
Location/Number of Hormones	**Names and Abbreviations**
Adrenal cortex (4)	Aldosterone, cortisol, dehydroepiandrosterone (DHEA), progesterone
Gonad (5)	Dehydroepiandrosterone (DHEA), progesterone, testosterone, dihydrotestosterone (DHT), estradiol
Kidney (1)	Calcitriol ($1,25\text{-}(OH)_2$-vitamin D)

TABLE 1-3.	Amine Hormones
Location/Number of Hormones	**Names and Abbreviations**
Adrenal medulla (2)	Epinephrine, norepinephrine
Thyroid (2)	Triiodothyronine (T_3), thyroxine (T_4)

secreted from the adrenal medulla, hypothalamus, thyroid gland, pineal gland, central nervous system (CNS), and gastrointestinal (GI) tract (Table 1-3). The characteristics of these hormones are shown in Table 1-4.

Peptides

Peptide hormone synthesis follows the typical sequence for protein synthesis: gene activation, DNA transcription, formation of messenger RNA (mRNA), and translation of mRNA

TABLE 1-4.	Hormone Characteristics	
Characteristic	**Peptides**	**Steroids**
Hormone synthesis	Typical sequence	Derived from cholesterol
Travel in circulation	Unbound	Bound to carrier proteins
Half-life	Short	Long
Solubility	Water	Lipid
Delivery	Injection or nasal	Oral
Membrane permeability	No	Yes
Receptor binding	Cell surface receptors	Intracellular receptors
Postreceptor binding action	Second messengers	Hormone–receptor complex

into protein. In general, an initial large preprohormone enters the endoplasmic reticulum. A signal sequence is cleaved; the remaining prohormone or hormone undergoes further modification, is packaged into vesicles, and delivered to the Golgi apparatus. Most of these hormones are stored in the gland in granules awaiting the appropriate stimulus for release. Occasionally, peptide hormones are altered further while in the storage granules.

Once released into the circulation, most peptide hormones travel unbound to carrier proteins. As these unbound hormones are subject to degradation by proteases, they tend to have short half-lives. Glycoproteins are peptides with one or more carbohydrate moieties. They are generally more stable and last longer in circulation than peptides. Due to the stomach acid and intestinal peptidases in the human GI system, most peptides are not given orally.

Peptide hormones are water soluble and cannot cross cell membranes easily. They bind to cell surface receptors, and most activate guanosine triphosphate (GTP)-binding proteins, which serve as on/off switches. Coupling of peptide hormones (first messengers) to cell surface receptors generates second messengers that set off a cascade of reactions, leading to changes in the phosphorylation state. For example, a combination of a peptide hormone with its cell surface receptor activates a GTP-binding protein. This results in increased or decreased adenylyl cyclase activity, which, in turn, increases or decreases the cyclic adenosine monophosphate (cAMP) formation. cAMP activates protein kinase A that initiates a phosphorylation cascade mediated by other kinases (Figure 1-3).

Another second messenger system involves the activation of phospholipase C via activation from the GTP-binding protein. Phospholipase C generates diacylglycerol that activates protein kinase C and initiates a phosphorylation cascade mediated by other kinases. Finally, activation of phospholipase C also generates inositol trisphosphate (IP_3) that increases cytosolic calcium by increasing calcium release from intracellular membranes (Figure 1-4).

Steroid Hormones

The basic steroid structure is derived from cholesterol. Steroid and steroid-type hormones are lipid soluble and must be carried in circulation attached to carrier proteins. They can be given orally, and, because they are lipid soluble, they can cross membranes and enter all cells.

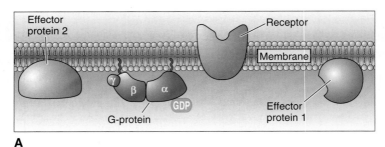

A

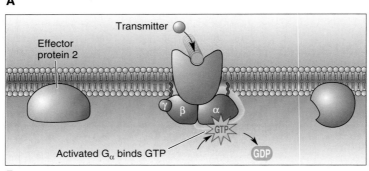

B

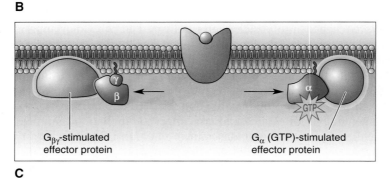

C

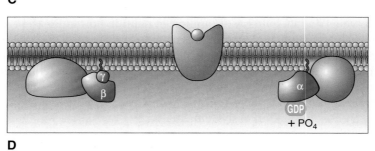

D

FIGURE 1-3. The basic mode of operation of G proteins. **(A)** In its inactive state, the α subunit of the G protein binds GDP. **(B)** When activated by a G protein–coupled receptor, the GDP is exchanged for GTP. **(C)** The activated G protein splits, and both the G (GTP) subunit and the G subunit become available to activate effector proteins. **(D)** The G subunit slowly removes phosphate (PO_4) from GTP, converting GTP to GDP and terminating its own activity. (From Bear MF, Connors BW, Parasido, MA. Neuroscience—Exploring the Brain. 2nd ed. Philadelphia, PA: Lippincott Williams & Wilkins; 2001.)

Steroid hormones bind to intracellular receptors that are located in the cytoplasm or nucleus. The intracellular receptors all have the same basic structure that includes hormone-binding and DNA-binding domains. These domains allow the hormone–receptor

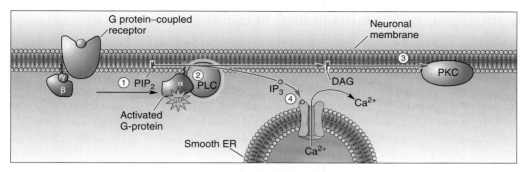

FIGURE 1-4. The basic mode of operation of a second messenger generated by the breakdown of the membrane phospholipid, phosphatidylinositol 4,5-biphosphate (PIP_2). 1) Activated G proteins stimulate the enzyme phospholipase C (PLC); 2) PLC splits PIP_2 into diacylglycerol (DAG) and inositol trisphosphate (IP_3); 3) DAG stimulates the downstream enzyme protein kinase C (PKC); 4) IP_3 stimulates the release of Ca^{2+} from intracellular stores. The Ca^{2+} can stimulate various downstream enzymes. (From Bear MF, Connors BW, Parasido, MA. Neuroscience—Exploring the Brain. 2nd ed. Philadelphia, PA: Lippincott Williams & Wilkins; 2001.)

complex to bind directly to DNA and alter the rate of initiation of gene transcription. The binding site on the target gene is known as a **hormone response element**.

Only a few hormone effects result from the altered transcription of genes binding hormone–receptor complexes directly (**primary response genes**). In this setting, changes can occur within 30 minutes. Most hormones act through **secondary response genes**. The hormone–receptor complex binds to primary response genes, initiating protein synthesis. The protein products then bind to the secondary response genes and initiate transcription. The process can take hours or days. Hormone–receptor complexes can also exert their effects by increasing mRNA stability.

The steroid-generated cascade of events can persist for days, even after the hormone–receptor complex releases from DNA. Steroid hormones are metabolized by the cytochrome P450 system in the liver. Their half-lives in plasma can be very long, especially for synthetic hormone preparations with added side chains.

The same hormone can affect different genes in different cells. Hormone action depends on the presence of other gene regulatory proteins (**transcription factors**) that can be specific to a particular cell. Response to steroid and steroid-type hormones is abnormal if the receptor is defective or if there are mutations in the genes to which the hormone–receptor complexes bind.

Amine Hormones

Amine hormones are derived from the amino acids tyrosine and tryptophan and include thyroid hormones (triiodothyronine [T_3] and thyroxine [T_4]) and catecholamines (dopamine, epinephrine, and norepinephrine). The thyroid hormones are secreted from the thyroid gland and behave similar to steroid hormones. They bind intracellular receptors, are bound to carrier proteins (thyroid-binding globulin and transthyretin), are not water soluble, and have a long half-life. The catecholamines act similar to peptide hormones. They bind cell surface receptors, are water soluble, are transported in blood plasma in solution, and have a very short half-life. Dopamine is stored in the kidney and the hypothalamus, whereas epinephrine and norepinephrine are stored in the adrenal medulla. The amine hormones derived from tryptophan are stored in nonendocrine glands and include melatonin (pineal gland) and serotonin (CNS and GI tract).

ENDOCRINE HOMEOSTASIS AND FEEDBACK REGULATION

Hormones may behave differently with diurnal variation and depending on the presence of receptors and other modulators. One hormone may produce one type of effect in the fetus; a different effect during childhood, puberty, or pregnancy; and still other effects in adults that may change with age. The gonadotropins (follicle-stimulating hormone and luteinizing hormone) are examples of hormones that are actively secreted in the fetus but shortly after birth return to dormant levels. They are reactivated with the onset of puberty.

Although the endocrine system interacts with many tissues and organ systems, it interacts primarily with the nervous system and the immune system. This interaction is most evident between the hypothalamus and the pituitary gland. Peptide hormones are secreted in a pulsatile fashion; normal pulse amplitude and duration are important for normal hormone action. There are diurnal rhythms to hormone secretion and rhythms that are tied to the sleep–wake cycle.

The goal of the endocrine system is to maintain homeostasis. Excess hormone down-regulates the number of receptors. Decreased receptor availability diminishes tissue response to the excess hormone. Hormone depletion usually upregulates receptors, whereas enhanced receptor availability increases the opportunity for tissue response.

Hormone secretion is regulated by a number of physiologic factors and feedback loops. Hormones are secreted in response to a signal. The hormone acts on a target tissue to produce a response. When this response has returned the initial signal to normal, hormone secretion decreases (Figure 1-5).

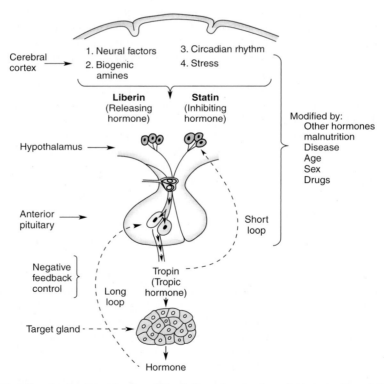

FIGURE 1-5. Negative feedback mechanism. Stimulation of a gland results in secretion of the gland's hormone. In order to prevent elevated levels of the specific hormone, the hormone feeds back in a negative fashion to inhibit further stimulation of the gland and further hormone release from the gland. (From Gornall AG, Luxton AW. Endocrine disorders. In: Gornall AG, ed. Applied Biochemistry of Clinical Disorders. 2nd ed. Philadelphia, PA: Lippincott; 1986, with permission.)

HORMONE EXCESS, DEFICIENCY, AND RESISTANCE

When control mechanisms fail, hormone excess and deficiency result in abnormal metabolism, water balance, blood pressure, growth, and reproduction. A high or low hormone level, however, does not always represent the primary problem.

An elevated hormone level can be an appropriate response to an acute and/or persistent stimulus (i.e., stress) or a deficiency state, or it can represent an appropriate attempt by a gland to overcome hormone resistance (an abnormality at the receptor or postreceptor level in target tissue). For example, an individual whose thyroid gland is not producing sufficient thyroid hormone will have an elevated thyrotropin (TSH) level. This elevated TSH level appears to be abnormal but is actually an appropriate response for an individual with a lower-than-normal concentration of thyroid hormone. Some individuals have polypeptide hormone receptors with abnormal GTP-binding proteins that constantly initiate hormone action whether the hormone is bound or not. Individuals with these receptors appear to have hormone excess.

A low hormone level might indicate a true deficiency or be an appropriate response to an abnormally low stimulus from a higher center. For example, a low thyroid hormone level may be the result of a thyroid gland failure or lack of TSH due to a defect of the pituitary gland. Usually, it is necessary to assess both the gland and target tissue response to find the true source of the problem.

CLINICAL ENDOCRINOLOGY

Hormones are secreted in response to a specific signal, but some hormones are not signal dependent and, therefore, do not vary according to chemical change. Circulating levels are usually undetectable unless a gland is removed completely. More sensitive hormone assays, such as automated immunoassay analyzers, reveal that in deficiency states, hormone levels are low but not zero.

Because peptide hormones are usually stored in glands until needed, the signal for secretion often elicits an initial burst of stored hormone into the circulation, followed by a decrease in the secretion of the hormone until the peptide synthetic machinery can be geared up. Hormone stimulation or suppression tests are often needed to assess gland capacity for a normal response.

Hormone replacement for deficiency states is becoming more and more sophisticated. Synthetic replacement hormones can be altered to prolong their half-lives in circulation and increase their potency. For hormone excess states, treatment is usually directed at the cause of the excess, and may require pharmacologic, surgical, or radioablative therapy.

In caring for the individual with a potential hormone abnormality, the measurement of the hormone concentration level must be interpreted in relationship to the clinical history and physical findings of the individual. Basal levels of hormones or peripheral effects of hormones must be interpreted with knowledge of the manner in which the hormone is released and controlled. In many cases, hormone levels must be interpreted in conjunction with another hormone or biochemical parameter. For example, the function of parathyroid hormone (PTH) is to maintain calcium homeostasis. An elevated serum PTH level must be evaluated in relationship to the serum calcium level. If the serum PTH level is elevated in an individual with a low serum calcium level, the serum PTH level is appropriately elevated. If, on the other hand, the serum PTH level is elevated in an individual with an elevated serum calcium level, the serum PTH level is inappropriately elevated.

Occasionally, urinary measurements are superior to serum or plasma tests for assaying the integrated release of some hormones. Imaging studies may be useful, especially in determining the source of hormone hypersecretion in some individuals.

CASE FOLLOW-UP

During stressful situations including fever, trauma, illness, sepsis, and anesthesia, the normal, physiologic response is for the hypothalamus to release corticotropin-releasing hormone that stimulates the anterior pituitary to release adrenocorticotropic hormone and, ultimately, stimulates the adrenal cortex to secrete cortisol (hydrocortisone). The finding that our patient has an elevated cortisol level during a stressful situation indicates an appropriate adrenal gland response. Our patient should be able to mount an appropriate cortisol response to stress if his hypothalamic–pituitary–adrenal axis feedback loop is intact. He does not require any treatment prior to the operation.

It is not routine to collect cortisol levels in those under stress or undergoing an operation. Because our patient was wearing a medical identification bracelet, there was the distinct possibility that he had adrenal insufficiency. A less-than-optimal cortisol level obtained during a stressful event should raise concern for adrenal insufficiency.

Our patient underwent surgery without event and maintained a normal blood pressure. Six months from the time of the accident, he was walking without difficulty.

REFERENCES and SUGGESTED READINGS

Cabrera-Vera TM, Vanhauve J, Thomas TO, et al. Insights into G protein stimulation, function, and regulation. Endocr Rev. 2003;24:765–781.

Habener JF. Genetic control of hormone formation. In: Wilson JD, Foster DW, Kronenberg HM, Larsen PR, eds. Williams Textbook of Endocrinology. 9th ed. Philadelphia, PA: W. B. Saunders; 1998:11–41.

Iiri T, Herzmark P, Nakamoto JM, van Dop C, Bourne HR. Rapid GDP release from Gsα in patients with gain and loss of endocrine function. Nature. 1994;371:164–168.

Johnson GL, Dhanasekaran N. The G-protein family and their interaction with receptors. Endocr Rev. 1989;10:317–331.

Kahn CR, Smith RJ, Chin WW. Mechanism of action of hormones that act at the cell surface. In: Wilson JD, Foster DW, Kronenberg HM, Larsen PR, eds. Williams Textbook of Endocrinology. 9th ed. Philadelphia, PA: W. B. Saunders; 1998:95–128.

Lefkowitz RJ. G-protein-coupled receptors: turned on to ill effect. Nature. 1993;365:603–604.

Linder ME, Gilman AG. G proteins. Sci Am. 1992; 267:56–61, 64–65.

Strader CD, Fong TM, Graziano MP, et al. The family of G protein-coupled receptors. FASEB J. 1995; 9:745–754.

CHAPTER REVIEW QUESTIONS

1. Which of the following is not a part of the endocrine system?

   A. Hypothalamus
   B. Adrenal cortex
   C. Ovary
   D. Cerebellum
   E. Thyroid gland

2. Which of the following is *not* a characteristic of most peptide hormones?

   A. Travel in the bloodstream bound to carrier proteins
   B. Have short half-lives
   C. Are water soluble

D. Bind to cell surface receptors

E. Exert their action through a secondary messenger system

3. Which of the following hormones is produced in both the adrenal cortex and testis?

A. Cortisol

B. Testosterone

C. Cortisone

D. Progesterone

E. Dihydrotestosterone

4. Which of the following hormones is not located in the hypothalamus?

A. Thyrotropin-releasing hormone (TRH)

B. Adrenocorticotropic hormone (ACTH)

C. Growth hormone–releasing hormone (GHRH)

D. Corticotropin-releasing hormone (CRH)

E. Gonadotropin-releasing hormone (GnRH)

5. A 32-year-old man has been diagnosed with a hormone deficiency. A peptide has been developed that will treat his condition. Which of the following statements about the therapy is true?

A. It has a long half-life.

B. It cannot be taken orally.

C. It is similar in structure to cholesterol.

D. It binds to carrier proteins.

E. It is permeable to most membranes.

CHAPTER REVIEW ANSWERS

1. The correct answer is D. The cerebellum is part of the nervous system and does not secrete any hormones. All of the other choices are found in the endocrine system.

The hypothalamus (**Choice A**), a gland in the central area of the skull, secretes four major peptides that trigger release of hormones from the pituitary gland. The adrenal cortex (**Choice B**) makes up 80% of the adrenal gland and secretes hormones, including mineralocorticoids, glucocorticoids, and androgens. The ovary (**Choice C**), a component of the female reproductive system, secretes estrogen and other hormones. The thyroid gland (**Choice E**), located in the anterior area of the neck, produces thyroid hormones.

2. The correct answer is A. Unlike steroid hormones, peptides are not bound to carrier proteins in circulation.

All of the other choices, short half-life (**Choice B**), water solubility (**Choice C**), bind to cell surface receptors (**Choice D**), and exert action through a secondary messenger system (**Choice E**) are true and characteristic of peptide hormones.

3. The correct answer is D. The enzyme cholesterol desmolase catalyzes the conversion of cholesterol to progesterone in the adrenal cortex, ovary, and testis.

Cortisol (**Choice A**) is also derived from cholesterol, but is only produced in the adrenal fasciculata of the adrenal cortex and not the gonads. Testosterone (**Choice B**) is synthesized and secreted from the testis. Although early precursor androgens (dehydroepiandrosterone and androstenedione) are synthesized and secreted from the adrenal reticularis, they are converted to testosterone in the periphery. Cortisone (**Choice C**) is not produced in either gland, but rather is the breakdown product of cortisol by the enzyme, 11-hydroxysteroid dehydrogenase. This reaction takes place in both the kidney and (to a smaller degree) the liver. Dihydrotestosterone (**Choice E**) is synthesized and secreted from the testis, but not from the adrenal gland. 5-α-Reductase is the enzyme that catalyzes the conversion of testosterone to dihydrotestosterone in the prostate, testes, and hair follicles.

4. The correct answer is B. Adrenocorticotropic hormone is located in the anterior pituitary gland and is stimulated by corticotropin-releasing hormone (CRH) from the hypothalamus.

All of the other hormones, thyrotropin-releasing hormone (**Choice A**), growth hormone–releasing hormone (**Choice C**), CRH (**Choice D**), and gonadotropin-releasing hormone (**Choice E**) are located in the hypothalamus.

5. The correct answer is B. Due to the stomach acid and intestinal peptidases, a peptide would not be able to serve its function and, therefore, cannot be taken orally.

The rest of the choices are all correct insofar as they are true statements regarding steroid hormones. Steroid hormones have a long half-life (**Choice A**), are similar in structure to cholesterol (**Choice C**), bind to carrier proteins (**Choice D**), and are permeable to most membranes (**Choice E**).

Hypothalamic and Pituitary Disorders

2

Sara D. Turbow
Briana C. Patterson

CASE

A 55-year-old man presents to the outpatient clinic complaining of increased sweating, hand stiffness, and palpitations. The symptoms developed gradually over the last 2 years. He does not smoke or take any medications. He reports drinking two glasses of red wine per week. His father has hypertension and has had a myocardial infarction. There is no family history of diabetes mellitus (DM) or thyroid disease.

His vital signs are as follows: temperature, 98.7°F; respiratory rate, 12 breaths per minute; blood pressure (sitting), 145/92 mmHg; and pulse, 90 beats per minute. On examination, he is overweight, has coarse facial features, large hands, and macroglossia. He denies any recent change in his appearance, but friends and family members who have not seen him in the past few months did not recognize him immediately.

This chapter initially reviews hypothalamic and pituitary endocrine physiology and then provides an overview of the congenital and acquired causes of hypothalamic–pituitary dysfunction to help the learner develop hypotheses that explore the etiology and pathophysiology of this man's condition.

OBJECTIVES

1. Describe the clinical and biochemical findings in an individual with hypothalamic–pituitary dysfunction.

2. List the congenital and acquired causes of hypothalamic–pituitary disorders.

3. Describe the evaluation and management of individuals with hypothalamic–pituitary disorders.

HYPOTHALAMIC AND PITUITARY GLAND PHYSIOLOGY

The pituitary gland is a central feature of the endocrine system, producing hormones that are released into the bloodstream. It receives signals from the brain and hypothalamus and responds by sending pituitary hormones to target glands. The target glands produce hormones that provide negative feedback at the level of the hypothalamus and pituitary. It is the feedback mechanism that enables the pituitary to regulate the amount of hormone released into the bloodstream by the target glands.

Hypothalamus

The hypothalamus can be thought of as the endocrine system's "central relay station." It gathers signals from the environment, the central nervous system, and from all over the body to integrate them and send information via hormones and neurotransmitters. The hypothalamus influences many aspects of bodily function, including arterial pressure, thirst and water conservation, temperature regulation, and body weight. Emotions, sleep, and instinctual control are also affected by the hypothalamus. The hypothalamic–pituitary axis, which is the focus of this section, controls the action of the thyroid gland, the adrenal glands, the gonads, and the production of growth hormone (GH); prolactin; thyroid-stimulating hormone (TSH); follicle-stimulating hormone (FSH); luteinizing hormone (LH); oxytocin; and vasopressin, also known as *antidiuretic hormone* (*ADH*).

The hypothalamus is located at the base of the brain between the cortex, the cerebellum, and the brainstem. The pituitary gland lies directly beneath the hypothalamus, resting in a depression of the base of the skull known as the sella turcica. The pituitary gland comprises the **adenohypophysis** (anterior lobe) and **neurohypophysis** (posterior lobe). The anterior lobe of the hypothalamus contains the neurons that produce hypothalamic-releasing hormones, which influence pituitary function. The hormones are released into a capillary plexus, known as the **hypophyseal portal system**, which signals the anterior pituitary gland prior to entering the systemic circulation, thereby enabling the hypothalamus to rapidly emit pulsatile signals to the pituitary gland (Figure 2-1). The releasing and inhibiting hypothalamic hormones are paired with the hormones from the anterior and posterior pituitary gland (Figure 2-2).

The posterior pituitary lobe receives inputs from the hypothalamus directly from hypothalamic nerves. Oxytocin and ADH are produced in the hypothalamic paraventricular and supraoptic nuclei as preprohormones and are transported in vesicles to the posterior pituitary via nerve projections.

The hypothalamus also plays an important role in the regulation of food intake. Hypothalamic control of appetite is mediated through neurotransmitters and neuropeptides. There are both orexigenic (appetite stimulating) and anorexigenic (appetite suppressing) peptides produced in the hypothalamus, and their production is influenced by nutrient availability and peripheral signals from the body, such as ghrelin, insulin, and leptin. The arcuate nucleus in the mediobasal hypothalamus plays an important role in regulating appetite. Neuropeptide Y (NPY) neurons in the arcuate

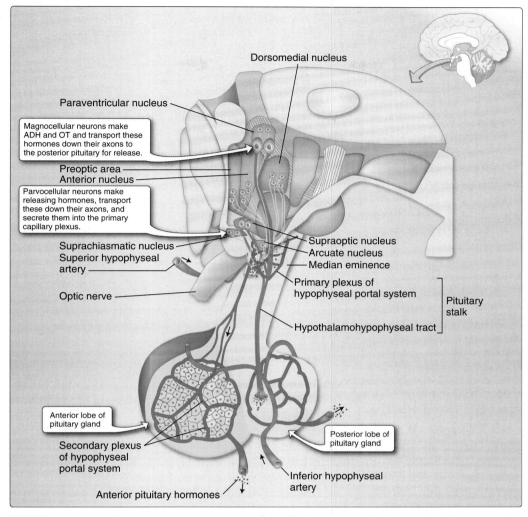

FIGURE 2-1. Hypothalamic control of the hypothalamic–pituitary axis. Endocrine function is regulated by the hypothalamic–pituitary system. (From Krebs C, Weinberg J, Akesson E. Lippincott's Illustrated Review of Neuroscience. Philadelphia, PA: Lippincott Williams & Wilkins; 2012.)

nucleus are inhibited by insulin and leptin. NPY release, which stimulates feeding, is increased when insulin and leptin levels are low and ghrelin levels are high. In contrast, proopiomelanocortin (POMC) neurons are activated by insulin and leptin and release α-melanocyte-stimulating hormone, which reduces appetite. Vagal input to the brainstem is stimulated in part by the gut hormone cholecystokinin, another important mediator of satiety. The incretin hormones and their relationship to obesity are discussed in Chapter 9.

Pituitary Gland: Anterior Lobe

The anterior pituitary lobe contains multiple cell types that synthesize a variety of hormones. The largest numbers of cells are the somatotrophs (50%), which secrete GH. Other cell types include corticotrophs, which produce adrenocorticotropic hormone ([ACTH] 20%); thyrotrophs, which produce TSH (5%); gonadotrophs,

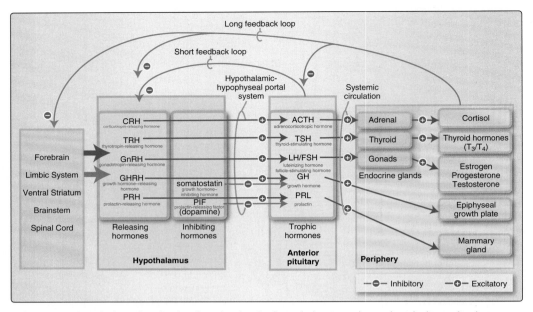

FIGURE 2-2. Regulation of endocrine function by the hypothalamus and anterior pituitary gland. (From Krebs C, Weinberg J, Akesson E. Lippincott's Illustrated Review of Neuroscience. Philadelphia, PA: Lippincott Williams & Wilkins; 2012.)

which produce LH and FSH (10%); and lactotrophs, which produce prolactin (15%) as shown in Figure 2-3. These hormones then exert their effects on target organs (Figure 2-4).

GH is important for postnatal growth and exerts its effects widely throughout the body. Despite its widespread action, the GH receptor is expressed mainly in the liver and mediates many effects through insulin-like growth factor 1 (IGF-1). Through both direct and indirect effects, GH causes epiphyseal growth, protein synthesis, lipolysis, decreased insulin sensitivity, and sodium retention (Figure 2-5). GH is secreted in a

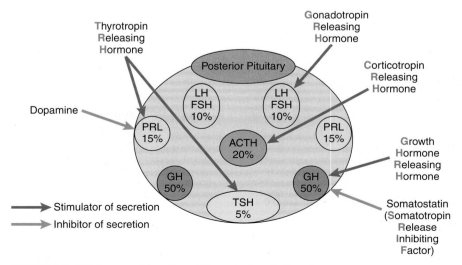

FIGURE 2-3. Cell types and location of the anterior pituitary hormones.

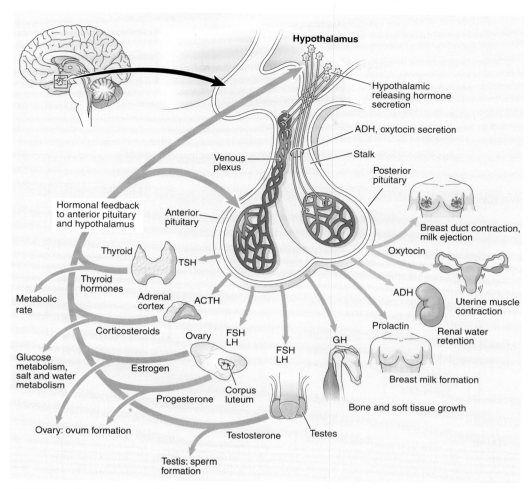

FIGURE 2-4. Hypothalamus, pituitary gland, and target organs. (From McConnell TH. The Nature Of Disease Pathology for the Health Professions, Philadelphia, PA: Lippincott Williams & Wilkins; 2007.)

pulsatile fashion with a short half-life. Fasting and hypoglycemia both cause an increase in the secretion of GH, whereas older age and obesity suppress its secretion (Figure 2-6). GH secretion is part of a negative feedback loop. It antagonizes the hypothalamus to decrease the release of growth hormone–releasing hormone (GHRH). IGF-1 inhibits pituitary GH secretion. Somatostatin, secreted by the hypothalamus, inhibits the release of GH from the pituitary gland.

ACTH stimulates production of glucocorticoids, mineralocorticoids, and adrenal androgens by the adrenal cortex and maintains the zona fasciculata and zona reticularis of the adrenal glands. ACTH release is mediated by corticotropin-releasing hormone (CRH), potentiated by ADH, and stimulated by physical and psychological stresses; its release is inhibited by circulating glucocorticoids. ACTH exhibits diurnal variation in secretion, with the highest levels early in the morning and the lowest levels in the late evening. The hypothalamic–pituitary–adrenal axis is discussed in detail in Chapter 10.

Thyroid hormone secretion is regulated by the circulating level of TSH, which is released by the anterior pituitary gland in response to thyrotropin-releasing hormone (TRH). TSH stimulates the release of thyroxine (T_4) and, to a lesser degree, triiodothyronine (T_3) by the thyroid gland. The physiologic effects of thyroid hormones are discussed

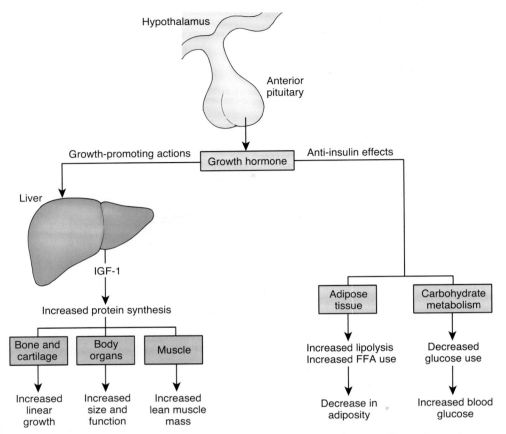

FIGURE 2-5. Effects of growth hormone. Growth-promoting and anti-insulin effects of growth hormone. IGF-1, insulin-like growth factor 1; FFA, free fatty acids. (Porth CM. Pathophysiology Concepts of Altered Health States. 7th ed. Philadelphia, PA: Lippincott Williams & Wilkins; 2005.)

in detail in Chapter 3. T_3 and T_4 act in a negative feedback loop at both the hypothalamus and the pituitary to decrease the release of TRH and TSH. Dopamine and somatostatin act on the anterior pituitary to inhibit TSH release, although their ultimate role in the physiology is not well understood. The hypothalamic–pituitary–thyroid axis is discussed in detail in Chapter 3.

FSH and LH are both produced by the gonadotrophs: 60% of these cells produce both hormones, 22% produce only FSH, and 18% produce only LH. LH and FSH act in the gonads of both males and females to increase sex hormone synthesis, spermatogenesis, development of ovarian follicles, and ovulation. LH and FSH are released in a pulsatile fashion and are highly regulated during the menstrual cycle, which is discussed in detail in Chapter 12. The hypothalamic–pituitary–gonadal axis is discussed in detail in Chapters 12 and 13.

Lactotrophs secrete prolactin that promotes breast differentiation, duct proliferation, glandular tissue development, milk protein synthesis, enzyme synthesis, and mammary gland development. Prolactin secretion is higher in females than in males, and the number of lactotrophs increases in response to elevated estrogen levels (as found during pregnancy). Prolactin secretion is also stimulated by TRH; therefore, patients with primary hypothyroidism who have high levels of TRH and TSH usually present with elevated prolactin levels. Concentrations are highest during sleep and lowest when awake. A number of environmental stimuli increase prolactin release; the most important is suckling. Prolactin release is inhibited by dopamine, somatostatin, and γ-aminobutyric acid (GABA).

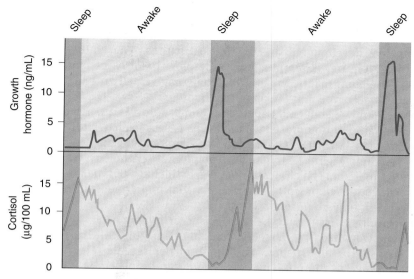

FIGURE 2-6. Circadian rhythms of physiologic growth hormone and cortisol. Fluctuations of serum growth hormone and cortisol levels are highest during the early morning hours. (Adapted from Coleman RM. 1986. Wide Awake at 3:00 A.M. by Choice or by Chance? New York, NY: W.H. Freeman. Figure 2.1.)

Pituitary Gland: Posterior Lobe

The posterior pituitary lobe produces neuropeptides when stimulated by hypothalamic neurons that originate in the supraoptic and paraventricular nuclei. Although it is these hypothalamic neurons that actually produce the hormones, they are often considered hormones of the posterior pituitary.

Oxytocin release is stimulated during breastfeeding and lactation. The physical signals sent to the hypothalamus during labor set off a positive feedback loop that enhances uterine contractility leading to rapid delivery of the baby and involution of the uterus after birth. Oxytocin aids in lactation by increasing contraction of the myoepithelial cells lining the breast ducts.

The major action of ADH is to increase water reabsorption by the kidney. It acts mainly in the distal convoluted tubules and the medullary collecting ducts, where, after binding to the vasopressin type 2 receptor, it signals the insertion of aquaporin-2 channels in the membrane to permit water reabsorption. The most potent stimulation for ADH release occurs with an increase in plasma osmolality or a decrease in blood volume, detected by osmoreceptors in the hypothalamus and the lamina terminalis. Other stimulatory factors include estrogen, progesterone, opiates, and nicotine. Alcohol and atrial natriuretic factor inhibit ADH release.

HYPOPITUITARISM

The endocrine deficits in hypopituitarism are variable, and may include GH deficiency, hypothyroidism, adrenal insufficiency, hypogonadism, and/or diabetes insipidus (DI). Hypopituitarism may be due to a defect in the pituitary gland (secondary insufficiency) or the hypothalamus (tertiary insufficiency). Deficiencies in the pituitary gland or hypothalamus are commonly referred to as *central hormone deficiencies* and not primary deficiencies, a term reserved for target organ defects. Hypopituitarism may be congenital or acquired and may affect only one hormone or multiple hormones. Each hormone deficiency is discussed in a general context in this chapter (most hormone deficiencies are discussed in more detail in other chapters).

Congenital Hypopituitarism

Congenital hypopituitarism may be caused by abnormalities in transcription factors that govern pituitary development and midline structures. The embryologic regulation of pituitary migration and differentiation is complex. In cases of hypopituitarism caused by a single gene abnormality, the affected gene may actually predict the constellation of specific deficits observed and the anatomic findings.

Several well-known congenital anomalies and syndromes are associated with pituitary deficits. For example, holoprosencephaly may be associated with isolated central DI. Septo-optic dysplasia (SOD), characterized by hypoplastic optic nerves and an absent septum pellucidum (Figure 2-7), may have no pituitary pathology, isolated GH deficiency, or panhypopituitarism. The clinical findings may include cleft palate, hypotelorism, nystagmus, seizures, developmental delay, and visual impairment. In other cases, intellectual development may be normal.

Anterior pituitary tissue may be hypoplastic or hyperplastic. The posterior pituitary tissue, usually visualized by magnetic resonance imaging (MRI) as a T1-weighted signal hyperintensity or bright spot, may be absent or ectopic (Figure 2-8). It should be noted that absence of the pituitary bright spot can be observed in normal subjects as well. Some infants will even demonstrate giant cell hepatitis associated with congenital pituitary defects.

The causes and radiographic findings of congenital hypopituitarism are listed in Table 2-1.

Acquired Hypopituitarism

Acquired hypopituitarism is caused by processes that damage the pituitary gland or hypothalamus and may present in childhood or adulthood. These may include neoplasms, surgery, radiation, inflammatory processes, trauma, and ischemic injury.

Neoplasms directly cause hypopituitarism when they are large enough to interfere with hypothalamic or pituitary function. Lesions may include craniopharyngioma, sellar/suprasellar germ cell tumors, and pituitary macroadenomas. In some instances,

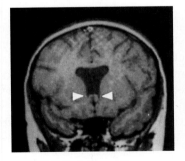

FIGURE 2-7. Septo-optic dysplasia. Coronal T1-weighted image shows absence of the septum pellucidum and squared-off frontal horns that have inferior points (*arrows*). (Eisenberg RL. An Atlas of Differential Diagnosis. 4th ed. Philadelphia, PA: Lippincott Williams & Wilkins; 2003.)

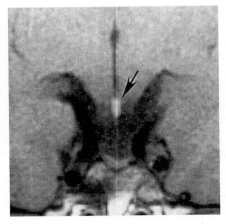

FIGURE 2-8. Posterior pituitary bright spot. (From Eisenberg RL. An Atlas of Differential Diagnosis. 4th ed. Philadelphia, PA: Lippincott Williams & Wilkins; 2003.)

TABLE 2-1.	**Etiology of Congenital Hypopituitarism**		
Etiology/ Defect	**Factor/ Condition**	**Hormone Deficiencies**	**Manifestations**
Transcription Factors	HESX1	GH, TSH, LH, FSH, ACTH, PRL	Pituitary hypoplasia Ectopic posterior pituitary
	POU1F1	GH, TSH, PRL	Pituitary hypoplastia (anterior)
	PROP1	GH, TSH, FSH, LH, ACTH (late)	Pituitary enlargement/ involution Partial empty sella
	SOX2	GH, FSH/LH	Pituitary hypoplasia (anterior) Ectopic posterior pituitary Midbrain defects
	TPIT	ACTH	Hypoplastic pituitary
Midline Defects	Holoprosencephaly	Variable	
	Septo-optic dysplasia	Variable	Absent septum pellucidum Absent or hypoplastic optic nerves
	Pierre-Robin sequence	Variable	Cleft palate, microagnathia, macroglossia
	Kallmann syndrome	FSH, LH	Anosmia, absence of puberty

Notes: GH, growth hormone; FSH, follicle-stimulating hormone; LH, luteinizing hormone; ACTH, adrenocorticotropic hormone; TSH, thyroid-stimulating hormone; PRL, prolactin.

hypopituitarism occurs after surgical or radioablative therapy of pituitary and hypothalamic lesions.

The effect of radiation on the pituitary is dose dependent and can range from subclinical findings to loss of multiple anterior pituitary functions (Table 2-2). These deficiencies are irreversible and often progressive. The pathophysiology of radiation-induced pituitary hypofunction is not well understood. It seems to be the result of neuronal injury rather than vascular injury to the hypothalamus or pituitary that results in ischemia and cell death. The pituitary may atrophy from decreased input of hypothalamic releasing factors or delayed direct effects of radiotherapy. Individuals with tumors that have compromised pituitary function prior to radiation experience more pituitary insufficiency than individuals without preexisting pituitary pathology who are treated with equivalent doses of radiation. Somatotrophs are the most radiosensitive cells; thyrotrophs and corticotrophs are most resistant. Low doses of radiation can result in precocious puberty in children, but higher doses are more likely to cause hypogonadism.

TABLE 2-2.	Hormone Defects Following Radiotherapy[a]
Radiotherapy Exposure	**Hormonal Abnormalities**
Total body irradiation (7–12 Gy)	Isolated GHD (usually prepubertal children only)
Total body irradiation (18–24 Gy)	GHD in <30% of prepubertal and pubertal children, may persist in adulthood Increased 24-h cortisol levels with normal ITT response Precocious puberty (girls)
Cranial irradiation (30–50 Gy, nonpituitary tumors)	GHD in 50–100% Precocious puberty (both sexes) (variable) Gonadotropin deficiency (20–50%) TSH deficiency (3–9%) ACTH deficiency (3%, often partial) Increased 24-h cortisol levels with normal ITT response Hyperprolactinemia (5–20%)
Skull base tumors/nasopharyngeal radiation (50–70 Gy)	GHD (almost all patients) Gonadotropin deficiency (20–50%) TSH deficiency (60%) ACTH deficiency (27–35%) Hyperprolactinemia (5–20%)
Pituitary adenoma treated with conventional radiotherapy (30–50 Gy)	GH deficiency (almost all patients) Gonadotropin deficiency (up to 60%) TSH deficiency (30%) ACTH deficiency (up to 60%) Hyperprolactinemia (5–20%)

Notes: GHD, growth hormone deficiency; ITT, insulin tolerance test; TSH, thyroid-stimulating hormone; ACTH, adrenocorticotropic hormone.
[a]Based on data from Darzy (2009).

The empty sella syndrome is a rare cause of hypopituitarism. Defects in the diaphragm of sella can allow the arachnoid and cerebrospinal fluid to herniate into the sella. This results in expansion of the sella and compression of the pituitary, leading to loss of pituitary function.

Traumatic brain injury may also result in hypopituitarism. Over half the patients with severe traumatic brain injury develop some form of pituitary dysfunction. The degree of hypopituitarism may be subtle or severe and relates to the severity of brain injury. The most common manifestations are dysfunction in GH and gonadotropin-releasing hormone (GnRH) cells. In some cases, traumatic brain injury may result in stalk transection with resultant loss of both anterior and posterior pituitary function.

Infiltrative lesions may also result in partial or complete loss of pituitary function. Hereditary hemochromatosis results in iron deposition in the pituitary gland that most commonly leads to gonadotropin deficiency. Lymphocytic adenohypophysitis is a rare but important cause of decreased pituitary function, which predominantly affects young women during pregnancy or in the peripartum period. It is an autoimmune disease of the pituitary gland that can present with varying degrees of pituitary hormonal impairment and/or with symptoms related to pituitary enlargement. Radiographic imaging shows enlargement of the pituitary gland mimicking an adenoma. Tuberculous granuloma is another infiltrative cause of hypopituitarism but is most commonly seen in the developing world. Individuals usually present with anterior pituitary dysfunction. In females, galactorrhea and amenorrhea are common, whereas decreased libido is seen in males. Imaging often reveals a sellar mass, and histology shows a central area of necrosis surrounded by macrophages, lymphocytes, plasma cells, and Langerhans cells. Sarcoidosis can also result in granulomatous lesions in the pituitary and hypothalamus. DI is the most common presentation of pituitary involvement with up to 90% of patients being affected. Wegener granulomatosis rarely involves the pituitary gland, but, when it does, it manifests as DI, with a presentation similar to that of sarcoidosis.

Langerhans cell histiocytosis (LCH) is characterized by an aberrant proliferation of Langerhans cells (a type of dendritic cell). In children, DI is the most common manifestation of LCH. The abnormal Langerhans cells infiltrate the pituitary gland, causing scarring that results in hypofunction. LCH can also cause the formation of anti-ADH antibodies that attack and destroy the ADH-producing cells of the pituitary gland. The destruction of these cells is often permanent, and ADH replacement therapy is needed.

Pituitary abscesses are rare but can be fatal. The most common presenting symptoms are headache, visual disturbances, meningismus, and fever. Up to 50% of individuals with pituitary abscesses have anterior pituitary hormone deficiencies. The most common of these are GH, FSH, and LH deficiencies.

Pituitary apoplexy is another rare but severe cause of hypopituitarism. It is caused by a sudden hemorrhage into a pituitary adenoma resulting in excruciating headache, diplopia, and cataclysmic hypopituitarism that results in cardiovascular collapse, loss of consciousness, and, potentially, sudden death. Treatment by surgical decompression of the pituitary can improve both the symptoms of hemorrhage and hypopituitarism.

During or shortly after childbirth, women who experience significant blood loss with or without hypovolemic shock may develop Sheehan syndrome, postpartum pituitary necrosis due to ischemic necrosis.

Individuals with hypopituitarism have highly variable pathologic findings that depend on the underlying causative process. In addition, there is an increase in mortality in children with associated pituitary deficiencies. Most of the deaths are due to adrenal insufficiency. The phenotype for neurodevelopmental outcomes in these patients with hypopituitarism is variable, depending on the associated cerebral anomalies. Even with a specific diagnosis, such as SOD, the prognosis is not clear. For example, visual and cognitive problems vary widely in this condition.

Treatment of GH deficiency in children can dramatically improve final adult height. The best results occur with early diagnosis and treatment. Treatment of adolescents and young adults also improves body composition (i.e., reduced visceral fat mass and increased muscle mass) and bone mineral density (BMD). In adults with severe GH deficiency, treatment with GH replacement therapy results in improvement in body composition, BMD, and quality of life. GH replacement therapy may also decrease the risk of cardiovascular events insofar as untreated adults with GH deficiency have an increased risk for congestive heart failure and acute myocardial infarction. Treatment of adults with mild or moderate deficiency is controversial due to the high cost of the drug and unclear evidence for substantial benefit.

Individual Pituitary Hormone Deficiencies

Individual hormone deficiencies that occur in hypopituitarism are presented in the order of predominant pituitary cell type in the anterior (GH deficiency, hypogonadotropic hypogonadism, central adrenal insufficiency, central hypothyroidism) and posterior (central DI) pituitary glands. Prolactin deficiency is discussed in Chapter 12.

Growth Hormone Deficiency

GH deficiency occurs when an insufficient amount of GH is produced to meet the body's metabolic demands. Interruption of GHRH input from the hypothalamus or impaired somatotroph function at the pituitary level may cause a loss of the normal, periodic, pulsatile secretion of GH. This results in a reduction in IGF-1 production from the liver.

Clinical Findings

In congenital cases, GH deficiency may be associated with hypoglycemia, jaundice, and micropenis (males). Most neonates with GH deficiency are not small at birth, insofar as many other factors are involved in the growth of the fetus. Most have poor linear growth in the first 2 years of life, but some may not demonstrate poor linear growth until age 4 years. The older child with GH deficiency usually has poor linear growth (subnormal height velocity for age) and a delayed bone age.

After childhood growth is complete, clinical findings of GH deficiency in the adult are more subtle but may include fatigue, weakness, loss of lean body mass, and increased fat mass.

Diagnostic Studies

GH deficiency is a clinical diagnosis requiring integration of growth data, history, risk factors, biochemical parameters, and radiologic imaging findings. Any child who has subnormal linear growth with adequate or excessive weight gain should be evaluated for GH deficiency. Unlike GH levels, IGF-1 and IGF-BP3 (binding protein 3) levels are stable throughout the day; collection of these serum levels may serve as useful screening tests. Decreased levels of IGF-1 and IGF-BP3, however, are not specific for GH deficiency, because they are also dependent upon nutritional status and bone age. They may also be low in states of chronic disease, impaired nutrition, or a constitutional delay of growth.

A bone age (Figure 2-9) is a useful tool in assessing children with growth disorders and short stature. The bone age will typically be delayed more than 2 standard deviations for chronologic age; however, this is not specific, as delayed bone age may be seen in children with a constitutional delay of growth (benign condition), chronic illness, or hypogonadism. Adults and children with GH deficiency may also have low BMD.

In addition to the growth data, physical findings, screening studies, and bone age, the diagnosis of GH deficiency is confirmed through provocative stimulation testing. Multiple protocols have been proposed, including those utilizing insulin-induced hypoglycemia, arginine, clonidine, L-dopamine, and glucagon. Insulin-induced hypoglycemia is considered the gold standard. All of these tests lack reproducibility, however, and none is completely specific for GH deficiency. The results of these tests must be integrated with the child's growth, historical, clinical, biochemical, and radiographic findings. In the individual with potential linear growth retardation, a GH-stimulated level ≥ 10 ng/mL is a normal response. In an individual who has completed linear growth, a GH-stimulated level ≥ 5 ng/mL is a normal response. Stimulation testing is discussed in detail in Chapter 19.

Neuroradiologic imaging of the hypothalamus and pituitary gland should be obtained in individuals with subnormal stimulated-GH levels to rule out a structural abnormality. Structural abnormalities may include abnormal development of the hypothalamus or pituitary gland, infiltrative lesions, or brain tumors.

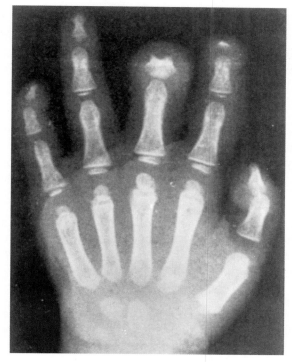

FIGURE 2-9. Bone age. (From Eisenberg RL. An Atlas of Differential Diagnosis. 4th ed. Philadelphia, PA: Lippincott Williams & Wilkins; 2003.)

Treatment

Treatment of GH deficiency requires injections of recombinant human GH. Doses are higher in children (0.3 mg/kg/week) in order to promote linear growth. Lower doses (0.06 mg/kg/week) are utilized after epiphyseal closure in order to avoid acromegalic changes. An active malignancy is a contraindication to treatment. In growing children, potential complications of GH replacement include worsening of scoliosis and slipped capital femoral epiphysis. Adult and pediatric patients may experience increased insulin resistance, swelling in the hands and feet, and pseudotumor cerebri.

Prognosis

A child who is untreated for GH deficiency will not achieve his/her appropriate, programmed final height. Untreated children achieve a final height standard deviation score (SDS) of –4 to –6. The long-term effects of GH deficiency on cardiovascular morbidity and mortality are unclear. Adults with GH deficiency have increased fat mass, decreased lean body and bone mass, are commonly overweight, and have elevated lipids. They also commonly have impaired quality of life.

GH treatment can reverse and reduce many of these abnormalities. Adult BMD is improved with continuous as opposed to discontinuous treatment; therefore, in the future, treatment may be routinely recommended for adults with severe GH deficiency. Most of these individuals tolerate therapy without difficulty, and less than 5% experience side effects.

Hypogonadotropic Hypogonadism

Hypogonadotropic hypogonadism occurs when an insufficient amount of estrogen (women) or testosterone (men) is produced because of a defect in gonadotropin secretion or effect. Decreased or abnormal secretion of GnRH, LH, and FSH result in impaired production of gonadal steroids and gametes in both sexes.

Clinical Findings

With onset of the deficiency in childhood, puberty may be absent or delayed. Infertility is a common presenting complaint in adults, in addition to amenorrhea or oligomenorrhea. Female patients may also complain of climacteric symptoms, such as sleep disturbances, vaginal dryness, or hot flashes. Male patients may experience sexual dysfunction, loss of libido, decreased energy, and decreased skeletal muscle mass. Both sexes are at risk for low BMD.

Congenital cases may present in infancy with a micropenis and/or cryptorchidism and may include anosmia as in patients with Kallmann syndrome (see Chapter 13). However, there may be no abnormalities at birth and some of these individuals will not manifest any symptoms or signs until they exhibit pubertal delay or infertility.

Diagnostic Studies

LH and FSH levels will be low in both sexes, and the typical changes that occur during puberty and the menstrual cycle will be absent. Testosterone levels will be low in males and estrogen levels will be low in females.

Treatment

Treatment typically involves replacement of the deficiencies in estrogen and progesterone in females and testosterone in males. Estrogen replacement may be administered orally or transdermally. Low doses are used in children in a slowly escalating fashion in order to mimic physiologic puberty and to allow for appropriate linear growth and the development of secondary sexual characteristics. Recombinant gonadotropins may be administered if fertility is desired. Testosterone may be administered by intramuscular or transdermal routes.

Prognosis

Administration of estrogen in the absence of progesterone should be avoided in postmenarchal females due to increased risk for endometrial hyperplasia. Side effects of testosterone include abnormalities in liver function and polycythemia. Females receiving hormone therapy are at increased risk for abnormal clotting.

For individuals with central hypogonadism, as long as replacement therapy is administered appropriately and laboratory studies are obtained if symptoms develop, most individuals will have an excellent prognosis. In those individuals who are not compliant with replacement therapy or have other serious medical conditions, prognosis may not be as favorable.

Central Adrenal Insufficiency

Central adrenal insufficiency occurs when an insufficient amount of cortisol is produced because of a defect in CRH or ACTH secretion or effect. Decreased stimulation of the adrenal glands from inadequate production of ACTH results in decreased secretion of cortisol, possibly resulting in adrenal gland atrophy. Mineralocorticoid production is spared in central adrenal insufficiency, insofar as mineralocorticoid secretion is primarily governed by the renin–angiotensin system (RAS).

Clinical Findings

Central adrenal insufficiency may present with fatigue, hypoglycemia, or hypotension. In contrast to primary adrenal insufficiency, in which both glucocorticoid and mineralocorticoid insufficiency occur, central adrenal insufficiency does not typically cause abnormalities in serum potassium but may result in hyponatremia due to the associated increase in ADH release in an attempt to retain free water.

Diagnostic Studies

These individuals have low morning cortisol levels and an impaired response to provocative testing. There are many provocative tests available to evaluate for central adrenal insufficiency, including insulin (gold standard), Cortrosyn (low or standard dose), glucagon, and metyrapone. Stimulation testing of the adrenal gland is discussed in detail in Chapter 19.

Treatment

Treatment of central adrenal insufficiency requires glucocorticoid replacement therapy. In children with growth potential, replacement should be with hydrocortisone (i.e., the deficient hormone). Individuals who have completed linear growth may benefit more from one of the synthetic glucocorticoids, prednisone or dexamethasone, because each may be taken once daily. Care must be taken to avoid excessive glucocorticoid administration, which could result in iatrogenic Cushing syndrome.

Prognosis

As long as replacement glucocorticoid therapy is administered properly, and dosing is increased during periods of increased stress, illness, or surgery, most individuals have an excellent prognosis. In those, however, who are not compliant with replacement therapy, do not absorb the medication effectively, or have another serious medical condition, prognosis may not be favorable.

Central Hypothyroidism

Central hypothyroidism occurs when impaired release of TRH from the hypothalamus or TSH from the pituitary gland results in a reduced production of thyroid hormone from the thyroid gland.

Clinical Findings

The signs and symptoms of central hypothyroidism are similar to primary hypothyroidism, except that a goiter is not present. Individuals of all ages may present with fatigue, constipation, cold intolerance, dry skin, or edema. Children, however, may experience growth arrest or pubertal arrest. Because neonates do not typically manifest many of the signs or symptoms of hypothyroidism until neurologic deficits are present, all newborns should undergo screening for thyroid hormone and TSH deficiency. The TSH level, however, may be in the normal range, and only newborn screening that includes T_4 measurement will identify individuals with central hypothyroidism.

Diagnostic Studies

The serum free T_4 (FT_4) and total T_4 levels are low, but the TSH level may be low, normal, or even mildly increased. TRH-stimulation testing was used in the past for the diagnosis of central hypothyroidism. The improved assays for TSH and T_4 make TRH-stimulation testing rarely necessary today.

Treatment

Treatment of central hypothyroidism requires levothyroxine. FT_4 and TSH levels should be monitored for adjustment of treatment.

Prognosis

The consequences of hypothyroidism are most severe when it presents in infancy. Untreated neonatal hypothyroidism results in irreversible cretinism with mental retardation; growth failure; puffy hands and face; and, commonly, deafness. Hypothyroidism that develops later in childhood is associated with slowed mentation, retarded bone development, decreased longitudinal growth, and delayed sexual maturation. These are reversible with thyroid replacement therapy.

For older children, adolescents, and adults, as long as replacement T_4 therapy is administered daily, and laboratory studies are obtained if symptoms develop, most individuals with hypothyroidism have an excellent prognosis. In those individuals who are not compliant with replacement therapy, do not absorb T_4 appropriately, or have another serious medical condition, prognosis may not be favorable.

Central Diabetes Insipidus

Diabetes insipidus (DI) is a condition characterized by excessive thirst and excretion of large amounts of severely diluted urine. Central DI is due to a defect in ADH secretion, whereas nephrogenic DI is due to an insensitivity of the kidneys to ADH. Central DI is caused by the interruption of ADH synthesis, transport, or release. In the absence of ADH, water permeability in the collecting ducts and distal convoluted tubules is unable to increase. Without the increase in permeability, water is not able to be reabsorbed into the bloodstream but rather is excreted in the urine, resulting in poorly concentrated, dilute urine.

Clinical Findings

Individuals with DI have polyuria and polydipsia. Urine specific gravity and urine osmolality may be low, even in the presence of dehydration, and the serum osmolality and serum sodium are elevated. Individuals may appear dehydrated, particularly infants and very young children who have impaired access to water and older children with impaired mobility, neurocognitive status, or impaired thirst mechanisms.

Diagnostic Studies

For untreated or individuals not well compensated, the diagnosis of DI is suspected in patients with polyuria, high serum sodium and osmolality, and inappropriately dilute urine. These findings must be differentiated from primary polydipsia and nephrogenic DI (resistant to ADH in patients with renal failure or genetic defects, or, those taking certain medications). The healthy child or adult should be capable of concentrating their urine to >600 mOsm/kg. In those with complete central DI, the maximum urine concentrating ability is ~100 mOsm/kg, whereas in partial central DI, the maximum urine concentrating ability is 300 to 600 mOsm/kg.

The water deprivation test is the modality of choice to evaluate an individual with possible DI. It is carried out as follows: all fluid intake is restricted, and serum osmolarity, urine osmolarity, and urine output are closely monitored for several hours. Individuals without DI will exhibit a reduction in urine output and an increase in urinary concentration in order to maintain normal serum sodium levels. Individuals with complete DI will fail to concentrate the urine appropriately and may experience clinically significant dehydration; therefore, body weight, vital signs, and electrolytes are closely monitored.

Individuals with only partial DI will exhibit some reduction in urine output and urine concentration but not as efficiently as in normal individuals. At the end of the test, if the individual continues to have urine output, increased serum osmolality, and decreased urine osmolality, arginine vasopressin or desmopressin acetate (DDAVP) should be administered. If this results in concentration of the urine, central DI is confirmed, and nephrogenic DI is excluded. Discussion of nephrogenic DI is beyond the scope of this chapter.

Treatment

Treatment of central DI includes replacement of vasopressin with desmopressin acetate. Delivery of the drug may be oral, intranasal, or subcutaneous. In critically ill patients, continuous infusion of vasopressin is advised. Individuals with an intact sense of thirst should have access to free water without limitation. Those with hypodipsia require a minimal daily fluid regimen to maintain adequate hydration and serum sodium levels.

Management of infants and neonates with administration of desmopressin may be difficult due to the risk for hyponatremia. These infants should be given supplemental free water or a thiazide diuretic.

Prognosis

Individuals who must take replacement therapy are at risk for developing hyponatremia or hypernatremia as a result of too much or too little drug intake. Most individuals with central DI and an intact thirst mechanism do not develop adverse effects from ADH deficiency or the replacement therapy. In those who do not have an intact thirst mechanism, the risk for dehydration is high, and the need for scheduling and documenting fluid intake is paramount.

PITUITARY HORMONE EXCESS STATES

Increased production of pituitary hormones is usually caused by a pituitary adenoma and less commonly by ectopic production of hypothalamic factors that stimulate the pituitary gland. Adenomas usually manifest between the fourth and seventh decades of life but may occur in children and younger adults. Microadenomas are defined as tumors less than 1 cm in diameter, whereas macroadenomas are tumors greater than 1 cm. Macroadenomas can cause local mass effects, including visual field abnormalities (classically bitemporal hemianopsia) and increased intracranial pressure (ICP). The most severe acute sequela of a pituitary adenoma is pituitary apoplexy.

Similar to pituitary hypofunction, the clinical manifestations of hyperpituitarism are dependent upon the hormones that are secreted in excess. For example, patients may exhibit hyperprolactinemia, acromegaly due to GH excess, or Cushing disease due to excess production of ACTH. Some pituitary adenomas are described as "nonfunctional." Prolactinomas, acromegaly, and nonfunctional adenomas are discussed in this chapter. Cushing disease is discussed in Chapter 10.

Other hormone-secreting pituitary adenomas are very rare. TSH-secreting adenomas make up less than 1% of adenomas. They are clinically recognizable by symptoms of hyperthyroidism, the presence of a goiter, and elevated TSH and T_4 levels. These tumors may also present with mass effects such as visual impairment if they are large. Treatment is surgical removal. Radiation and somatostatin analogues may be needed if surgery is unsuccessful in controlling the symptoms. Some patients may require radioactive iodine thyroid ablation to control their symptoms.

Gonadotropin-secreting pituitary adenomas secrete FSH and LH variably, but many patients do not even have elevated serum levels of these hormones. Because they lack a recognizable clinical syndrome, these tumors most often present with mass effects. Therapy is generally surgical with adjunctive radiotherapy.

Nonfunctioning pituitary adenomas make up 25% to 30% of all pituitary adenomas. They may be composed of a variety of cell types. The cell type is established by immunohistochemical staining for hormones. These tumors generally present with mass effects. They may present with hypopituitarism if they grow so large that they impinge on the pituitary stalk.

Pituitary carcinomas are rare and make up less than 1% of all pituitary tumors. They are usually functional and secrete ACTH or prolactin. Pituitary carcinomas are much more aggressive than pituitary adenomas and may exhibit local recurrence and/or metastases.

Hyperprolactinemia

Hyperprolactinemia is the presence of abnormally elevated levels of prolactin in the blood. Normal levels range from 3 to 24 ng/mL and 3 to 18 ng/mL, in women and men, respectively. Hyperprolactinemia is most commonly caused by a prolactin-secreting adenoma (prolactinoma). Other causes include previous cranial radiation therapy, structural interruption of dopaminergic input to the pituitary that inhibit prolactin release (e.g., nonfunctional pituitary adenoma or parasellar tumors), or medications. Medications that cause hyperprolactinemia include antipsychotics, antidepressants, antihypertensives, and metaclopromide. Pregnancy, lactation, stress, exercise, primary hypothyroidism, and renal insufficiency may also increase prolactin levels.

Another cause of apparently elevated prolactin levels is the presence of macroprolactinemia, which results from prolactin circulating in the blood in a dimeric or polymeric form. In most individuals, prolactin circulates in the monomeric form but occasionally may be present in dimeric or polymeric forms. For individuals with a preponderance of the polymeric forms, the assay for prolactin may be spuriously high, but prolactin itself is not actually elevated.

Pathology

Prolactinomas (Figure 2-10) are the most commonly recognized pituitary adenomas, accounting for 30% of all pituitary tumors. These neoplasms are more common in women

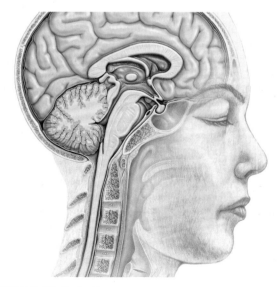

FIGURE 2-10. Prolactinoma.

and are often less than 1 cm in females. Macroprolactinomas (tumors > 1 cm) occur more often in males. Gender differences in prolactinomas may reflect sexually dimorphic differences in tumor biology. Some macroprolactinomas are invasive, invading the cavernous sinus. Routine histologic study of a prolactinoma reveals small, uniform cells with round nuclei and scanty cytoplasm. Electron microscopy reveals the secretory granules in the lactotrophs, which can be immunohistochemically stained to show that they contain prolactin. Macroprolactinomas may increase in size and result in a mass effect, whereas microprolactinomas seldom enlarge.

Pathophysiology

Gonadal dysfunction occurs in 90% of women with prolactinomas. The excess prolactin inhibits normal secretion of LH and FSH and the midcycle LH surge, leading to a lack of ovulation. It also inhibits the positive feedback effect of estrogen on gonadotropin secretion, so patients with prolactinomas are often estrogen deficient. Over the long term, this can result in decreased BMD and other effects of low estrogen.

Clinical Findings

Although the majority of symptoms of prolactinomas are different between men and women, both genders develop galactorrhea. In women, presenting complaints may include amenorrhea, oligomenorrhea, or infertility due to hypogonadism. In men, impotence, infertility, and decreased libido are usually present. Macroprolactinomas may present with changes in the visual fields, classically a bitemporal hemianopsia, or symptoms of increased ICP.

Diagnostic Studies

The elevated serum prolactin level is diagnostic, and dynamic endocrine function tests are not necessary. If macroprolactinemia is suspected, serum should be precipitated with polyethylene glycol to identify this variant.

For individuals with prolactinomas, the serum prolactin level will often correlate with the size of the tumor. Serum prolactin levels greater than 250 mcg/L indicate a prolactinoma. If the levels are above 500 mcg/L, a macroprolactinoma may be present, whereas if the levels are less than 250 mcg/L, a microprolactinoma is usually present, but medications, as described above, may also be the cause of the elevation in serum prolactin. Hypothalamic and pituitary stalk lesions can also present with mild to moderate elevation of prolactin levels (usually less than 100 mcg/L) due to interruption of dopamine reaching the lactotroph cells in the pituitary gland. When a prolactinoma is suspected, an MRI of the pituitary gland will confirm its presence.

Treatment

Treatment depends on the size of the tumor and its mass effect on the sella turcica. Dopamine-receptor agonists, bromocriptine and cabergoline, are usually the first-line therapy, regardless of tumor size. Cabergoline is more effective at reducing prolactin levels; however, not all patients will respond to medications. Surgery is an option if these medications fail, or if the patient has symptoms of pituitary apoplexy or evidence that the prolactinoma is expanding. Radiotherapy is indicated for patients with tumors resistant to medication, who have failed surgery, or are not candidates for surgery, or if the prolactinoma is invasive. Treatment of prolactinomas that occur during pregnancy or in the postmenopausal woman involves special considerations that is beyond the scope of this chapter.

Prognosis

Cabergoline normalizes prolactin levels in 95% of patients with microadenomas. The majority of these patients will also have a reduction in tumor size and normalization of gonadal function. Cabergoline normalizes prolactin levels in 77% of patients with macroadenomas and often shrinks these lesions as well.

Prognosis is less favorable in medication-resistant prolactinomas. Approximately half of surgically treated tumors recur, and two-thirds of patients treated with radiotherapy maintain elevated prolactin levels.

Acromegaly

Acromegaly results when the anterior pituitary gland produces excess GH after epiphyseal closure whereas gigantism results when the anterior pituitary gland produces excess GH before epiphyseal closure. Acromegaly occurs much more frequently than gigantism and, therefore, only acromegaly is discussed in this section. Pituitary adenomas composed of somatotrophs cause GH excess and acromegaly. They are the second most common type of pituitary adenoma, following prolactinomas.

Pathology

These typically nonmalignant tumors demonstrate isolated somatotrophs on histology or occasionally are mixed with galactotrophs. GH-producing adenomas are more commonly macroadenomas. They may extend dorsally and impinge on the optic chiasm or laterally and invade the cavernous sinus.

Pathophysiology

In 40% of these tumors, a mutation in the α-subunit of the stimulatory G protein confers constitutive activation of cyclic adenosine monophosphate. This results in a loss of expression of a proapoptotic, growth-arresting protein, while simultaneously overexpressing the pituitary tumor-transforming gene. Together, these cause cellular proliferation and increased secretion of GH. Secretion usually remains pulsatile, but the frequency, duration, and amplitude of the GH pulses increase.

The excessive GH results in increased IGF-1 production from the liver, which promotes DNA, RNA, and protein synthesis and leads to most of the clinical symptoms. The carbohydrate intolerance and insulin resistance that may occur with these tumors are most likely due to the excess GH, and not the excess IGF-1.

Clinical Findings

GH-producing tumors are far more common in adults than in children. In adults, these tumors result in acromegaly (Figures 2-11 and 2-12), which is characterized by progressive growth of the soft tissues of the face and the bones of the hands and feet, cardiac dysfunction and atherosclerosis, organomegaly, and thyroid dysfunction. These individuals may also develop carbohydrate intolerance and diabetes. Increasing size of the hands and feet as well as coarsening of the facial features are common early signs. Many patients do not notice these signs because the growth occurs so slowly. Over time, a degenerative arthritis may also develop.

Systemic manifestations of individuals with acromegaly include increased sweating, heat intolerance, decreased energy with increased sleep requirement, and weight gain. Cardiomegaly occurs in 15% of patients and hypertension in 25%. Arrhythmias may

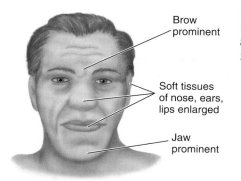

Brow prominent

Soft tissues of nose, ears, lips enlarged

Jaw prominent

FIGURE 2-11. Acromegaly. (From Bickley LS, Szilagyi P. Bates' Guide to Physical Examination and History Taking. 8th ed. Philadelphia, PA: Lippincott Williams & Wilkins; 2003.)

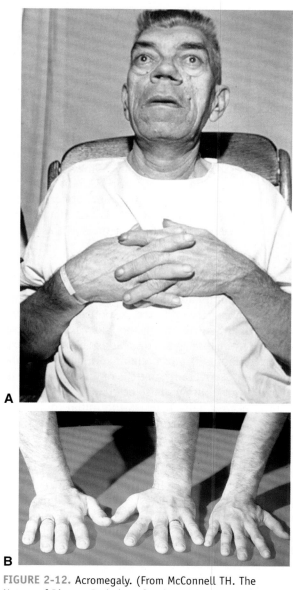

A

B

FIGURE 2-12. Acromegaly. (From McConnell TH. The Nature of Disease Pathology for the Health Professions. Philadelphia, PA: Lippincott Williams & Wilkins; 2007.)

occur in association with the increase in heart size. Impaired glucose tolerance is common and occurs in more than 50% of patients.

In children, whose growth plates have not yet closed, GH-producing tumors, while rare, result in gigantism. In these children, abnormally tall stature may coexist with other features of acromegaly.

Diagnostic Studies

Acromegaly is not always an obvious diagnosis, and a high index of suspicion is needed to identify it. Normally, GH release is cyclical, so measurement of random GH levels may not be diagnostic. In normal individuals, basal fasting GH levels are elevated to twice the upper limit. IGF-1 has been used as a marker of disease activity in acromegaly for over a decade. IGF-1 is an ideal screening test insofar as it has a long half-life of 18 to 20 hours, and the levels remain stable throughout the day. Despite these advantages in the use of IGF-1 for diagnosis, multiple physiologic factors affect IGF-1 levels and need to be taken into account. IGF-1 is affected by age, gender, and the presence of malnutrition; and liver and renal failure lower IGF-1 levels. On the other hand, normal pregnancy and adolescence are associated with elevated IGF-1 levels. The current international consensus for the diagnosis of acromegaly recommends a nadir GH of more than 1 μg/L for diagnosis in conjunction with clinical suspicion and high IGF-1 levels. Measurement of GH during an oral glucose tolerance test (OGTT) is the preferred method to diagnose acromegaly. The standard OGTT consists of the administration of 75 g of glucose with GH measurements at various time points for up to 120 min. GH levels should decline to less than 1 ng/mL if the highly sensitive assay is used. In acromegalic patients, GH levels may increase, decrease, or remain unchanged but will not decrease to the level of a normal individual.

When acromegaly is suspected by clinical and biochemical findings, an MRI of the brain is necessary to determine the size of the tumor and identify if adjacent structures are compromised. Visual field testing is advised for most of these individuals.

Treatment

Surgery and resection of the pituitary adenoma is the preferred treatment for acromegaly; however, factors such as tumor size, expected response to therapy, and the health of the patient may influence the initial treatment modality. In general, microadenomas are more likely to have a complete response to surgical excision, resulting in an appropriate reduction of GH secretion in about 80% of patients. Surgical cure rates are lower for the more common macroadenomas. Overall, surgical outcomes are best if a surgeon with vast experience in removing these tumors is selected.

Medical management is occasionally used as the initial therapy for acromegaly and where surgical treatment has failed to normalize IGF-1 and GH levels. Octreotide, an analogue of somatostatin, is the drug of choice. Sustained-release formulations are available that can be given every 2 to 4 weeks. Octreotide therapy, though effective in decreasing GH and IGF-1 levels, is less effective in reducing tumor size. It may have a role, however, in the pre-operative management of these individuals to reduce tumor size.

Pegvisomant is a GH-receptor antagonist; it does not reduce GH levels or decrease the size of the tumor but is effective in reducing IGF-1 levels in about 90% of patients. Some experts have suggested a strategy that administers both octreotide and pegvisomant simultaneously.

Radiotherapy is used for invasive GH tumors that are not amenable to complete resection or if medical management fails. After radiotherapy, years are required before GH levels normalize, thus limiting its usefulness in correcting the systemic symptoms.

Prognosis

Untreated patients and those with refractory disease have impaired quality of life and increased mortality due to cardiovascular disease, respiratory disease, and colon cancer.

For individuals who are successfully treated, there is not only cessation of bone growth, but also reduction in the soft tissue of the extremities, increased energy, and reversal of heat and glucose intolerance. Successful treatment reduces excess mortality and improves the quality of life as well.

CASE FOLLOW-UP

Initial laboratory evaluation reveals TSH, 2.45 mIU/mL; FT$_4$, 1.1 ng/dL; IGF-1, 1,145 ng/mL; fasting glucose, 116 mg/dL. The patient's symptoms and elevated IGF-1 level suggest a diagnosis of acromegaly. A GH-suppression test is performed in a lab that uses a highly sensitive GH assay. The nadir GH level is 4.5 ng/mL. Serum glucose levels are also measured during the suppression test, and the 2-hour glucose level is 160 mg/dL. The results of this test confirm the diagnosis of acromegaly and associated glucose intolerance.

The patient requires additional evaluation, however. An MRI of the brain is performed, and reveals a 1.0-cm pituitary adenoma. Visual field testing is normal. An echocardiogram is performed that demonstrates slight left ventricular dilatation, normal ejection fraction, and a high systolic output. These cardiac findings are acceptable for the patient to undergo surgical removal of the tumor.

He is treated with a transphenoidal resection of the adenoma and has an uncomplicated recovery. Follow-up testing demonstrates normalization of IGF-1, resolution of impaired glucose tolerance, and reduction in the left ventricular cavity size. The GH and IGF-1 levels are monitored every 6 months to assess for recurrence.

REFERENCES and SUGGESTED READINGS

Ayuk J, et al. Growth hormone and its disorders. Postgrad Med J. 2006;82:24–30.

Balasubramanian R, Dwyer A, Seminara SB, Pitteloud N, Kaiser UB, Crowley WF, Jr. Human GnRH deficiency: a unique disease model to unravel the ontogeny of GnRH neurons. Neuroendocrinology. 2010;92(2):81–99.

Carpinteri R, et al. Inflammatory and granulomatous expansive lesions of the pituitary. Best Prac Clin Endo Met. 2009;23:639–650.

Chrousos, G. Seminars in Medicine of the Beth Israel Hospital, Boston. The hypothalamic-pituitary axis and immune mediated inflammation. N Engl J Med.1995;332:1351.

Colao, A. The prolactinoma. Best Prac Res Clin Endo Met. 2009;23:575–596.

Darzy KH, Shalet SM. Hypopituitarism following radiotherapy. Pituitary. 2009;12(1):40–50.

Dworakowska D, et al. The pathophysiology of pituitary adenomas. Best Prac and Res Clin Endo Met. 2009;23:525–541.

Feinberg E, et al. The incidence of Sheehan's syndrome after obstetric hemorrhage. Fertil Steril 2005;84:975–979.

Fitzgerald P, Dinan TG. Prolactin and dopamine: what is the connection? A review article. J Psychopharmacol. 2008;22(2 suppl):12–19.

Gimpl G, Fahrenholz F. The oxytocin receptor system: structure, function, and regulation. Physiol Rev. 2001;81:629–683.

Karavitaki N, et al. Non-adenomatous pituitary tumors. Best Prac Res Clin Endo Met. 2009; 23:651–665.

Lombardi G, et al. Acromegaly and the cardiovascular system. Neuroendocrinology. 2006;83:211–217.

Melmed S. Current treatment guidelines for acromegaly. J Clin Endocrinol Metab. 1998;83:2646–2652.

Melmed S. Acromegaly. N Engl J Med. 2006; 355:2558–2573.

Melmed S, Casanueva FF, Hoffman AR, Kleinberg DL, Montori VM, Schlechte JA, et al. Diagnosis and treatment of hyperprolactinemia: an Endocrine Society clinical practice guideline. J Clin Endocrinol Metab. 2011;96(2):273–288.

Mills JL, Schonberger LB, Wysowski DK, Brown P, Durako SJ, Cox C, et al. Long-term mortality in the United States cohort of pituitary-derived growth hormone recipients. J Pediatr. 2004;144(4):430–436.

Molitch ME. Drugs and prolactin. Pituitary. 2008;11(2):209–218.

Neggers SJ, van der Lely AJ. Combination treatment with somatostatin analogues and pegvisomant in acromegaly. Growth Horm IGF Res. 2011;21(3):129–133.

Romero CJ, Nesi-Franca S, Radovick S. The molecular basis of hypopituitarism. Trends Endocrinol Metab. 2009;20(10):506–516.

Sherlock M, Woods C, Sheppard MC. Medical therapy in acromegaly. Nat Rev Endocrinol. 2011;7(5):291–300.

Sibal L, et al. Pituitary apoplexy: a review of clinical presentation, treatment, and outcome in 45 cases. Pituitary. 2004;7:157–163.

Taback SP, Dean HJ. Mortality in Canadian children with growth hormone (GH) deficiency receiving GH therapy 1967–1992. The Canadian Growth Hormone Advisory Committee. J Clin Endocrinol Metab. 1996;81(5):1693–1696.

Thomas JD, Monson JP. Adult GH deficiency throughout lifetime. Eur J Endocrinol. 2009;161(suppl 1): S97–S106.

Torbenson M, Hart J, Westerhoff M, Azzam RK, Elgendi A, Mziray-Andrew HC, et al. Neonatal giant cell hepatitis: histological and etiological findings. Am J Surg Pathol. 2010;34(10):1498–1503.

van Bunderen CC, van Nieuwpoort IC, Arwert LI, Heymans MW, Franken AA, Koppeschaar HP, et al. Does growth hormone replacement therapy reduce mortality in adults with growth hormone deficiency? Data from the Dutch National Registry of Growth Hormone Treatment in adults. J Clin Endocrinol Metab. 2011;96(10):3151–3159.

CHAPTER REVIEW QUESTIONS

1. A 6-year-old boy is referred for evaluation of short stature. Current height is at −2.5 SDS for age and gender. Review of the growth chart indicates normal linear growth for the first 3 years of life, and poor linear growth for the past 3 years with a height velocity of only 3 cm/year. Free T_4 is low at 0.6 ng/dL. Cortisol is normal. After replacement with thyroid hormone, a GH-stimulation test is performed and the peak GH level is low. What is the next best step in the management of this patient?

   A. Initiate GH therapy with daily injections of recombinant human GH.
   B. Obtain an MRI of the brain.
   C. Evaluate for celiac disease as an occult cause of poor growth.
   D. Measure the IGF-1 level.
   E. Obtain a bone age to determine growth potential.

2. A 21-year-old female presents with secondary amenorrhea after normal menarche at age 12 years and 9 years of uneventful menses. As part of the evaluation, her prolactin level is 55 mcg/L and her urine HCG test is negative. Possible etiologies for amenorrhea in this woman include all of the following except:

   A. Risperidone therapy
   B. Microprolactinoma
   C. Occult hypothyroidism
   D. Prior cranial X-ray therapy (XRT)
   E. Hyperthyroidism

3. A previously healthy 40-year-old female presents with headaches, bilateral hemianopsia, and coarsening facial features. She is found to have high IGF-1 levels and an abnormal glucose suppression test with GH levels that fail to adequately suppress. A 2-hour glucose level of 194 mg/dL is also noted during the GH-suppression test. An MRI of the brain identifies a 2.5-cm adenoma in the pituitary gland with impingement

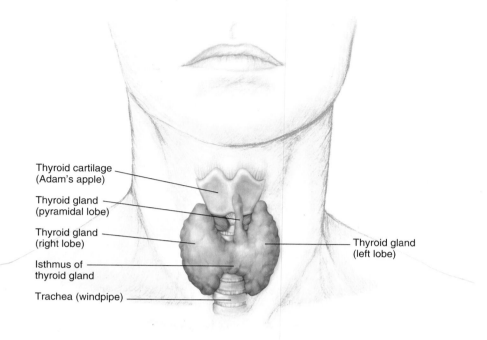

Thyroid cartilage
(Adam's apple)

Thyroid gland
(pyramidal lobe)

Thyroid gland
(right lobe)

Isthmus of
thyroid gland

Trachea (windpipe)

Thyroid gland
(left lobe)

FIGURE 3-1. Thyroid anatomy labeled. (Asset provided by Anatomical Chart Co.)

follicles are C cells, or parafollicular cells, that are derived from neural crest cells and are responsible for secreting **calcitonin**, a calcium-modulating hormone.

The thyroid gland is derived from the foramen cecum, an epithelial proliferation at the base of the tongue. By week 7 of embryologic development, the thyroid gland has migrated from its initial position at the posterior pharynx to its permanent adult anatomic location just anterior to the trachea. It maintains a connection with the foramen cecum through the **thyroglossal duct**, which normally involutes. If the thyroglossal duct persists, it takes the form of midline cysts that are found along the path of the thyroid decent. These cysts are known as **thyroglossal duct cysts**. Aberrant thyroid tissue can also be found anywhere along the path of thyroid descent.

THYROID GLAND PHYSIOLOGY

The physiology of the thyroid gland involves synthesis, regulation, transport, and action of thyroid hormones. Individuals with a normal-functioning thyroid gland despite abnormal clinical and/or biochemical abnormalities are also described.

Thyroid Hormone Synthesis

Synthesis of the thyroid hormones involves a number of steps (Figure 3-2). The first step begins with the adequate ingestion of iodine. Approximately 1 g of iodine per week is needed to ensure adequate thyroid hormone synthesis. Iodine is absorbed through the gastrointestinal tract and travels through the bloodstream bound to serum proteins, usually albumin. Once it arrives at the thyroid gland, it is taken up by basal iodine pumps on the thyroid follicular cells. These pumps concentrate the iodine in the thyroid gland to 30 times

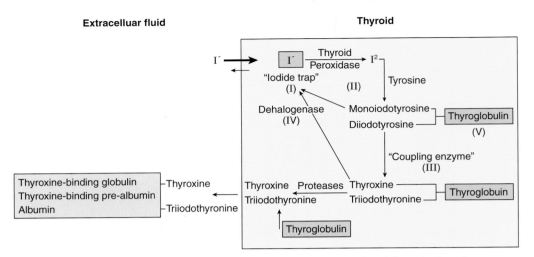

FIGURE 3-2. Thyroid hormone synthesis. The roman numerals correspond to defects in thyroxine synthesis resulting in thyroid dyshormonogenesis. (MacDonald MG, Seshia MMK, et al. Avery's Neonatology Pathophysiology & Management of the Newborn. 6th ed. Philadelphia, PA: Lippincott Williams & Wilkins; 2005.)

the blood iodine level. The iodine is then transported to the apical membrane, is oxidized with hydrogen peroxide by an apical peroxidase enzyme, and becomes highly reactive.

The second step in thyroid hormone synthesis is the production of thyroglobulin. Thyroglobulin is a glycoprotein that is the backbone for thyroid hormone synthesis. Each thyroglobulin molecule contains approximately 70 tyrosine amino acids that can be iodinated and coupled to form thyroid hormone. Once thyroglobulin is synthesized in the endoplasmic reticulum and modified by the Golgi apparatus, it is transported to the apical membrane.

There, thyroglobulin and the oxidized iodine meet and combine in an organification reaction via the iodinase enzyme. The result is a thyroglobulin glycoprotein with multiple iodinated tyrosine amino acids. These tyrosine amino acids are first iodized to monoiodotyrosine (MIT) and then to diiodotyrosine (DIT). Over time, the iodotyrosines are coupled by ester linkages. The coupling of two DITs forms thyroxine (T_4), whereas the coupling of one DIT with one MIT forms triiodothyronine (T_3). T_4 usually represents about 90% of thyroid hormone formation; the remainder is T_3.

The thyroid gland stores large amounts of thyroid hormone in the colloid matrix in the form of iodinated thyroglobulin. When there is need for thyroid hormone, thyroid epithelial cells ingest colloid by endocytosis from their apical borders. These colloid-laden endosomes fuse with lysosomes. Proteases within these lysosomes break down the iodinated thyroglobulin into individual T_3 and T_4 molecules that are then able to diffuse through the basement membrane and into the bloodstream.

The thyroid gland produces nearly 20 times more T_4 than T_3, but T_3 is the more active form of the hormone and produces the majority of the clinical effects. T_4 is peripherally converted to T_3 by removing one iodine molecule via a deiodinase enzyme from a T_4 molecule.

Regulation of Thyroid Hormone

Thyroid hormone regulation serves as the paradigm for the hypothalamic–pituitary–target organ axis regulation. Thyrotropin-releasing hormone (TRH) is secreted from the hypothalamus to stimulate the pituitary, which in turn releases thyrotropin, or thyroid-stimulating hormone (TSH). Thyrotropin then stimulates the thyroid gland to release T_4, which provides negative feedback at the thyroid gland, pituitary gland, and hypothalamus (Figure 3-3).

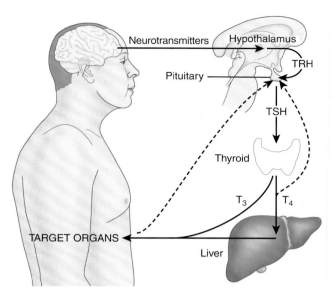

FIGURE 3-3. Hypothalamic–pituitary–thyroid axis. Thyroid-releasing hormone (TRH) from the hypothalamus stimulates the pituitary gland to secrete thyroid-stimulating hormone (TSH). TSH stimulates the thyroid gland to produce and secrete thyroid hormones (T_4 and T_3). High circulating levels of T_3 and T_4 inhibit further TRH and TSH secretion and thyroid hormone production through a negative feedback mechanism (*dashed lines*). (From Smeltzer SC, Bare BG. Textbook of Medical-Surgical Nursing. 9th ed. Philadelphia, PA: Lippincott Williams & Wilkins; 2000.)

TRH is a tripeptide secreted from the hypothalamus. The stimulation of TRH release is complex, but it can be stimulated by cold temperatures and inhibited by stress and anxiety. TSH is a glycoprotein secreted from the anterior pituitary gland. TSH stimulates a G protein receptor on thyroid follicular epithelium, leading to increased levels of cyclic adenosine monophosphate (cAMP) within follicular cells. cAMP serves as a second messenger; overall, cAMP stimulates immediate release of thyroid hormone, increases synthesis of thyroid hormone, and increases the number and size of thyroid cells.

High levels of thyroid hormone serve as a negative feedback to the hypothalamus and pituitary, inhibiting both TRH and TSH secretion. When thyroid hormone levels exceed 1.75 times the normal, TSH becomes undetectable. Additionally, a high proportion of T_3/T_4 can inhibit both TRH and TSH release.

Thyroid Hormone Transport

Upon release from the thyroid gland, T_4 and T_3 travel through the bloodstream bound tightly to plasma proteins, most commonly thyroxine-binding globulin (TBG). Changes in the level of TBG can dramatically affect the total level of thyroid hormone in the circulation, but does not alter the amount of free thyroid hormone. High estrogen states, such as pregnancy, cause a dramatic increase in TBG and cause large derangement in total thyroid hormone concentrations, but without any signs or symptoms of thyrotoxicosis. Alternatively, high androgen states cause a decrease in the level of TBG, leading to low levels of total thyroid hormone without any change in the free thyroid hormone level or signs of hypothyroidism. Nephrotic syndrome can also cause a decrease in TBG, because it results in an increase in the renal excretion of protein.

Target Organ Action

The thyroid hormone exerts its target organ effects by diffusing into the target cells and binding to nuclear thyroid hormone receptors. This hormone-binding step forms hormone–receptor complexes that bind to hormone-response elements in promoter regions of target genes. The binding of these complexes serves to promote or to suppress the gene transcription and thus alter its cellular function.

Thyroid hormone has a wide variety of physiologic effects. Its four most basic functions are: 1) stimulation of metabolism (the basal metabolic rate), 2) enhancement of autonomic reflexes (sympathetic tone), 3) promotion of tissue growth, and 4) promotion of tissue maturation. The effect of thyroid hormone on basal metabolic rate is best depicted by its effect on cellular metabolic activity. Thyroid hormone increases both the synthesis and the degradation of proteins, leading to an overall heightened metabolic activity. It also increases carbohydrate and fat metabolism, without having an anabolic effect, and stimulates the number and activity of mitochondria, leading to an increase in adenosine triphosphate (ATP) production.

The effect of thyroid hormone on the autonomic nervous system is complex, including its indirect upregulation of sympathetic activity. For example, it has been shown that patients with hyperthyroidism have increased concentration of β-adrenergic receptors in the heart that produces both inotropic and chronotropic effects on myocardial tissue.

Thyroid hormone is necessary for total body growth and maturation but is most apparent in bone maturation. A child who secretes excess thyroid hormone will grow at a faster rate than his or her peers. The brain is similarly dependent on thyroid hormone for growth and maturation. Without sufficient thyroid hormone, the central nervous system (CNS) will not develop properly and may result in **cretinism**. In this condition, the neonate does not produce a sufficient amount of thyroid hormone during the critical CNS development period, causing developmental delay and lifelong intellectual disability.

Biochemical Testing

Thyroid function is assessed by quantification of serum TSH, total T_4 (TT_4), and free T_4 (FT_4). TT_4 is a measurement of T_4 bound to TBG, whereas FT_4 measures only the active hormone. Due to rare abnormalities in thyroid hormone transport, FT_4 is usually the recommended T_4 level to measure. Stimulation testing of the pituitary and thyroid gland can be performed using TRH; it is discussed in more detail in Chapter 19.

Euthyroid States: Abnormal Clinical Findings

A goiter is an enlargement of the thyroid gland (Figure 3-4). It is commonly present in individuals with thyroid disease. An individual with a goiter may be **hypothyroid**, **hyperthyroid**, or **euthyroid**.

Goiters can form for a variety of reasons but are most commonly seen in individuals with autoimmune thyroid disease. Specific causes of goiter are discussed later in detail, with their individual processes. An isolated goiter rarely causes symptoms and generally does not require treatment. Large goiters that result in compression of adjacent structures, typically the trachea or esophagus, may require surgical removal or reduction.

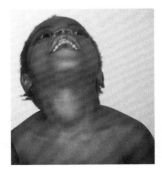

FIGURE 3-4. Goiter. This child with an enlarged thyroid gland (goiter) has Graves disease. Patients with Graves disease typically have a goiter with smooth texture upon palpation. (Sadler T. Langman's Medical Embryology. 9th ed. Image Bank. Baltimore, MD: Lippincott Williams & Wilkins; 2003.)

Goiters may also occur because of abnormal formation or secretion of thyroid hormone. When thyroid hormone synthesis is impaired, thyroid hormone levels are low; resulting in negative feedback to the hypothalamus and pituitary and leading to increased secretion of TSH by the pituitary gland. The increased levels of TSH cause hypertrophy and hyperplasia of thyroid follicular cells. Over time, and with prolonged TSH stimulation, the thyroid gland can enlarge and may be detected on physical examination. The hypertrophied thyroid gland may produce enough hormone to overcome the underlying thyroid hormone deficiency and prevent the individual from developing hypothyroidism.

Euthyroid States: Abnormal Biochemical Findings

A number of genetic abnormalities of the iodothyronine-binding serum proteins have been described. All of these abnormalities are evident at birth, and treatment is not necessary because the FT_4 and TSH levels are normal, and these individuals are clinically euthyroid. Once an individual is diagnosed with one of these disorders, however, physicians must realize that TT_4 levels should not be collected when assessing thyroid function but, rather, only FT_4 levels. The TBG conditions are inherited in an X-linked manner and include complete and partial TBG deficiency (low TT_4) and TBG excess (elevated TT_4).

A condition known as the **euthyroid sick syndrome**, or **low T_3 syndrome**, is another condition in which individuals have abnormal thyroid function studies but are clinically euthyroid. These patients are usually seen in the intensive care unit and are very ill, because extreme illness promotes conversion of T_4 to reverse T_3, rather than T_3 (hence the name "low T_3 syndrome"), but, in actuality, it may actually cause any of the thyroid function studies to be abnormal. These patients do not require thyroid replacement therapy.

HYPOTHYROIDISM

Hypothyroidism results from a lack of thyroid hormone available to the body's tissues and organ systems. Depending on the location of the defect, hypothyroidism is classified as primary or central and may be congenital or acquired. The most common cause of congenital hypothyroidism is the absence of the thyroid gland. The most common cause of acquired hypothyroidism is the autoimmune disease known as **Hashimoto thyroiditis**.

Clinical Manifestations

The major clinical manifestations of hypothyroidism in adults are present regardless of etiology. The signs and symptoms are directly related to the four core functions of thyroid hormone mentioned above. More than 90% of patients with hypothyroidism complain of lethargy, weakness, slow speech, and dry skin. Fatigue, cold intolerance, and hoarseness occur commonly. A complete list of the signs and symptoms of hypothyroidism are shown in Box 3-1.

Weight gain is a very common initial complaint of hypothyroidism, but is not a common cause of obesity. Weight gain in individuals with hypothyroidism is modest and rarely exceeds 10% of a person's body weight. The weight gain is primarily due to accumulation of glycosaminoglycans, hyaluronic acid, and interstitial edema, not adipose tissue. This results in the characteristic nonpitting edema of the hands, feet, and periorbital fossa. This edema is the most likely cause for the increased incidence of peripheral entrapment syndromes such as carpal tunnel syndrome. A similar pathophysiologic explanation has been proposed for the high incidence of subclinical pleural and pericardial effusions seen with hypothyroidism.

BOX 3-1.	Clinical Manifestations of Hypothyroidism

General
Cold intolerance
Fatigue
Hoarse voice
Weight gain

Cardiovascular
Bradycardia
Diastolic hypertension
Pericardial effusions

Dermatologic
Coarse skin
Dry/brittle hair

Gastrointestinal
Constipation

Hematologic
Anemia, normocytic

Pulmonary
Pleural effusions

Musculoskeletal
Entrapment syndromes
(carpal tunnel)
Muscle weakness

Neurologic
Delayed recovery of
reflexes

Reproductive
Menstrual irregularities

Hypothyroidism has a profound effect on the cardiovascular system. Cardiac output is significantly depressed due to a reduction in both heart rate and cardiac contractility. The reduction in cardiac output together with an increase in peripheral vascular resistance results in a narrowed pulse pressure. These cardiovascular manifestations are due to the decrease in sympathetic tone that is characteristic of hypothyroidism.

Anemia is common in the individual with hypothyroidism and is due to the overall hypometabolic state and less tissue demand for oxygen. This causes a decrease in erythropoietin production and leads to a mild normochromic normocytic anemia.

Neurologic symptoms are also prominent in hypothyroidism and range from fatigue and lethargy to memory difficulty and psychiatric disturbances. The mechanism of action of these symptoms may be attributable to an overall hypometabolic state of the CNS. Several studies have shown a reduction in cerebral blood flow and a segmental decrease in glucose uptake. Delayed deep tendon reflexes are not due to a neurologic deficit but, instead, to a delay in muscle contraction and relaxation.

Sexual function is often disturbed with hypothyroidism and includes decreased libido, erectile dysfunction, and menstrual irregularities, most commonly menorrhagia. In children, hypothyroidism is characterized by sexual immaturity and delayed puberty. Paradoxically, there are rare cases of hypothyroid-induced precocious puberty. This is thought to be due to excessively high levels of TSH cross-stimulating sex hormone production. Causes of precocious puberty are discussed in detail in Chapter 14.

Goiter is a common feature of primary hypothyroidism, but is not present with all of the etiologies of hypothyroidism. It is due to high levels of TSH causing hypertrophy of the thyroid gland. It is most commonly seen in Hashimoto thyroiditis, iodine deficiency, and drug-induced hypothyroidism.

Diagnostic Studies

The diagnosis of hypothyroidism is based on simple laboratory tests. Primary hypothyroidism is confirmed by an elevated TSH level together with a low FT_4 level, regardless of the T_3 level; however, it is important to note that an elevated TSH is the most sensitive of all the thyroid hormone tests. For this reason, TSH is often used as a screening test for thyroid dysfunction. High levels of TSH can occur in isolation, without a depression of T_3 or T_4 levels. This phenomenon is referred to as **subclinical hypothyroidism** and is not associated with clinical symptoms. It is not uncommon, affecting nearly 5% of individuals in the United States. In mild hypothyroidism, T_3 levels often remain normal despite low levels of T_4, due to upregulation of peripheral deiodinases and increased peripheral conversion of T_4 to T_3.

Central hypothyroidism, either due to a deficiency of TRH or TSH, is confirmed by a low FT_4 level with a low or normal TSH level. A TSH level that remains in the normal range despite a low FT_4 level is clearly abnormal and indicates an abnormality with either TRH or TSH.

Treatment

Treatment of hypothyroidism requires exogenous replacement of thyroid hormone, regardless of the etiology. Synthetic thyroid hormone is available in the form of levothyroxine, and dosing is based on age and weight (Table 3-1). Neonates and infants require a higher dose per weight or body surface area as compared to older children, adolescents, and adults. Elderly patients require a lower dose, and pregnant women require a higher dose. Surgical removal of the thyroid gland is only required for cosmetic purposes or in cases of compression caused by a large goiter but is rarely performed in individuals with hypothyroidism.

The plasma half-life of T_4 is 7 to 10 days, so daily administration of replacement hormone does not cause large fluctuations in the plasma concentration of T_4. Peripheral conversion of T_4 to T_3 supplies the active hormone. For individuals with primary hypothyroidism, the dose of levothyroxine is adjusted gradually until the serum TSH level is within the normal range. For central hypothyroidism, the dose of levothyroxine is adjusted gradually until the serum FT_4 level is within the normal range. Adjustments in the dose should be made in 4- to 6-week intervals, after steady-state concentrations of the hormone are attained.

Prognosis

The consequences of hypothyroidism are most severe when it presents in infancy. Untreated neonatal hypothyroidism results in irreversible **cretinism** that includes mental retardation; growth failure; puffy hands and face; and, commonly, deaf-mutism. Hypothyroidism that develops later in childhood is associated with slowed mentation, retarded bone development, decreased longitudinal growth, and delayed sexual maturation. These are reversible with thyroid hormone replacement therapy.

Most older children, adolescents, and adults with hypothyroidism have an excellent prognosis, as long as replacement T_4 is taken consistently and laboratory studies are

TABLE 3-1.	Dosing of Levothyroxine
Patient	Average Dose (mcg/kg)
Neonate	10–15
Ages 2–12 mo	5–10
Ages 1–3 y	2–5
Child	1–3
Adolescent	1–3
Adult	1–2

collected routinely and if symptoms develop. In those, however, who are not compliant with replacement therapy, do not absorb the medication effectively, or have other serious medical conditions, prognosis may not be favorable. Individuals may develop a serious, life-threatening condition known as **myxedema coma**, which is discussed in detail at the end of this section.

PRIMARY HYPOTHYROIDISM: CONGENITAL CAUSES

Congenital hypothyroidism occurs in approximately 1 in 4,000 newborns and is twice as common in females. The vast majority of cases are due to thyroid dysgenesis, in which the thyroid gland does not form at all (**agenesis**), partially forms (**hypogenesis**), or forms in a different location (**ectopia**). The remaining causes of primary congenital hypothyroidism are rare and include dyshormonogenesis and a transient form during pregnancy that results from maternal blocking antibodies and medications that cross the placenta. Defects causing dyshormonogenesis are generally inherited in an autosomal recessive pattern and can involve a deficiency at any step of thyroid hormone synthesis. The most common deficiency involves a mutation in the thyroid peroxidase gene and affects 1 in 40,000 newborns. The most common presentation of this syndrome is a newborn with a goiter and an elevated TSH level. Newborns with thyroid gland dysgenesis do not present with a goiter. Abnormalities in thyroid embryogenesis may also account for congenital hypothyroidism, but these individuals do not usually present until later in life. When an individual has an ectopic thyroid gland, the gland may initially function adequately but typically fails soon after birth. A child born with a persistent thyroglossal duct (Figure 3-5), which normally involutes prior to birth, may develop an infected cyst of the duct. Surgical removal of the duct is then necessary. Occasionally with duct removal, a majority of the thyroid gland is removed, and the child develops hypothyroidism.

Cretinism is a historic term that refers to the constellation of deficits seen in children with untreated hypothyroidism. Clinical features are due to a lack of neuronal development and bone growth. Children with untreated hypothyroidism have profound and irreversible cognitive deficits, short stature, and coarse facial features. Other features in the neonate include feeding difficulty, failure to thrive, jaundice, hypotonia, large tongue, umbilical hernia, and congenital heart defects.

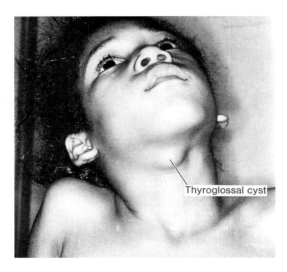

Thyroglossal cyst

FIGURE 3-5. Thyroglossal duct cyst. The cyst, a remnant of the thyroglossal duct, may be located anywhere along the migration pathway of the thyroid gland. Thyroglossal duct cysts are commonly found behind the arch of the hyoid bone. An important diagnostic characteristic is their midline location. (From Bickley LS, Szilagyi P. Bates' Guide to Physical Examination and History Taking. 8th ed. Philadelphia, PA: Lippincott Williams & Wilkins; 2003.)

Congenital hypothyroidism is rarely evident at birth but leads to devastating conse-quences if left untreated. For this reason, thyroid screening is a part of neonatal screening throughout the world. Fortunately, if hypothyroidism is found and treated within the first few weeks of life, the devastating clinical consequences may be avoided. Administration of simple exogenous T_4 replacement is the only treatment needed.

PRIMARY HYPOTHYROIDISM: ACQUIRED CAUSES

The five causes of acquired hypothyroidism include Hashimoto thyroiditis, iodine defi-ciency, pharmacologic agents, thyroid gland removal, and TSH receptor antibodies; the most common is Hashimoto thyroiditis.

Hashimoto Thyroiditis

Hashimoto thyroiditis, or *chronic lymphocytic thyroiditis*, is due to autoimmune destruc-tion of the thyroid gland. It is the most common cause of hypothyroidism in the United States and in parts of the world with sufficient dietary iodine. It occurs in 4 out of 1,000 women and 1 out of 1,000 men.

Etiology

The average age of onset is the fifth decade of life. Risk factors include those of auto-immune disease: female gender, family history of autoimmune disease, and a personal history of autoimmune disease. Individuals carrying human leukocyte antigen (HLA)-DR 3, 4, and 5 genotypes have been shown to be associated with higher risks of the disease. Radiation, pregnancy, and certain drugs may increase the risk of Hashimoto thyroiditis.

Pathology

The histopathology of Hashimoto thyroiditis is unique. The gross specimen is pale in color, diffusely enlarged, and firm. Microscopy shows lymphocytic infiltration and the development of germinal centers within the thyroid gland. Epithelial cells with abundant eosinophilic cytoplasm, known as **Hürthle cells,** are characteristic of Hashimoto thy-roiditis. They form in response to follicular injury. There is often an increase in fibrotic interstitial tissue that does not extend beyond the thyroid capsule, known as **atrophic thyroiditis**; it is the severe end histologic stage of Hashimoto thyroiditis.

Pathophysiology

The autoimmune thyroid destruction is primarily mediated by the cellular arm of the immune system and can be classified as a type IV hypersensitivity reaction. Cytotoxic T cells and cytokine release are primarily responsible for inducing thyroid cell apoptosis and follicular destruction. Humoral immunity and antibody-mediated destruction play a secondary role in the pathogenesis and are thought to be insufficient in isolation to induce clinically significant disease. Clinical signs of hypothyroidism generally do not appear until more than 90% of the thyroid tissue has been destroyed. The pathophysiol-ogy of autoimmune disorders is discussed in detail in Chapter 16.

Clinical Findings

Clinical manifestations of Hashimoto thyroiditis include all of the core features of hypo-thyroidism: fatigue, weight gain, nonpitting edema, dry skin, decreased hair and nail growth, and other signs and symptoms listed in Box 3-1. The classic goiter of Hashimoto thyroiditis, with a bosselated or pebbly texture, often, is the only presenting feature that points to the specific diagnosis.

Diagnostic Studies

The diagnosis of hypothyroidism due to Hashimoto thyroiditis is characterized by an elevated TSH level, a low FT_4 level, and antithyroid antibodies. Antithyroperoxidase (TPO) is present in 90% of cases of Hashimoto thyroiditis, but other antithyroid antibodies (including antithyroglobulin [Tg]) can also be diagnostic. If the suspected diagnosis is still not established, fine-needle aspiration (FNA) of the thyroid may be necessary to confirm the histologic appearance. Autoimmune destruction of the thyroid gland occurs over many years; therefore, an individual may have antithyroid antibodies but still have normal TSH and FT_4 levels. Furthermore, due to the destruction of the thyroid gland by lymphocytic infiltration, occasionally an excessive amount of thyroid hormone may leak from the gland and result in an elevated FT_4 level and suppressed TSH level. This is known as the **Hashi thyrotoxic phase** and may last up to 6 weeks. Individuals experiencing this do not always need treatment for hyperthyroidism but, ultimately, will need thyroid replacement therapy for hypothyroidism.

Treatment

Treatment of Hashimoto thyroiditis is identical to that for other types of hypothyroidism and consists of exogenous replacement of thyroid hormone with levothyroxine.

Prognosis

Prognosis is excellent with timely recognition and replacement with exogenous T_4. Individuals with Hashimoto thyroiditis do not appear to be at increased risk for thyroid cancer; they are, however, at risk for developing other endocrine and nonendocrine autoimmune diseases. Autoimmune polyglandular syndromes are discussed in detail in Chapter 16.

Iodine Deficiency and Goitrogens

Iodine deficiency is an extremely rare condition in the United States because most foods and salt are supplemented with iodine. It does, however, affect nearly 200 million people worldwide. Iodine deficiency occurs in areas that are mountainous, including the Alps, Himalayas, and Andes, where the soil is depleted of iodine stores resulting in low iodine intake. The term **endemic goiter** is reserved for goiter due to iodine deficiency that is present in over 10% of the population (Figure 3-6).

The clinical features of iodine deficiency are often limited to the presence of a goiter alone, because iodine deficiency only rarely leads to overt hypothyroidism. The elevated levels of TSH and resultant goiter are often able to accommodate for the iodine deficiency, with FT_4 levels remaining in the normal range. If iodine levels are severely depressed or absent, the hypertrophied gland cannot overcome this lack of iodine, and overt hypothyroidism may result.

There is significant variation in the rate of goiter development in regions that have similar levels of iodine deficiency. This variation is thought to be due, in part, to the presence of **goitrogens** in the diet. Goitrogens are substances that interfere with iodine uptake and therefore thyroid hormone synthesis. Foods grown in soils that contain either

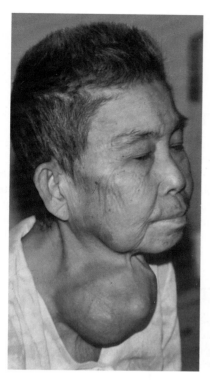

FIGURE 3-6. Endemic goiter. The lumpy appearance of this unusually large goiter and lack of exophthalmos in this individual living in a region of dietary iodine deficiency is a nodular, nontoxic, endemic goiter due to iodine deficiency. (Reprinted with permission from Rubin E. Pathology. 4th ed. Philadelphia, PA: Lippincott Williams and Wilkins; 2005.)

natural goitrogens or goitrogens from industrial wastes may accumulate enough of these iodine-blocking compounds to cause goiters and hypothyroidism. Common goitrogens include broccoli, brussels sprouts, cabbage, cauliflower, kale, cassava, bamboo shoots, sweet potatoes, and turnips.

The treatment of iodine deficiency consists of supplemental iodine in the diet. Increased levels of iodine will not cause a long-standing goiter to regress but may induce regression early in the disease course. Thyroid hormone replacement is necessary if overt hypothyroidism has developed, but will have minimal effect on goiter size.

Pharmacologic Agents

Certain medications can also cause hypothyroidism by inhibiting TRH, TSH, or thyroid hormone synthesis. Glucocorticoids and dopamine inhibit TRH secretion. Lithium inhibits thyroid hormone synthesis. Amiodarone inhibits T_4 and T_3 entry into the peripheral tissues. The antithyroid drugs used to treat hypothyroidism, propylthiouracil (PTU) and methimazole, inhibit thyroid hormone synthesis. Individuals with abnormal thyroid function studies who are taking any of these medications may not necessarily need thyroid replacement therapy. The individual's clinical status together with thyroid function studies must be assessed prior to initiating therapy, if needed.

Thyroid Gland Removal

Ablation of the thyroid gland, surgically or with radioactive iodine therapy, may cause hypothyroidism. Radioactive iodine (I-131) damages thyroid cell DNA and may cause hypothyroidism that develops in weeks to years. External radiation to the neck may also cause hypothyroidism.

Thyroid-stimulating Hormone Receptor Antibodies

Hypothyroidism due to inhibitory TSH receptor antibodies is extremely rare. Individuals present with a goiter due to the low production of thyroid hormone with elevated TSH secretion.

CENTRAL HYPOTHYROIDISM: CONGENITAL CAUSES

The majority of congenital hypothyroidism is primary hypothyroidism, but 5% to 10% is secondary, due to a central cause. The most common of these is hypopituitarism, in which several of the pituitary hormones fail to develop. This is most commonly the result of a genetic mutation that results in panhypopituitarism. In addition to panhypopituitarism, central hypothyroidism occurring in isolation without other pituitary hormone deficiencies may be due to transient hypothyroxinemia of the premature infant, mutations of the gene coding for the β-subunit of TSH, and mutations of the gene coding for TRH or the TRH receptor.

CENTRAL HYPOTHYROIDISM: ACQUIRED CAUSES

Acquired causes of central hypothyroidism may also be due to pituitary or hypothalamic diseases. The acquired forms are usually associated with other pituitary hormone deficiencies, including brain tumors affecting the hypothalamus and/or pituitary or head trauma resulting in infarction of the central structures.

The etiology of central hypothyroidism is discussed in more detail along with other acquired causes of hypopituitarism in Chapter 2.

The thyroid gland is usually capable of producing some T_4 and T_3 in the absence of TSH, so central hypothyroidism is usually not as severe as primary hypothyroidism.

All of the causes of hypothyroidism are shown in Table 3-2.

Serious Consequence of Hypothyroidism: Myxedema Coma

Myxedema coma is a rare, but life-threatening complication of hypothyroidism in which individuals manifest extreme symptoms of thyroid hormone deficiency. It is most common in elderly individuals and those with long-standing untreated hypothyroidism. There is often a precipitating factor, such as trauma, infection, medications (e.g., sedative hypnotics and anesthetics), or prolonged exposure to the cold. Diagnosis of myxedema coma is made by recognition of clinical features and a low serum FT_4 level. Treatment should not, however, be delayed while waiting for laboratory conformation of a low FT_4 level, because there is a 20% mortality rate without treatment.

Clinical features of myxedema coma are characterized by the most extreme manifestations of hypothyroidism. Additional features include altered mental status, hypothermia, bradycardia, hypotension, hyponatremia, hypoventilation, and seizures. The altered mental state of myxedema coma ranges from lethargy and stupor to coma. The hypoventilation may be severe and can lead to hypoxia and hypercapnea.

Treatment of myxedema coma requires parenteral thyroid hormone replacement. It is important that the thyroid hormone is delivered intravenously because the absorption of drugs is decreased in the severely hypothyroid state. Corticosteroids must also be administered because there is an increased incidence of concomitant adrenal dysfunction. Supportive care is needed to combat hypothermia, bradycardia, hypotension, and hypoventilation. It is often necessary to intubate the individual in order to stabilize vital signs.

Condition	FT$_4$	TT$_3$	TSH	Pathology
TABLE 3-2. Hypothyroidism: Biochemical Findings and Pathology				
Primary (congenital)				
Dysgenesis	↓	↓	↑	All or some absence of gland
Dyshormonogenesis	↓	↓	↑	Defect in thyroid hormone synthesis
Transient	↓	↓	↑	Maternal factors
Primary (acquired)				
Hashimoto thyroiditis	↓	↓	↑	Autoimmune (lymphocyte)-mediated
TSH receptor antibodies	↓	↓	↑	Antibodies to the TSH receptor
Iodine deficiency	↓	↓	↑	Inability to synthesize T$_4$ and T$_3$
Goitrogens	↓	↓	↑	Inhibits synthesis of T$_4$ and T$_3$
Medications	↓	↓	↓/N	Inhibits release/synthesis of TRH, TSH, T$_4$, and T$_3$
Ablation	↓	↓	↑	^{131}I radioablation or thyroidectomy
Central (congenital)				
Hypopituitarism	↓	↓	↓/N	Anomalous HT/Pit development
Isolated TSH deficiency	↓	↓	↓	Abnormal β-subunit of TSH
Central (acquired)				
Hypopituitarism	↓	↓	↓/N	CNS space-occupying lesions affecting HT/Pit

Notes: ↓, low; ↑, high; N, normal; FT$_4$, free thyroxine; TT$_3$, total triiodothyronine; TSH, thyroid-stimulating hormone (thyrotropin); TRH, thyrotropin-releasing hormone; HT, hypothalamus; Pit, pituitary gland.

HYPERTHYROIDISM

Thyrotoxicosis results from the effects of excess thyroid hormone on peripheral tissues. **Hyperthyroidism**, the more specific term, is used to describe a state of thyrotoxicosis that is due to the overproduction of thyroid hormone by the thyroid gland. The most common cause of hyperthyroidism is Graves disease (also referred to as **autoimmune hyperthyroidism**). Other causes of hyperthyroidism are multinodular goiter, adenoma, thyroiditis, and exogenous thyroid hormone (Table 3-3).

TABLE 3-3.	Hyperthyroidism: Biochemical Findings and Pathology				
Condition	FT$_4$	TT$_3$	TSH	Uptake	Pathology
Graves disease	↑	↑	↓	↑	TSH-receptor stimulating antibodies
Multinodular goiter	↑	↑	↓	↑	Mutation of TSH-receptor signaling pathway involving iodine-deficient thyroid tissue
Toxic adenoma	↑	↑	↓	↑/↓	Mutation of TSH-receptor signaling pathway involving normal thyroid tissue
Thyroiditis	↑	↑	↓	↓	Inflammation of thyroid gland— infectious
Struma ovarii	↑	↑	N/↓	N/↓	Ovarian teratoma with thyroid tissue
TSH-secreting tumor	↑	↑	N/↑	N/↓	Increased secretion of TSH
Drugs	↑	↑	↑/N/↓	↓/N/↑	Stimulate thyroid hormone synthesis/release
Exogenous	↑	↑	↓	↓	Ingestion of levothyroxine

Notes: ↓, low; ↑, high; N, normal; FT$_4$, free thyroxine; TT$_3$, total triiodothyronine; TSH, thyroid-stimulating hormone (thyrotropin); TRH, thyrotropin-releasing hormone; HT, hypothalamus; Pit, pituitary gland.

Clinical Manifestations

The clinical manifestations of thyrotoxicosis are consistent for all thyrotoxic disease states, regardless of etiology (Box 3-2). These signs and symptoms can be directly traced to the four core functions of the thyroid hormone.

The rate of metabolism increases with excess thyroid hormone as the result of increases in the rates of both the synthesis and the degradation of biologic molecules, including protein, lipids, and carbohydrates. During the thyrotoxic state, the rate of degradation increases more than the rate of synthesis, resulting in a net catabolic effect. The consequences include weight loss and muscle weakness despite increased appetite and adequate caloric intake.

Cardiovascular manifestations are among the first clinical consequences of the thyrotoxic state. Excess sympathetic nervous system (SNS) stimulation together with increased peripheral oxygen demand secondary to the increased metabolic rate leads to increased cardiac output. This increase in cardiac output is initially due to an increase in heart rate and contractility but later results from an increase in stroke volume. Total peripheral resistance decreases in order to supply more oxygen to peripheral tissues. The increase in cardiac output with a concurrent decrease in total peripheral resistance leads to the wide pulse pressure characteristic of the thyrotoxic patient.

The SNS is stimulated by unknown mechanisms in the thyrotoxic state, but it is believed that thyroid hormone likely plays a permissive role in the SNS, insofar as there are no signs of direct upregulation of the SNS, and levels of epinephrine, norepinephrine, and their metabolites remain unchanged. This increased **sympathetic tone** in the thyrotoxic state leads to increases in heart rate, respiratory rate, the thyroid stare, and lagging

---

BOX 3-2.   **Clinical Manifestations of Thyrotoxicosis**

General
- Anxiety
- Diaphoresis
- Fatigue
- Hair loss
- Heat intolerance
- Insomnia
- Irritability
- Weight loss

Cardiovascular
- Arrhythmias
- Sinus tachycardia
- Systolic hypertension

Dermatologic
- Pretibial myxedema
- Thin skin
- Onycholysis

Gastrointestinal
- Frequent bowel movements

Hematologic
- Anemia, normocytic

Pulmonary
- Pleural effusions

Musculoskeletal
- Muscle aches
- Osteoporosis
- Weakness

Neurologic
- Brisk reflexes
- Fine tremor

Ophthalmologic
- Lid lag
- Thyroid stare

Reproductive
- Menstrual irregularities

---

of the upper eyelid. Stimulation of the SNS results in nervousness, irritability, hyperactivity, and fatigue; psychosis has also been observed in the thyrotoxic state.

Symptoms of thyrotoxicosis can also be attributed to altered tissue growth and maturation including integumentary effects such as smooth skin, onycholysis, and osteoporosis.

Treatment

Currently, there is a variety of treatment options for thyrotoxicosis, none of which is ideal. There are three pathways for treatment: medical therapy, radioactive iodide ablation, and surgical excision. None of these options addresses the underlying pathophysiology of hyperthyroidism, nor do they provide an ideal physiologic solution. Therefore, the treatment regimens vary widely, and the clinician must determine the best solution for a given individual.

Medical therapy is the treatment both early in the course of chronic hyperthyroidism and during an acute onset when life threatening. The thionamides, PTU, carbimazole, and its metabolite methimazole, are the key drugs of chronic medical therapy. They act to reduce the production of thyroid hormone by inhibiting thyroperoxidase, the enzyme responsible for oxidizing iodine. The thionamides also reduce levels of antithyroid antibodies by an unknown mechanism. PTU is unique in that it also inhibits peripheral deiodinase, thereby inhibiting the peripheral conversion of T_4 to the more active T_3. It usually takes 6 to 8 weeks before these drugs render a hyperthyroid individual euthyroid. One advantage of thionamides is that they are titratable and their effects can be monitored by simple blood tests. The typical side effects of thionamides are mild and include rash, urticaria, arthralgias, and a lupus-like syndrome. More severe side effects are quite rare but include fulminant hepatitis and agranulcytosis. These serious complications occur in less than 0.3% of patients and generally occur within the first few months of initiating therapy. Due to an increase in hepatic failure in children and adolescents using PTU for hyperthyroidism, methimazole is the only approved medical therapy for individuals younger than age 18 years with hyperthyroidism.

Iodine-containing solutions, such as potassium iodine and Lugol solution, function to inhibit the release of preformed thyroid hormone from the thyroid gland. Iodine-containing solutions have a very rapid onset of action, making them good choices for acute management of life-threatening thyrotoxicosis. Unfortunately, the suppressive effects of iodine solutions wane over time, making them a poor choice for long-term management. The primary negative effect of iodine solutions is that they saturate the iodine-binding receptors, thereby decreasing the efficiency of thionamides and radioactive iodine. Side effects of iodine solutions tend to be mild and include acneform rash, conjunctivitis, sialadenitis, rhinitis, and vasculitis.

β-Blockers are often used in the acute treatment of thyrotoxicosis because they have a fairly rapid onset of action. They act to counter the effect of increased sympathetic autonomic activity and are useful in treating the adrenergic symptoms such as tachycardia. Dexamethasone is also useful in the acute treatment of severe thyrotoxicosis and thyroid storm. It rapidly decreases peripheral levels of T_3 by inhibiting the release of thyroid hormone and by inhibiting peripheral conversion of T_4 to T_3. It also has immunosuppressant effects that can target the underlying disease process.

Radioactive iodine ablation of thyroid tissue is commonly used in the United States as definitive treatment for hyperthyroidism. Originally, there were attempts to titrate the dose of radioactive iodine to spare enough thyroid tissue to render the patient euthyroid. Unfortunately, these precise titrations proved unsuccessful and often led to treatment failure, requiring additional radioiodine (^{131}I) treatments or permanent hypothyroidism. Currently, most physicians target total thyroid ablation and use **add-back** thyroid hormone replacement. It takes several months for ^{131}I to take full effect, and individuals with hyperthyroidism often need medical suppression therapy during this time. This treatment time lag obviates the use of ^{131}I as an acute treatment for hyperthyroidism. There is a small risk of a thyrotoxic crisis during iodine radioablation because of the release of preformed thyroid hormone with its inflammatory response and destruction of the thyroid tissue. This risk is greatly reduced by achieving a euthyroid state with medical therapy prior to ^{131}I ablation. Pregnancy and breastfeeding are absolute contraindications to ^{131}I therapy insofar as ^{131}I can cause destruction of the neonate's thyroid tissue. Caution should be used with ^{131}I when treating a patient with ophthalmopathy, because ^{131}I has been shown to worsen the ophthalmologic complications of Graves disease.

Surgical excision is the least commonly used treatment of thyrotoxicosis. Surgery is recommended only when other treatment options have failed or when the hyperthyroid individual is experiencing symptoms from a mass effect of the goiter, such as tracheal compression or difficulty swallowing. Both complete thyroidectomy and subtotal thyroidectomy have been performed. The treatment success is similar to that of other treatment modalities, and the recurrence rate appears to be equal to ^{131}I ablation. Thyrotoxic crisis after surgery is uncommon but can often be avoided by pretreatment with thionamide and iodine therapy. Other complications include bleeding, infection, recurrent laryngeal nerve damage, and hypoparathyroidism.

Prognosis

If recognized and treated early, the prognosis for thyrotoxicosis is good. Depending on the therapy, there is a chance for remission, reversion to the hypothyroid state, or relapse. Depending on the etiology of an individual's hyperthyroidism, different treatments have different rates for remission, recurrence, or reversion to hypothyroidism.

Most older children, adolescents, and adults with hyperthyroidism have an excellent prognosis, as long as medical therapy is taken consistently, or definitive therapy is chosen, and laboratory studies are collected routinely and/or if symptoms develop. In those, however, who are not compliant with replacement therapy, do not absorb the medication effectively, or have other serious medical conditions, prognosis may not be favorable. Individuals may develop a serious, life-threatening condition known as **thyroid storm**, which is discussed in detail at the end of this section.

Graves Disease

Graves disease is the most common cause of thyrotoxicosis. It accounts for 50% to 80% of all cases and affects 1% to 2% of the population. It affects females 10 times more commonly than males. The peak age of onset is between ages 20 to 50 years, with an onset prior to puberty rare. Risk factors for Graves disease include personal or family history of autoimmune disease, HLA-B8 genotype, smoking, high iodine intake, or use of iodine-containing medications (such as amiodarone).

Pathology

The thyroid gland in Graves disease is usually diffusely enlarged. The histology is characterized by follicular hyperplasia, intracellular colloid droplets, cell scalloping, a reduction in follicular colloid, and a patchy lymphocytic infiltration.

Pathophysiology

The pathophysiology of Graves disease is quite unique, in that it is an autoimmune disease that does not destroy the tissue but, instead, results in hyperfunctioning of the gland. Graves disease is a classic type 2 hypersensitivity reaction characterized by the formation of thyrotropin receptor antibodies (TRABs), which are directed toward the TSH receptors. Unlike antibodies that lead to destruction of their targets, these autoantibodies stimulate the TSH receptor via the cAMP pathway in the same manner as TSH. This autoantibody stimulation leads to overproduction of thyroid hormone in the absence of TSH stimulus. Ultimately, this overproduction leads to signs and symptoms of thyrotoxicosis. The stimulus for initiation of Graves disease and the creation of TRAbs remains unknown, but both viral illnesses and acutely stressful states appear to play a role.

Clinical Findings

Clinical manifestations of Graves disease include all of the core features of thyrotoxicosis (see Box 3-2) as well as some signs and symptoms specific to Graves disease. A diffusely enlarged thyroid gland is a classic finding in Graves disease (see Figure 3-4). The goiter is generally symmetrically enlarged to two to three times the normal size, rubbery to firm in texture, and may be accompanied by an arterial bruit or *thrill*.

In addition to the thyroid stare and lid lag characteristic of thyrotoxicosis, there are distinct ocular manifestations that are unique to Graves disease. **Proptosis or exophthalmos**, the forward displacement of the eyes within the orbit, is the most common ocular manifestation (Figure 3-7). It is the result of increased volume of retrorbital tissue secondary to infiltration by monocytes, inflammation, and fibrosis. It is often accompanied by periorbital edema and corneal injection. Generally, this ocular manifestation causes only mild discomfort but may be cosmetically significant. Ocular manifestations of Graves disease can progress to serious complications that result in diplopia and optic nerve compression. Although there are no separate risk factors for Graves ophthalmopathy, smoking appears to slightly increase the risk of severe disease, and ^{131}I may make the underlying ophthalmopathy worse.

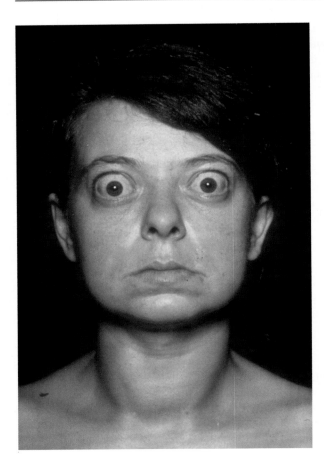

FIGURE 3-7. Exophthalmos. The abnormal protrusion of the eyeball within the orbit in a patient with Graves disease. (Sandoz Pharmaceutical Corporation.)

Approximately 5% of individuals with Graves disease have associated **infiltrative dermopathy**, or **pretibial myxedema**, most commonly seen in patients with significant ophthalmopathy. Indurated, pinkish purple plaques are characteristic of the dermopathy, which is often found on the anterior shins. Pretibial myxedema is the result of inflammation and fibrosis within the dermis. This fibrosis compresses the dermal lymphatics and leads to localized nonpitting lymphedema.

Diagnostic Studies

Graves disease is generally suspected clinically and confirmed by laboratory testing. The presence of a goiter or ophthalmopathy with low TSH and elevated FT_4 levels is diagnostic. In rare cases, the FT_4 will be normal, whereas T_3 will be significantly elevated. The presence of TRAbs may be helpful in the diagnosis of unclear cases but is not necessary for the diagnosis of Graves disease. [123]I uptake studies are rarely necessary for the diagnosis but, when obtained, show uniformly increased uptake of iodine throughout the thyroid gland.

Treatment

Treatment of Graves disease is outlined above. Individuals with Graves disease treated medically have a 25% remission rate within 2 years. Unfortunately, the relapse rate is between 30% to 40%, making medical therapy less attractive than definitive therapy with radioablation using ^{131}I or thyroidectomy.

Prognosis

With timely recognition and treatment, prognosis is excellent. However, in those who develop severe ophthalmopathy, eye muscle fibrosis, leading to diplopia and, rarely, blindness, may occur. In those with severe ophthalmopathy, a thyroidectomy should be chosen as definitive therapy because medical and radioablative therapy tend to cause the ophthalmopathy to worsen.

Graves disease is of particular concern during pregnancy, because the immunoglobulin G (IgG) TSH receptor antibodies readily cross the placenta. The antibodies can stimulate excessive production of thyroid hormone in the fetus or neonate. Neonatal Graves disease occurs in less than 5% of pregnant women with Graves disease, but, when it does occur, neonates are born with low birth weight; ravenous appetite; tachycardia; hypertension; and occasionally, with exophthalmos and a goiter. These neonates are treated with methimazole but typically only need therapy for the 4 to 8 weeks it takes the IgG antibodies to leave the neonate's system.

Toxic Multinodular Goiter

Toxic multinodular goiter (MNG), also known as **Plummer disease**, is the second most common cause of hyperthyroidism and usually affects individuals in the sixth decade of life. Hyperthyroidism occurs in approximately 10% of patients with long-standing nontoxic MNG due to low iodine intake. A portion of their thyroid tissue develops automaticity and begins to secrete thyroid hormone in the absence of the TSH signal. This automaticity is typically the result of a somatic mutation in the TSH-receptor signaling pathway, causing the continuous activation of the TSH-receptor pathway. The thyrotoxicosis of toxic MNG is often insidious in onset and relatively mild in symptomatology. Only the core symptoms of thyrotoxicosis will be present, and, unlike with Graves disease, there is no associated dermopathy or ophthalmopathy. For these reasons, it is necessary to check a TSH level yearly in individuals with nontoxic MNG to ensure that they have not developed automaticity within the thyroid gland. ^{123}I uptake scans will show a single area of increased uptake, with suppression of the remaining thyroid. Rarely, there is more than one focus of automaticity, and multiple areas of increased uptake may be present. The T_4 and T_3 levels are elevated, and the TSH level is suppressed. Treatment options for MNG are the same as for Graves disease.

Toxic Adenoma

The third most common cause of hyperthyroidism is a toxic adenoma, which usually develops slowly in the fourth to sixth decades of life. These adenomas rarely cause symptoms of thyrotoxicosis before reaching 3 cm in diameter. Toxic adenomas, like toxic MNGs, are caused by somatic mutations of the TSH-receptor signaling pathway, which lead to increased automaticity of the thyroid tissue. However, unlike toxic MNGs, the automaticity develops in an otherwise normal thyroid gland. The excess T_4 and T_3 secreted by the nodule results in suppression of TSH. A radioactive scan reveals a single **hot nodule**. These individuals are ideal for ^{131}I therapy because most of the gland is already suppressed and will not take up the ^{131}I; therefore, only the nodule would be destroyed. After the nodule is destroyed, TSH is no longer suppressed, and the rest of the gland resumes normal function. The incidence of hypothyroidism is much lower than with ^{131}I therapy for Graves disease or MNG.

Thyroiditis

Thyroiditis, or inflammation of the thyroid gland, encompasses a diverse group of disease processes that are similar only because they result in inflammation of the thyroid gland. These diseases are due to a variety of etiologies, including autoimmune phenomena, infection, postinfectious reactions, and postradiation. Other causes of hyperthyroidism due to thyroiditis include subacute lymphocytic and Riedel syndrome.

Acute Infectious Thyroiditis

Acute infectious thyroiditis is the result of a bacterial or fungal infection of the thyroid gland. Common pathogens include *Staphylococcus*, *Pneumococcus*, and *Mycobacterium tuberculosis*. *Candida* and *Aspergillus* are less commonly implicated pathogens. Acute infectious thyroiditis is an uncommon cause of thyroiditis, usually occurring in the immunocompromised individual, in patients with underlying thyroid disease, or in patients with anatomic thyroid anomalies.

Clinical features of acute infectious thyroiditis include local pain and tenderness over the thyroid gland that often radiates over the entire neck or into the ear. There is often associated pain with swallowing. Individuals frequently have fever, chills, and regional lymphadenopathy. Acute infectious thyroiditis is frequently associated with a thyrotoxic state, which is transient and due to the release of preformed thyroid hormone. Radioactive iodine scans show diffuse, decreased uptake of iodine during the infection.

Antibiotics are the mainstay of treatment for acute infectious thyroiditis. The most commonly used antibiotics include penicillin and ampicillin. The prognosis for acute infectious thyroiditis is excellent, and nearly all patients return to the euthyroid state without complications.

De Quervain Thyroiditis (Subacute Granulomatous Thyroiditis)

Subacute granulomatous thyroiditis is the most common cause of a painful thyroid gland and occurs much more frequently than acute infectious thyroiditis. The pathogenesis is not fully understood, but it is believed to be the result of a viral infection. Commonly implicated viruses include *coxsackie virus*, *mumps*, and *adenovirus*. It occurs more frequently in women and most commonly in middle age. There is often a recent history of an upper respiratory infection.

The primary clinical feature is pain within the thyroid gland. This pain can be associated with an enlargement of the thyroid gland itself. Transient thyrotoxicosis occurs in approximately 50% of patients. The thyrotoxicosis is often followed by a transient period of hypothyroidism prior to a return to the euthyroid state. The entire disease course occurs over several months. Diagnosis is generally clinical, but can be aided by radionucleotide studies that show a decreased uptake of [123]I. Histologic examination demonstrates granulomas within the thyroid parenchyma and numerous multinucleated giant cells.

Treatment of subacute granulomatous thyroiditis is supportive and consists of nonsteroidal antiinflammatory drugs for pain control. If the patient becomes overtly symptomatic during the transient thyrotoxic state, β-blockers are the treatment of choice; thionamides do not play a role in treatment. Minimal doses of levothyroxine can be given if the patient becomes symptomatic during the hypothyroid state; however, the doses should be low enough to ensure that the TSH is able to recover to baseline.

Subacute Lymphocytic Thyroiditis (Painless Thyroiditis)

Subacute lymphocytic thyroiditis occurs frequently in the postpartum period and is characterized by painless enlargement of the thyroid gland. It is thought to be a variant of autoimmune thyroiditis, insofar as anti-TPO antibodies are often present. Like subacute granulomatous thyroiditis, subacute lymphocytic thyroiditis involves a transient period of thyrotoxicosis followed by a transient period of hypothyroidism. Over 80% of patients return to the euthyroid state within months of disease onset.

Diagnosis of subacute lymphocytic thyroiditis is made by its clinical manifestations that can be aided by radionucleotide studies showing decreased uptake of ^{123}I. Histologic examination demonstrates lymphocytic infiltrate and a paucity of germinal follicles within the thyroid parenchyma. Treatment is similar to subacute granulomatous thyroiditis, with β-blockers for the thyrotoxic period and levothyroxine for the hypothyroid period. Individuals with subacute lymphocytic thyroiditis should receive lifelong monitoring of thyroid function because nearly 30% will eventually develop hypothyroidism.

Riedel Thyroiditis

Riedel thyroiditis is a rare form of fibrosing thyroiditis that occurs most frequently in middle-aged women. The etiology is unknown, but the disease presents with extensive fibrosis of the thyroid gland extending beyond the thyroid capsule. This fibrosis leads to a hard and noncompressible thyroid gland. Symptoms of Riedel thyroiditis are primarily due to compression of adjacent structures including the trachea and esophagus. Occasionally, Riedel thyroiditis is accompanied by overt hypothyroidism. Various treatment options have been explored and include corticosteroids and chemotherapeutic regimens. Currently, the most commonly employed treatment regimen is surgical decompression by separating the thyroid gland along the isthmus.

Other Causes of Thyrotoxicosis

Ectopic thyroid tissue can cause thyrotoxicosis. Most commonly, ectopic thyroid tissue is the result of failed embryologic migration of a lingual thyroid or functioning thyroid carcinoma metastasis. Rarely, thyrotoxicosis can be the initial presentation of an ovarian teratoma, which contains functioning thyroid tissue. This latter phenomenon is known as **struma ovarii**.

Excess TSH is an exceedingly rare cause of thyrotoxicosis and is usually due to autonomous TSH secretion by a pituitary adenoma. In this condition, the aberrantly elevated TSH causes excess thyroid hormone production, and there is no pathology within the thyroid gland itself. The excess TSH leads to a Graves-like picture with a diffusely enlarged rubbery thyroid. However, these individuals do not develop dermopathy or ophthalmopathy.

Increased levels of iodine can rarely lead to iodine-induced hyperthyroidism. This occurs only when the thyroid tissue has underlying automaticity. Although not definitively proven, the theory is that the autonomous thyroid tissue previously did not have sufficient iodine to produce excess thyroid hormone; therefore, when the individual was iodine deficient, he or she remained asymptomatic. Once increased levels of iodine are introduced, the automaticity picks up and causes excess thyroid hormone production.

Iatrogenic overdosing of thyroid hormone replacement is a common cause of thyrotoxicosis. In addition, there are numerous drugs that can lead to thyrotoxicosis by a variety of mechanisms. The most notable of these is amiodarone, a commonly used antiarrhythmic agent that leads to thyroid dysfunction in up to 10% of individuals.

Serious Consequence of Hyperthyroidism: Thyroid Storm

Thyroid storm is a rare complication of thyrotoxicosis in which the hyperthyroid individual manifests life-threatening symptoms of thyrotoxicosis. It occurs in less than 10% of patients hospitalized with thyrotoxicosis but carries 20% mortality. It occurs most commonly in the context of Graves disease but can be seen with other thyrotoxic conditions. A major stressor, such as serious illness, surgery, trauma, or childbirth, often precipitates thyroid storm. It is the result of decreased physiologic reserve and is caused by the body's inability to accommodate the chronically elevated levels of thyroid hormone, even though the levels of thyroid hormone are not markedly elevated.

Thyroid storm is an exceptionally difficult diagnosis to make because the chief clinical features are the same as the most extreme manifestations of thyrotoxicosis. In addition to the signs and symptoms commonly associated with thyrotoxicosis, fever, arrhythmias, and altered mental status occur. The altered mental status of thyroid storm ranges from lethargy and stupor to psychosis. This difficulty in diagnosis is not clinically significant insofar as all extreme thyrotoxic states should be treated expeditiously in the same manner.

Treatment of thyroid storm is similar to treatment of other thyrotoxic states, with attempts to target the synthesis, release, peripheral conversion, and target organ effects of thyroid hormone. This is accomplished by a combination of a thionamide, iodine solution, and dexamethasone. The goal of treatment is to bring thyroid hormone levels to normal within 48 hours. If this combination of drugs is unsuccessful in lowering thyroid hormone levels, dialysis and plasmaphoresis can be undertaken as a last resort. The β-blocker propranolol is used to treat the target organ effects of thyroid storm but does not contribute to the lowering of thyroid hormone. Treatment of the precipitating event is also vital to the treatment of the thyroid storm, and empiric antibiotics should be started if underlying infection is suspected. Supportive care is also necessary and includes fluids, cooling blankets, and antipyretics. With proper treatment, improvement is generally seen within 2 days, and full recovery is seen in 1 week.

THYROID NODULES

Thyroid nodules are exceedingly common and occur in 1% to 10% of adults in the United States. They are generally asymptomatic and are detected on palpation during routine physical examination. To be palpable, thyroid nodules must exceed 1 cm in diameter.

Solitary Thyroid Nodule

Greater than 95% of all thyroid nodules are benign and represent thyroid cysts, toxic adenomas, or scar tissue. The thyroid nodule provides a significant diagnostic challenge insofar as malignancy must be excluded. Features of thyroid nodules that favor malignancy include male gender, younger age, solitary occurrence, history of external neck radiation, and decreased uptake on ^{123}I scan.

The work-up of an individual with a solitary thyroid nodule starts with the determination of the TSH level. If the TSH level is low, usually indicating a thyrotoxic state, malignancy is unlikely, and tissue diagnosis is often unnecessary. These patients undergo diagnostic ^{123}I scan to determine if tissue diagnosis is necessary. Patients with an area of decreased uptake on ^{123}I scan, also referred to as a **cold nodule**, need further diagnostic work-up to exclude malignancy. Patients with an area of increased uptake, also referred to as a **hot nodule**, are extremely unlikely to have underlying malignancy, and treatment can proceed as in other cases of thyrotoxicosis. If the TSH is normal or if the diagnostic ^{123}I scan shows a cold nodule, a fine needle aspiration (FNA) biopsy is indicated to exclude malignancy. An algorithm for work-up of a thyroid nodule is shown (Figure 3-8).

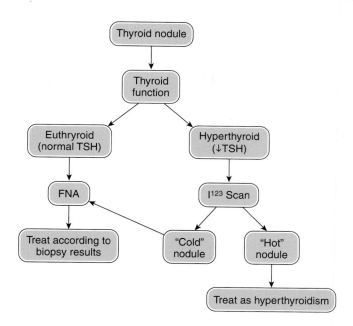

FIGURE 3-8. Algorithm for the evaluation of a thyroid nodule.

THYROID CANCER

Thyroid neoplasms are a rare form of malignancy accounting for less than 1.5% of all malignancies; however, thyroid neoplasms do represent the most common endocrine malignancy, with 15,000 diagnosed in the United States annually. Fortunately, thyroid neoplasms typically represent indolent disease and have a 20-year survival rate of nearly 90%. The types of thyroid neoplasms include follicular adenoma, papillary carcinoma, follicular carcinoma, medullary carcinoma, anaplastic carcinoma, and lymphoma.

Thyroid Neoplasms

The incidence of thyroid neoplasm is greater among women than men and generally peaks around the sixth decade. Thyroid neoplasms in younger patients are associated with worse prognosis. Other features associated with poor prognosis include larger tumor burden (>4 cm), extension beyond the thyroid capsule, distant metastasis, previous neck irradiation, and anaplastic histology. Thyroid neoplasms are staged according to the TNM (tumor, nodes, metastasis) staging system for both prognosis and treatment purposes.

Follicular Adenoma

Follicular adenomas are the most common benign neoplasm of the thyroid gland. They typically present as asymptomatic, unilateral, painless thyroid masses. They are typically less than 3 cm in diameter, but can reach up to 10 cm in diameter. When follicular adenomas become exceedingly large, an uncommon occurrence, they can cause compressive symptoms including hoarseness and respiratory compromise. Follicular adenomas are typically nonfunctional and appear as a cold nodule on diagnostic radioiodine ^{123}I scans. Rarely, they are functional and appear as hot nodules on diagnostic radioiodine ^{123}I scans. These hot nodules are referred to as **toxic adenomas** and were discussed previously (see Thyrotoxicosis section).

Follicular adenomas are derived from thyroid follicular epithelium. On microscopy, there are numerous uniform-appearing follicles without increased mitotic activity. Hürthle cells, a variant of follicular cells with brightly eosinophilic cytoplasm, can be seen in some specimens of follicular adenomas, but do not impart any clinical significance. On gross specimen, follicular adenomas appear as solitary spherical lesions completely encircled by a thick fibrous capsule. The presence of an intact capsule is what distinguishes the follicular adenoma from follicular carcinoma. Any breakdown of capsule integrity causes the lesion to be classified as follicular carcinoma. Despite the similarity between follicular adenomas and carcinomas, less than 10% of all follicular adenomas undergo malignant transformation. So, they are often treated conservatively.

Papillary Carcinoma

Papillary carcinoma is the most common form of thyroid neoplasms and represents 85% of all cases of thyroid malignancy. Papillary carcinoma affects women more frequently than men and most frequently between ages 25 and 50 years. The incidence of papillary carcinoma has been increasing over the past several decades for reasons that have not been fully elucidated, but it may be due to increases in iodizing radiation exposure. Papillary carcinoma can be solitary or multifocal and appear as encapsulated lesions on gross pathologic examination. On microscopic examination, numerous papillae emanating from a single fibrovascular stalk are evident. There are characteristic empty-appearing nuclei due to dispersed chromatin within the nuclei. These nuclei are often referred to as **orphan Annie eye nuclei** in reference to the 1930s' comic series in which Orphan Annie was drawn without pupils (Figure 3-9). Psammoma bodies are commonly found in papillary carcinoma and are useful in distinguishing them from other types of thyroid cancer insofar as they are not seen in follicular, anaplastic, or medullary thyroid cancer.

Metastasis is common at presentation of papillary carcinoma and is primarily by lymphatic spread. Metastasis to the cervical lymph nodes occurs in 50% of cases. Cervical metastasis is often the initial presentation of papillary carcinoma and on biopsy is referred to as **lateral aberrant thyroid**. This finding should not be confused with a benign ectopic thyroid because it is actually metastatic tissue. Interestingly, the finding of cervical lymph node metastasis does not significantly affect the prognosis of the disease. Overall, papillary thyroid carcinoma carries an excellent prognosis, with a 10-year survival rate exceeding 95%.

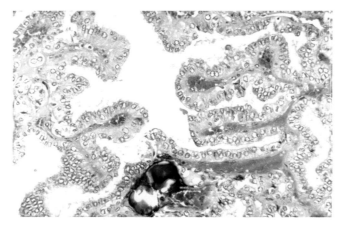

FIGURE 3-9. Papillary carcinoma of the thyroid gland. Branching papillae are lined by neoplastic columnar epithelium containing clear nuclei. A calcospherite or psammoma body is evident. (Image from Rubin E, Farber JL. Pathology. 3rd ed. Philadelphia, PA: Lippincott Williams & Wilkins; 1999.)

Follicular Carcinoma

Follicular carcinoma is the second most common form of thyroid neoplasm, comprising 5% to 15% of all cases of thyroid malignancy. Like other thyroid neoplasms, follicular carcinoma affects a preponderance of women, with women being affected three times more frequently than men. The average age of diagnosis is slightly higher than in papillary carcinoma and generally affects patients between ages 40 and 60 years. There is a slightly increased risk for follicular carcinoma in places of iodine deficiency. Follicular carcinoma generally presents as a slowly enlarging thyroid mass that appears cold on ^{123}I scan.

On microscopic examination, a follicular carcinoma is difficult to distinguish from a follicular adenoma because numerous uniform-appearing follicles characterize both. Hürthle cells can be seen in both follicular carcinomas and follicular adenomas. The only distinguishing feature is the presence of capsular invasion with a follicular carcinoma. Because of this marked similarity, it is often impossible to differentiate between follicular adenoma and follicular carcinoma based on FNA, and an excisional biopsy is necessary to fully determine if there is capsular integrity.

Follicular carcinoma tends to metastasize via hematogenous spread. Common sites of metastasis include bone, liver, and lung. Prognosis for follicular carcinoma is typically good, with a 10-year survival of 60% to 80%.

Medullary Carcinoma

Medullary carcinoma comprises 5% of all thyroid neoplasms and is associated with multiple endocrine neoplasia (MEN) 2A or MEN 2B in approximately 30% of cases. Sporadic cases occur in patients in their sixth and seventh decades, whereas cases associated with MEN syndromes tend to occur earlier in life. Medullary carcinoma typically presents as a slowly enlarging solitary thyroid mass, but can be multiple or bilateral, especially in cases associated with MEN syndromes. MEN syndromes are discussed in detail in Chapter 17.

Medullary carcinoma is distinct from other thyroid neoplasms insofar as it is a tumor of parafollicular C cells, rather than thyroid follicular cells. These tumors are often functional and secrete calcitonin. Despite the presence of increased calcitonin, clinically significant hypocalcemia is rare. The increased amount of secreted calcitonin is significant in that it forms the basis for amyloid deposits within the thyroid tissue. Microscopically, medullary carcinoma is distinguished by its numerous calcitonin secretory granules and extracellular amyloid deposits. The treatment of medullary thyroid carcinoma is distinct from other types of thyroid cancer insofar as the parafollicular cells are not responsive to ^{131}I treatments. Despite this, prognosis remains favorable in medullary carcinoma, with a 10-year survival rate of 70% to 80%.

Anaplastic (Undifferentiated) Carcinoma

Anaplastic carcinoma is a rare form of thyroid cancer that comprises less than 5% of all thyroid cancers. It differs from other types of thyroid neoplasms in that it is rapidly progressive, aggressive, and carries an extremely poor prognosis. Anaplastic carcinoma tends to affect the elderly population more frequently than other thyroid cancers, with the average age of diagnosis between ages 60 and 70 years. Up to 25% of patients with anaplastic carcinoma have a prior history of well-differentiated thyroid neoplasm. The microscopic evaluation of anaplastic carcinoma is widely variable but includes highly anaplastic cells with spindle cells, giant cells, and mixed cellularity.

The clinical presentation is more characteristic than with other thyroid neoplasms. Individuals typically present with a rapidly enlarging, bulky neck mass. Compressive symptoms are common and include dyspnea, cough, and hoarseness. Local invasion and pulmonary metastasis are both common at the time of diagnosis. The prognosis of anaplastic carcinoma is dismal, with a median survival of only 5 months.

Thyroid Lymphoma

Thyroid lymphoma is a B-cell lymphoma that occurs almost exclusively in the setting of Hashimoto thyroiditis. It is an entity distinct from other types of thyroid neoplasms and is treated as a lymphoma rather than as a primary thyroid neoplasm.

Treatment Principles

The treatment for thyroid neoplasms is surgical excision. Total thyroidectomy is the modality of choice for patients with thyroid cancer. In rare cases of very low-risk carcinomas, a partial thyroidectomy or lobectomy can be undertaken. Lymph node dissection or radical neck dissections are sometimes performed in conjunction with thyroidectomy if lymphatic metastasis is suspected.

With the exception of medullary carcinoma, after an individual with thyroid cancer undergoes a thyroidectomy, any remaining thyroid tissue is destroyed by ^{131}I ablation. This postoperative radiation serves two purposes. First, ^{131}I ablation destroys neoplastic cells. Neoplastic cells tend to take up iodine at lower rates than normal thyroid tissue; however, if given in high enough doses, the ^{131}I is able to destroy the neoplastic cells. Second, it allows for postablation surveillance. When all normal thyroid tissue is destroyed, there should be no remaining endogenous thyroid function. If endogenous thyroid function returns at any time, it would represent a neoplastic recurrence. This endogenous function is measured by serum thyroglobulin levels. If thyroglobulin levels remain stable or undetectable, it is unlikely that there is a recurrence of neoplasm.

The final part of the treatment regimen is aggressive exogenous thyroid hormone replacement, which is done to keep TSH at low-normal levels. TSH can stimulate growth of neoplastic cells; therefore, it is desirable to keep TSH levels as low as possible without causing adverse effects. Levothyroxine is, therefore, given at higher-than-usual doses for its negative feedback that keeps TSH low and prevents potential malignant thyroid tissue not removed during surgery from being stimulated.

CASE FOLLOW-UP

Laboratory tests reveal the following: elevated TSH (28.4 µIU/L), low TT4 (3.0 µg/dL), and low FT4 (0.5 ng/dL). Anti-Tg and anti-TPO antibodies are positive. The electrocardiogram shows sinus bradycardia and low voltage.

Our patient's signs and symptoms suggest hypothyroidism, which is confirmed by the biochemical findings of a low FT4 and elevated TSH. The elevated TSH shows that the hypothyroidism is due to failure of the thyroid gland and that the hypothalamic–pituitary portion of the axis is intact. The presence of antibodies establishes the etiology of her hypothyroidism as Hashimoto thyroiditis.

Based on her weight, she is prescribed levothyroxine (1 to 2 mcg/kg/day) and returns to clinic for repeat labs in 4 to 6 weeks. Her dose will be adjusted, if necessary, based on the laboratory findings.

REFERENCES and SUGGESTED READINGS

Abduljabbar MA, Afifi AM. Congenital hypothyroidism. J Pediatr Endocrinol Metab. 2012;25(1–2): 13–29.

Alexander EK, Marqusee E, Lawrence J, Jarolim P, Fischer GA, Larsen PR. Timing and magnitude of increases in levothyroxine requirements during pregnancy in women with hypothyroidism. N Engl J Med. 2004;351:241–249.

Bahn RS. Graves' ophthalmopathy. N Engl J Med. 2010;362:726–738.

Bartalena L. The dilemma of how to manage Graves' hyperthyroidism in patients with associated orbitopathy. J Clin Endocrinol Metab. 2011;96:592–599.

Beroukhim RS, Moon TD, Felner EI. Neonatal thyrotoxicosis and conjugated hyperbilirubinemia. J Maternal-Fetal Neonatal Med. 2003;13:426–428.

Bhowmick SK, Dasari G, Levens KL, Rettig KR. The prevalence of elevated serum thyroid stimulating hormone in childhood/adolescent obesity and of autoimmune thyroid diseases in a subgroup. J Natl Med Assoc. 2007;9(7):773–776.

Brent GA. Graves' disease. N Engl J Med. 2008;358:2594–2605.

Chung DC, Maher MM, Faquin WC. Case 37-2006: a 19-year-old woman with thyroid cancer and lower gastrointestinal bleeding. N Engl J Med. 2006;355:2349–2357.

Cooper DS. Antithyroid drugs. N Engl J Med. 2005;352:905–917.

De Felice M, Di Lauro R. Thyroid development and its disorders: genetics and molecular mechanisms. Endocr Rev. 2004;25:722–746.

Eastman CJ. Screening for thyroid disease and iodine deficiency. Pathology. 2012;44(2):153–159.

Farwell AP. Thyroid hormone therapy is not indicated in the majority of patients with the sick euthyroid syndrome. Endocr Pract. 2008;14(9):1180–1187.

Fauci AS, Harrison TR. Chapter 335: Disorders of the thyroid gland. In: Harrison's Principles of Internal Medicine. New York: McGraw-Hill, Medical Division; 2008:2224–2247.

Felner EI. A newborn with a goiter and thyroid dyshormonogenesis. J Maternal-Fetal Neonatal Med. 2002;12:207–208.

Felner EI, White PC, Dickson BA. Secondary hypothyroidism in siblings as a result of a single base deletion in the TSH-Beta subunit. J Pediatr Endocrinol Metabol. 2004;17(4):669–672.

Hegedus L. The thyroid nodule. N Engl J Med. 2004;351:1764–1771.

Lin JD, Chao TC, Huang B, Chen ST, Chang HY, Hsueh C. Thyroid cancer in the thyroid nodules evaluated by ultrasonography and fine-needle aspiration cytology. Thyroid 2005;15.7:708–717.

Moore, KL, Agur AMR, Dalley AF. Essential Clinical Anatomy. Philadelphia, PA: Lippincott Williams & Wilkins; 2011.

Ross DS. Radioiodine therapy for hyperthyroidism. N Engl J Med. 2011;364:542–550.

Sadler TW, Langman J. Langman's Medical Embryology. Philadelphia, PA: Lippincott Williams & Wilkins; 2006.

Singer PA, Cooper DS, Levy EG. Treatment guidelines for patients with hyperthyroidism and hypothyroidism. Standards of Care Committee, American Thyroid Association. JAMA. 1995; 273:808–812.

Toft AD. Subclinical hypothyroidism. N Engl J Med. 2001;345(7):512–516.

CHAPTER REVIEW QUESTIONS

1. A 34-year-old male who recently had surgery to remove a pheochromocytoma is found to have bilateral thyroid nodules on a follow-up physical examination. A fine-needle aspirate (FNA) confirms the presence of thyroid neoplasm. The histology likely shows:

   A. Numerous well-demarcated follicles cells
   B. Hürthle cells
   C. Extracellular amyloid deposits
   D. Psammoma bodies
   E. Empty-appearing nuclei

2. A healthy 27-year-old pregnant female of 20-weeks gestation, with no symptoms of thyroid disease, is participating in a research study. She has a battery of labs including TSH, TBG, FT_4, and TT_4. What changes, if any, would you expect to see in her laboratory values?

	TSH	TBG	FT$_4$	TT$_4$
A.	Normal	Normal	Normal	Normal
B.	Normal	↑	Normal	Normal
C.	Normal	↑	Normal	↑
D.	↑	↑	↑	↑
E.	↓	Normal	↓	↓

3. A previously healthy 42-year-old female complains of a 6-month history of increased fatigue and anxiety. She states that she feels jittery all the time and occasionally feels her heart beating rapidly in her chest. She also noticed a 10-lb weight loss, despite an increase in appetite. Her family history reveals that her twin sister has type 1 diabetes but the rest of her family is in good health. She is afebrile and on physical examination, she has a pulse of 103 beats per minute, respiratory rate of 21 breaths per minute, and blood pressure of 142/82 mmHg. She has proptosis and increased thickness in the neck. What would you expect to see on a ^{123}I scan?

    A. Diffusely increased uptake
    B. Diffusely decreased uptake
    C. Solitary hot nodule
    D. Solitary cold nodule
    E. Multiple hot nodules and an otherwise normal thyroid scan

4. A 64-year-old male noticed a 2-cm nodule on the lateral portion of his neck along the sternocleidomastoid muscle when he was shaving. A biopsy of the lesion shows thyroid tissue. This thyroid tissue most likely represents:

    A. Thyroglossal duct cyst
    B. Ectopic thyroid tissue
    C. Follicular carcinoma
    D. Papillary carcinoma
    E. Medullary carcinoma

5. A 75-year-old male with a history of atrial fibrillation, hypertension, diabetes, and depression feels increasing fatigue over the past 3 months. He noticed some mild muscle weakness and weight gain despite normal exercise and appetite. His primary care physician checks a TSH level and is surprised to find that it is markedly elevated. What drug is likely responsible for this thyroid abnormality?

    A. Hydrochlorothiazide
    B. Sertraline
    C. Metformin
    D. Propranolol
    E. Amiodarone

CHAPTER REVIEW ANSWERS

1. The correct answer is C. This patient likely has medullary thyroid carcinoma in the setting of MEN 2, insofar as he has a history of a pheochromocytoma and presents with bilateral thyroid carcinoma, an unusual finding in the absence of hereditary tumor syndromes. He should also be evaluated for hyperparathyroidism, as that is also a component of the MEN 2 triad. The histologic examination of medullary thyroid carcinoma shows multiple secretory granules (containing calcitonin) and extracellular amyloid deposits, which are made primarily of calcitonin protein.

Numerous well-demarcated follicles (**Choice A**) can be seen both in follicular adenomas and in follicular carcinoma. They are nonspecific and cannot help distinguish between these two entities. Hürthle cells are follicular cells with abundant eosinophilic cytoplasm (**Choice B**). They can be found in Hashimoto thyroiditis, follicular adenoma, and follicular carcinoma. They are nonspecific and cannot be used to make a pathologic diagnosis. Psammoma bodies (**Choice D**) are laminar calcified lesions seen in papillary thyroid carcinoma. They are almost pathognomonic for papillary carcinoma. Empty-appearing nuclei (**Choice E**) or "Orphan Annie nuclei" are commonly seen in papillary carcinoma and represent diffuse chromatin within the nuclei of neoplastic cells.

----

2. The correct answer is C. Pregnancy is a high estrogen state. Increased levels of estrogen cause an increase in the overall level of TBG. The body accommodates for the increased TBG by increasing the total thyroid hormone released. The increased thyroid is immediately bound up by the excess TBG. There is no change in the FT_4 level. Because FT_4 is the only metabolically active form of thyroid hormone, there are no symptoms of thyrotoxicosis and the TSH level remains normal. Thus, despite elevated total body thyroid hormone, the patient remains clinically euthyroid.

----

3. The correct answer is A. This patient likely has Graves disease. Not only because it is the most common etiology for thyrotoxicosis but also because there are several additional clinical features present. She is the typical age and gender for an autoimmune disease such as Graves disease and has a positive family history of autoimmune disease. Finally, while some ocular manifestations (thyroid stare and lid lag) are common in all types of thyrotoxic states, proptosis is specific to Graves disease. The typical radioiodine scan seen in Graves disease shows a diffusely increased uptake of ^{123}I.

Diffusely decreased uptake (**Choice B**) is not the typical radioiodine scan in thyrotoxic state. It occasionally can be seen in subacute thyroiditis after the initial release of preformed thyroid hormone. A solitary hot nodule (**Choice C**) is the characteristic radioiodine scan of a toxic adenoma. While this could be the cause of her thyrotoxicosis, it is much less likely than Graves disease. A solitary cold nodule (**Choice D**) is a common radioiodine scan finding seen with thyroid neoplasms, cysts, or scar tissue. However, it is generally found with the euthyroid state and would not account for thyrotoxicosis. Multiple hot nodules and an otherwise normal scan (**Choice E**) is the characteristic radioiodine scan of a toxic multinodular goiter. While this could be the cause of thyrotoxicosis, it is much less likely than Graves disease.

----

4. The correct answer is D. This patient likely has papillary thyroid carcinoma with metastasis to the cervical lymph nodes. Up to 50% of patients have lymph node metastasis at the time of diagnosis. The finding of a palpable lymph node is often the presenting feature of papillary thyroid cancer. This phenomenon is sometimes referred to as **lateral aberrant thyroid**. Despite the presence of metastasis, the prognosis remains excellent in these individuals.

A thyroglossal duct cyst (**Choice A**) occurs along the path of thyroid descent, from the foramen cecum at the base of the tongue, to the final resting point of the thyroid. They are always a midline structure and are never found in the lateral aspect of the neck. Ectopic thyroid tissue (**Choice B**) can occur anywhere along the path of the thyroid descent from the foramen cecum at the base of the tongue, as far down as the anterior mediastinum. They are always midline structures. Follicular carcinoma (**Choice C**) spreads by hematogenous routes and does not typically present as a lymph node metastasis. Medullary carcinoma (**Choice E**) is a neoplasm of the parafollicular C cells and would not appear as thyroid tissue on biopsy.

----

5. The correct answer is E. There are numerous medications that can cause thyroid dysfunction including amiodarone, lithium, and sulfonamides. Amiodarone is the most deleterious drug that affects the thyroid, insofar as it can cause both hypothyroidism and thyrotoxicosis. TSH levels should be obtained regularly when an individual is on long-term amiodarone therapy. The mechanism of amiodarone toxicity is complex, but is related to its high iodine content.

Although use of propranolol (**Choice D**) may mimic some of the symptoms of hypothyroidism (i.e., bradycardia) it would not elevate the TSH level. The other choices, hydrochlorothiazide (**Choice A**), a diuretic; sertraline (**Choice B**), an antidepressant; and metformin (**Choice C**), an antihyperglycemic agent, do not have any known effects on thyroid function or thyroid biochemical studies.

Hypocalcemia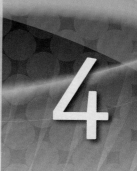

David L. Gutteridge
Eric I. Felner

CASE

The mother of a 1-week-old baby boy notices that his extremities jerk for about a minute. Despite holding his extremities, she observes that he still has the jerking motion. He was awake during the event, but, shortly after the jerking stopped, he fell asleep. According to his mother, the baby was born by vaginal delivery at term without complications. He was discharged home from the newborn nursery 24 hours after delivery. He has been breast-feeding every 2 hours without difficulty. When obtaining his vital signs, the nurse notes that when inflating the blood pressure cuff, he develops a carpal spasm of his hand. On physical exam, he is noted to have hyperreflexia in all extremities but no other neurologic abnormalities. There is no family history of epilepsy or other neurologic problems.

Initial laboratory evaluation reveals a low serum calcium level (4.5 mg/dL) and an elevated serum phosphate level (11.1 mg/dL). The serum parathyroid hormone (PTH) level is pending.

This chapter reviews calcium and phosphate physiology and the etiology, pathophysiology, and management of hypocalcemia to help the reader determine the etiology of this child's hypocalcemia. We summarize the work-up and provide a therapeutic plan to promote a better understanding of the diagnosis. This chapter is organized as follows: 1) basic physiology of calcium and phosphorous homeostasis involving the renal, skeletal, and endocrine systems; 2) the many causes of hypocalcemia; and 3) metabolic bone diseases associated with hypocalcemia and hypophosphatemia. Chapter 5 focuses on hypercalcemia.

OBJECTIVES

1. Develop a differential diagnosis for a patient with hypocalcemia.

2. Discuss the clinical and laboratory findings in a patient with hypocalcemia.

(continues)

(*continued*)

PHYSIOLOGY: CALCIUM AND PHOSPHORUS HOMEOSTASIS

Calcium is a major extracellular ion. It is critically important for many bodily functions. Extracellular calcium is essential for blood clotting, myocyte contraction, nerve conduction, hormone secretion, and bone strength. Intracellular calcium regulates cell secretion, motility, and differentiation. Calcium ions are cofactors for several enzymes and act as intracellular second messengers. Calcium homeostasis is tightly regulated because of its critical importance. Despite changes in dietary intake, renal excretion, and the demands of pregnancy, extracellular calcium concentration fluctuates very little. The intracellular calcium concentration, on the other hand, can change dramatically due to the release of calcium from intracellular stores or the influx of extracellular calcium. The extracellular calcium is maintained at a level 1,000-fold greater than the intracellular calcium.

The recommended daily adult intake of calcium (1,000 to 1,500 mg) differs only slightly from that for children and adolescents (800 to 1,200 mg) but significantly when compared with infants (400 to 600 mg). Calcium can be found in a variety of foods, including dairy products (e.g., milk and cheese) and green vegetables (e.g., broccoli, okra, and kale). The calcium from food is absorbed into the bloodstream by the duodenum via specialized calcium transporters. About 40% of the calcium in the blood is bound to proteins, primarily albumin. The other 60% exists either complexed to sulfate and phosphate anions (~10%) or in its free ionized form (~50%). The normal total concentration of these three forms is 8.5 to 10.5 mg/dL. Free calcium is the only active form and is regulated by the body's hormones. Therefore, any significant change in the free calcium level can have a significant impact on calcium activity in the body.

When measuring total serum calcium levels it is important to remember that the level represents bound calcium and free calcium. If a serum free calcium level is not measured, a correction for an abnormal albumin level must be made. For every 1 g/dL drop in serum albumin below 4 g/dL, measured serum calcium decreases by 0.8 mg/dL. Therefore, to correct for a serum albumin level <4 g/dL, 0.8 mg/dL should be added to the serum total calcium level for every 1 g/dL decrease in serum albumin. Without this correction, a normal serum total calcium level may appear to be low. The corrected serum total calcium level can be calculated using the following formula:

$$\text{Corrected serum total calcium level} = [(4.0 - \text{serum albumin}) \times 0.8] + \text{measured serum total calcium level}.$$

TABLE 4-1.	Serum Calcium and Phosphorus Parameters	
Parameter	Calcium	Phosphorus
Total serum concentration (mg/dL)	8.5–10.5	2.5–4.5[a]
Serum ionized concentration (mg/dL)	4.1–4.7	2.1–3.8
Bound to plasma proteins (%)	40	15
Total body stores in bone (%)	99	85
Extracellular:intracellular concentrations	1,000:1	1:10

[a]For the first year of life: 4.0–8.0 mg/dL.

Phosphorus (or phosphate) is a major intracellular anion. It is required for the generation of adenosine triphosphate (ATP), is an essential component of cell membrane phospholipids, and directly regulates enzyme action and protein function. Together, calcium and phosphate make up hydroxyapatite, the major component of bone matrix. Unlike calcium, extracellular phosphate is not as tightly regulated, and therefore, the plasma concentration of phosphate varies widely. Dairy products and red meat serve as major sources of phosphorus in the diet. The kidneys are responsible for regulating plasma phosphate concentration. A diet consistently low in phosphate can increase the reabsorptive potential of the renal tubules. The major differences between calcium and phosphate in serum and bone are shown in Table 4-1.

Regulators of Calcium Balance

PTH and vitamin D are the hormones that primarily affect calcium homeostasis. Other factors, including calcium-sensing receptors (CaSRs), calcitonin, magnesium, fibroblastic growth factor-23 (FGF23), osteoblasts, osteoclasts, and renal function also contribute to calcium and phosphate balance.

PTH is the major hormone that regulates calcium homeostasis. It is produced by chief cells in the parathyroid glands. Chief cells have CaSRs on their surface that sense extracellular concentrations of calcium. PTH secretion and production are acutely responsive to any change in the concentration of serum free calcium (Figure 4-1). This change is recognized by CaSRs on the parathyroid cells. The major function of PTH is to correct hypocalcemia by acting directly on bone and the kidney, and indirectly on the intestine. In bone, PTH interacts with receptors on osteoblasts that result in cytokine release. The cytokines then activate osteoclasts, which release calcium and phosphate from bone through the process of resorption. In the kidney, PTH increases phosphate excretion and calcium reabsorption in the distal tubule. PTH also stimulates the activity of the renal enzyme 1α-hydroxylase, which then converts the inactive 25-(OH)-vitamin D_3 to the active 1,25-$(OH)_2$-vitamin D_3. In the small intestine, 1,25-$(OH)_2$-vitamin D_3 increases both calcium and phosphate absorption.

Vitamin D is produced by the effect of sunlight on the skin. It is a generic term used to refer to several metabolites of vitamin D_3. Vitamin D_3, also referred to as cholecalciferol, is a soluble prohormone produced in the epidermis. 1,25-dihydroxy-vitamin D_3 (calcitriol) is the active metabolite of vitamin D_3. It is the final metabolite produced in the vitamin D pathway (Figure 4-2). It regulates calcium and phosphate homeostasis

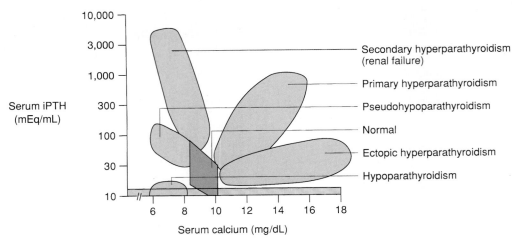

FIGURE 4-1. Parathyroid hormone release as a function of extracellular calcium. When calcium concentrations fall below the normal range, there is a steep increase in the secretion of parathyroid hormone (PTH). Low levels of the hormone are secreted even when blood calcium levels are high. Serum calcium levels are low in patients with hypoparathyroidism, psuedohypoparathyroidism, and secondary hyperparathyroidism. Serum calcium levels are elevated in patients with hyperparathyroidism. The figure depicts PTH release from cells cultured in vitro in differing concentrations of calcium. (After Clark OH, Way LW. Thyroid and parathyroid. In: Way LW, ed. Current Surgical Diagnosis and Treatment. 8th ed. Norwalk, CT: Appleton & Lange; 1989:249.)

by crossing cell membranes and binding to vitamin D receptors in the nucleus. Endogenously, all vitamin D levels exist in the form of vitamin D_3, whereas vitamin D added as a dietary supplement comes from plants and yeast in the form of vitamin D_2 (**ergocalciferol**). Vitamin D_2 and its metabolites have the same biologic activity as vitamin D_3.

Vitamins D_2 and D_3 travel in the blood bound to the vitamin D-binding protein. In the liver, vitamin D is 25-hydroxylated by the cytochrome P450-like enzyme to 25-hydroxyvitamin D_3 (**calcidiol**) and binds to vitamin D-binding proteins and albumin. This hydroxylation step is poorly regulated. Therefore, any amount of vitamin D can be converted to calcidiol, the major storage form of the hormone. The best determinant of the status of vitamin D in the bloodstream is to measure the serum calcidiol level, because it reflects vitamin D stores.

Eventually, calcidiol is transported to the renal tubules where it is further hydroxylated to the active form, calcitriol, by the 1α-hydroxylase enzyme. The action of this enzyme is tightly regulated by several feedback loops. A decrease in ionized calcium results in an increase in PTH that then stimulates renal 1α-hydroxylase activity. Calcitriol also regulates its own production. If it is present in a low concentration, it can stimulate its own synthesis.

The major role of vitamin D on the small intestine is to increase calcium and phosphate absorption, which is mediated by the active vitamin D hormone, calcitriol. For vitamin D_3 to be effective it must progress through the metabolic pathway, converting to calcitriol, and calcitriol must interact with its receptor.

The **CaSRs** are located on the surfaces of the chief cells and are responsible for sensing the extracellular level of calcium. Three distinct intracellular processes regulate activation of the CaSRs. The first is its effect on the CaSR based on the intracellular calcium level. Elevated intracellular calcium levels, sensed by the CaSR, result in a decrease in PTH release. Low intracellular calcium levels result in an increase in PTH release. The

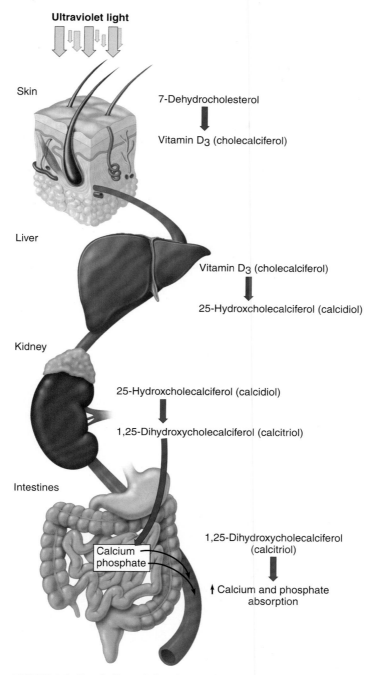

Ultraviolet light

Skin

7-Dehydrocholesterol

Vitamin D$_3$ (cholecalciferol)

Liver

Vitamin D$_3$ (cholecalciferol)

25-Hydroxcholecalciferol (calcidiol)

Kidney

25-Hydroxcholecalciferol (calcidiol)

1,25-Dihydroxycholecalciferol (calcitriol)

Intestines

Calcium phosphate

1,25-Dihydroxycholecalciferol (calcitriol)

↑ Calcium and phosphate absorption

FIGURE 4-2. Metabolism of vitamin D and the regulation of serum calcium. (From Premkumar K. The Massage Connection Anatomy and Physiology. Baltimore: Lippincott Williams & Wilkins; 2004.)

second is through gene transcription. Activation of the CaSR influences *prepro-PTH* gene transcription that causes a decrease in the rate of PTH synthesis. The third is the CaSR effect on cell proliferation.

Calcitonin is secreted primarily by parafollicular C cells of the thyroid gland in response to an increase in extracellular calcium. Its main action is to suppress osteoclastic activity.

Calcitonin and PTH check and balance each other in order to maintain calcium homeostasis. It is unclear, however, if calcitonin has a significant effect on plasma calcium. Thyroid C cells secrete calcitonin in response to acute changes in plasma calcium. Calcitonin secretion, in response to chronic hypercalcemia, however, is not as reliable. For example, patients undergoing a total thyroidectomy lose all of their thyroid C cells, but do not develop hypercalcemia. Similarly, those with medullary carcinoma of the thyroid have extremely high levels of plasma calcitonin, but do not develop hypocalcemia.

Magnesium is necessary for both PTH synthesis and secretion. Patients with magnesium deficiency develop hypocalcemia due to a reduction in PTH synthesis and secretion.

Fibroblastic growth factor 23 (FGF23), a protein encoded by the *FGF23* gene, is a member of the FGF family that is responsible for phosphate metabolism. It is usually expressed in bone and connective tissue and inhibits renal tubular phosphate transport by acting mainly in the proximal convoluted tubule. It also inhibits the 1α-hydroxylase enzyme, preventing the conversion of calcidiol to calcitriol (Figure 4-3). FGF23 is a substrate for the X-linked, phosphate-regulating endopeptidase homologue (*PHEX*) enzyme. This enzyme is primarily active in bones and teeth and is responsible for the cleavage and inactivation of *FGF23*.

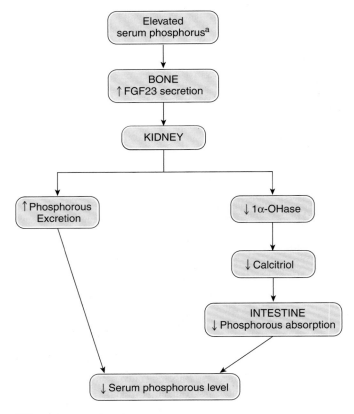

a Normal serum phosphorous range:

Birth–10 days:	5.4–9.0 mg/dL
10 days–1 year:	4.5–6.7 mg/dL
2–11 years:	4.5–5.5 mg/dL
>12 years:	2.7–4.5 mg/dL

FIGURE 4-3. Serum phosphate-lowering effects of FGF23.

Osteoblasts and **osteoclasts** are instrumental in controlling the amount of bone tissue. Osteoblasts form bone and osteoclasts resorb bone. Osteoclasts are activated via the receptor activator nuclear factor κ-B ligand (RANKL). Osteoclastic activity is triggered via the osteoblasts' surface-bound RANKL activating the osteoclasts' surface-bound receptor activator of nuclear factor κ-B (RANK).

The **renal system** plays a major role in calcium and phosphorus homeostasis. This chapter reviews only the endocrine biochemical parameters of individuals with hypocalcemia due to renal failure and not other renal conditions.

HYPOCALCEMIA

Hypocalcemia may occur as a congenital or acquired abnormality. It may also be permanent or transient.

Signs and Symptoms

Hypocalcemia affects multiple organ systems. Neurologically it can cause neuromuscular irritability, seizures, tremors, muscle cramping, tetany, and parethesias. In the ocular system, it causes cataracts, papilledema, and pseudotumor cerebri. In the cardiovascular system, it causes prolongation of the QT interval and nonspecific T-wave changes on the echocardiogram. Increased neuromuscular activity of the gastrointestinal (GI) tract causes diarrhea.

The two classic physical examination findings of hypocalcemia are **Chvostek Trousseau** and **signs (Figure 4-4A,B)**. The Chvostek sign is evident by repetitive twitching of the nose and lips when the facial nerve is tapped at the angle of the jaw along the

A

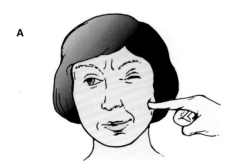

FIGURE 4-4. Signs of hypocalcemia. **(A)** Chvostek sign. **(B)** Trousseau sign in a woman with hypocalcemia. (From Nettina, SM. The Lippincott Manual of Nursing Practice. 7th ed. Lippincott Williams & Wilkins; 2001.)

B

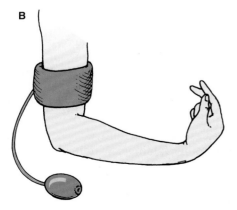

masseter muscle. The Trousseau sign manifests as a carpal spasm after inflation of an arm blood pressure cuff above the systolic blood pressure for 2 to 3 minutes.

Treatment

The majority of patients with hypocalcemia are treated with both calcium and vitamin D (D_2, D_3, or 1,25-dihydroxy-vitamin D). For hypocalcemia due to vitamin D deficiency, cholecalciferol is substituted for calcitriol. Neonates and infants require 50 to 100 mg/kg/day of elemental calcium and 0.25 to 1.00 mcg/day of calcitriol. Older children and adults require 1 to 2 g/day of calcium carbonate and 0.25 to 0.5 mcg/day of calcitriol. Because calcium supplementation is extremely variable, frequent monitoring of the serum calcium level is necessary to determine the ideal dose required during the initial months of treatment.

HYPOCALCEMIA WITH LOW OR NORMAL PARATHYROID HORMONE LEVELS

This section reviews congenital and acquired causes of hypocalcemia and its relationship to a low or normal serum PTH level.

Congenital Causes

Congenital causes include hypoparathyroidism, a CaSR defect, and magnesium deficiency.

Parathyroid Dysgenesis

Congenital hypoparathyroidism is due to agenesis or dysgenesis of the parathyroid glands.

Etiology

Absent or dysfunctional parathyroid glands cause PTH deficiency. The most common cause of congenital hypoparathyroidism is the DiGeorge sequence, a genetic condition caused by a mutation in chromosome 22 (22q deletion) that results in dysgenesis of the pharyngeal pouches (Figure 4-5). In addition to possible parathyroid maldevelopment, abnormal physical facial features, thymus development, and cardiovascular structures may be present. It has a prevalence of 1:4,000.

Pathology

The parathyroid glands are usually small or absent but may be normal in size.

Pathophysiology

In the absence of the parathyroid glands and its hormone, PTH, there is no stimulus available to increase extracellular calcium. Without PTH, serum levels of calcium cannot be maintained because calcium is unable to be **resorbed** from bone, absorbed in the intestines, or **reabsorbed** from the renal tubules.

Clinical Findings

In addition to the characteristic clinical features associated with hypocalcemia, individuals with DiGeorge sequence (22q deletion) have other findings including ear malrotation, microagnathia, upturned nose, flat nasal bridge, hypertelorism, thymic-related abnormalities, and aortic arch abnormalities (Figure 4-6). These findings, specific for the 22q deletion, are the result of failure of the pharyngeal pouches to develop or form properly

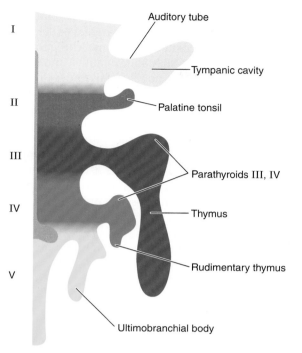

I

II

III

IV

V

Auditory tube

Tympanic cavity

Palatine tonsil

Parathyroids III, IV

Thymus

Rudimentary thymus

Ultimobranchial body

FIGURE 4-5. Pharyngeal pouches. Schematic diagram of the pharyngeal pouches in a human embryo of 6 weeks. Five pairs of pouches give rise to many important structures of the head, neck, and chest. A wide spectrum of congenital malformations results from abnormalities of the pharyngeal pouches. (From Rubin R, Strayer DS. Rubin's Pathology: Clinicopathologic Foundations of Medicine. 5th ed. Philadelphia: Lippincott Williams & Wilkins; 2008.)

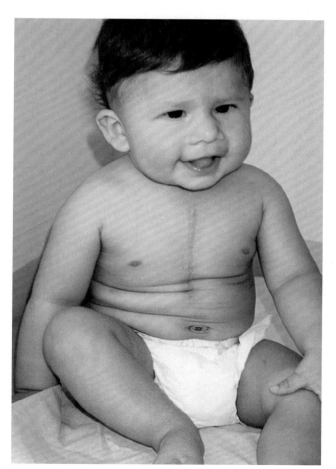

FIGURE 4-6. DiGeorge sequence. The surgical scar on the chest suggests open heart surgery. Repair of a truncus arteriosus or an interrupted aortic arch are common cardiovascular abnormalities in DiGeorge sequence. Note the characteristic facial features: hypertelorism, low-set ears, hypoplastic mandible, and upward bowing of the upper lip. (From Roberts R. Atlas of Infectious Diseases, Mandell G (series ed.), Catherine M. Wilfert. © 1998 Current Medicine, Inc.)

during embryogenesis. Characteristic facial features result from developmental failure of the first and second pouches. The thymus develops from the third pharyngeal pouch and failure of its development increases the risk of T-cell-mediated infections. The parathyroid glands arise from the third and fourth pouches. Aortic arch abnormalities and other cardiovascular abnormalities occur when the fourth and fifth pouches fail to develop.

Diagnostic Studies

The diagnosis of hypocalcemia due to hypoparathyroidism is based on a low serum calcium level and a low, or inappropriately normal, serum PTH level. In the setting of hypocalcemia, a normal serum PTH level is inappropriate. The CaSR, in response to hypocalcemia, should trigger PTH release to raise the serum calcium level. Therefore, a normal serum PTH level during hypocalcemia indicates that the parathyroid glands are not functioning optimally. The serum phosphate level is also elevated due to the absence of PTH.

Prognosis

In most cases of congenital hypocalcemia due to hypoparathyroidism, early diagnosis and treatment make the prognosis excellent. In patients with the DiGeorge sequence, prognosis is generally not related to calcium status (as that is generally not difficult to manage) but rather to the thymic and/or cardiovascular manifestations.

Treatment

Individuals with hypoparathyroidism and absent or low serum levels of PTH usually require both calcium and calcitriol supplementation. This is necessary because upregulation of the 1α-hydroxylase enzyme does not occur in the absence of PTH. Low endogenous calcitriol and reduced intestinal absorption of calcium are the results of the absence of PTH.

Calcium-Sensing Receptor Defect

A defect in the CaSR is caused by a mutation of the *CaSR* gene.

Etiology

More than 50 activating (gain-of-function) mutations of the *CaSR* gene have been identified. They are all inherited in an autosomal dominant pattern.

Pathology

The parathyroid glands may be of normal or slightly smaller size.

Pathophysiology

The CaSR is activated by an increased extracellular calcium concentration that decreases PTH release and renal tubular calcium reabsorption. When ionized calcium concentrations fall, CaSR activation also falls, leading to increased PTH release and renal tubular calcium reabsorption.

A gain of function mutation of the *CaSR* gene increases CaSR sensitivity to calcium, causing an increase in calcium ion suppression of PTH release, and decreasing renal tubular reabsorption of calcium. This impairment of PTH secretion, coupled with renal calcium and magnesium wasting, results in hypocalcemia, hypocalciuria, hyperphosphatemia, and hypomagnesemia.

Clinical Findings

This condition clinically appears very similar to hypoparathyroidism. There are no obvious physical abnormalities present.

Diagnostic Studies

The diagnosis of hypocalcemia due to a *CaSR* gene defect is based on a low serum calcium level and a low, or inappropriately normal, PTH level. In addition, the serum phosphate level is usually elevated, and the serum magnesium level is low. It is very difficult to differentiate this condition from hypoparathyroidism due to parathyroid gland dysgenesis. In children with congenital hypocalcemia due to hypoparathyroidism who do not have DiGeorge sequence, genetic testing for a *CaSR* gene deletion can be performed in those with a strong family history. Further pursuit of the exact etiology may not be necessary insofar as management is similar in both conditions.

Treatment

The treatment is similar to that for hypoparathyroidism due to parathyroid gland dysgenesis in the acute state, but after initial stabilization, the calcitriol (or any vitamin D metabolite) dose should be minimized because of the risk of worsening hypercalciuria, or promoting the development of nephrolithiasis, nephrocalcinosis, or renal impairment. In rare instances, patients will also require magnesium supplementation.

Prognosis

With proper replacement and frequent monitoring, the prognosis is excellent.

Magnesium Deficiency

Several inherited conditions (i.e., Gitelman and Bartter syndromes) are associated with excessive urinary loss of magnesium.

Etiology

Gene mutations of proteins involving the intestinal absorption of magnesium have also been identified. In these conditions, primary hypomagnesemia causes secondary hypocalcemia.

Pathology

The parathyroid glands are normal in size.

Pathophysiology

Profound hypomagnesemia results from both impaired intestinal absorption and renal reabsorption of magnesium. The low magnesium level inhibits the synthesis and secretion of PTH that results in hypocalcemia and hyperphosphatemia.

Clinical Findings

These individuals exhibit the typical features of hypocalcemia. Symptoms begin in infancy, and patients usually present with generalized seizures. Differentiation between the inherited and acquired forms of hypomagnesemia is based on the magnesium level (much lower in the inherited form), clinical presentation (more overt in the inherited form), and a positive family history.

Diagnostic Studies

The diagnosis of hypocalcemia due to primary hypomagnesemia is based on low serum calcium and magnesium levels and a low or normal serum PTH level.

Treatment

These individuals require lifelong, high-dose (0.4 to 3.9 mmol/kg/day) oral magnesium supplementation. Acutely, they also require intravenous magnesium and calcium, as well as calcitriol supplementation. Once the magnesium level stabilizes, calcium and calcitriol are usually not necessary.

Prognosis

Prognosis is dependent on the time of diagnosis. If the diagnosis is made early, there is little likelihood of developing severe neurologic impairment.

Transient Neonatal Hypocalcemia

Neonates can be born with a transient form of hypocalcemia that is due to maternal hypercalcemia. The mother may have hypercalcemia secondary to hyperparathyroidism, gestational diabetes, or excessive vitamin D intake. Prior to birth, the elevated maternal calcium crosses the placenta. Shortly after birth, the elevated serum calcium in the neonate feeds back at the level of the parathyroid gland, inhibiting neonatal PTH secretion. Within age 1 to 2 weeks, these neonates develop hypocalcemia and hyperphosphatemia that appear clinically and biochemically similar to hypoparathyroidism. Within 8 to 12 weeks of treatment with calcium and calcitriol, however, serum calcium and phosphate levels return to the normal range, and remain in the normal range even after the supplements are discontinued.

Acquired Causes

Acquired causes include autoimmune hypoparathyroidism, vitamin D deficiency, a variety of pharmacologic agents, and renal failure.

Autoimmune Hypoparathyroidism

Acquired hypoparathyroidism is most commonly due to autoimmune destruction of the parathyroid glands.

Etiology

Autoimmune hypoparathyroidism usually occurs as part of the autoimmune polyglandular syndrome type 1 (APS1) (see Chapter 14).

Pathology

The parathyroid glands are inflamed and ultimately shrink in size or involute.

Pathophysiology

In the absence of parathyroid glands and, therefore PTH, there is no stimulus for increasing extracellular calcium. Without PTH, serum levels of calcium cannot be maintained because calcium is unable to be **resorbed** from bone, **absorbed** in the intestines, or **reabsorbed** from the renal tubules.

Clinical Findings

These patients exhibit the typical features of hypocalcemia. The onset of symptoms usually occurs in the first or second decade of life.

Diagnostic Studies

The diagnosis of hypocalcemia due to hypoparathyroidism is based on a low serum calcium level and a low, or inappropriately normal, PTH level. In addition, the serum phosphate level is elevated due to the inability to promote phosphaturia in the absence of PTH. In those with gene mutation-proven APS1 and hypoparathyroidism, less than 50% have antibodies to parathyroid tissue or the CaSR. Although the presence of these antibodies may be helpful in confirming the diagnosis, they are generally not necessary.

Treatment

Individuals with hypoparathyroidism usually require both calcium and calcitriol supplementation.

Prognosis

In most cases of autoimmune hypoparathyroidism, treatment of hypocalcemia is relatively simple. Prognosis is dependent on the individual's other APS1-related conditions.

Iatrogenic Hypoparathyroidism

The most common iatrogenic cause of hypocalcemia is the surgical removal of the parathyroid glands during a thyroidectomy.

Etiology

The majority of patients undergoing a total thyroidectomy or multiple parathyroid gland removal develop a decrease in serum calcium level shortly after the operation. About 25% develop hypocalcemia, with less than 5% being permanent.

Pathology

If the patient undergoes a parathyroidectomy, the parathyroid glands are absent. If the patient undergoes a thyroidectomy, the parathyroid glands may be absent (if removed or damaged) or normal.

Pathophysiology

In the absence of parathyroid glands and PTH, there is no stimulus for increasing extracellular calcium. Without PTH, serum levels of calcium cannot be maintained because calcium is unable to be *resorbed* from bone, *absorbed* in the intestines, or *reabsorbed* from the renal tubules. Hypocalcemia that develops after total thyroidectomy could be due to devascularization of the parathyroid glands, accidental removal or destruction of one or more of the glands, or hematoma formation around the glands during or after surgery.

Clinical Findings

These individuals exhibit the typical features of hypocalcemia. The onset of symptoms usually occurs within 8 hours of the surgery.

Diagnostic Studies

The diagnosis of hypocalcemia secondary to surgical removal or compromise of the parathyroid glands is based on the history, a low serum calcium level, and a low, or inappropriately normal, PTH level. In addition, the serum phosphate level is usually elevated due to the absence of PTH and its ability to promote phosphaturia.

Treatment

Those with iatrogenic hypoparathyroidism usually require both calcium and calcitriol supplementation.

Prognosis

In most cases of iatrogenic hypoparathyroidism, treatment of hypocalcemia is relatively simple. Prognosis is dependent on compliance with the administration of calcium and calcitriol supplementation. The hypocalcemia that develops in these patients is usually transient. The calcium level returns to normal and remains in the normal range off therapy in less than 4 weeks. However, it is important to monitor these patients insofar as overtreatment may result in hypercalciuria leading to nephrocalcinosis, renal function impairment, and soft tissue calcification.

Acquired Magnesium Deficiency

In addition to the inherited forms of hypomagnesemia, individuals may also develop hypomagnesemia. Acquired hypomagnesemia may be secondary to inadequate intake, intracellular shifts (i.e., treatment of diabetic ketoacidosis or refeeding syndrome), GI loss (i.e., chronic diarrhea, alcohol intake, malabsorption syndrome, steatorrhea, vomiting, or nasogastric suction), or renal loss (extracellular fluid volume expansion or due to medications). Differentiation between the inherited and acquired forms of hypomagnesemia is based on magnesium level (much lower in the inherited form), clinical presentation (more overt in the inherited form), and a positive family history.

HYPOCALCEMIA WITH ELEVATED PARATHYROID HORMONE LEVELS

This section reviews congenital and acquired causes of hypocalcemia and its relationship to an elevated serum PTH level.

Congenital Causes

Hypocalcemia and hyperphosphatemia in the presence of an elevated PTH level may occur if there is a defect in the PTH receptor or an abnormality in the secondary messenger system.

Pseudohypoparathyroidism

The term **pseudohypoparathyroidism (PHP)** encompasses a group of heterogeneous disorders whose common feature is impaired signaling of a variety of hormones (primarily PTH) that activate cAMP-dependent pathways via the α-subunit of the stimulatory G protein (Gsα). The three main forms of PHP are PHP-1a, PHP-1b, and pseudopseudohypoparathyroidism (PPHP).

Etiology

The PTH level is elevated because the parathyroid glands oversecrete PTH in an attempt to compensate for the hypocalcemia. Individuals with PPHP do not develop hypocalcemia. They do, however, have the same gene mutation as those with PHP. Both PHP and PPHP are inherited in autosomal dominant fashion and are usually not diagnosed until late in the first or early part of the second decade of life.

Pathology

Due to the increase in PTH secretion, the parathyroid glands may be larger than usual.

Pathophysiology

Heterozygous inactivating mutations within the Gsα-encoding region of the *GNAS* gene are found in patients with PHP-1a. These patients also show resistance to other hormones and exhibit a constellation of physical features known as **Albright hereditary** osteodystrophy (AHO). Patients who exhibit features of AHO without evidence for hormone resistance have PPHP and also carry heterozygous inactivating Gsα mutations. Maternal inheritance of the *GNAS* gene mutation results in PHP-1a (AHO plus hormone resistance). Paternal inheritance of the same mutation, on the other hand, results in PPHP (AHO without hormone resistance). This mode of inheritance for hormone resistance is explained by the predominantly maternal expression of Gsα in certain tissues, including renal proximal tubules. Patients with PHP-1b lack coding Gsα mutations, but display epigenetic defects of the *GNAS* locus. Their most consistent defect is the loss of imprinting at the exon A/B differentially methylated region. Therefore, patients with PHP-1b have abnormal biochemical parameters but do not have features of AHO. The Gsα subunit is also necessary for other hormones, such as thyrotropin, follicle-stimulating hormone, and luteinizing hormone.

Clinical Findings

The biochemical features of PHP-1a and PHP-1b are similar to those of hypoparathyroidism with the one exception that in PHP, PTH levels are elevated. The clinical features of AHO include short stature, round faces, brachydactyly (usually shortened fourth or fifth metacarpals or metatarsals), obesity, dental hypoplasia, and subcutaneous calcifications (Figure 4-7A,B). These individuals are also likely to have a below-normal IQ. Many individuals with PHP have other hormone abnormalities and frequently develop clinical features of hypothyroidism and hypogonadism.

Diagnostic Studies

Patients with PHP-1a and PHP-1b have hypocalcemia, hyperphosphatemia, and elevated serum PTH levels. Patients with PPHP have normal serum calcium, phosphate, and PTH levels. Patients with PHP-1a and PPHP, on radiographs of the hands, may show shortening of the distal phalanx of the thumb and/or any of the metacarpals or metatarsals. The most common radiographic finding is a short fourth metacarpal (see Figure 4-8B). Patients with PHP-1b have a normal physical appearance.

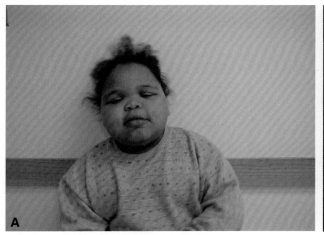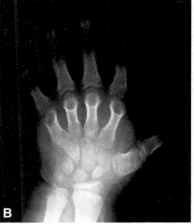

FIGURE 4-7. Albright hereditary osteodystrophy. An 8-year-old girl with pseudohypoparathyroidism type 1a. **(A)** Note the characteristic facial features: round facies, flat nasal bridge, upturned nostrils, and upward bowing of the upper lip. **(B)** The radiograph of her hand reveals the characteristic shortness of all metacarpal bones. (Photograph taken by Eric Felner, MD, MSCR and Radiograph from the Department of Radiology, Tulane University School of Medicine.)

Treatment

The treatment for PHP-1a and PHP-1b is identical to the treatment for hypoparathyroidism. Supplementation with both calcium and calcitriol is necessary in these patients because upregulation of the 1α-hydroxylase enzyme does not occur in the absence of PTH. Low endogenous calcitriol and reduced intestinal absorption of calcium is the result of absent PTH. Supplementation is not needed for patients with PPHP.

Prognosis

Little is known of the long-term outcomes of PHP because the condition is rare. The underlying cause of PHP is incurable. The majority of these patients require lifelong calcium and calcitriol supplementation. Patients with PHP-1a are also at increased risk for other hormone deficiencies that require Gsα. These patients should have a thorough evaluation to search for all potential hormone deficiencies and they must be treated appropriately.

Acquired Causes

Acquired causes of hypocalcemia include vitamin D deficiency, rickets, and osteomalacia as well as pharmacologic agent-induced hypocalcemia and hypocalcemia from renal failure.

Vitamin D Deficiency

People of all age groups are at risk for developing vitamin D deficiency. Children and older adults are at the highest risk for complications. Infants and young children with vitamin D deficiency may develop growth retardation and skeletal deformities. Adults, whose growth plates are fused, may develop osteomalacia. Vitamin D deficiency occurs because of a defect in supply or processing of vitamin D. Low dietary intake, inadequate sunlight exposure, and malabsorption are examples of a defective supply. Processing defects of vitamin D include deficiency of the 25-hydroxylase enzyme (due to liver disease or gene mutation), deficiency of the 1α-hydroxylase enzyme (due to kidney disease or gene mutation), or abnormalities associated with the vitamin D receptor.

Rickets

Chronic vitamin D deficiency in childhood results in rickets, which is characterized by the formation of disordered excess cartilage, poor bone formation at the epiphyseal growth plate, and poor mineralization of osteoid in cortical and trabecular bone.

Etiology

Vitamin D deficiency is a biochemical abnormality, but rickets is a radiographic abnormality. All causes of rickets are due to a deficiency in one of the forms of vitamin D, with the exception of hypophosphatemic rickets.

Pathology

The cortical and trabecular bones are demineralized and soft.

Pathophysiology

A defect may occur at a number of sites in the vitamin D metabolism pathway (see Figure 4-2), which prevents the formation or action of calcitriol. Without calcitriol, the intestinal **absorption** of calcium and phosphate is reduced, resulting in oversecretion of PTH and bone **resorption**. Despite the poor intestinal absorption of calcium, initially, the increase in bone resorption maintains the serum calcium in the normal range. Phosphate levels, however, continue to decrease because of both the phosphaturic effect of increased PTH secretion and the persistent poor intestinal absorption of phosphate. The latter is due to the deficiency in vitamin D. Eventually the bone becomes devoid of calcium, and the serum calcium level falls. The serum calcium and phosphate levels will continue to decrease until calcitriol (or cholecalciferol) is administered. The rachitic findings seen in these children with vitamin D deficiency are the result of the resorptive effects of PTH as well as the loss of bone calcium and phosphate.

Clinical Findings

Infants with rapidly growing bones develop widened cranial sutures, soft calvaria prone to deformity, bulging costochondral junctions (rachitic rosary on the anterior chest), wrist enlargement, and delayed eruption of teeth (Figure 4-8). Older children develop bowed legs (genu varum) or knock-knees (genu valgum) due to pressure on weak growth plates in weight-bearing bones. In children with the very rare form of vitamin D-resistant rickets, additional clinical features include growth retardation and alopecia.

Diagnostic Studies

Rickets is characterized by radiographic findings that include widened, irregular, and cupped metaphyses (Figure 4-9A–C). Radiography is used to assess the extent of the skeletal deformity. Regardless of the biochemical findings, the diagnosis of rickets is confirmed by specific radiographic findings.

For any form of vitamin D deficiency, children usually have hypophosphatemia and, eventually, hypocalcemia. The serum calcium, phosphate, PTH, and vitamin D levels depend on the underlying cause of the vitamin D deficiency (Table 4-2). For example, in nutritional vitamin D deficiency, serum vitamin D and 25-hydroxy-vitamin D levels are low, but the serum calcitriol level may be low, normal, or high. The elevated calcitriol levels in some children with nutritional vitamin D deficiency rickets remains a puzzling phenomenon. Hypocalcemia and increased PTH secretion may cause an increase in calcitriol production despite a low level of calcidiol, but only if there is at least a minimal

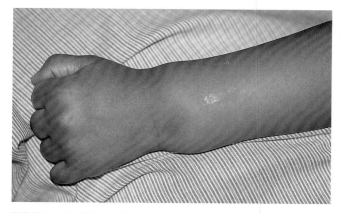

FIGURE 4-8. Rickets. This infant's arm shows the characteristic widening of the wrist caused by flaring at the end of the radius and ulna. (From Fleisher GR, Ludwig S, Baskin MN. Atlas of Pediatric Emergency Medicine. Philadelphia: Lippincott Williams & Wilkins; 2004.)

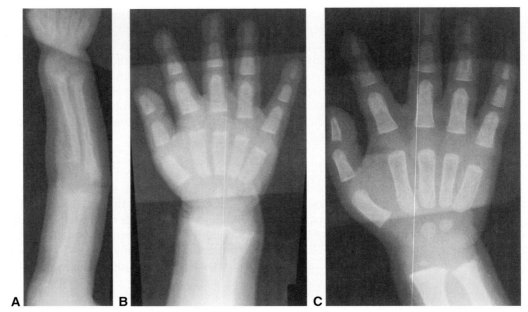

FIGURE 4-9. Radiograph of an infant with rickets. Radiographic images of the upper extremity from an 11-month-old boy breast-fed since birth. **(A)** Note the profound demineralization of the skeleton, with frayed, irregular cupping at the end of the metaphysis with a poorly defined cortex. There is also retardation of skeletal maturation. **(B)** Same patient with some healing 4 weeks after vitamin D supplementation. Severe rachitic changes are evident. Periosteal cloaking, both of the metacarpals and of the radius and ulna, is evidence of healing. **(C)** Complete healing 8 months after treatment. There is reappearance of the provisional zone of calcification.

amount of calcidiol available. In those with virtually no calcidiol, calcitriol levels should be low. The range of calcitriol levels in those with nutritional vitamin D deficiency could possibly be explained by a timing issue. Those children with elevated calcitriol levels may be early in the course of vitamin D deficiency compared to those with low levels. Given more time, eventually all children with nutritional vitamin D deficiency will have low levels of calcitriol.

Treatment

Hypocalcemia due to vitamin D deficiency is best treated with an improved diet, more sunlight exposure, and supplementation with calcium and some form of vitamin D. Nutritional vitamin D deficiency can be treated with cholecalciferol, ergocalciferol, or calcidiol. Individuals with a deficiency of the 25-OHase enzyme are treated with calcidiol or calcitriol. Those with 1α-OHase deficiency are treated with calcitriol. Those with the rare condition of vitamin D resistance are treated with very large doses of calcium but usually cannot maintain adequate calcium and phosphate levels.

Prognosis

The prognosis of children with hypocalcemia due to vitamin D deficiency is very good if the diagnosis is made early in the course of the disease (see Figure 4-9). Other than vitamin-D-resistant rickets, in which the individuals usually have poor bone mineralization due to chronic hypocalcemia and hypophosphatemia, the prognosis is good with replacement of the appropriate form of vitamin D.

Hypophosphatemic Rickets

The most common form of hypophosphatemic rickets is the inherited, X-linked dominant disorder, hypophosphatemic rickets (XHR). The other form is an autosomal dominant disorder (ADHR).

Etiology

The incidence of XHR is estimated to affect 1 in 20,000 live births.

Pathology

Unmineralized osteoid accumulates along the trabeculae within cancellous bone.

Pathophysiology

Hypophosphatemic rickets is the only form of rickets in which there is not a defect in vitamin D metabolism. XHR is due to an inactivating mutation in the *PHEX* gene. As the *PHEX* gene cleaves and inactivates FGF23, an inactivating mutation of the *PHEX* gene results in overproduction of FGF23. Increased activity of FGF23 results in renal phosphate wasting (see Figure 4-3). ADHR is due to an activating mutation of the *FGF23* gene that also results in overproduction of FGF23 and renal phosphate wasting. Mesenchymal tumors that cause hypophosphatemia do so by a similar mechanism that results in overproduction of FGF23.

Clinical Findings

The clinical findings are similar to other forms of rickets and include short stature, genu varum or valgum that begins when the infant begins to walk, metaphyseal flaring, rachitic rosary, frontal bossing, and dental decay.

Diagnostic Studies

Hypophosphatemic rickets is characterized by radiographic findings that include widened, irregular, and cupped metaphyses. Although serum levels of total and free calcium are normal, hypophosphatemia is marked, due to urinary wastage from a substantially decreased renal tubular resorption of filtered phosphate. Although serum concentrations of PTH and calcidiol are normal, calcitriol levels are inappropriately low for the degree of hypophosphatemia.

Treatment

Individuals with hypophosphatemic rickets do not develop hypocalcemia and are not vitamin D deficient. They are treated with large doses of phosphorous and occasionally calcitriol to help maximize phosphate *absorption* in the intestine.

Prognosis

If the diagnosis and treatment are begun early, the prognosis for children with hypophosphatemic rickets is very good. Many of these children are short at age 5 years, but with proper treatment, their growth rate improves. Most untreated adults are hypophosphatemic but clinically asymptomatic, except for dental abnormalities and degenerative hip disease. Heterozygous females with XHR are less symptomatic than hemizygous males, but both males and females with ADHR have similar clinical courses.

Osteomalacia

In adults, epiphyseal growth plates are fused. Therefore, those with severe vitamin D deficiency develop a defect in bone mineralization known as **osteomalacia**.

Etiology

Osteomalacia is a disease in which insufficient mineralization leads to softening of the bones. This is usually caused by a deficiency of vitamin D. Similar to rickets, osteomalacia is a radiographic diagnosis. It differs from rickets in that it occurs in fused epiphyseal growth plates whereas rickets affects immature epiphyseal growth plates.

Pathology

The cortical and trabecular bones are demineralized and become soft, similar to that in children with rickets.

Pathophysiology

The pathophysiology of osteomalacia is similar to that of rickets.

Clinical Findings

The major clinical finding in patients with osteomalacia is diffuse bone pain. The pain may appear similar to that of arthritis, but in osteomalacia, the pain is between the joints of the long bones and not at the joint, as in those with arthritis. Individuals with osteomalacia may also have weakness and gait instability.

Diagnostic Studies

The diagnostic biochemical studies are similar to those of rickets, but the radiographic findings are not as obvious in osteomalacia because the adult skeleton is metabolically less active. The bones have thin cortices, and indistinct, fuzzy trabeculae with a ground-glass appearance (Figure 4-10).

Treatment

The treatment is the same as for rickets.

Prognosis

If diagnosed early, and treatment is followed correctly, the prognosis for adults with hypocalcemia due to vitamin D deficiency is very good.

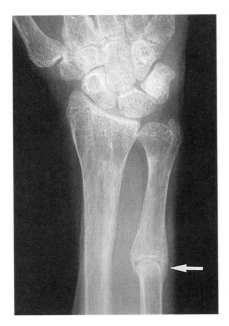

FIGURE 4-10. Wrist radiograph of a patient with osteomalacia. It shows the distinctive malacial changes including the generalized decrease in density, coarsened trabecular patterns, loss of cortical definition, and the pseudofracture (*arrow*). (From Yochum TR, Rowe LJ. Yochum and Rowe's Essentials of Skeletal Radiology. 3rd ed. Philadelphia, PA: Lippincott Williams & Wilkins; 2004.)

Pharmacologic Agent-Induced

There are a number of agents that can lower the serum calcium level. It is important to review the patient's history to determine whether there was exposure to a drug or agent prior to the development of hypocalcemia.

Bisphosphonates, fluoride, mithramycin, and calcitonin cause hypocalcemia by suppressing osteoclastic activity thereby decreasing calcium release from bones. The anticonvulsants, phenytoin and phenobarbital, cause hypocalcemia by accelerating the degradation of vitamin D to water-soluble forms and increasing urinary loss of vitamin D. Loop diuretics cause hypocalcemia by inhibiting renal calcium reabsorption. Transfusion with citrated blood may result in hypocalcemia because the citrate complexes with calcium and lowers the serum calcium. Contrast dyes that contain the calcium-chelating agent ethylenediaminetetraacetic acid (EDTA) can also cause hypocalcemia.

Renal Failure

Hypocalcemia may develop in individuals with compromised or failed renal function. These individuals usually have secondary hyperparathyroidism because the PTH compensates for the low serum calcium level. There are many mechanisms of hypocalcemia in these individuals including inability to produce calcitriol, inability to reabsorb calcium, and inability to excrete phosphorous. The elevated phosphate can also complex with calcium, further lowering the serum calcium level.

The differential diagnosis and biochemical abnormalities associated with each cause of hypocalcemia are shown in Table 4-2. An algorithm for the evaluation of an individual with hypocalcemia is shown in Figure 4-11.

TABLE 4-2. Causes of Hypocalcemia					
Etiology	Serum Level				
	Mg	Pho	PTH	25-D$_3$	1,25-D$_3$
Hypoparathyroidism Agenesis/dysgenesis *CaSR* defect Autoimmune	N	↑	↓/N	N	↓/N
Mg deficiency	↓	↑	↓	N	↓
PHP-1a or PHP-1b	N	↑	↑	N	↓/N

Vitamin D deficiency
   Vitamin D$_3$ deficiency
   25-α-OHase deficiency
   1-α-OHase deficiency
   1,25-(OH)$_2$-Vitamin D$_3$
   resistance
	
	N
	N
	N
	N
		
		↓
		↓
		↓
		↓
			
			↑
			↑
			↑
			↑
				
				↓
				↓
				N
				N
					
					↓/N/↑
					↓
					↓
					↑

Osteoclastic agents	N	N	↓/N	↑	↑
Anticonvulsants	N	↓	↑	↓	↓
Furosemide/citrates/EDTA	N	N	↑	↑	↑

Notes: EDTA, ethylenediaminetetraacetic acid; Mg, magnesium; Pho, phosphorous; PTH, parathyroid hormone; 25-D$_3$, 25-hydroxy vitamin D$_3$; 1,25-D$_3$, 1,25-dihydroxy vitamin D$_3$; N, normal; ↓, low; ↑, high.

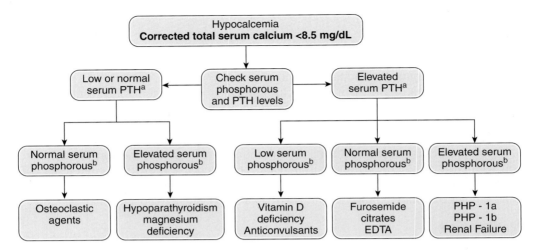

a Normal PTH reference range: 10–65 pg/mL
b Normal serum phosphorous range:
    Birth–10 days: 5.4–9.0 mg/dL
    10 days–1 year: 4.5–6.7 mg/dL
    2–11 years: 4.5–5.5 mg/dL
    >12 years: 2.7–4.5 mg/dL

FIGURE 4-11. Algorithm for the evaluation of hypocalcemia.

CASE FOLLOW-UP

The differential diagnosis for neonates who present with seizures due to hypo-calcemia and hyperphosphatemia is either hypoparathyroidism or renal failure. The hypoparathyroidism may be due to agenesis or dysgenesis of the parathyroid glands, an activating mutation of the *CaSR* gene, transient hypoparathyroidism, or PHP type 1a or 1b. Serum blood urea nitrogen (7 mg/dL) and creatinine (0.4 mg/dL) levels are normal, making renal failure less likely. Regardless of the etiology, the child is appropriately treated with intravenous (IV) calcium gluconate, oral calcium carbonate, and calcitriol.

Further questioning of the mother confirms that she was healthy throughout pregnancy and the baby has not taken any medications since he was born. After 1 day of treatment, his serum total calcium level is still low but improving (7.1 mg/dL), and his serum phosphate level is still elevated (10.2 mg/dL). IV calcium gluconate is discontinued, but oral calcium carbonate and calcitriol supplementation is maintained.

On the second day of treatment, the serum PTH level (6 pg/mL [normal = 10 to 60 pg/mL]), collected when his total calcium level was 4.5 mg/dL, is low, confirming hypoparathyroidism.

On closer inspection, he has mild hypertelorism and slight posterior rota-tion to his ears. Although no abnormalities were detected on cardiovascular examination, because of the low PTH level, an echocardiogram was performed, revealing an interrupted aortic arch. Genetic studies confirmed a deletion of chromosome 22, consistent with DiGeorge sequence.

Follow-up appointments are scheduled with the cardiologist and immunolo-gist the following week.

REFERENCES and SUGGESTED READINGS

Asadi F. Hypomagnesemia: an evidence-based approach to clinical cases. IJKD. 2010;4(1):13–19.

Asari R, Passler C, Kaczivck K, Scheuba C, Niederle B. Hypoparathyroidism after total thyroidectomy: a prospective study. Arch Surg. 2008;143(2):132–137.

Garabedin M, Vainsel M, Mallet E, Guillozo H, Toppet M, Grimberg R, et al. Circulating vitamin D metabolite concentrations in children with nutritional rickets. J Pediatr. 1983;103(3):381–386.

Giovannucci E, Liy Y, Hollis BW, Rimm EB. 25-Hydroxyvitamin D and risk of myocardial infarction in men. Arch Intern Med. 2008;168(11):1174–1180.

Holick M. Vitamin D deficiency. N Engl J Med. 2007;357(3):266–281.

Hudson JQ. Secondary hyperparathyroidism in chronic kidney disease: focus on clinical consequences and vitamin D therapies. Ann Pharmacother. 2006;40(9):1584–1593.

Juppner H, Bastepe M. Different mutations within or upstream of the GNAS locus cause distinct forms of pseudohypoparathyroidism. J Pediatr Endocrinol Metab. 2006;19(suppl 2):641–646.

Mantovani G. Clinical review: Pseudohypoparathyroidism: diagnosis and treatment. J Clin Endocrinol Metab. 2011;96(10):3020–3030.

Marx S. Hyperparathyroid and hypoparathyroid disorders. N Engl J Med. 2000;343(25): 1863–1875.

Peterlik M, Cross HS. Vitamin D and calcium insufficiency-related chronic diseases: molecular and cellular pathophysiology. Eur J Clin Nutr. 2009;63(12):1377–1386.

Prie D, Friedlander G. Genetic disorders of renal phosphate transport. N Engl J Med. 2010;362(25): 2399–2409.

Saliba W, El-Haddad B. Secondary hyperparathyroidism: pathophysiology and treatment. JABFM. 2009;22(5):574–581.

Shoback D. Hypoparathyroidism. N Engl J Med. 2008;359(4):391–403.

CHAPTER REVIEW QUESTIONS

1. You are asked to see a 2-year-old boy with short stature and leg bowing. Serum studies obtained include calcium 9.0 mg/dL (normal = 8.5 to 10.5 mg/dL), phosphate 1.0 mg/dL (normal = 2.5 to 4.0 mg/dL), PTH 55 pg/mL (normal = 10 to 65 pg/mL), 25-hydroxy-vitamin D_3 30 pg/mL (normal = 20 to 40 pg/mL), and 1,25-dyhydroxy-vitamin D_3 20 pg/mL (normal = 20 to 50 pg/mL). Radiographic studies show metaphyseal flaring and cupping. Which of the following statements is true regarding his diagnosis?

   A. Rickets is not present.
   B. The etiology of the problem involves FGF23.
   C. The 1α-hydroxylase enzyme is absent.
   D. The calcitonin level is increased.
   E. Poor nutrition is the main problem.

2. All of the following conditions can be associated with hypocalcemia and hyperphosphatemia except:

   A. A defect in the α-subunit of the stimulatory G protein
   B. An inactivating mutation of the CaSR
   C. Hypomagnesemia
   D. Surgical removal of the thyroid gland
   E. Autoimmune destruction of the parathyroid glands

3. A 12-year-old boy presents to the emergency room with tetany involving his right arm. Serum studies obtained include calcium 6.0 mg/dL (normal = 8.5 to 10.5 mg/dL), phosphate 7.0 mg/dL (normal = 2.5 to 4.5 mg/dL), PTH 175 pg/mL (normal = 10 to 60 pg/mL), 25-hydroxy-vitamin D_3 35 pg/mL (normal = 20 to 40 pg/mL), and 1,25-dihydroxy-vitamin D_3 15 pg/mL (normal = 20 to 50 pg/mL). What is the diagnosis?

A. Nutritional vitamin D deficiency
B. XHR
C. PHP
D. 1α-Hydroxylase deficiency
E. DiGeorge sequence

4. A 57-year-old man has a routine check-up with his internist. Although the man is asymptomatic and has no obvious findings on his physical exam, the internist orders routine blood work to be performed. All of the results are in the normal reference range except for total calcium, which is 7.9 mg/dL. What is the best explanation?

A. Osteomalacia is present.
B. Thyroidectomy was recently performed.
C. The 1α-hydroxylase enzyme is absent.
D. The serum albumin level is low, and a corrected total calcium is normal.
E. The Gsα is defective.

5. You are asked to consult on a 36-year-old African American woman who 8 hours earlier underwent a total thyroidectomy for the treatment of thyroid cancer. She complains of numbness around the lips, and her hands are twitching. On examination, her temperature is 97.5°F, heart rate is 80 bpm, and blood pressure is 100/60 mmHg in both arms. Her head, eyes, ears, neck, and throat exam reveals occasional twitches of her lips when you tap her cheek. Her neck is covered in a sterile dressing and her lungs are clear. The remainder of the examination is normal. Which of the following serum values would be most likely in this patient?

	Total Calcium (mg/dL)	Albumin (g/dL)	Parathyroid hormone (pg/mL)	Calcitriol (pg/mL)
Normal values	8.5–10.5	3.5–4.5	10–65	10–60
A.	6.5	1.5	100	70
B.	11.0	1.5	100	5
C.	6.1	3.5	5	5
D.	7.5	2.0	100	103
E.	10.1	3.0	5	103

CHAPTER REVIEW ANSWERS

1. The correct answer is B. Based on the radiographic findings, the child has rickets. With the exception of hypophosphatemia, all of his laboratory values are in the normal range. This indicates that he has hypophosphatemic rickets, which is due to renal phosphate wasting and likely related to overactivity of FGF23, a protein responsible for inhibiting renal tubular phosphate transport. All other choices are incorrect.

The radiographic findings confirm rickets; therefore, to state that rickets is not present (**Choice A**) is incorrect. A deficiency of the 1α-hydroxylase enzyme (**Choice C**) would result in an inability to convert 25-hydroxy-vitamin D_3 to 1,25-dihydroxy-vitamin D_3. He has normal serum levels of 25-hydroxy-vitamin D_3, 1,25-dihydroxy-vitamin D_3, PTH, and calcium. If this child had deficiency of the 1α-hydroxylase enzyme, by age 2 years, he should have low serum calcium and 1,25-dihydroxy-vitamin D_3 levels and increased PTH levels. He would not have an elevated calcitonin level (**Choice D**) since he does not have hypercalcemia. If this child had poor nutrition (**Choice E**), he would be expected to have a low 25-hydroxy-vitamin D_3 level.

---

2. The correct answer is B. An inactivating mutation will make the CaSR less sensitive to extracellular calcium, increasing PTH, and causing hypercalcemia and hypocalciuria. An activating mutation of the CaSR will make it more sensitive to extracellular calcium, inhibiting PTH secretion. All of the other choices are consistent with hypoparathyroidism associated with hypocalcemia and hyperphosphatemia.

A mutation in the α-subunit of the G-protein (**Choice A**) is the defect in PHP-1a and PHP-1b. Although the condition involves an elevated PTH level, these patients have hypocalcemia and hyperphosphatemia because despite the increased activity of PTH, without a functional G-protein mechanism, hormone function does not occur. Hypomagnesemia (**Choice C**) inhibits synthesis and secretion of PTH, causing hypocalcemia and hyperphosphatemia. About 25% of patients undergoing a thyroidectomy (**Choice D**) develop hypoparathyroidism with less than 5% of those being permanent. Autoimmune destruction of the parathyroid glands (**Choice E**) occurs in autoimmune polyglandular syndrome type 1 and is the most common cause of acquired, permanent hypoparathyroidism.

---

3. The correct answer is C. All of the findings described in the scenario point to PHP. Hypocalcemia with hyperphosphatemia is consistent with hypoparathyroidism. His PTH level being above the normal range and his calcitriol level being slightly below the normal range are consistent with PHP. His physical features are not described, but if he is normal in appearance, then PHP-1b would be most likely.

The biochemical features of nutritional vitamin D deficiency (**Choice A**) include hypophosphatemia, normocalcemia, or hypocalcemia, elevated PTH, and low calcidiol levels. The biochemical features of XHR (**Choice B**) include hypophosphatemia due to renal phosphate wasting. All other parameters including serum calcium, PTH, and vitamin D levels are usually in the normal range. A deficiency of the 1α-hydroxylase enzyme (**Choice D**) results in an inability to convert 25-hydroxy-vitamin D_3 to 1,25-dihydroxy-vitamin D_3. Reduced 1,25-dihydroxy-vitamin D_3 leads to hypophosphatemia and elevated serum PTH levels. In the DiGeorge sequence (**Choice E**), patients develop hypocalcemia secondary to hypoparathyroidism but with low, or inappropriately normal, PTH levels.

---

4. The correct answer is D. An asymptomatic individual with a mildly reduced total calcium level and no physical findings likely does not have a calcium-related abnormality. The total calcium level reflects the amount of calcium that is bound to protein. If either the calcium level or the albumin level was low, the total calcium level could be low. In this individual without evidence of a calcium abnormality, it is more likely that a low albumin level is present.

Osteomalacia (**Choice A**) is the radiographic finding in adults with chronic vitamin D deficiency. Their most common biochemical features include hypophosphatemia, low calcidiol levels, and normocalcemia or hypocalcemia. If the individual recently underwent a thyroidectomy (**Choice B**) and his reduced calcium was related to the surgery, either the history or physical exam (with a neck scar) should have been evident. In addition, patients who develop hypocalcemia due to a thyroidectomy would have transient or permanent hypoparathyroidism with hyperphosphatemia. A deficiency of the 1α-hydroxylase enzyme (**Choice D**) would result in an inability to convert 25-hydroxy-vitamin D_3 to 1,25-dihydroxy-vitamin D_3. Serum PTH levels would be elevated, and hypophosphatemia would be present. If the Gsα is defective (**Choice E**) the patient would have abnormal physical features (PHP-1a or PPHP) and/or hypocalcemia, hyperphosphatemia, and elevated PTH levels (PHP-1a or PHP-1b).

---

5. The correct answer is C. This woman recently had parathyroid surgery and is experiencing signs and symptoms of hypoparathyroidism. The laboratory findings confirm hypoparathyroidism with low serum calcium, PTH, and calcitriol levels. The serum albumin level is lower than normal, but, even after correcting the calcium to 6.5 mg/dL [6.1 + (4.0 − 3.5) × 0.8], true hypocalcemia is present.

A total serum calcium of 6.5 mg/dL, that, after correction for a low serum albumin (1.5 g/dL) is 8.5 mg/dL [6.5 + (4.0 − 1.5) × 0.8], is not true hypocalcemia. In addition, elevated PTH and calcitriol levels are not expected in a patient with hypoparathyroidism (**Choice A**). Biochemical findings indicative of hyperparathyroidism (**Choice B**) are not consistent with this woman's presentation and diagnosis of hypoparathyroidism. A normal total serum calcium level after correction for the low albumin level, together with elevated serum PTH and calcitriol levels (**Choice D**), is not consistent with hypoparathyroidism. It may be seen in the early stages of nutritional vitamin D deficiency and poor nutrition, because calcitriol levels are occasionally elevated in the early course of nutritional vitamin D deficiency but not in hypoparathyroidism. Hypercalcemia with an appropriately decreased PTH level but elevated calcitriol (**Choice E**) is most consistent with hypercalcemia due to excess PTH-related peptide or an infiltrative condition such as sarcoidosis.

Hypercalcemia 5

David L. Gutteridge
Eric I. Felner

CASE

A 61-year-old woman is seen in the primary care clinic complaining of back and left lower leg pain. She does not recall any recent trauma. She has had increased urinary frequency and constipation during the past month and 2 weeks ago passed a kidney stone. She has had recurrent nephrolithiasis for more than 20 years, but states that she is healthy and is not taking any medications. Her family history is remarkable for her mother, who died of breast cancer at 55 years of age, and her father, who died of a myocardial infarction at 60 years of age. Her vital signs are normal and include temperature, 98°F; pulse, 85 beats per minute; respiratory rate, 14 breaths per minute; and blood pressure, 127/68 mmHg in both arms. Physical examination is unremarkable. Her strength is good in all extremities, cerebellar and vestibular function is normal, reflexes are normal, and her cranial nerves are intact.

A routine chemistry profile is significant for an elevated serum calcium level (12.5 mg/dL) and a low serum phosphate level (1.1 mg/dL). All other biochemical parameters are normal. A urinalysis is negative for glucose, blood, protein, nitrites, and leukocyte esterase.

This chapter reviews the etiology, pathophysiology, evaluation, and management of hypercalcemia to help the learner determine the etiology of this woman's hypercalcemia. We summarize the work-up and develop a therapeutic plan at the end of the chapter to give the learner a better understanding of the diagnosis.

OBJECTIVES

1. List the various causes of hypercalcemia.

2. Discuss the clinical and laboratory findings in a patient with an endocrine cause of hypercalcemia.

3. Describe the evaluation and management of a patient with hypercalcemia.

(continues)

OVERVIEW

Hypercalcemia results from either excessive bone **resorption** or increased calcium absorption from the intestine coupled with inadequate renal excretion of the excess calcium. It most often presents as an abnormal laboratory measurement in individuals who are asymptomatic or have vague symptoms (e.g., weakness, pain, fatigue) that might be attributed to other conditions. The first step in the evaluation for hypercalcemia is to determine whether the serum calcium level is not falsely elevated from dehydration, hemoconcentration, or hyperalbuminemia. As shown in the previous chapter, for abnormal levels of serum albumin, this is accomplished by calculating the corrected serum calcium level using the following formula:

$$\text{Corrected serum total calcium level} = [(4.0 - \text{serum albumin}) \times 0.8] + \text{measured serum total calcium level}$$

Signs and Symptoms

Hypercalcemia is described as the disease of the "-ones" because many of the symptoms rhyme with stone (i.e., moans, groans, and bone pain). Most patients with hypercalcemia are asymptomatic and it is usually discovered by routine measurement of the serum calcium level. In the past, prior to routine measurement of serum chemistry levels during clinic visits, patients usually presented with bone pain and kidney stones. The symptoms and signs are a reflection of the patient's age; the underlying disease; associated medical disorders; and the degree, duration, and rate of development of the hypercalcemia. In a young individual who gradually develops mild to moderate hypercalcemia, it may be well tolerated with minimal symptoms, whereas hypercalcemia that develops acutely may be associated with overt symptoms. In the elderly patient, mild elevations in serum calcium manifest more readily. Most symptoms reflect disturbances in the renal, gastrointestinal (GI), cardiovascular, neuromuscular, and central nervous systems.

    Hypercalcemia impairs the concentrating ability of the kidney that causes polyuria and polydipsia by stimulating the cation receptor on the basolateral surface of thick ascending limb cells in the loop of Henle. This leads to inhibition of the rat outer medulla potassium channel (ROMK) that regulates the sodium/potassium/chloride (Na/K/2Cl) channel. ROMK closure leads to inhibition of the Na/K/2Cl channel and results in saline diuresis and a reduction in medullary osmolality. The latter effect leads to an inability to reabsorb large volumes of water, even in the presence of antidiuretic hormone (ADH). The hypercalcemia causes an effect similar to a loop diuretic that leads to an osmotic diuresis and a subsequent resistance to ADH. This is similar to nephrogenic diabetes insipidus. Electrolytes are wasted in the urine and the reduction of medullary hypertonicity reduces the kidney's capacity to absorb free water resulting in polyuria. The resulting dehydration promotes nephrocalcinosis and nephrolithiasis. GI symptoms are common and include gastroesophageal reflux and constipation. Cardiovascular manifestations are due to increased cardiac repolarization that results in a short QT interval on electrocardiogram. Patients may become hypertensive unless their plasma volume decreases due to the dehydration from the renal effects and possibly, become hypotensive. Disturbances in the neuromuscular system include weakness, nausea, emesis, depression, and confusion. Impairment in cognitive function is also common, particularly in older adults. The common symptoms of joint and bone pain are due to calcium deposition and fractures.

Treatment

The most important principle in the therapy for patients with hypercalcemia is to maintain adequate hydration, insofar as dehydration develops commonly. Patients should discontinue any medications that could potentially cause hypercalcemia and avoid immobilization if possible. No treatment is necessary for asymptomatic individuals with mild hypercalcemia.

For symptomatic patients or those with severe hypercalcemia, medical or surgical treatment may be necessary. Medical therapy should target at least one of the mechanisms outlined in Table 5-1: 1) inhibit osteoclastic activity, thereby decreasing release of

TABLE 5-1.	Medical Treatment of Hypercalcemia	
	Acute or Chronic	**Mechanism of Action**
Calcitonin	Acute	Inhibits bone resorption
Oral phosphate	Acute	Binds to calcium and inhibits intestinal absorption of calcium
Bisphosphonates	Chronic	Inhibits osteoclastic activity
Gallium nitrite	Chronic	Inhibits osteoclastic activity
Mithramycin	Chronic	Inhibits osteoclastic activity
Normal saline	Both	Promotes calciuresis
Loop diuretics	Both	Natriuresis promotes calciuresis
Glucocorticoids	Both	Inhibits tumor cytokines and intestinal absorption of calcium
Dialysis	Both	Calcium-free dialysate inhibits intestinal absorption of calcium

calcium from bone; 2) increase urinary excretion of calcium; and 3) decrease intestinal absorption of calcium.

Causes

Primary hyperparathyroidism and hypercalcemia of malignancy account for >90% of hypercalcemia in ambulatory patients. Other causes include familial hypocalciuric hypercalcemia (FHH), granulomatous diseases, thyrotoxicosis, adrenocortical insufficiency, immobilization, pharmacologic agents, excess intake of vitamins and minerals, and immobilization. In the hospital setting, a variety of solid and hematologic malignancies are the most common causes of hypercalcemia. In this chapter, the causes of hypercalcemia are presented with relation to parathyroid hormone (PTH). Pharmacologic agents are presented separately because some pharmacologic agents that cause hypercalcemia are associated with normal or elevated levels of serum PTH, and others are associated with low serum PTH levels. Renal failure is also discussed separately due to the fact that patients with renal failure do not have an endocrine abnormality. The etiologies of hypercalcemia with their appropriate serum and urine level values are shown in Table 5-3.

HYPERCALCEMIA WITH NORMAL OR ELEVATED PARATHYROID HORMONE

Primary hyperparathyroidism is the most common cause of hypercalcemia that is associated with normal or elevated serum PTH levels.

Primary Hyperparathyroidism

Primary hyperparathyroidism is due to overproduction of PTH from one or more of the parathyroid glands. The annual incidence is approximately 10 per 100,000 people and the prevalence is 300 per 100,000 of the general population. It occurs four times more frequently in women than men. The peak incidence occurs between ages 60 and 70 years.

Sporadic Primary Hyperparathyroidism

The most common cause of primary hyperparathyroidism is a single, sporadically occurring parathyroid adenoma that accounts for 85% of the cases. The remainder is due to parathyroid hyperplasia in multiple parathyroid glands (15%) and parathyroid carcinoma (<1%).

Pathology

Benign parathyroid adenomas are infrequently small and difficult to locate even at surgical exploration. They are well encapsulated, soft, yielding yellow-to-tan-to-red lesions due to hemosiderin. The cells are arranged in large islands or broad bands (Figure 5-1A,B).

Pathophysiology

Solitary parathyroid adenomas are monoclonal or oligoclonal tumors. The underlying genes that develop mutations in hyperparathyroidism have been identified only in a minority of tumors. Many of the known and unknown genes that have mutated in parathyroid tumors are probably tumor-suppressor genes and contribute to the formation of the tumor through a sequential inactivation of both copies of the gene. Primary hyperparathyroidism is characterized by a shift in the set point for suppression of PTH secretion, such that the level of increased hormone secretion is inappropriate for the level of calcium. The normal ability to suppress PTH in the presence of elevated calcium

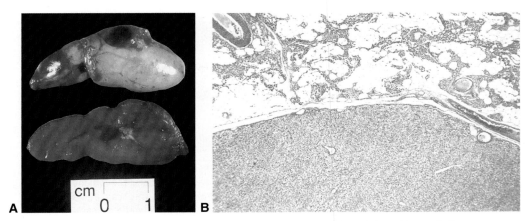

FIGURE 5-1. Parathyroid adenoma. **(A)** External (*top*) and cross-sectional views (*bottom*) show a tan, fleshy tumor. **(B)** The tumor consists of sheets of neoplastic chief cells and is separated from normal parenchyma by a thin capsule. (From Rubin R, Strayer DS. Rubin's Pathology: Clinicopathologic Foundations of Medicine, 5th ed. Philadelphia, PA: Lippincott Williams & Wilkins, 2008.)

is lost. Excess PTH results in an increase in bone remodeling and an increased release of calcium that contributes to hypercalcemia. In the kidney, excess PTH lowers tubular phosphate reabsorption that augments phosphaturia and contributes to the development of hypophosphatemia. In addition, tubular reabsorption of calcium is increased. The net effect on urinary excretion of calcium, however, is balanced by the increased filtered load of calcium as a function of the degree of hypercalcemia. Both excess PTH and hypophosphatemia stimulate calcitriol production that augments intestinal absorption of calcium.

Clinical Findings

More than 50% of patients with hypercalcemia are asymptomatic and the diagnosis is made fortuitously. Of the patients who are symptomatic, most have subtle neurobehavioral symptoms (i.e., fatigue, weakness) and up to 25% have calcium nephrolithiasis. Less than 5% of calcium stone formers, however, have primary hyperparathyroidism. Renal stones tend to occur in young patients with primary hyperparathyroidism, with a peak incidence in the third and fourth decades. In addition, 30% to 50% of patients with primary hyperparathyroidism have hypertension and may develop cardiac calcifications and left ventricular hypertrophy. About 25% of patients have osteopenia or osteoporosis in cortical and trabecular bone. Although the risk of bone fractures in patients with mild hyperparathyroidism is similar to that in normal individuals, the presence of hyperparathyroidism significantly increases the risk of fracture in several bones, particularly the vertebrae.

Diagnostic Studies

When making the diagnosis of primary hyperparathyroidism, a thorough history is paramount. A detailed physical examination is usually not revealing, but appropriate biochemical tests may uncover the problem. The diagnosis is based on an elevated serum calcium level and inappropriately normal or elevated serum PTH level. Mild-to-moderate hypophosphatemia is present in 50% of patients and is caused by a lowered renal threshold for phosphorus reabsorption due to an excess of PTH. The urinary calcium excretion varies from normal to elevated depending on the: 1) level of serum calcium, 2) filtered load of calcium by the kidney, 3) intestinal absorption of calcium, 4) dietary intake,

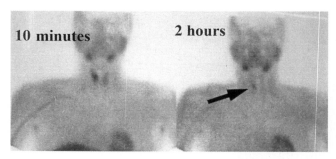

FIGURE 5-2. Sestamibi scan of a patient with a parathyroid adenoma. The radionuclide is present in both thyroid and parathyroid tissue on the 10-minute film; however, by 2 hours, the radionuclide has washed out of the thyroid and remains only in the right parathyroid glands. This scan shows a right upper parathyroid adenoma (*arrow*). (From Mulholland MW, Maier RV, et al. Greenfield's Surgery Scientific Principles and Practice. 4th ed. Philadelphia, PA: Lippincott Williams & Wilkins, 2006.)

and 5) effect of PTH on tubular reabsorption of calcium. Technetium-99m sestamibi is the gold standard for imaging parathyroid glands in patients with suspected hyperparathyroidism. The MIBI portion of the ligand is the biologic tracer that accumulates in the mitochondria of cells. Adenomas are hypermetabolic; so they have higher ratios of mitochondria-rich cells than the surrounding tissue, allowing for good contrast in the concentrations of tracer accumulation. Imaging with a sestamibi scan helps to localize adenomas (Figure 5-2). Imaging studies for hyperparathyroidism are discussed in detail in Chapter 20.

Treatment

For asymptomatic patients with primary hyperparathyroidism as well as those with only minimal symptoms, no treatment is necessary. For symptomatic patients, patients younger than 50 years of age, and patients with osteoporosis or impaired kidney function, surgical removal of the adenoma or the hyperplastic glands is the definitive treatment. Indications for surgery in asymptomatic patients with primary hyperparathyroidism include:

- Serum calcium >11.5 mg/dL
- Creatinine clearance reduced by 30%
- Bone mineral density T-score <-2.5
- Age <50 years

For patients who are poor surgical candidates but have symptomatic hypercalcemia, medical therapy should include bisphosphonate therapy to inhibit osteoclast activity and reduce bone turnover. Calcimimetics are given to patients with secondary hyperparathyroidism, but because they act by reducing PTH release from the parathyroid glands, they are now being evaluated for use in patients with primary hyperparathyroidism.

Prognosis

For patients who undergo surgical removal, the complication rate is low. Complications for the procedure include iatrogenic hypoparathyroidism, development of a hematoma at the incision site, or damage to one or both recurrent laryngeal nerves. Patients with severe and symptomatic hyperparathyroidism who do not undergo surgical treatment are at increased risk for developing the classic bone disease of osteitis fibrosa cystica, which results in pain, osteoporosis, and pathologic fractures.

Syndromes of Hereditary Primary Hyperparathyroidism

Primary hyperparathyroidism due to hyperfunction of multiple parathyroid glands is inherited in about 20% of patients. Individuals with any of these hereditary syndromes may present with isolated hyperparathyroidism, or in addition to other abnormalities.

Syndromes of hereditary primary hyperparathyroidism include multiple endocrine neoplasia (MEN) 1, MEN 2A, FHH, neonatal severe primary hyperparathyroidism (NSPH), and hyperparathyroidism-jaw tumor syndrome (HJTS). Each syndrome raises special issues for diagnosis and management (Table 5-2). MEN syndromes are discussed in detail in Chapter 17.

Familial Hypocalciuric Hypercalcemia

FHH is characterized by asymptomatic lifelong hypercalcemia with low urinary calcium excretion. It is inherited as an autosomal dominant trait and caused by inactivating germline mutations of the *CaSR* gene. Under physiologic conditions, the CaSR is activated by a decrease in extracellular calcium concentration that causes an increase in both PTH release and renal tubular calcium reabsorption. When ionized calcium concentrations rise, CaSR activation should normally decrease, resulting in a decrease in PTH secretion and renal tubular calcium reabsorption.

An inactivating (loss of function) mutation of the *CaSR* gene decreases CaSR sensitivity to calcium. This results in a decrease in calcium ion suppression of PTH release, and an increase in renal tubular reabsorption of calcium. This impairment of PTH suppression causes an elevation in the serum calcium level and reduces renal calcium wasting.

The diagnosis of hypercalcemia due to FHH is based on an elevated serum calcium level, a low urine calcium level (calcium/creatinine <0.01), and an inappropriately normal or elevated serum PTH level. The serum magnesium may be slightly elevated and serum phosphate level may be slightly low. Genetic testing for a *CaSR* gene mutation can be performed in those with a positive family history for hypercalcemia.

Individuals with FHH have a benign clinical course and do not require treatment. Those who have undergone a subtotal parathyroidectomy will continue to have hypercalcemia. Those who undergo a total parathyroidectomy will develop hypoparathyroidism and iatrogenic hypocalcemia and require lifelong calcium and vitamin D replacement therapy. With proper recognition and minimal intervention, the prognosis is excellent.

Neonatal Severe Primary Hyperparathyroidism

NSPH is a rare and potentially lethal disorder. Affected neonates have enlargement of all parathyroid glands, very high serum PTH levels, and very high serum calcium levels. It is caused by homozygous inactivating germline mutations of the *CaSR* gene.

Hyperparathyroidism-Jaw Tumor Syndrome

HJTS is characterized by hyperparathyroidism, cement-ossifying fibromas of the jaw, renal cysts, Wilms tumor, and renal hamartomas. By the fifth decade of life, almost 80% of patients with this syndrome have hyperparathyroidism, and about 10% of those have a parathyroid carcinoma. Often, at the first presentation of hyperparathyroidism, only one parathyroid adenoma is present, but multiple adenomas can occur simultaneously or at different times. The disorder is caused by a mutation of an unknown gene on chromosome 1q24 and is inherited as an autosomal dominant trait.

TABLE 5-2.	Hereditary Primary Hyperparathyroidism				
	FHH	**MEN 1**	**MEN 2A**	**NSPH**	**HJTS**
Inheritance pattern	AD	AD	AD	AR	AD
Age of onset of hypercalcemia	Birth	Third decade	Seventh to eighth decade	Birth	Third to fourth decade
Serum PTH	N/↑	↑	↑	↑↑	↑
Number of parathyroid glands	Multiple	Multiple	Multiple	Multiple	Multiple
Parathyroid gland enlargement	Minimal	5x normal	Minimal	10x normal	Minimal
Pathophysiologic defect	Monoallelic-inherited inactivation of the *CaSR* gene decreases the sensing of serum calcium by parathyroid cells and renal tubules	Sequential inactivation of the *MEN1* gene leads to the growth of one or more neoplastic clones in parathyroid glands	Inactivating mutation of the *RET* proto-oncogene leads to the growth of one or more neoplastic clones in parathyroid glands	Biallelic inactivation of the *CaSR* gene impairs calcium sensing in parathyroid cells more than monoallelic inactivation	Inactivating mutation of an unknown gene on chromosome 1q24
Treatment	None	Surgery	Pharmacotherapy or surgery	Surgery	Surgery

Notes: FHH, familial hypocalciuric hypercalcemia; MEN, multiple endocrine neoplasia; NSPH, neonatal severe primary hyperparathyroidism; HJTS, hyperparathyroidism-jaw tumor syndrome; AD, autosomal dominant; AR, autosomal recessive; N, normal; ↑, high (11.6–15.5 mg/dL); ↑↑, very high (>15.5 mg/dL).

HYPERCALCEMIA WITH LOW PARATHYROID HORMONE

The most common causes of hyperparathyroidism and low serum PTH levels include malignancy, granulomatous diseases, and renal failure.

Hypercalcemia Associated with Malignancy

Malignancy-associated hypercalcemia accounts for 10% of all causes of hypercalcemia. It is the most common cause of hypercalcemia in hospitalized patients and is the second (after primary hyperparathyroidism) most common cause of hypercalcemia.

Etiology

Tumors usually cause hypercalcemia by producing factors that affect bone resorption. More than 50% of malignancy-associated hypercalcemia is due to production of a peptide that is structurally homologous to PTH, known as **PTH-related peptide (PTHrp)**. The other causes of malignant hypercalcemia include local osteolysis by direct bone invasion, bone destruction, and ectopic production of calcitriol.

Pathophysiology

PTHrp is a protein secreted by some cancer cells leading to humeral hypercalcemia of malignancy. It is produced commonly in patients with squamous cell carcinoma, breast or prostate cancer, and occasionally in patients with myeloma. PTHrp shares 8 of the first 13 amino acids as PTH; therefore, it can bind to the same receptor, the type 1 PTH receptor (PTHR1) resulting in activation of the G protein-secondary messenger system. PTHrp is larger than PTH and contains between 139 and 173 amino acids, compared to 84 in PTH. PTHrp shares many actions with PTH and promotes hypercalcemia by binding to the PTH receptor, thus promoting hypercalcemia and hypophosphatemia. Increased PTHrp leads to increased calcium resorption from bone, and reduced calcium excretion and phosphate reabsorption from the kidney.

The mechanisms of hypercalcemia secondary to malignancy involve increased osteoclastic activity. For example, individuals with multiple myeloma may develop increased osteoclastic bone resorption caused by potent cytokines expressed or secreted locally by the myeloma cells (receptor activator of nuclear factor-κB ligand [RANKL], macrophage inflammatory protein [MIP]-1α, and tumor necrosis factors [TNFs]) or overexpressed by other cells in the local microenvironment. The bone resorption in turn leads to efflux of calcium into the extracellular fluid.

Hypercalcemia that is due to bone destruction by invasive tumor metastases is most likely due to local tumor production of cytokines or due to PTHrp. In addition, lymphomas may produce excessive vitamin D (calcitriol) by excessive conversion of cholecalciferol to calcitriol due to increased 1α-hydroxylase activity by the tumor cells leading to hypercalcemia.

Clinical Findings

The clinical findings are similar to those of patients with hypercalcemia described at the beginning of this chapter.

Diagnostic Studies

If hypercalcemia is due to PTHrp, the diagnosis of malignancy-induced hypercalcemia is established by the presence of a malignant disorder and by laboratory evidence of elevated serum calcium, low serum PTH, and measureable PTHrp levels. The serum phosphate level is usually low. If the hypercalcemia is due to excessive conversion of cholecalciferol to calcitriol, then elevated levels of calcitriol may be present.

Treatment

Parathyroid surgery is not an option in hypercalcemia-associated malignancy because this condition is not related to a primary parathyroid abnormality. Calcitonin has been used to suppress osteoclastic activity, but the effect is weak and transient. Bisphosphonates that consistently inhibit osteoclastic activity are the preferred agents. Through inhibition of tumor cytokine release and intestinal calcium absorption, glucocorticoids prevent excess production of calcium, due to increased osteoclastic activity, and calcitriol, from bone tumors such as multiple myeloma. If hypercalcemia is severe and accompanied by renal failure, dialysis may be required.

Prognosis

Unfortunately, prognosis is not related to hypercalcemia but to the malignancy. In most patients, hypercalcemia of malignancy is usually a late and terminal condition associated with a poor prognosis. If the tumor load can be minimized, the hypercalcemia will either resolve or respond to bisphosphonate therapy.

Granulomatous Diseases

Hypercalcemia commonly occurs in patients with granulomatous diseases.

Etiology

The most common granulomatous diseases that cause hypercalcemia are sarcoidosis and tuberculosis. Granulomatous diseases that cause hypercalcemia are shown in Box 5-1. The primary abnormality is due to increased intestinal calcium absorption induced by high serum calcitriol concentrations, although a calcitriol-induced increase in bone resorption may also contribute.

Pathophysiology

Normally, the conversion of 25-hydroxyvitamin D_3 to 1,25-dihydroxyvitamin D_3 occurs via the 1α-hydroxylase enzyme in the proximal tubule of the kidney that is under physiologic control of PTH and fibroblast growth factor 23 (FGF23). Hypercalcemia normally suppresses the release of PTH and therefore the production of 1,25-dihydroxyvitamin D_3.

BOX 5-1.	Hypercalcemia Due to Granulomatous Diseases	
Sarcoidosis	Candidiasis	Silicone-induced
Tuberculosis	Leprosy	granulomas
Berylliosis	Crohn disease	Catscratch disease
Coccidiomycosis	Histiocytosis X	Wegener granulomatosis
Histoplasmosis		

The hypercalcemia that occurs in patients with granulomatous diseases is the result of ectopic production of calcitriol by alveolar macrophages. Increased calcitriol production results in increased intestinal absorption of calcium and phosphorous despite PTH suppression. Macrophage 1α-hydroxylase does not respond to the suppressed PTH and is also not downregulated by high calcitriol levels.

Clinical Findings

Most patients are asymptomatic, but those with symptomatic hypercalcemia have symptoms that are similar to those described at the beginning of this chapter.

Diagnostic Studies

The diagnosis is based on the presence of a granulomatous disease coupled with elevated serum calcium and calcitriol levels and an elevated urinary calcium level. Due to the elevated calcitriol level, increased intestinal absorption of phosphate occurs, and the serum phosphate level may also increase. Serum PTH levels are suppressed.

Treatment

Patients with hypercalcemia due to a granulomatous disease respond best to glucocorticoid therapy because these steroids inhibit intestinal calcium absorption. In sarcoidosis, in particular, glucocorticoids prevent and suppress inflammation caused by mechanical, chemical, infectious, and immunologic stimuli. They repress many inflammatory genes. Regardless of which granulomatous disease a patient has, successful treatment of the underlying granulomatous disease will usually correct the hypercalcemia. For patients who do not respond to therapy for the granulomatous condition, symptomatic treatment with fluid as well as the agents listed in Table 5-1 should be considered.

Prognosis

Prognosis is not related to the hypercalcemia but to the granulomatous disease. If the granulomatous disease is treated effectively, calcium levels will normalize. Exposure to excessive sunlight may worsen hypercalcemia and hypercalciuria because it increases cholecalciferol stores.

HYPERCALCEMIA ASSOCIATED WITH OTHER ENDOCRINE CONDITIONS

Hypercalcemia is associated with both thyrotoxicosis and adrenal insufficiency.

Thyrotoxicosis

Mild hypercalcemia may be seen in many patients with thyrotoxicosis. Increased bone resorption caused by increased circulating levels of thyroxine and triiodothyronine is believed to be responsible for the hypercalcemia. The diagnosis of thyrotoxicosis is confirmed by elevated free thyroxine and triiodothyronine levels and suppressed TSH levels. Patients present with mild-to-moderate hypercalcemia and low serum PTH and calcitriol levels. Successful treatment of thyrotoxicosis will resolve the hypercalcemia, unless there is concomitant primary hyperparathyroidism.

Adrenal Insufficiency

Hypercalcemia is commonly seen with adrenal insufficiency especially during an adrenal crisis. The underlying pathophysiology is unclear; however, volume contraction and hemoconcentration may be the cause. The hypercalcemia usually normalizes with volume and glucocorticoid replacement.

HYPERCALCEMIA ASSOCIATED WITH NONENDOCRINE CONDITIONS

Hypercalcemia is also associated with nonendocrine conditions that include pharmacologic agents, excess levels of vitamins and minerals, and immobilization.

Pharmacologic Agents

There are a number of therapeutic agents including thiazides, lithium, and theophylline that can raise the serum calcium level. It is important to carefully review the patient's history to determine whether there was an exposure to a drug or agent prior to the development of hypercalcemia.

Thiazide Diuretics

Thiazide diuretics act on the distal convoluted tubule and decrease renal calcium excretion by 50 to 150 mg/day by an unknown mechanism. Although this rarely causes hypercalcemia in patients with normal calcium metabolism, it can result in hypercalcemia in patients with increased bone resorption and in those with even mild hyperparathyroidism.

Lithium

Patients receiving lithium commonly develop mild hypercalcemia because lithium increases the set point for PTH suppression by calcium. Hypercalcemia almost always resolves if therapy with lithium is discontinued.

Theophylline

Theophylline, a drug that is occasionally given to asthmatic patients, may also cause hypercalcemia. The theophylline level in these patients is usually above the normal therapeutic level and the hypercalcemia resolves when the theophylline level returns to the normal range. The mechanism of action is unknown. Treatment of asthma has changed significantly in the past 20 years and theophylline is rarely used today.

Vitamin and Mineral Toxicity

Excessive intake of vitamin A or D can result in hypercalcemia. The milk-alkali syndrome is a rare condition caused by ingestion of large amounts of calcium together with sodium bicarbonate.

Vitamin A

Vitamin A taken in large doses (more than 50,000 IU/day) can cause hypercalcemia as a result of increased osteoclast bone resorption. It is usually seen in patients taking excessive amounts of retinoic acid derivatives for treatment of acne. The most likely mechanism is that vitamin A acts directly on bone, causing stimulation of osteoclastic resorption or inhibition of osteoblastic formation, or both.

Vitamin D

Both cholecalciferol and calcitriol circulate in blood partially bound to the vitamin-D-binding protein. Individuals ingesting a large amount of vitamin D (converted to cholecalciferol in the liver) or cholecalciferol itself displace calcitriol from the binding protein, resulting in increased free calcitriol levels. The total calcitriol level may be low because calcitriol production is inhibited. Elevated free calcitriol levels will cause hypercalcemia because of increased intestinal calcium absorption and increased bone resorption. The hypercalcemic episode is rare in patients taking vitamin D, but if it occurs, it is usually prolonged, due to the prolonged half-life of vitamin D, and often requires therapy with corticosteroids and bisphosphonates together with the usual nonspecific therapy for hypercalcemia.

Another form of vitamin D intoxication occurs when calcitriol is used excessively in the treatment of hypoparathyroidism and for the hypocalcemia in secondary hypoparathyroidism for patients with renal insufficiency. In these patients, the total calcitriol level in the serum is increased. The hypercalcemia is transient if calcitriol is discontinued because of calcitriol's short half-life. Maintaining adequate hydration is usually all that is necessary for correction of the hypercalcemia.

Calcium and Sodium Bicarbonate

The milk-alkali syndrome is usually seen in individuals who ingest calcium carbonate in over-the-counter antacid preparations and in those who use it for the treatment and prevention of osteoporosis. Features of the syndrome include hypercalcemia, renal failure, and metabolic alkalosis. The exact pathophysiologic mechanism is unknown. The amount of calcium ingested may be as little as 2 to 3 g/day but is typically between 6 to 15 g/day. Therapy requires rehydration, diuresis, and stopping calcium and antacid ingestion. If diuresis is impractical because of renal failure, dialysis against a dialysate with a low calcium concentration is effective. Renal failure usually resolves in short-term cases, but may persist in chronic cases.

Immobilization

Long-term immobilization may cause hypercalcemia in patients whose underlying bone resorption is elevated. This occurs in children and adolescents, patients with Paget disease, in those with mild primary and secondary hypoparathyroidism, and in mild hypercalcemia of malignancy. These patients are at risk for osteopenia. There is recent evidence that bisphosphonates may diminish hypercalcemia and the development of osteopenia, but resumption of weight bearing is essential for complete resolution of hypercalcemia and hypercalciuria.

| TABLE 5-3. | Causes of Hypercalcemia | | | | |

Etiology	Serum				Urine
	Pho	PTH	25-D$_3$	1,25-D$_3$	Ca
Primary hyperparathyroidism (sporadic)	↓	↑	N	↑	↑ or N
Primary hyperparathyroidism (hereditary)					
FHH	N	↑ or N	N	N	↓
MEN 1	↓	↑	N	↑	↓
MEN 2A	↓	↑	N	↑	↓
NSPH	↓	↑	N	↑	↑ or N
HJTS	↓	↑	N	↑	↑ or N
Malignancy					
PTHrp	↓	↓	N	↑	↓
Calcitriol	↑	↓	N	↑	↑
Tumor cytokines	↑	↓	N	↓	↑
Tumor invasion	↑	↓	N	↓	↑
Granulomatous diseases	↑	↓	N	↑	↑
Thyrotoxicosis	↑	↓	N	↓	↑
Adrenocortical insufficiency	↑	N or ↓	N	N	N
Pharmacologic agents					
Hydrochlorothiazide	N	N	N	N	↑
Lithium	N	↑	N	N	↑
Theophylline	N	N	N	N	N
Vitamin or mineral ingestion					
Vitamin D	↑	↓	↑	↑*	↑
Vitamin A	↑	↓	N	↓	↑
Sodium bicarbonate	N	↓	N	N or ↓	↑
Immobilization	↑	↓	N	N	↑

Notes: Pho, phosphorous; PTH, parathyroid hormone; 25-D$_3$ cholecalciferol (25-hydroxy vitamin D$_3$); 1,25-D$_3$ calcitriol (1,25-dihydroxy vitamin D$_3$); N, normal; L, low; H, high. *The total calcitriol level is low, but the free is high.

FHH, familal hypocalcuric hypercalcemia; MEN, multiple endocrine neoplasia; NSPH, neonatal severe primary hyperparathyroidsm; HJTS, hyperparathyroidism-jaw tumor syndrome; PTHrp, parathyroid hormone-related peptide.

CASE FOLLOW-UP

Our patient has the characteristic symptoms and biochemical findings of hypercalcemia. Prior to performing an extensive work-up, a number of conditions can be removed from the many potential etiologies. She denies taking any medications, so drugs such as thiazides, lithium, or theophylline can be ruled out. Because she has symptoms of hypercalcemia, it is unlikely that she has FHH.

(*continues*)

CASE FOLLOW-UP (*continued*)

She denies any pulmonary symptoms making it less likely that she has a granulomatous disease such as sarcoidosis or tuberculosis as a cause of hypercalcemia.

Additional biochemical studies and tests are ordered to help determine the etiology of hypercalcemia. Since the serum PTH and vitamin D levels are not available immediately, a chest radiograph is ordered to rule out a pulmonary lesion such as a malignancy or granulomatous disease. An electrocardiogram is ordered to determine whether the QT interval is shortened, a common finding in a patient with hypercalcemia.

The results of the serum biochemical studies are:

Calcium	12.9 mg/dL (normal = 8.5 to 10.5 mg/dL)
Albumin	4.1 g/dL (normal = 3.5 to 5.5 g/dL)
Phosphate	1.7 mg/dL (normal = 2.7 to 4.5 mg/dL)
PTH	194 pg/mL (normal = 10 to 60 pg/mL)
25-hydroxyvitamin D_3	35 ng/mL (normal = 30 to 90 ng/mL)
1,25-dihydroxyvitamin D_3	85 pg/mL (normal = 20 to 70 pg/mL)
Free thyroxine	1.4 ng/dL (normal = 0.9 to 1.6 ng/dL)
Thyroid-stimulating hormone	2.1 µIU/L (normal = 0.5 to 4.2 µIU/L)

Her chest radiograph is normal without evidence for pulmonary disease. Her electrocardiogram is also normal without evidence for an abnormal QT interval.

The elevated PTH level, in the face of hypercalcemia, narrows the cause to primary hyperparathyroidism. Without a family history, an extremely elevated serum calcium level, bone tumors, or other endocrine disease, the inherited forms of primary hyperparathyroidism can be ruled out. Based on her age, symptoms, and markedly elevated serum PTH level, the most likely diagnosis is sporadic primary hyperparathyroidism.

Prior to scheduling surgery, a 24-hour urine is collected and the calcium/creatinine ratio is determined. The ratio is 0.4; therefore, FHH can be ruled out, insofar as it is usually <0.01 in individuals with FHH. A sestamibi scan is performed that shows significant uptake in the left inferior parathyroid gland.

She is scheduled to have a minimally invasive parathyroidectomy the following week. Prior to surgery she is instructed to maintain adequate hydration.

The operation is uneventful and the left inferior parathyroid gland is removed successfully. Within 15 minutes, intraoperative PTH levels normalize.

One week after surgery her biochemical studies have returned to normal and her back and leg pain have completely resolved. Her polyuria, dysuria, and constipation have almost dissipated.

REFERENCES and SUGGESTED READINGS

Ambrogini E, Cetani F, Cianferotti L, et al. Surgery or surveillance for mild asymptomatic primary hyperparathyroidism: a prospective, randomized clinical trial. J Clin Endocrinol Metab. 2007;92(8):3114–3121.

Bargren AE, Repplinger D, Chen H, Sippel RS. Can biochemical abnormalities predict symptomatology in patients with primary hyperparathyroidism? J Am Coll Surg. 2011;213(3):410–414.

Carlson D. Parathyroid pathology hyperparathyroidism and parathyroid tumors. Arch Pathol Lab Med. 2010;134:1639–1644.

Hudson JQ. Secondary hyperparathyroidism in chronic kidney disease: focus on clinical consequences and vitamin D therapies. Ann Pharmacother. 2006;40(9): 1584–1593.

Jacobs TP, Bilezikian JP. Rare causes of hypercalcemia. J Clin Endocrinol Metab. 2005;90:6316–6322.

Khan AA, Bilezikian JP, Kung AW, et al. Alendronate in primary hyperparathyroidism: a double-blind, randomized, placebo-controlled trial. J Clin Endocrinol Metab. 2004;89(7):3319–3325.

Marcocci C, Cetani F. Primary hyperparathyroidism. NEJM. 2011;365(25):2389–2397.

Marx S. Hyperparathyroid and hypoparathyroid disorders. NEJM. 2000;343(25):1863–1875.

Polyzois Makras P, Papapoulos SE. Medical treatment of hypercalcaemia. Hormones. 2009;8(2):83–95.

Porepa M, Punthakee X, Weinstein J. Accounting for polyuria. Univ Tor Med J. 2001;79(1):61–64.

Rao DS, Phillips ER, Divine GW, Talpos GB. Randomized controlled clinical trial of surgery versus no surgery in patients with mild asymptomatic primary hyperparathyroidism. J Clin Endocrinol Metab. 2004;89(11):5415–5422.

Szalet A, Mazch H, Freund HR. Lithium-associated hyperparathyroidism: report of four cases and review of the literature. Eur J Endocrinol. 2009;160: 317–323.

CHAPTER REVIEW QUESTIONS

1. Which one of the following is *not* a treatment option for acute hypercalcemia?

   A. Intravenous fluid
   B. Calcitonin
   C. Calcitriol
   D. Alendronate
   E. Furosemide

2. An asymptomatic 70-year-old man comes to you for evaluation of hypercalcemia. His calcium level is 10.5 mg/dL (normal range is 8.5 to 10.5 mg/dL) and his albumin is 3.2 g/dL (normal = 3.5 to 5.0 g/dL). His referring physician checked a PTH level and found it to be 51 pg/mL (normal = 10 to 60 pg/mL). What is your next step?

   A. Repeat serum calcium and 24-hour urine calcium in 1 year.
   B. Send to surgery for parathyroidectomy.
   C. Obtain a bone scan looking for metastasis.
   D. Order a bone mineral density test.
   E. Treat with a bisphosphonate.

3. A previously healthy 73-year-old man has had excruciating back and leg pain over the past 2 weeks. He has also had a 10-lb weight loss but no other symptoms. Routine serum laboratory studies include a calcium of 12.4 mg/dL (normal = 8 to 10.5 mg/dL) and an albumin of 4.0 g/dL (normal = 3.5 to 4.5 g/dL). All of the following would be included in the differential diagnosis of his condition *except*:

   A. Parathyroid cancer
   B. Elevated PTHrp
   C. Overdose of furosemide
   D. Sarcoidosis
   E. Systemic malignancy

4. In a patient with hypercalcemia due to sarcoidosis, which of the following laboratory tests would be seen?

   A. Elevated serum PTH, elevated calcitriol, and low cholecalciferol levels
   B. Elevated serum calcium and phosphorus levels with a suppressed calcitriol level
   C. Positive PTHrp, elevated cAMP levels in the urine, and elevated serum PTH level
   D. Elevated serum albumin, low serum calcium, and elevated urine phosphorus levels
   E. High serum calcium, low PTH, and high calcitriol

5. A 21-year-old woman comes to your clinic with a history of having a low phosphorus level on several occasions. She suffers from chronic bone pain, constipation, and polyuria. Her fasting phosphorus level is 1.6 mg/dL (normal = 3.0 to 4.5 mg/dL). Which of the following is *most likely* to be found on her laboratory testing?

A. Serum calcium level of 6.5 mg/dL (normal = 8.5 to 10.5 mg/dL)
B. Low urine phosphate level
C. Serum PTH level of 200 pg/mL (normal = 10 to 65 pg/mL)
D. Serum calcitriol level of 55 pg/mL (normal = 10 to 60 pg/mL)
E. Serum TSH level of 0.01 μIU/L (normal = 0.5 to 4.5 μIU/L)

CHAPTER REVIEW ANSWERS

1. The correct answer is C. There are many options for medical treatment in a patient with hypercalcemia. Calcitriol (1,25-dihydroxy-vitamin D_3) is the active form of vitamin D and causes an increase in intestinal absorption of both calcium and phosphorous. Calcitriol is the correct answer because it is the only choice that would make hypercalcemia worse.

Intravenous fluid (**Choice A**) is an appropriate treatment for hypercalcemia since it lowers the serum calcium through hemodilution. Calcitonin (**Choice B**) is a hormone secreted by the parafollicular C cells of the thyroid gland in response to an increase in extracellular calcium. It acts mainly by suppressing osteoclasts and opposes PTH. Alendronate (**Choice D**) is a bisphosphonate that acts by inhibiting osteoclast activity. Furosemide (**Choice E**) is a loop diuretic that causes a decrease in serum calcium by increasing urinary calcium. Furosemide blocks the transport of sodium to the loop of Henle. Since calcium is reabsorbed because of a favorable electrochemical gradient via sodium and chloride reabsorption, calcium reabsorption is inhibited and excretion in the urine occurs.

2. The correct answer is A. After correction for his mildly low albumin, this man still has mild hypercalcemia [(4 − 3.2) × 0.8 + 10.5 = 11.14]. The finding that he is asymptomatic and has a normal serum PTH level makes it less likely that he needs further work-up or treatment. Reevaluating him in a year is the best choice of the available options.

He does not need surgery for a parathyroidectomy (**Choice B**) at this time since he is asymptomatic and likely does not have primary hyperparathyroidism. It is also unlikely that he has a form of malignancy causing his mild hypercalcemia, and ordering a bone scan to evaluate for metastases (**Choice C**) is unnecessary at this time. Ordering of a bone mineral density test (**Choice D**) is unnecessary because it is unlikely that he has osteopenia or osteoporosis given the fact that he has hypercalcemia rather than hypocalcemia. Treatment with a bisphosphonate (**Choice E**) is incorrect because he is asymptomatic and will not achieve any symptomatic benefit from a bisphosphonate and would be at risk for bisphosphonate side effects.

3. The correct answer is C. The findings described are consistent with the symptoms of hypercalcemia as he has symptoms of back pain, an elevated serum calcium level, and a normal serum albumin. An overdose of furosemide would result in hypocalcemia due to the inhibition of sodium, chloride, and calcium reabsorption in the loop of Henle.

Parathyroid cancer (**Choice A**) and an elevated PTHrp (**Choice B**) would result in symptomatic hypercalcemia with hypophosphatemia. Sarcoidosis (**Choice D**) usually causes symptomatic hypercalcemia through increased production of calcitriol by macrophages.

Systemic malignancy (**Choice E**) also frequently causes symptomatic hypercalcemia with a low serum PTH level. In addition to the hypercalcemia and low serum PTH, those with malignancy and production of PTHrp will have a low serum phosphate level, whereas those with increased production of calcitriol, cytokines, or local bone destruction will have an elevated phosphate level.

---

4. The correct answer is E. Individuals with a granulomatous disease, such as sarcoidosis, develop hypercalcemia because alveolar macrophages produce excess calcitriol (1,25-dihydroxy-vitamin D_3) by upregulation of 1α-hydroxylase. The macrophage 1α-hydroxylase does not respond to suppressed serum PTH and is also not downregulated by elevated levels of calcitriol. Therefore, the biochemical findings in individuals with hypercalcemia due to sarcoidosis include hypercalcemia, hyperphosphatemia, elevated calcitriol levels, and a suppressed serum PTH.

Elevated PTH causing elevated calcitriol and low cholecalciferol levels (**Choice A**) is incorrect because the serum PTH would be suppressed if the hypercalcemia were due to sarcoidosis. Calcitriol would be elevated, but cholecalciferol would be normal. Elevated serum calcium and phosphorus levels, with a suppressed calcitriol level (**Choice B**), would be incorrect because the calcitriol level would be increased in sarcoidosis. The presence of PTHrp, elevated urine cAMP levels, and an elevated serum PTH level (**Choice C**) is incorrect because granulomatous diseases do not produce PTHrp as tumors do. Urine cAMP levels would be elevated in conditions where serum PTH or PTHrp levels are elevated. Since hypercalcemia of sarcoidosis is due to increased calcitriol production, serum PTH levels would be suppressed, not elevated. Elevated serum albumin, low serum calcium, and elevated urine phosphorus levels (**Choice D**) would be incorrect because a low serum calcium level with an elevated albumin level would be seen in hypocalcemia, not hypercalcemia. With a suppressed PTH level, as expected in sarcoidosis, urine phosphate levels would be low, not elevated.

---

5. The correct answer is C. The woman has symptoms of hypercalcemia. In association with hypophosphatemia, the most likely cause for her symptoms is primary hyperparathyroidism. The abnormally elevated serum PTH results in hypercalcemia, hypophosphatemia, and increased bone resorption leading to bone pain and fractures. Hypercalcemia causes constipation and polyuria.

A low serum calcium level of 6.5 mg/dL (**Choice A**) is not correct since the woman has symptoms suggestive of hypercalcemia. A low urine phosphate level (**Choice B**) is not expected in the presence of an elevated serum PTH level since elevated PTH levels cause increased calcium reabsorption and increased phosphate excretion from the kidney. A serum calcitriol level of 55 pg/mL (**Choice D**) would not be expected in a patient with hyperparathyroidism since PTH upregulates the 1α-hydroxylase enzyme that promotes increased calcitriol production. A serum TSH level of 0.01 μIU/L (**Choice E**) would not be expected to cause this woman's findings since thyrotoxicosis may cause hypercalcemia due to the bone resorptive effects of excessive thyroid hormone, but, both serum calcium and phosphate levels would be elevated.

Glucose Metabolism and Hypoglycemia

6

Anna L. Lipowska
Eric I. Felner

CASE

A 4-year-old boy presents to the emergency department with a history of a seizure lasting 2 minutes. According to his mother, the boy was playing inside at home when he began sweating and trembling. He reported feeling dizzy, had difficulty speaking, and suddenly fell to the ground and began shaking. In the emergency department an intravenous (IV) line is placed in the boy, and blood samples are obtained and sent to the laboratory.

Our patient's birth history is unremarkable. His family history reveals that his father had a heart attack last year, and his mother has insulin-dependent diabetes. The boy is on a regular diet and does not take any medications. The mother appears nervous, does not want to answer any questions asked by the physician, and reports that she is in a hurry to get home because her husband will be getting home from work soon.

Some of the blood test results are available and reveal a low serum glucose (21 mg/dL), normal serum sodium (138 mEq/L), and normal serum calcium (10.0 mg/dL). Other biochemical studies including serum ketones, cortisol, insulin, and growth hormone (GH) levels are not yet available.

This chapter reviews the physiology of glucose metabolism, which plays such a vital role in understanding the pathophysiology of hypoglycemia and hyperglycemia, followed by reviews of the etiology, evaluation, and treatment of hypoglycemia to help the learner develop hypotheses that focus on the etiology of this child's hypoglycemia. A summary of the work-up and a therapeutic plan are provided at the end of this chapter to give the learner a better understanding of hypoglycemia, which is divided into nonketotic and ketotic categories.

OBJECTIVES

1. List and categorize the causes of hypoglycemia.

2. Recognize the clinical and laboratory findings in an individual with hypoglycemia.

CHAPTER OUTLINE

Physiology
  Glucose Transition from Intrauterine
    to Extrauterine Life
  Regulation of Blood Glucose
  Fuel Metabolism (Carbohydrates)
  Fuel Metabolism (Fats)
  Insulin Secretion after Glucose
    Delivery
  Hormonal Effects
  Counterregulation
Hypoglycemia
  Etiology
  Symptoms
  Evaluation
  Treatment
Nonketotic Hypoglycemia
  Hyperinsulinism (Congenital)

(continues)

(*continued*)

OBJECTIVES

3. Develop a differential diagnosis for an individual who presents with hypoglycemia.

4. Describe the evaluation and management of an individual with hypoglycemia.

PHYSIOLOGY

After the newborn period, the occurrence of hypoglycemia is abnormal and demands immediate investigation and treatment. Fasting and random blood glucose levels in infants, children, and adults are maintained within a relatively small normal range of 70 and 100 mg/dL and less than 180 mg/dL, respectively. Blood glucose levels in neonates are lower, ranging from 45 to 80 mg/dL. The following section describes the mechanisms involved in normal glucose homeostasis.

Glucose Transition from Intrauterine to Extrauterine Life

The transition from the intrauterine state of glucose sufficiency to the sudden state of starvation, induced by umbilical cord clamping, results in a series of adaptations to extrauterine life. Once this transition is complete, the mechanisms of glucose homeostasis are similar throughout life. The most important difference between infants, children, and adults is the rate of glucose utilization. The change in glucose utilization, dependency on gluconeogenesis, glycogenolysis, and fatty acid oxidation in infants and children is greater than that in adolescents and adults. Thus, many disorders of hypoglycemia manifest after early infancy with the natural progression to longer feeding intervals later in life. Unfortunately, this is also a time when the developing brain is very susceptible to hypoglycemic damage.

For individuals with a known cause of hypoglycemia, such as insulin-treated diab mellitus (DM), the focus should be on immediate treatment followed by adjustment of insulin dosage to prevent further hypoglycemia. For noninsulin-treated individuals and in those without a definite cause for hypoglycemia, the initial treatment should be followed by collection of critical blood samples that may help determine the etiology of hypoglycemia so that treatment can be implemented quickly.

Regulation of Blood Glucose

Insulin is produced and stored in the β-cells of the pancreatic islets and released in response to elevated blood glucose levels. Insulin production begins when preproinsulin is synthesized in the rough endoplasmic reticulum and delivered to the Golgi apparatus where a series of prohormone convertases cleave it into mature insulin and C-peptide. Insulin and C-peptide are then stored in secretory granules until their release into the circulation. Once in circulation, insulin binds to the tyrosine kinase insulin receptors on target cells. This stimulates translocation of glucose transport proteins (GLUTs) from the Golgi apparatus to the plasma membrane, facilitating cellular uptake of glucose. Each cell type has a different GLUT transporter to handle glucose transport/uptake. Some transporters, such as the GLUT-2 transporters, are found on pancreatic β-cells and in hepatocytes, are insulin-independent, and respond to the presence of glucose in circulation. Other glucose transporters, such as GLUT-4, are located in striated muscle and adipose tissue, are insulin-dependent, and are expressed in response to circulating insulin. Glucose transporters allow for maintenance of appropriate glucose concentration in response to insulin release and peripheral glucose uptake into cells (Table 6-1).

TABLE 6-1.	Glucose Transporters	
Transporter	**Location**	**Function**
GLUT 1	Erythrocytes and endothelial cells of barrier tissues (i.e., blood-brain barrier)	Responsible for the low level of basal glucose uptake required to sustain respiration in cells
GLUT 2	Pancreatic β-cells, renal tubular cells, small intestinal epithelial cells, and liver cells	*Liver*: Bidirectionality required to uptake glucose for glycolysis and release of glucose during gluconeogenesis *Pancreatic β cells*: Free-flowing glucose required so that the intracellular environment of these cells can accurately gauge the serum glucose levels *Intestine*: All three monosaccharides transported from intestinal mucosal cell into portal circulation
GLUT 3	Neurons and placenta	Allows transport even during times of low glucose concentrations
GLUT 4	Striated muscle and adipose tissue	Only insulin-regulated glucose transporter and responsible for insulin-regulated glucose storage

Fuel Metabolism (Carbohydrates)

Processes such as gluconeogenesis, glycogenolysis, and fatty acid oxidation are important biochemical processes involved in glucose (energy) production. Maintenance of a constant blood glucose level is essential for all of the body's organs, particularly for the central nervous system (CNS). This is because the brain can neither synthesize nor store the amount of glucose required for normal cellular function. In the postabsorptive state, systemic glucose balance is maintained and hypoglycemia and hyperglycemia are prevented by dynamic, minute-to-minute regulation of endogenous glucose production by the liver and kidneys and, by glucose utilization by the peripheral tissues. Glucose production is a result of gluconeogenesis and glycogenolysis. Gluconeogenesis causes noncarbohydrate precursors, such as lactate, alanine, and glycerol, to be converted to glucose. Excess glucose is polymerized to glycogen that is mainly stored in the liver and muscle. Glycogenolysis breaks down glycogen to individual glucose units for mobilization during times of metabolic need. These steps depend on the interaction of various mechanisms, including glucoregulatory hormones (insulin, glucagon, and other counterregulatory hormones) and gluconeogenic substrate supply (lactate, glycerol, and amino acids). In addition, paracrine mediators and the autonomic nervous system (ANS) also have a significant regulatory role in glucose metabolism.

Between meals, the body balances glucose levels through gluconeogenesis, glycogenolysis, and fatty acid oxidation. When glucose levels fall to unexpectedly low levels, other sources of metabolic fuel are harnessed.

Gluconeogenesis is the synthesis of glucose from noncarbohydrate substrates such as glycerol, lactate, and amino acids. This process occurs mainly in the liver and muscle; the remainder in the kidneys. The 3 most important gluconeogenic precursors are glycerol, generated from lipolysis (in the liver), and lactate and amino acids, from muscle. The kidneys play an important role in patients with hepatic failure, providing the body with an additional supply of glucose. In the renal cortex, glutamine is the gluconeogenesis precursor. The process begins in the mitochondria and ends in the cytosol of the cell.

Glycogenolysis is the process of glycogen breakdown that generates glucose. Glycogen, a polysaccharide, is composed of glucose monomers. As glucose molecules are separated through hydrolysis, the polysaccharide is phosphorylated, forming glucose-6-phosphate, an important substrate in glycolysis. Glycogen phosphorylase is the main regulatory enzyme in this process. Glycogenolysis occurs in both liver and muscle tissues.

Fuel Metabolism (Fats)

Free fatty acids (FFAs) are another available energy source that the liver and muscle tissues can oxidize for energy. From fatty acids, the liver can produce ketone bodies, an alternate energy supply for the brain. Ketone body homeostasis results from the interaction of insulin, glucagon, catecholamines, and thyroid hormones. Insulin lowers ketone body concentrations by three independent mechanisms: 1) inhibition of lipolysis lowering FFA availability for ketogenesis, 2) restraint of ketone body production within the liver, and 3) enhanced peripheral ketone body utilization. With elevated insulin concentrations or defects in fatty acid oxidation, ketone concentrations are low. Increased concentrations of glucagon, catecholamines, and thyroid hormone increase ketogenesis by stimulating lipolysis and by increasing intrahepatic ketogenesis.

In fatty acid oxidation and ketone body formation, initially triacylglycerol, one of the body's key fuel storage reserves, is broken down into glycerol and FFAs in the adipocytes. The unesterified fatty acids are exported out of the adipocytes; transported in the plasma bound to albumin; and, ultimately, enter the liver and muscle tissues. Glycerol serves as an important gluconeogenic precursor. In hypoglycemic patients, this process saves essential glucose stores for the brain, while providing an alternate supply of energy for other tissues.

In tissues requiring energy, fatty acids undergo β-oxidation in the mitochondria to provide adenosine triphosphate (ATP), nicotinamide adenine diphosphate (NAD[H]), and acetyl coenzyme A (CoA). Fatty acids are then converted to a CoA derivative by fatty acyl CoA synthetase. The resulting product is transported across the inner mitochondrial membrane by the carnitine shuttle. This process involves two critical enzymes, carnitine palmitoyltransferases I (CPT-1) and II (CPT-2), which, when defective, results in the inability to use fatty acids as metabolic fuel. Once inside the mitochondrial matrix, β-oxidation produces acetyl CoA in a series of steps with a significantly high energy yield. The first of step in this process requires acyl CoA dehydrogenase. A deficiency of this enzyme, most often the medium-chain acyl-CoA dehydrogenase (MCAD), results in decreased fatty acid oxidation.

Excess acetyl CoA in the liver mitochondria can be converted into the ketone bodies, acetoacetate and β-hydroxybutyrate, which serve as an additional energy source for the brain and peripheral tissues. Ketone bodies are then oxidized in the tissues to generate energy. High levels can be detected in the blood (ketonemia) and in the urine (ketonuria). If their quantity gets high enough, ketoacidosis can result.

High plasma ketone body concentrations are found in patients with diabetic ketoacidosis (DKA), during states of starvation, and with various hypoglycemic states. In each of these conditions, tissues do not receive the necessary glucose supply. In some cases of hypoglycemia, such as in conditions associated with increased circulating insulin levels, there is no increased ketone body production. Because ketone body concentrations are relatively easy to measure, and the number of conditions resulting in nonketotic hypoglycemia is very small (i.e., hyperinsulinemia and defects in fatty acid oxidation), it is easy to classify hypoglycemic disorders into two broad categories: nonketotic and ketotic.

Insulin Secretion after Glucose Delivery

Following a meal, glucose levels in the blood increase. Multiple factors regulate the level of glucose in the blood, but insulin and glucagon are the most important. Glucose is taken up by the pancreatic β-cells through GLUT-2 (Figure 6-1). It is metabolized in the β-cells, resulting in increased production of ATP. This, in turn, increases the ATP/adenosine diphosphate ratio that closes potassium channels in the cell membrane and depolarizes the cell. As potassium channels close and cell depolarization occurs, calcium channels in the cell membrane open and allow calcium to flow into the cell. As pancreatic calcium accumulates, insulin is secreted into the bloodstream by the β-cells. Circulating insulin acts on fat, muscle, and liver cells by binding to a receptor on the plasma membrane of the cells. This stimulates intracellular signaling pathways that ultimately cause translocation of glucose transporters to the cell membrane. These transporters increase glucose uptake into the cell. In fat and muscle cells, glucose normally serves as an important source of energy, which can be converted into a stored form of energy as either fat or glycogen. The liver cells produce glucose either by gluconeogenesis or by the breakdown of glycogen. The binding of insulin to its receptor on liver cells leads to increased synthesis of glycogen and inhibition of glucose production by liver cells. After a meal, glucose levels will gradually fall. Once a certain glucose threshold is reached, glucagon is released from pancreatic α-cells and acts primarily on the liver to increase glucose production, either by the breakdown of glycogen to glucose or by *de novo* synthesis of glucose. This results in an increase in circulating glucose levels. The liver responds to fluctuations in the circulating glucose levels and regulates its release into the bloodstream. Through this balancing of insulin and glucagon secretion, glucose levels in the circulation are typically maintained within a narrow range.

During meals, insulin concentrations reach peaks of 50 to 100 μ/mL. This activates glycogen synthesis, enhances peripheral glucose uptake, and inhibits gluconeogenesis

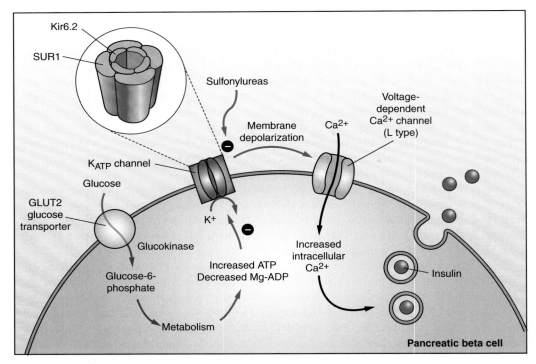

FIGURE 6-1. Regulation of insulin secretion from the β cell. In the basal state, the plasma membrane of the cell is hyperpolarized, and the rate of insulin secretion from the cell is low. When glucose is available, it enters the cell via GLUT2 transporters in the plasma membrane and is metabolized to generate intracellular ATP. ATP binds to and inhibits the plasma membrane K+/ATP channel. Inhibition of the K+/ATP channel decreases plasma membrane K+ conductance. The resulting depolarization of the membrane activates voltage-gated Ca^{2+} channels and thereby stimulates an influx of Ca^{2+}. Ca^{2+} mediates fusion of insulin-containing secretory vesicles with the plasma membrane, leading to insulin secretion. The K+/ATP channel, an octamer composed of Kir6.2 and SUR1 subunits, is the target of several physiologic and pharmacologic regulators. (From Gloyn et al. NEJM. 2004;350(18):1838–1849.)

and glycogenolysis. Simultaneously, lipid synthesis is activated, and lipolysis and keto-genesis are curtailed. During fasting, insulin levels drop to 5 to 10 μ/mL. The fall in insulin reverses the metabolic pathways and ensures that there is an adequate supply of glucose, fatty acids, and ketones.

Hormonal Effects

The hormones involved in the regulation of hepatic glucose production are insulin and the counterregulatory hormones glucagon, epinephrine, cortisol, and GH. Insulin is the main glucoregulatory hormone; it inhibits hepatic glucose production and stimulates peripheral glucose uptake in insulin-sensitive tissues, primarily muscle. In the liver, insu-lin directs glucose-6-phosphate to glycogen by increasing the activity of glycogen syn-thase and decreasing the activity of glycogen phosphorylase, thereby stimulating the breakdown of glycogen to glucose. Insulin also prevents gluconeogenesis by inhibiting gene transcription and expression of phosphoenolpyruvate carboxykinase (PEPCK), the rate-limiting step in hepatic gluconeogenesis, and by increasing the transcription of pyru-vate kinase, the main glycolytic enzyme.

Decreased insulin secretion is the first defense against falling plasma glucose levels, and glucagon is the primary counterregulatory hormone. Epinephrine is not normally critical but becomes essential when glucagon is deficient, as in patients with diabetes. Hypoglycemia develops or progresses when both glucagon and epinephrine are deficient and insulin is present despite actions of other hormones, neurotransmitters, and substrates. Cortisol, GH, glucagon, and epinephrine are involved in the defense against prolonged, as opposed to short-term, hypoglycemia, but neither GH nor cortisol is critical to the correction of hypoglycemia.

Glucagon activates glycogenolysis and gluconeogenesis and increases hepatic glucose production within minutes. Epinephrine is secreted in response to falling plasma glucose levels. It stimulates hepatic glucose production and limits glucose utilization. The actions of epinephrine are both direct and indirect and are mediated through α- and β-adrenergic receptors. α-Adrenergic limitation of insulin secretion allows the hyperglycemic response to occur. β-Adrenergic stimulation causes glucagon secretion to occur. Epinephrine directly increases hepatic glycogenolysis and gluconeogenesis. The hyperglycemic effects of cortisol and GH do not occur for several hours and are due to activation of gluconeogenesis.

Counterregulation

The response to hypoglycemia, or counterregulation of insulin, occurs in stages based on the plasma glucose concentration (Table 6-2). The first response to hypoglycemia is a reduction in insulin secretion that promotes gluconeogenesis, glycogenolysis, and lipolysis and a reduction in glucose uptake. Insulin secretion is inhibited when the plasma glucose falls below 80 mg/dL (4.4 mmol/L), signaling the need for endogenous glucose production. The next response to hypoglycemia is the secretion of glucagon and epinephrine when the plasma glucose falls below 65 mg/dL (3.6 mmol/L). These hormones increase gluconeogenesis and glycogenolysis in the liver and activate the lipase enzyme. The last response to hypoglycemia is an increase in the secretion of cortisol and GH that occurs when the plasma glucose falls below 60 mg/dL (3.3 mmol/L).

During hypoglycemia, insulin production and secretion is inhibited, whereas counterregulatory hormone secretion is accelerated. These counterregulatory hormones attempt to raise an individual's blood glucose level. If a hormone does not follow its predicted physiologic response, hormone deficiency should be suspected; therefore, it is imperative to measure these hormone levels at the time an individual has hypoglycemia. By

TABLE 6-2.	Hypoglycemia Counterregulation	
Glucose Level Threshold mg/dL (mmol/L)	Bodily Defenses	Symptoms
80 (4.4)	Insulin inhibition	—
65 (3.6)	Glucagon secretion	—
65 (3.6)	Epinephrine secretion	—
60 (3.3)	Cortisol and growth hormone secretion	Hunger
55 (3.1)	—	Neuroglycopenia
50 (2.8)	—	Cognitive dysfunction

understanding the physiologic mechanisms that occur during hypoglycemia, any hormone that is not at its expected level during hypoglycemia may be the cause of the pathology.

HYPOGLYCEMIA

A healthy individual's normal fasting blood glucose level ranges from 70 to 100 mg/dL (3.9 to 5.6 mmol/L). In patients treated for diabetes with insulin or oral agents, hypoglycemia is defined by a blood glucose level below 70 mg/dL (3.9 mmol/L), whereas in healthy individuals, hypoglycemia is defined by a blood glucose level <50 mg/dL (3 mmol/L). The Whipple triad is a collection of three criteria that suggest an individual's symptoms result from hypoglycemia and include: 1) symptoms associated with hypoglycemia, 2) a low blood glucose level during the time of symptoms, and 3) resolution of these symptoms once the blood glucose is raised to the normal range.

Hyperglycemia, on the other hand, is defined by a fasting blood glucose level above 100 mg/dL. As discussed in Chapters 7 and 8, individuals with fasting blood glucose levels of 101 to 125 mg/dL (5.6 to 6.9 mmol/L) have impaired fasting glucose, whereas those with fasting blood glucose levels above 125 mg/dL are categorized as having DM. Infants, children, and adolescents have similar glucose levels as adults, but neonates' glucose levels are much lower. The normal fasting serum glucose in the neonate ranges from 45 to 80 mg/dL. Hypoglycemia in the neonate is usually defined by a serum glucose level less than 45 mg/dL.

Etiology

The etiology for hypoglycemic disorders is extensive but is best classified based on the presence or absence of ketones. At the end of the chapter, the etiology of hypoglycemia (Tables 6-3 and 6-4) and an algorithm for evaluating an individual with hypoglycemia (Figure 6-2) is shown.

Symptoms

Clinical symptoms of hypoglycemia do not usually appear until the serum glucose level falls below 60 mg/dL (3.3 mmol/L), although some individuals may experience symptoms earlier (see Table 6-2). Evidence of cognitive dysfunction is usually apparent when arterial glucose is below 50 mg/dL (2.8 mmol/L). Symptoms can largely be categorized as autonomic or neuroglycopenic.

ANS symptoms are due to the secretion of catecholamines and include sweating, anxiety, nausea, trembling, and feelings of warmth. Because the brain is unable to store glycogen or synthesize glucose, it relies on a continuous blood supply of glucose. If an individual develops hypoglycemia for a prolonged period, irreversible brain damage may occur. Hypoglycemia-induced brain injury affects the following structures in a sequential order: 1) middle layers of the cerebral cortex and hippocampus, 2) basal ganglia and anterior thalamus, and 3) brainstem and spinal cord. The neuroglycopenic symptoms are due to a deprivation of brain glucose and include dizziness, tiredness, headache, confusion, difficulty speaking, and the inability to concentrate. More severe cognitive dysfunction results in seizures, coma, and death.

Evaluation

The hypoglycemic state can be life threatening, and the patient should be evaluated without delay. Prior to the administration of glucose, an immediate blood glucose sample at the time of presentation is a crucial component for the evaluation of hypoglycemia.

Evaluation should begin with a detailed history with attention to specific areas regarding the timing of symptoms, description of symptoms, exacerbating factors, underlying ailments, use of pharmacologic agents, and family history as well as a physical examination.

Because biochemical tests should be ordered prior to providing glucose, rather than attempting to pinpoint the etiology prior to collecting blood samples, it is best to order tests that evaluate the individual's glucose homeostasis mechanisms. Initial biochemical tests performed at the time of hypoglycemia should include blood levels sent for serum glucose, insulin, cortisol, GH (in infants and children), and ketones. Once the absence or presence of ketosis is established, a more focused evaluation should be followed. In the absence of ketosis, and based on the age of the individual as well as the history, collection of serum C-peptide and carnitine levels as well as urine sulfonylurea and organic acids should be considered. In the presence of ketosis, collection of lactate and ethanol levels should be considered.

Prolonged fasting studies are often recommended if a hypoglycemic disorder is suspected without a definite etiology or if the individual claims to have had symptoms of hypoglycemia that are not documented biochemically. The fasting test will allow the examiner to determine whether proper bodily defenses exist in response to a hypoglycemic state. Traditionally, in adults, the fast lasts 72 hours. In children, however, the time is limited to 24 hours. If the subject experiences hypoglycemic symptoms accompanied by low serum glucose level during the study, the critical sample should be collected and the fast should be terminated. A healthy patient without a hypoglycemic disorder will respond to the fasting study with a decrease in insulin and increase in serum glucagon, epinephrine, cortisol, and GH levels. Additionally, C-peptide levels should be low, and ketone levels should increase. In the healthy individual with normal glucose homeostatic mechanisms, the fast should not induce hypoglycemia.

Treatment

Regardless of the cause, individuals with hypoglycemia are initially treated with glucose to normalize their blood glucose level. If the hypoglycemic individual is not conscious enough to swallow oral glucose, IV glucose should be administered. Individuals with diabetes should have an emergency glucagon kit available. If the individual is unconscious or experiences a seizure, glucagon should be administered subcutaneously or intramuscularly. Glucagon provides a temporary rise in glucose through its stimulation of gluconeogenesis. For individuals with disorders of gluconeogenesis or who have ingested alcohol or salicylates, glucagon should not be administered. Following the administration of glucose, blood glucose levels should be closely monitored. Long-term therapy is based on the etiology of the hypoglycemia.

As discussed in the remainder of this chapter, treatment for chronic hypoglycemia should include: 1) nutritional supplementation regulating carbohydrate, fat, and protein intake; 2) pharmacotherapy such as sulfonylurea receptor (SUR) antagonists and somatostatin; and 3) surgery including total or partial pancreatectomy or tumor excision.

NONKETOTIC HYPOGLYCEMIA

Nonketotic hypoglycemia is due to either an increase in insulin secretion or a defect in fatty acid oxidation. Excessive insulin secretion during hypoglycemia may be due to endogenous or exogenous hyperinsulinism. In hyperinsulinemic nonketotic hypoglycemia, the body's first defense system fails as insulin levels do not drop in response to low plasma glucose concentrations. Elevated insulin levels inhibit lipolysis, gluconeogenesis, and glycogenolysis. In addition, insulin secretion inhibits glucagon secretion, the second defense mechanism in individuals with hypoglycemia. Hyperinsulinism may occur as a congenital or acquired condition.

Defective fatty acid metabolism may occur as an enzyme deficiency or as an inability to shuttle fatty acids from cytosol to mitochondria and *vice versa*.

Hyperinsulinism (Congenital)

Congenital causes of hypoglycemia that are due to genetic mutations of the K_{ATP} channel, glutamate dehydrogenase (GDH), or glucokinase (GCK) are known as **persistent hypoglycemia due to hyperinsulinism of infancy (PHHI)**. Other congenital causes include overgrowth syndromes, such as hyperinsulinism associated with the infant of a diabetic mother and Beckwith-Wiedemann syndrome (BWS).

Shortly after birth, neonates with hyperinsulinism experience lethargy, irritability, feeding difficulties, and tachypnea. Later, more specific neurogenic and neuroglycopenic symptoms develop. Symptoms are especially severe during fasting periods; therefore, a part of the treatment regimen focuses on diet regulation. The main goal of treatment is to normalize glucose concentrations, which, depending on the cause of the hyperinsulinism, may be accomplished by diet, medical therapy, or surgery.

Persistent Hypoglycemia due to Hyperinsulinism of Infancy

Pancreatic β-cells normally release insulin in response to elevated glucose levels. Glucose that is transported into the β-cell with the GLUT-2 transporter initiates a number of events that lead to insulin secretion in the following sequence: 1) closure of the K_{ATP} channel, 2) decreased potassium efflux, 3) β-cell depolarization, 4) opening of voltage-gated calcium channels, 5) influx of calcium into the cell, and (6) release of insulin. During hypoglycemia, the K_{ATP} channel remains open, ultimately preventing insulin secretion. Activating mutations of the genes coding for the K_{ATP} channel, GDH, or GCK can cause hyperinsulinism (see Figure 6-3). PHHI is usually diagnosed in the first few weeks of life. This condition can be transient or severe and has an incidence of 1:40,000. Other names for this condition are *nesidioblastosis*, *β-cell hyperplasia*, and *β-cell dysmaturation syndrome*. Genetic testing can be performed to confirm the diagnosis.

Gene mutations that cause PHHI most commonly affect the K_{ATP} channel, which is composed of α- (Kir6.2) and β- (SUR1) subunits (see Figure 6-1). In neonates with an activating mutation of the *ABCC8* gene (coding for the SUR1 subunit) or *KCNJ11* gene (coding for the Kir6.2 subunit), the K_{ATP} channel remains constantly closed, causing membrane depolarization, calcium-channel opening, and insulin secretion, regardless of the glucose level. Mutations may be inherited in an autosomal recessive fashion, as a paternal point mutation with clonal loss of heterozygosity, or in an autosomal dominant pattern. Over 100 mutations of the *ABCC8* gene have been identified and account for approximately 60% of all causes of PHHI. Only four mutations of the *KCNJ11* gene have been identified and account for approximately 15% of all causes of PHHI. These infants develop severe hypoglycemia shortly after birth. The severity of the hypoglycemia is usually determined by the pattern of inheritance. Neonates with an autosomal recessive mutation, the most common form, have a severe, diffuse pattern of hyperinsulinism. Those with a mutation due to a clonal loss of heterozygosity have focal changes and have a less severe form. Those with the autosomal dominant form usually have very mild disease and may not require therapy.

Activating mutations involving the GDH enzyme cause hyperinsulinism. The resultant hypoglycemia is usually less severe than the autosomal recessive K_{ATP} channel mutation. GDH is a mitochondrial matrix enzyme found in both the β-cell and the liver, is activated by leucine, and is necessary for the oxidation of glutamate. In the β-cell, the oxidation of glutamate results in increased levels of α-ketoglutarate and ATP, promoting the secretion of insulin. Neonates with this mutation are unable to oxidize glutamate in the liver and also are unable to eliminate ammonia; therefore, hypoglycemia with hyperammonemia is diagnostic of GDH deficiency. Leucine sensitivity has been previously described to cause hypoglycemia insofar as it stimulates insulin release by allosterically activating GDH. Whether leucine itself actually causes hypoglycemia or only in those with a GDH mutation is not known.

Only one family has been identified as having PHHI due to a mutation of the *GCK* gene. GCK is a key enzyme in glucose metabolism and provides the principal control for insulin secretion. GCK acts as a glucose sensor, and, therefore, an activating mutation of the gene coding for GCK prevents the inhibition of insulin until the serum glucose is below 40 mg/dL, rather than 80 mg/dL. Like mutations of the gene for GDH, this form of PHHI is less severe than the autosomal recessive form of mutations of the K_{ATP} channel.

Overgrowth Syndromes

Maternal diabetes is the most common cause of overgrowth in infants who are large for gestational age. Even in the absence of symptoms or a family history, the birth of an excessively large infant (macrosomia) should lead to the evaluation of maternal (or gestational) diabetes. The pregnant woman who develops hyperglycemia during pregnancy (gestational diabetes) places the newborn at risk for a number of complications. Hyperglycemia in the last trimester increases the risk of macrosomia and hypoglycemia in the newborn infant. Fetal macrosomia (>90th percentile for gestational age or >4,000 g in the term infant) occurs in 15% to 45% of diabetic pregnancies and is most commonly observed as a consequence of maternal hyperglycemia. When macrosomia is present, the infant appears puffy, fat, and, often, hypotonic. The neonate may present with hypoglycemia within the first few hours of life. Although the infant is generally asymptomatic, symptoms may include jitteriness, irritability, apathy, poor feeding, high-pitched or weak cry, hypotonia, or frank seizure activity. Hypoglycemia that requires intervention may persist for as long as 1 week. Hypoglycemia is caused by hyperinsulinemia due to hyperplasia of fetal pancreatic β-cells secondary to maternal hyperglycemia. During fetal life, maternal glucose crosses the placenta, stimulating fetal secretion of insulin and β-cell hyperplasia. Due to inhibition of the continuous supply of glucose after birth, and the inhibitory effect of insulin on gluconeogenesis, glycogenolysis, and lipolysis, the neonate develops hypoglycemia because of insufficient substrate. Fetal insulin release due to maternal hyperglycemia that occurs during labor significantly increases the risk of neonatal hypoglycemia. The overall risk of hypoglycemia for the infant of a mother with gestational hyperglycemia is 25% to 40%. Macrosomic and preterm infants are at the highest risk.

BWS is a congenital overgrowth disorder characterized by an increased risk of cancer and congenital features. The syndrome is characterized by five defining features including: 1) macroglossia, 2) macrosomia, 3) midline abdominal wall defects, 4) ear creases or pits, and 5) neonatal hypoglycemia. Half of the newborns with BWS have hypoglycemia that is due to hyperinsulinism and β-cell hyperplasia. Most have a gene mutation on chromosome 11. The proximity of the mutation to the insulin gene may play a role in the development of hypoglycemia. Most newborns with BWS and hypoglycemia are asymptomatic and usually only have hypoglycemia for the first week of life.

Diagnostic Testing

For infants with congenital hypoglycemia due to hyperinsulinism, and who do not respond to nutrition or medical therapy, an intraarterial calcium infusion study with transhepatic vein sampling may identify a focal or diffuse pattern of excess insulin secretion. In this study, calcium is injected into selected arteries to stimulate insulin release from various parts of the pancreas, which can be measured by sampling blood from their respective veins (see Chapter 19). If the insulin levels are consistently elevated across all veins, then the hyperinsulinism is diffuse. If, on the other hand, insulin levels are significantly elevated in one vein when compared with the others, a focal area of insulin secretion is likely. Positron emission tomography (PET) scanning using the tracer 18-fluoro-dopa (18F DOPA) is an excellent test to differentiate focal from diffuse disease because it enables detection of hyperfunctional islet pancreatic tissue. It, however, is only approved in a few of centers in the world.

Treatment

It is often difficult to determine the exact etiology of neonatal hypoglycemia because some newborns with hypoglycemia normalize their blood glucose levels either without an intervention or, with mild increases in oral feeds. Therefore, treatment of congenital hyperinsulinism should always start with a conservative approach, which begins with increasing delivery of oral feeds and, if necessary, providing IV glucose. Newborns not responding to increased nutrition may benefit from diazoxide or octreotide. Diazoxide improves glucose by activating K_{ATP} channels and counteracting the persistent insulin release. It inhibits insulin secretion by binding to the sulfonylurea receptor (SUR) and preventing closure of the potassium channel. Octreotide, a somatostatin analog, improves glucose by inhibiting insulin secretion from the β-cell. Neonates responding to nutritional and/or medical therapy may possibly discontinue therapy within a few years. Neonates with focal hyperinsulinism should be treated with surgery to remove the affected portion of the pancreas. Alternatively, diffuse hyperplasia may require a subtotal or near-total pancreatic resection.

For the specific causes of PHHI, the autosomal recessive K_{ATP} channel mutations result in a diffuse, severe form of hyperinsulinism. Treatment usually requires a near-total pancreatectomy. For the clonal loss of heterozygosity in which the hyperinsulinism is usually focal, surgical management involves a partial pancreatectomy removing the focal area of insulin secretion. Autosomal dominant mutations of the K_{ATP} *channel* gene, *GDH* gene, and *GCK* gene can usually be managed with diazoxide and/or nutritional therapy.

Hyperinsulinism (Acquired)

The acquired causes of hyperinsulinism occur rarely in neonates or children and are due to insulinomas, nonislet cell insulin-producing tumors, reactive hypoglycemia, and pharmacologic agents and, in individuals with diabetes.

Insulinomas

An insulinoma is a benign or malignant tumor of the pancreas that is derived from β-cells and oversecretes insulin. Because secretion of insulin by an insulinoma is not properly regulated by glucose, the tumor will continue to secrete insulin, resulting in fasting hypoglycemia, regardless of the individual's serum glucose level.

Genetics and Epidemiology

Insulinomas are rare neuroendocrine tumors with an incidence estimated at 2.5 new cases per million persons per year and are one of the most common types of tumor arising from the pancreas. Over 99% of insulinomas originate in the pancreas with rare cases from ectopic pancreatic tissue. Between 5% and 10% are associated with multiple endocrine neoplasia type I (MEN1). More than 90% of insulinomas are small (<2 cm), but those associated with MEN1 are more likely to be large and malignant. Insulinomas associated with MEN1 usually appear around the fourth decade of life, whereas sporadic insulinomas occur in the sixth decade. MEN syndromes are discussed in detail in Chapter 17.

Symptoms

Individuals with an insulinoma commonly develop repeated neuroglycopenic symptoms, particularly with exercise or prolonged fasting. Severe hypoglycemia may result in seizures, coma, and permanent neurologic damage. Symptoms resulting from the catecholaminergic response to hypoglycemia are not as common. Sudden weight gain is usually seen due to the frequent ingestion of glucose.

Diagnostic Testing

In the setting of hypoglycemia, endogenous insulin production is normally suppressed. A 72-hour fast, usually supervised in a hospital setting, can be performed to determine if insulin levels fail to suppress, which is a strong indicator of the presence of an insulin-secreting tumor. Once the blood glucose level drops below 50 mg/dL (2.7 mmol/L) or when the patient develops symptoms of hypoglycemia, a blood sample is collected and measured for serum glucose, insulin, ketones, and C-peptide levels. The fast is stopped at that point, and the hypoglycemia treated with IV glucagon and IV dextrose or calorie-containing food or drink. Elevated insulin levels with a low glucose, elevated C-peptide level, and negative serum ketones indicate an insulin-producing tumor. Within 30 minutes of the administration of IV glucagon, serum glucose should increase by >25 mg/dL because in individuals with hyperinsulinism, glycogen storage is increased. Glucagon stimulates glycogenolysis thereby increasing serum glucose. If biochemical testing indicates an insulin-producing tumor, localization of the tumor may be performed using ultrasound, computed tomography (CT) scan, or magnetic resonance imaging (MRI) techniques. CT detects 70% to 80% of the tumors, MRI detects 85%, and endoscopic pancreatic ultrasounds have a 90% sensitivity rate.

Depending on treatment, if the tumor cannot be localized by imaging studies, an intra-arterial calcium infusion study with transhepatic vein sampling may identify the location of the tumor. Calcium is injected into selected arteries to stimulate insulin release from various parts of the pancreas, which can be measured by sampling blood from their respective veins.

Treatment

The definitive management of an insulinoma is surgical removal. This may involve removing most or part of the pancreas. Medications such as diazoxide and somatostatin can be used to block the release of insulin for patients who are not surgical candidates or who otherwise have inoperable malignant tumors.

Most patients with benign insulinomas are cured with surgery. Persistent or recurrent hypoglycemia after surgery may occur in patients with multiple tumors. Approximately 2% of patients develop DM after pancreatic surgery and removal of an insulinoma.

For insulin-producing carcinomas, streptozotocin, doxorubicin, and fluorouracil are chemotherapeutic options. Tumors that metastasize with intrahepatic growth may require hepatic arterial occlusion or embolization.

Nonislet Cell Tumors

Nonislet cell tumors, such as hepatoblastomas, Wilms tumor, and Hodgkin disease can also cause hypoglycemia. These tumors are large and mesenchymal in origin. They release insulin-like growth factor (IGF)-2 that, when secreted in excessive amounts, stimulates the IGF-1 receptor and cross-activates the insulin receptor, causing hypoglycemia. These tumors are rarely completely resectable. Excision of a portion of the tumor may, however, resolve the hypoglycemia. Unlike in individuals with an islet cell tumor, insulin levels are appropriately suppressed with hypoglycemia. The diagnostic biochemical finding is an elevated IGF-2 level. If an individual with a nonislet cell tumor has hypoglycemia and is unable to undergo surgery or does not respond to surgery, medical therapy with diazoxide, hydrocortisone, or GH may improve blood glucose levels.

Reactive Hypoglycemia

Reactive hypoglycemia is characterized by symptoms of hypoglycemia that occur 2 to 4 hours after a carbohydrate-rich meal. The high carbohydrate intake triggers an excessive insulin release from pancreatic β-cells. Once glucose disposal has occurred, however, insulin levels remain elevated, resulting in hypoglycemia. Although the diagnosis is made after an oral glucose tolerance test, rarely do these individuals have fasting hypoglycemia. Most endocrinologists discredit the existence of this entity or at least express skepticism as to whether reactive hypoglycemia exists. This form of hypoglycemia occurs predominately in adolescent females. Individuals suspected of having this diagnosis should avoid simple carbohydrates. If simple carbohydrates are ingested, protein, fat, and frequent feedings should be implemented. Medical therapy has proven to be of little benefit.

Drug-induced Hypoglycemia

Insulin and sulfonylureas are the most common causes of pharmacologic agent-induced hypoglycemia. Hypoglycemia may occur in individuals with diabetes and in those who receive the medications surreptitiously. Individuals who develop hypoglycemia from exogenous insulin or sulfonylurea therapy have elevated serum levels of insulin. Unlike individuals who develop hypoglycemia from an insulin-producing tumor, those receiving exogenous insulin have negative C-peptide levels, because pharmacologic insulin does not contain the C-peptide. Individuals with hypoglycemia due to sulfonylurea therapy have elevated C-peptide levels and the presence of sulfonylurea in the urine.

Treatment requires correction of the serum glucose with administration of glucose, orally or IV. If the medication was taken without being prescribed, a psychiatric evaluation is necessary to determine the motivation and prevent recurrences.

Diabetes Mellitus

The challenge in caring for the patient with diabetes is balancing ideal glycemic control with minimizing the risk of hyperglycemia and hypoglycemia. The average patient with type 1 DM (T1DM) develops hypoglycemia twice a week and at least one episode of severe hypoglycemia a year. Approximately 3% of patients with T1DM die from hypoglycemia. Patients with type 2 DM (T2DM) have less hypoglycemic episodes early in their course, but, as the illness progresses, hypoglycemia increases in frequency. Of T2DM patients treated with insulin for more than 5 years, 25% experience severe hypoglycemia each year. Overall, insulin-treated T2DM patients have one-third the hypoglycemic episodes of T1DM patients.

The treatment regimen for drug-induced hypoglycemia in diabetic patients has two approaches. Initially, the acute hypoglycemic state should be treated with oral or IV glucose and glucagon. The most important challenge, however, is the prevention of future episodes. Medications should be tailored to the patient's capabilities and needs and should remain flexible. Frequent self-monitoring should be encouraged, especially after a hypoglycemic spell. Patients should also learn to become aware of a potential hypoglycemic episode when their glucose concentration falls below 70 mg/dL (3.9 mmol/L) and to prepare to correct the lowered blood glucose levels.

Disorders in Fatty Acid Oxidation

The human body relies on fatty acid oxidation as an energy source during the fasting state and when under stress. Deficiency in any of the enzymes in the fatty acid pathway will result in the inability to generate ketones as an energy source and, during the fasting state or, when carbohydrate intake is decreased, may result in hypoglycemia.

Medium-Chain Acyl-Coenzyme A Dehydrogenase Deficiency

Medium-chain acyl-CoA dehydrogenase deficiency (MCADD), which normally functions to oxidize medium-chain fatty acids, is the most common enzyme disorder in fatty acid oxidation. It is an inborn error of metabolism, inherited as an autosomal recessive trait. It is a mutation of the *ACADM* gene on chromosome 1p31. One in 15,000 people are affected with this disorder. MCADD most often affects children and presents between ages 3 to 24 months with a peak incidence at 15 months. Caucasian individuals of Northern European or American descent are most commonly affected.

The usual presentation is sleepiness, irritable mood, behavioral changes, and lack of appetite. Because this metabolic crisis may be initiated by an infection, diarrhea, vomiting, and fever may be seen on the initial presentation. If the illness is not treated quickly, it can progress to seizures, breathing problems, and coma. MCADD is a known cause of sudden infant death syndrome in the United States.

The key to the treatment is to avoid fasting periods, insofar as reliance on fatty acid oxidation for energy would be futile in an individual with MCADD. Individuals with MCADD should maintain a diet high in carbohydrates and low in fat. Supplementation with L-carnitine is occasionally recommended to increase energy production.

Carnitine Deficiency

The failure to shuttle fatty acids from the cytosol to the mitochondria for β-oxidation can also result in nonketotic hypoglycemia. The carnitine shuttle is composed of CPT-1 in the outer mitochondrial membrane and CPT-2 in the inner membrane.

Carnitine deficiency is usually the result of an inadequate intake of carnitine in the diet or an enzyme deficiency that impedes carnitine metabolism. Approximately 75% of a person's carnitine supply comes from the diet, mainly from meat, fish, and dairy products. Acquired carnitine deficiency may be due to diets that lack these food groups. Inherited carnitine deficiency is due to a deficiency of the CPT enzyme. The *CPT-1* gene is located on chromosome 1, and the *CPT-2* gene is located on chromosome 11. These deficiencies are inherited in autosomal recessive fashion.

Individuals with CPT-1 deficiency present with metabolic encephalopathy. CPT-2 deficiency is the most common inherited disorder of lipid metabolism affecting the skeletal muscle of adults. It is divided into three subtypes based on tissue-specific symptomatology and age of onset. Symptoms include muscle weakness and stiffness due to muscle fiber necrosis and are commonly provoked by prolonged exercise and periods of starvation.

Treatment is similar to disorders of fatty acid-enzyme deficiency, and patients must avoid fasting and strenuous exercise. The patient's diet is the fundamental treatment focus. Consuming a carnitine-rich diet can help control the disorder, and patients should maintain a constant intake of carbohydrates while keeping fat intake to a minimum. Individuals should also refrain from prolonged periods of exercise.

Jamaican Vomiting Sickness

Jamaican vomiting sickness is an acquired disorder of fatty acid oxidation. It originates from ingesting unripe akee fruit, which produces the toxin hypoglycin. Hypoglycin interferes with fatty acid oxidation by inhibiting medium- and short-chain acyl-CoA dehydrogenase enzymes, resulting in hypoglycemia. Hypoglycemia should be treated immediately and individuals instructed to abstain from eating unripe akee fruit.

KETOTIC HYPOGLYCEMIA

Ketotic hypoglycemia encompasses all other disorders that respond physiologically to hypoglycemia by increasing lipolysis and ketogenesis. These include substrate-limited disorders, maple syrup urine disease (MSUD), hormone deficiencies, glycogen-storage diseases (GSDs), gluconeogenesis disorders, pharmacologic agent-induced disorders, and systemic illness.

Substrate-Limited Disorders

Ketotic hypoglycemia due to limited substrate is a common form of childhood hypoglycemia. This condition usually presents between ages 18 months and 5 years and spontaneously remits by age 9 years. It rarely occurs in adolescents or adults. Hypoglycemic episodes typically occur during periods of illness when food intake is limited. The classic presentation is a child who eats poorly or completely avoids the evening meal, is difficult to arouse the following morning, and seizes or becomes comatose by mid-morning.

The diagnosis is confirmed during a documented episode of hypoglycemia by a serum glucose level that is less than normal (age-dependent) and associated with suppressed serum insulin and alanine levels and elevated serum levels of cortisol, GH, and ketones.

Alanine is the major gluconeogenic amino acid precursor. Its formation and release from muscle during periods of caloric restriction are enhanced by the presence of a glucose-alanine cycle and by *de novo* formation from other substrates, principally branched-chain amino acid catabolism, within the muscle. Therefore, the cause of substrate-limited hypoglycemia may be a defect in any of the complex steps of protein catabolism, including oxidative deamination of amino acids, transamination, alanine synthesis, or alanine efflux from muscle.

Most children with this condition are smaller than age-matched controls and often have a history of neonatal hypoglycemia. Therefore, any decrease in muscle mass may compromise the supply of gluconeogenic substrate at a time when glucose demands are already high and, thereby, predispose to the rapid development of hypoglycemia. The presence of ketones represents an attempt to switch to an alternate fuel supply. The spontaneous remission by age 9 years might be explained by a combination of an increase in muscle bulk with a resultant increase in the supply of endogenous substrate and a relative decrease in glucose requirement with aging.

Treatment consists of frequent feedings of a high-carbohydrate diet, especially during illnesses. If the child is ill or is not adhering to an appropriate carbohydrate-rich diet, testing the urine for ketones may be useful insofar as ketosis usually precedes hypoglycemia by several hours. If the child will not take high-carbohydrate liquids or solids or does not tolerate them, the child should be admitted to the hospital for IV glucose administration.

Maple Syrup Urine Disease (Branched-Chain Ketonuria)

Hypoglycemia may occur in individuals with the autosomal recessive condition of MSUD. This autosomal recessive condition is the result of a deficiency of the branched-chain α-keto acid oxidative decarboxylase enzyme complex, resulting in the accumulation of leucine, isoleucine, and valine in plasma and the urinary excretion of keto acids that impart the characteristic odor of maple syrup. Reports of individuals with MSUD who present with hypoglycemia usually have low insulin concentrations, disregarding the possibility that the elevated leucine level stimulates insulin release in these patients. In addition, the presence of ketones also dispels the possibility of elevated insulin levels. The most likely cause for the hypoglycemia in these individuals is due to the deficiency of alanine and glutamine, primary gluconeogenic amino acid substrates utilized by humans. The elevated branched-chain amino acids are associated with depressions in alanine and glutamine levels. When branched-chain amino acids are corrected by dietary therapy, concentrations of alanine, glutamine, and glucose are normal. This condition affects 1 in 180,000 infants. Manifestations of affected infants include lethargy, vomiting, muscular hypertonia, convulsions, and hypoglycemic episodes, which are due to interference with production of alanine insofar as it is a gluconeogenic substrate. Treatment is dietary to maintain appropriate levels of branched chain amino acids.

Hormone Deficiency

Hypoglycemia may be associated with hormone deficiencies. Cortisol deficiency (due to adrenocorticotropic hormone deficiency) is the most common and may be associated with GH deficiency. Both of these conditions are discussed in more detail in Chapters 2 and 10. Although cortisol deficiency may result in hypoglycemia as a primary disorder, the most common cause of cortisol deficiency in a pediatric patient is hypopituitarism. Other less common hormone abnormalities include deficiencies in glucagon and epinephrine. Individuals who develop hypoglycemia from one of these hormone deficiencies do so because of an inability to increase hepatic glucose production from gluconeogenesis or glycogenolysis. In addition to clinical findings associated with the hormone deficiency, the diagnosis can be made biochemically with a suppressed insulin level at the time of hypoglycemia and an inappropriately low level of the hormone in question. Once the diagnosis is established, exogenous treatment of the deficient hormone should prevent future recurrences.

Glycogen-Storage Diseases

GSD may cause persistent hypoglycemia in the newborn period although it is commonly not recognized until late infancy or childhood. Most infants present with failure to thrive and hepatomegaly. There are five types of GSD that cause hypoglycemia, but type I GSD (i.e., glucose-6-phosphatase deficiency) is the most common. The other four types occur much less commonly and include types III, VI, IX, and 0.

Deficiency of the enzyme that hydrolyzes glucose-6-phosphate to free glucose, the final step in both the glycogenolytic and gluconeogenic pathways, results in severe hypoglycemia in early infancy. In its classic form, children develop hepatomegaly that results in a protuberant abdomen. Metabolic acidosis is common and is caused by marked lactic acidosis and mild ketosis. Affected children display a remarkable tolerance to their hypoglycemia with serum glucose levels in the 20 to 50 mg/dL range. These children usually do not develop the classic symptoms of hypoglycemia, reflecting the adaptation of the CNS to excess lactate. Biochemical testing reveals a low serum glucose, a suppressed insulin level, appropriate elevation of counterregulatory hormone levels, and an elevated lactate level. Enzyme studies on liver tissue, obtained by biopsy, may pinpoint the exact diagnosis. The elevated counterregulatory hormone response is responsible for most of the metabolic abnormalities including: 1) lactic acidosis, due to increase in gluconeogenesis and glycogenolysis; 2) hyperlipidemia, due to increased lipolysis; and 3) hyperuricemia, due to hyperglucagonemia that causes depletion of hepatic ATP and inorganic phosphate. This is a consequence of ATP consumption during glycogenolysis and decreased renal clearance of urate. Treatment involves frequent feedings (i.e., every 2 hours during the day and continuously overnight) of glucose (8 mg/kg/minute) and uncooked cornstarch (every 4 to 6 hours).

Gluconeogenesis Disorders

There are several rare enzyme defects in gluconeogenesis that cause hypoglycemia. The most common enzyme deficiency is fructose 1-phosphate aldolase. Other deficiencies include fructose 1,6-diphosphatase, PEPCK, and pyruvate carboxylase. In fructose 1-phosphate aldolase deficiency, infants and children exposed to dietary fructose present with acute vomiting, abdominal pain, and diarrhea that may progress to hypoglycemia, shock, and liver failure. Immediate treatment with IV glucose may reverse all of the symptoms of hypoglycemia. All fructose-containing foods must be avoided.

The other enzyme defects of gluconeogenesis are less severe, and prevention involves avoiding the fasting state. These conditions should be suspected in individuals with fasting hypoglycemia and the acute onset of symptoms with the ingestion of fructose. Lactic acidosis is usually present. Enzyme studies on liver tissue can confirm the diagnosis.

Pharmacologic Agent-Induced Disorders

Several nonislet cell-activating agents can cause hypoglycemia. Ethanol causes hypoglycemia by inhibiting gluconeogenesis, cortisol secretion, and GH secretion. It also delays the epinephrine response to hypoglycemia. Ethanol inhibits gluconeogenesis because the first step in its metabolism is the oxidation of ethanol to acetaldehyde, catalyzed by alcohol dehydrogenase and requires the coenzyme NAD. Because NAD is a cofactor critical for the entry of most precursors into the gluconeogenic pathway, depletion of it to metabolize ethanol inhibits gluconeogenesis. Salicylates cause hypoglycemia through inhibition of gluconeogenesis and fatty acid oxidation. Although many drugs have been implicated, there is very little quality evidence to support the association between most drugs and hypoglycemia.

Systemic Disorders

Hypoglycemia can also be caused by systemic disorders that result in malnutrition and by hepatic disease that inhibits gluconeogenesis, glycogenolysis, and fatty acid oxidation. Treatment involves IV glucose administration, usually in the form of total parenteral nutrition.

TABLE 6-3.	Nonketotic Hypoglycemia: Biochemical Findings and Treatment				
Condition	**Insulin**	**C-peptide**	**Cortisol**	**GH**	**Treatment**
Hyperinsulinism					
K_{ATP} mutation (AR)	↑	↑	↑	↑	Surgery
K_{ATP} mutation (CLH)	↑	↑	↑	↑	Surgery
K_{ATP} mutation (AD)	↑	↑	↑	↑	Nutrition, diazoxide
GDH mutation	↑	↑	↑	↑	Diazoxide
GK mutation	↑	↑	↑	↑	Diazoxide
Insulinoma	↑	↑	↑	↑	Surgery
Nonislet cell secretion	↓	↓	↑	↑	Surgery
Commercial insulin	↑	↓	↑	↑	Lower the dose in diabetics or discontinue
Sulfonylurea	↑	↑	↑	↑	Lower the dose in diabetics or discontinue
Fatty acid oxidation defect					
MCADD	↓	↓	↑	↑	Avoid periods of prolonged fasting
Carnitine deficiency	↓	↓	↑	↑	Avoid fasting and L-carnitine
CPT-1 deficiency	↓	↓	↑	↑	Avoid fasting
CPT-2 deficiency	↓	↓	↑	↑	Avoid exercise and fasting
Akee fruit	↓	↓	↑	↑	Avoid unripe Akee fruit

Notes: KATP, ATP-dependent potassium channel; AR, autosomal recessive; AD, autosomal dominant; CLH, clonal loss of heterozygosity; GDH, glutamate dehydrogenase; GK, glycerol kinase; MCADD, medium-chain acyl-coenzyme A dehydrogenase deficiency; CPT-1 and -2, carnitine palmitoyltransferases.

TABLE 6-4.	Ketotic Hypoglycemia: Biochemical Findings and Treatment				
Condition	Insulin	C-peptide	Cortisol	GH	Treatment
Substrate limited	↓	↓	↑	↑	Avoid periods of prolonged fasting; Eat frequently
Maple syrup urine Disease	↓	↓	↑	↑	Avoid branched-chain amino acids
Hormone deficiency					
Glucagon	↓	↓	↑	↑	Glucagon replacement[a]
Epinephrine	↓	↓	↑	↑	—
Cortisol	↓	↓	↓	↑	Cortisol replacement
Growth hormone	↓	↓	↑	↓	GH replacement
Glycogen-storage disorder	↓	↓	↑	↑	Avoid fasting and consume corn starch
Disorder of gluconeogenesis	↓	↓	↑	↑	Avoid fasting and consume fructose
Pharmacologic agent	↓	↓	↑	↑	Stop agent
Systemic illness	↓	↓	↑	↑	Improve nutrition

[a]Only replace glucagon if hypoglycemia is due to deficiencies of both glucagon and epinephrine.

CASE FOLLOW-UP

After receiving IV glucose for 30 minutes, our patient's blood glucose level increased to 75 mg/dL. He was able to recognize his mother and responded appropriately to questions. While awaiting results of the other biochemical tests, his mother was questioned further. She stated that her son had never experienced seizures or symptoms of hypoglycemia. She also stated that his appetite had been appropriate and that he had not been ill recently. Our patient was admitted to the hospital for observation. The IV dextrose administration was discontinued after an hour, and he was allowed to eat a regular diet. Blood glucose levels were obtained before meals, at bedtime, and in the middle of the night. All levels remained in the normal range.

Twenty-four hours after admission, our patient appeared well without any signs or symptoms of hypoglycemia. The results from the initial blood sample obtained on presentation were as follows:

Glucose	21 mg/dL
Cortisol	28 mcg/dL (normal = >17 mcg/dL)
GH	18 ng/mL (normal = > 9.9 ng/mL)
Ketones	Negative
Insulin	49 µIU/L (normal = < 5 during hypoglycemia)

(continues)

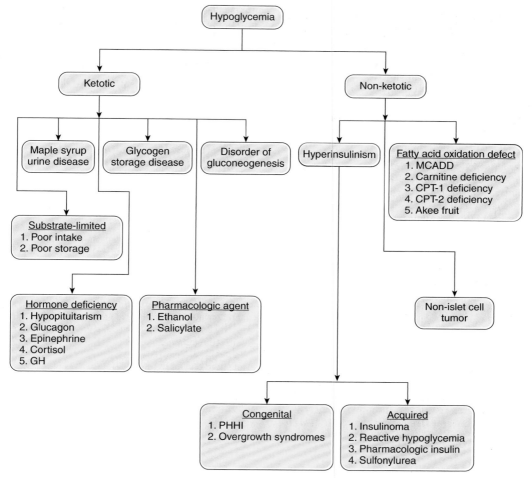

FIGURE 6-2. Algorithm for determining etiology of hypoglycemia.

CASE FOLLOW-UP (*continued*)

The diagnosis in our patient with nonketotic hypoglycemia and an elevated insulin level is limited to endogenous insulin secretion (due to an insulinoma) or exogenous insulin administration (due to injection of insulin). A C-peptide level obtained simultaneously with an elevated insulin level and low glucose level will differentiate between these two conditions.

Because a C-peptide was not obtained and because our patient experienced no problems while in the hospital, a diagnosis of an insulinoma is unlikely.

Throughout the child's stay in the hospital, his mother appeared nervous and expressed a desire to leave as soon as possible. She has diabetes and takes insulin injections daily. After further questioning, his mother admitted to giving him an injection of insulin about 3 hours before he developed the seizure. She used it as a punishment because he had not cleaned his room. Child Protective Services was called to evaluate the situation.

REFERENCES and SUGGESTED READING

Agus MSD, Steil GM, Wyphil D, et al. Tight glycemic control versus standard care after pediatric cardiac surgery. N Engl J Med. 2012;367(13):1208–1219.

Andresen BS, Dobrowolski SF, O'Reilly L, et al. Medium-chain acyl-CoA dehydrogenase (MCAD) mutations identified by MS/MS-based prospective screening of newborns differ from those observed in patients with clinical symptoms: identification and characterization of a new, prevalent mutation that results in mild MCAD deficiency. Am J Hum Genet. 2001;68:1408–1418.

Brent J. Fomepizole for ethylene glycol and methanol poisoning. N Engl J Med. 2009;360(21):2216–2223.

Cryer PE. Glucose counterregulation: the prevention and correction of hypoglycemia in humans. Am J Physiol. 1993;264:E149–E155.

Cryer PE, Axelrod L, Grossman AB, et al. Evaluation and management of adult hypoglycemic disorders: an Endocrine Society clinical practice guideline. J Clin Endocrinol Metab. 2009;94:709–728.

Fodor E, Hellerud, Hulting J, et al. Glycerol kinase deficiency in adult hypoglycemic academia. N Engl J Med. 2004;364:1838–1849.

Gloyn AL, Pearsen ER, Antcliff JF, et al. Activating mutations in the gene encoding the ATP-sensitive potassium-channel subunit Kir6.2 and permanent neonatal diabetes. N Engl J Med. 2011;350:1781–1782.

Guettier JM, Kam A, Chang R, et al. Localization of insulinomas to regions of the pancreas by intra-arterial calcium stimulation: the NIH experience. J Clin Endocrinol Metab. 2009;94:1074–1080.

Hermanides J, Bosman RJ, Vriesendorp TM, et al. Hypoglycemia is associated with intensive care unit mortality. Crit Care Med. 2010;38:1430–1434.

Kauhanen S, Seppänen M, Minn H, et al. Fluorine-18-L-dihydroxyphenylalanine (18F-DOPA) positron emission tomography as a tool to localize an insulinoma or beta-cell hyperplasia in adult patients. J Clin Endocrinol Metab. 2007;92:1237–1244.

Lteif, A. Hypoglycemia in Infants and Children. Endocrinol Metab Clin. 1999;28(3):619–646.

Murad MH, Coto-Yglesias F, Wang AT. Drug-induced hypoglycemia: A systematic review. J Clini Metb Endocrinol. 2009;94:741–745.

Noone TC, Hosey J, Firat Z, Semelka RC. Imaging and localization of islet-cell tumours of the pancreas on CT and MRI. Best Pract Res Clin Endocrinol Metab. 2005;19:195–211.

Rice G, Brazelton T, Maginot K, Srinivasan S, Hollman G, Wolff IA. Medium-chain acyl-CoA dehydrogenase deficiency in a neonate. N Engl J Med. 2007;357(17):1781.

Service, FJ. Hypoglycemic disorders. N Engl J Med. 1995;332(17):1144–1152.

Service, FJ. Classification of hypoglycemic disorders. Endocrinol Metab Clin. 1999;28(3):501–517.

The NICE-SUGAR Study Investigators. Intensive versus conventional glucose control in critically ill patients. N Engl J Med. 2009;360:1283–1297.

The NICE-SUGAR Study Investigators. Hypoglycemia and risk of death in critically ill patients. N Engl J Med. 2012;367(12):1108–1118.

Vaidya A, Kaiser UB, Levy BD, Loscalzo J. Lying low. N Engl J Med. 2011;364(9):871–875.

CHAPTER REVIEW QUESTIONS

1. A 3-year-old girl has a generalized tonic–clonic seizure shortly after awakening in the morning. Her serum glucose was noted to be 22 mg/dL. Which of the following would not be a normal physiologic response?

   A. Elevated cortisol level
   B. Elevated glucagon level
   C. Tachycardia and sweating
   D. Elevated insulin level
   E. Elevated ketones

2. A 65-year-old man is referred to you because of spells of confusion that were relieved by eating. He was well until approximately 6 months ago, when he developed episodes of confusion, occasionally associated with a cold sweat. Drinking a cola usually reduced the symptoms. Most mornings he wakes up confused. Recently, he has had to set his alarm clock to eat at 3:00 a.m. to prevent these episodes. In the past 6 months he gained 25 lbs, and twice he was found comatose by his family. EMTs were called and his blood glucose by fingerstick was low (< 30 mg/dL on both occasions). He is 5 ft 8 in tall, weighs 203 lbs, and has no other remarkable physical findings. At presentation, his laboratory findings are as follows: serum glucose, 52 mg/dL; insulin, 42 IU/mL (normal = 5 to 15 IU/mL); GH, 15 ng/mL (normal = 0 to 10 ng/mL); IGF-1,

39 μM (normal = 10 to 50 μM); and IGF-2, 110 μM (normal = 60 to 120 μM). Which of the following is the most likely diagnosis?

A. Insulinoma
B. Adrenal insufficiency
C. Acromegaly
D. Reactive hypoglycemia
E. Substrate-limited hypoglycemia

3. A 15-month-old female presents with a serum glucose of 23 mg/dL and has MCADD. All of the following statements regarding her condition are true except:

A. Her insulin level is low.
B. She is unable to produce ketones.
C. She is unable to shuttle large-chain fatty acids from cytoplasm to mitochondria.
D. She has fasting hypoglycemia.
E. The most appropriate chronic treatment is prevention (i.e., avoid fasting).

4. A 13-month-old boy is difficult to arouse the morning after his parents had a "blow-out" Fourth of July party at their home. He is a healthy child but over the past 3 days had been running a low grade fever (100.6°F), was congested, and, although he was taking fluids appropriately, had been eating only a small amount of food. In the Emergency Department, his labs are as follows: serum glucose (33 mg/dL), Na (140 mEq/L), K (4.5 mEq/L), Cl (100 mEq/L), CO_2 (21 mEq/L), serum ketones (negative), and insulin (0 IU/mL). Which of the following is the most likely cause of his hypoglycemia?

A. Alcohol consumption
B. Disorder of fatty acid oxidation
C. GSD
D. Hyperinsulinism
E. Adrenal insufficiency

5. A 33-year-old man has a seizure. His blood glucose level immediately following the seizure is 22 mg/dL, and his simultaneously obtained serum ketone level is elevated. Which of the following is the most likely cause of his hypoglycemia?

A. Hyperinsulinism
B. Sulfonylurea ingestion
C. Carnitine deficiency
D. Insulinoma
E. Adrenal insufficiency

CHAPTER REVIEW ANSWERS

1. The correct answer is D. During hypoglycemia, normal physiologic responses include inhibition of insulin secretion, stimulation of counterregulatory hormone secretion, increased hepatic glucose production through gluconeogenesis and glycogenolysis, and increase in ketone production through oxidation of fatty acids. In this scenario of hypoglycemia, the insulin should have been inhibited resulting in low serum insulin level. Hormones, such as cortisol, glucagon, GH, and epinephrine, stimulate gluconeogenesis and glycogenolysis. In addition, during hypoglycemia, other energy-producing mechanisms, such as ketogenesis, should also be increased.

An elevated cortisol level (**Choice A**) should be expected during hypoglycemia insofar as this is a counterregulatory hormone promoting increased glucose production through stimulation of glycogenolysis. An elevated glucagon level (**Choice B**) would also be expected as this counterregulatory hormone increases glucose production through its effects on glycogenolysis and gluconeogenesis. Tachycardia and sweating (**Choice C**) are ANS symptoms that may be due to hypoglycemia and would be expected in this child with hypoglycemia. Elevated ketones (**Choice D**) are the expected normal response due to fatty acid oxidation and ketogenesis that occurs in low-glucose states.

---

2. The correct answer is A. An elevated insulin level with a very low blood glucose level and symptoms of hypoglycemia relieved by fasting are characteristic of an insulinoma.

Individuals with hypoglycemia due to adrenal insufficiency have suppressed insulin levels. (**Choice B**) Acromegaly (**Choice C**) or excess GH secretion results in hyperglycemia rather than hypoglycemia. The insulin level in acromegalic patients may be elevated due to insulin resistance, but the glucose level is normal or elevated, not low. Individuals with reactive hypoglycemia (**Choice D**) usually experience hypoglycemia after a simple carbohydrate-rich meal. Insulin levels may be elevated when hypoglycemia is present, but these individuals do not experience excessive weight gain nor do they have fasting hypoglycemia. Individuals with substrate-limited hypoglycemia (**Choice E**) develop hypoglycemia after prolonged fasting but usually do not develop hypoglycemia shortly after eating. In addition, insulin levels in individuals with substrate-limited hypoglycemia are suppressed.

---

3. The correct answer is C. Individuals with MCADD usually present between ages 3 and 24 months, with the average age of presentation being 15 months. Deficiency of the medium acyl dehydrogenase enzyme prevents the complete oxidation of medium-chain fatty acids. This prevents production of an alternative energy source, such as ketones, during a period of hypoglycemia. These individuals usually present at a young age during periods of limited food intake, especially during an illness. Since large chain acyl dehydrogenase (LCAD) is not affected in this condition, large-chain fatty acids are capable of shuttling between cytoplasm and mitochondria. These individuals have normal carnitine levels and normal function of their CPT-1 and CPT-2 enzymes.

Her insulin level is low (**Choice A**) because she is able to mount an appropriate inhibition of insulin during a period of hypoglycemia. She is unable to generate ketones (**Choice B**) as this enzyme deficiency prevents complete fatty acid oxidation and ultimate generation of ketones. She has fasting hypoglycemia (**Choice C**) because she is unable to develop the alternative energy source from fatty acid oxidation. The only treatment for this condition is to avoid fasting (**Choice E**) and prevent the need for fatty acids as an energy source.

---

4. The correct answer is B. A disorder in fatty acid oxidation causes hypoglycemia when decreased glucose intake occurs, typically in an infant or child. Due to the inability to generate ketones, these individuals are unable to utilize an alternative energy source. During hypoglycemia, the body attempts to increase energy-releasing processes, such as gluconeogenesis, glycogenolysis, lipolysis, ketogenesis, protein catabolism, and amino acid oxidation. Due to the boy's current illness, he has been taking in far less calories over the past 24 hours.

Alcohol consumption (**Choice A**) causes ketotic hypoglycemia directly because ethanol requires nicotinamide adenine dinucleotide (NAD) as a cofactor for its metabolism, and gluconeogenesis is inhibited. It also indirectly causes hypoglycemia by inhibiting cortisol and GH secretion, as well as delaying epinephrine response. A GSD (**Choice C**) causes ketotic hypoglycemia through the inability to completely break down glycogen into glucose. Hyperinsulinism (**Choice D**) causes nonketotic hypoglycemia and individuals have elevated insulin levels. There is usually a history of symptoms and increased glucose intake. Adrenal insufficiency (**Choice E**) causes ketotic hypoglycemia because of cortisol's effect on gluconeogenesis and glycogenolysis.

5. The correct answer is E. Adrenal insufficiency is usually defined by both glucocorticoid (i.e., cortisol) and mineralocorticoid (i.e., aldosterone) deficiency. Ketotic hypoglycemia is unlikely in the presence of insulin excess or a defect in fatty acid oxidation. Hormone deficiencies cause ketotic hypoglycemia. Adrenal insufficiency is the most likely answer since all of the other choices result in nonketotic hypoglycemia.

Hyperinsulinism (**Choice A**) inhibits ketone production. Sulfonylurea ingestion (**Choice B**) increases insulin secretion from the β-cell and inhibits ketone production. Carnitine deficiency (**Choice D**) prevents shuttling of large-chain fatty acids from the cytoplasm to the mitochondria, preventing fatty acid oxidation and inhibiting ketone production. An insulinoma (**Choice E**) would secrete excess insulin and inhibit ketone production.

Type 1 Diabetes Mellitus

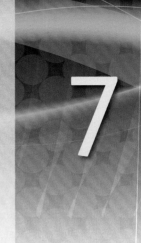

Dane Todd
Guillermo E. Umpierrez

CASE

A 19-year-old female college student was brought to the emergency room after being found unresponsive by her roommate. During the past month, she experienced increasing thirst and having to urinate frequently. The day prior to presentation, the patient complained of feeling hot, having lower back pain, frequently urinating, and vomiting four times. She spent most of the afternoon drinking a lot of liquids. Her vital signs are as follows: temperature 97.5°F, heart rate 120 beats per minute, respiratory rate 32 per minute, and blood pressure 80/60 mmHg in both arms. She is 165 cm tall and weighs 50 kg. On physical examination, she is lethargic but responsive to voice. She answers questions by nodding her head. She has dry mucous membranes and a fruity breath odor. She is taking deep breaths at a labored and rapid pace. Her lungs are clear to auscultation. Her serum glucose level is 545 mg/dL.

This chapter reviews the epidemiology, pathophysiology, clinical presentation, complications, and general treatment of patients with type 1 diabetes mellitus permitting the reader to determine the etiology of this patient's hyperglycemia. We summarize the evaluation and provide a therapeutic plan at the end of the chapter to give the reader a better understanding of the diagnosis. The following chapter focuses on type 2 diabetes mellitus.

OBJECTIVES

1. Describe the autoimmune process and progression of β-cell destruction.

2. Discuss the clinical and laboratory findings in a patient with type 1 diabetes mellitus.

3. List the complications of diabetes mellitus.

CHAPTER OUTLINE

Overview
  Epidemiology
  Pathophysiology
  Genetic Susceptibility
  Autoimmunity
  Environmental Factors
  Clinical Presentation
  Diagnostic Studies
  Management
  Complications
    Acute Complications
    Diabetic Ketoacidosis
    Chronic Complications

OVERVIEW

Type 1 diabetes mellitus (T1D) is a chronic autoimmune disease in which the β-cells of the pancreatic islets are destroyed, resulting in severe insulin deficiency. This **autoimmune destruction** is irreversible and the disease, so far, is incurable. By the time symptoms appear, the β-cell mass (BCM) has almost completely been destroyed. Due to insulin deficiency, patients require exogenous insulin for survival and to prevent long-term complications that can cause substantial disability and shorten lifespan.

Epidemiology

T1D accounts for 5% to 10% of the total cases of diabetes worldwide. It is the most common type of diabetes in youth and accounts for more than 85% of all cases in patients aged less than 20 years. Data from large epidemiologic studies worldwide indicate that the incidence of T1D has been increasing by 2% to 5% with a prevalence of 1 in 300 in the United States by age 18 years. In the United States, it affects more than 150,000 children under age 18 years, and there are 13,000 new cases diagnosed each year. The age of onset of T1D follows a bimodal incidence pattern with the first peak occurring between ages 5 and 7 years and a second occurring between ages 10 and 14 years (Figure 7-1). *puberty* The incidence of T1D in adults is lower than in children, although approximately one-fourth of individuals with T1D are diagnosed as adults. Up to 10% of adults initially diagnosed with type 2 diabetes mellitus (T2D) have antibodies associated with T1D. β-Cell destruction in adults appears to occur at a much slower rate than in children with T1D, often delaying the need for insulin therapy at the time of diagnosis. In contrast to many other autoimmune diseases, in which the number of females affected is far greater than males, T1D affects males and females equally.

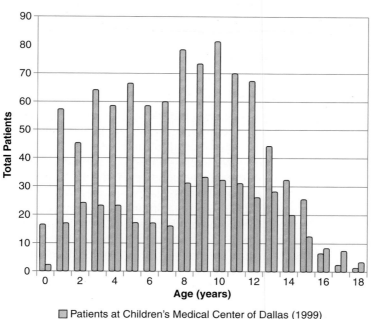

FIGURE 7-1. Histogram of age of onset of type 1 diabetes mellitus in total patients at Children's Medical Center of Dallas (1999) and patients from the Human Biological Data Interchange.

Pathophysiology

T1D is a multifactorial disease caused by a combination of events in genetically susceptible individuals (Figure 7-2). Although the pathophysiology of T1D is not completely understood, it results from three mechanisms that lead to islet cell destruction: genetic susceptibility, autoimmunity, and environmental insult(s). An environmental insult, such as a virus or allergen, in genetically susceptible individuals, induces the production of autoantibodies to β-islet cells. This autoimmune reaction creates **autoreactive T cells** that destroy β-islet cells, and cause a progressive and predictable loss of insulin-secretory function. The serum autoantibodies serve as a marker of the autoimmune disease. The autoantibodies are typically present years before the diagnosis of T1D is made because T1D does not manifest clinically until 80% to 90% of β-islet cells have been destroyed (Figure 7-3).

Genetic Susceptibility

T1D has a multifactorial inheritance pattern that is influenced by genetic and environmental risk factors. Several genes contribute to T1D susceptibility. The genes that have shown the strongest association with T1D include those coding for the major histocompatibility complex (MHC) class II proteins, specifically human leukocyte antigen (HLA) on chromosome 6. Two susceptibility haplotypes in the HLA class II region DR3 (HLA-DR3) and HLA-DR4 are now considered the principal susceptibility markers for T1D and are present in about 90% of patients with T1D. Approximately 40% to 50% of familial clustering in T1D is attributable to allelic variation in the HLA region. The remaining genetic risk is due to a variety of diverse genes, each having a small individual impact on susceptibility. The non-HLA genes that have the most impact on T1D susceptibility are the variable nucleotide tandem repeat (VNTR) region of the *INS* gene and the *cytotoxic T-lymphocyte associated-4* (*CTLA-4*) gene.

Although the majority of T1D cases occur in individuals without a family history of the disease, T1D is influenced by genetic factors. Individuals with a first-degree relative with T1D have a 1 in 20 lifetime risk of developing T1D, compared to a 1 in 300 lifetime risk for the general population. Monozygotic twins have a concordance rate of >60%, whereas dizygotic twins have a concordance rate of only 6% to 10%.

Autoimmunity

The presence of autoantibodies against multiple islet antigens predicts the development of T1D (Table 7-1). Although many individuals are genetically predisposed to the development of T1D, the disease does not occur until there is autoimmune destruction of the β-cells. A number of theories have been proposed to explain the trigger for autoimmunity against the β-islet cells of the pancreas; however, the specific mechanism responsible has yet to be elucidated. Autoantibodies against the islet cell (ICA), insulin (IAA), glutamic acid decarboxylase (GAD65), and insulinoma antigen-2 (IA-2) are the primary markers of the autoimmune process. Autoantibodies appear to develop sequentially. IAA is usually the first expressed autoantibody, especially in young children. Family members who express IAA, GAD65, and ICA-512 have a 75% 5-year risk of T1D compared to a 25% 5-year risk in relatives who express only one of these autoantibodies. These autoantibodies are important markers of disease, but they do not appear to have an etiologic role in the development of T1D. Autoantibodies are present in 70% to 80% of patients newly diagnosed with T1D, as compared to less than 1% of the general population and 3% to 4% of relatives of patients with T1D, respectively. The younger a person is when the autoantibodies are discovered, the more likely they will develop T1D, especially in the presence of multiple autoantibodies.

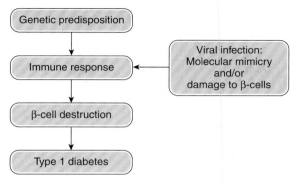

FIGURE 7-2. Theoretical mechanism for the pathophysiology of type 1 diabetes mellitus.

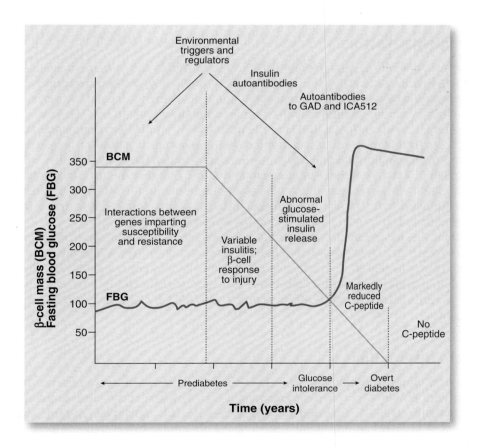

FIGURE 7-3. Progression of β-cell destruction in type 1 diabetes mellitus (T1D). T1D develops from an initial genetic susceptibility to defective recognition of β-cell epitopes and ends with essentially complete β-cell destruction. An environmental event likely triggers the immune attack, and individuals with specific genetic markers (HLA-DR3 and HLA-DR4) are particularly susceptible to the autoimmune disease. Individuals with islet cell antibodies and normal blood glucose levels are in a prediabetes state. The rate of decline in β-cell mass (BCM) determines the length of time between onset of β-cell destruction and eventual hyperglycemia due to loss of >90% of functioning islet cells. (From Rubin R, Strayer DS. Rubin's Pathology: Clinicopathologic Foundations of Medicine. 5th ed. Philadelphia, PA: Lippincott Williams & Wilkins; 2008.)

TABLE 7-1.	Major Autoantibodies in Type 1 Diabetes Mellitus	
Autoantibody	Targeted Against	Percentage of Patients with T1D with Antibody Present at Time of Diagnosis
GAD-65	Glutamic acid decarboxylase	80
ICA	Cytoplasmic proteins in the β-cell	70–90
IAA	Insulin autoantibodies	70
IA-2A	Tyrosine phosphatase	55–75

Environmental Factors

Several environmental factors operate early in life to trigger the immune-mediated process in individuals genetically susceptible to T1D. Studies involving migration patterns and monozygotic twins provide evidence that nongenetic environmental factors, such as nutrition and infectious agents, may play a role in the development of T1D. Cow's milk, breastfeeding, gluten, and vitamin D are the most widely studied environmental factors. Some studies have shown an association between a shortened period of breastfeeding, early exposure to cow's milk, and early introduction of gluten to the infant's diet with the development of T1D. Vitamin D supplementation during infancy, on the other hand, has been associated with a decreased risk of islet autoimmunity in the offspring and reduced risk for childhood T1D. Despite these intriguing associations, there is little firm evidence for the significance of nutritional factors in the etiology of T1D.

Infectious agents and mediators of inflammation, such as prenatal rubella and enteroviral infections, have been proposed to induce β-cell autoimmunity. Widespread vaccination has greatly decreased the incidence of fetal rubella and consequently the presence of T1D due to fetal rubella. Although direct virus-induced β-cell injury is rarely severe enough to cause T1D, the viral infection may cause mild β-cell injury and subsequent antigen release.

Clinical Presentation

The classical clinical presentation of T1D is characterized by an acute onset of hyperglycemia with polyuria, polydypsia, and weight loss. Polyuria is the most common presenting symptom (96%), followed by weight loss (61%) and fatigue (52%). Vaginal candidiasis (females) and occasional blurry vision are among other common symptoms. When the serum glucose concentration exceeds the renal threshold for glucose reabsorption (>180 mg/dL), glycosuria results, and an osmotic diuresis leads to polyuria. Persistent polyuria leads to hypovolemia and results in increased thirst (polydypsia). The combination of polyuria and polydypsia may manifest as nocturia, bedwetting, and increased frequency of wet diapers in infants. Weight loss is due to a loss of calories from excessive glycosuria and impaired glucose uptake into skeletal muscle. This prompts the body to utilize amino acids and adipose tissue for energy. If the diagnosis and treatment are delayed, approximately 30% of patients with newly diagnosed T1D present in a state of diabetic ketoacidosis (DKA).

Diagnostic Studies

An expert committee of the American Diabetes Association (ADA) recommended dividing T1D into two major clinical classes. Type 1 is subdivided into type 1A (immune-mediated) and type 1B (nonimmune-mediated diabetes with severe insulin deficiency). The diagnosis of type 1A diabetes is established if there are clinical and biochemical findings of hyperglycemia in the presence of one or more insulin or islet autoantibodies. Other types of diabetes are categorized as T2D, which results from a progressive insulin secretory defect in association with insulin resistance (see Chapter 8). Gestational diabetes occurs in women who develop diabetes during pregnancy. There are other subtypes of diabetes with clinical and biochemical features of hyperglycemia not due to an autoimmune process or insulin resistance [e.g., genetic defects in β-cell function or insulin action, diseases of the exocrine pancreas (such as cystic fibrosis), and drug- or chemical-induced diabetes (corticosteroids, treatment of AIDS, or after organ transplantation)].

The diagnosis of diabetes can be made using either an oral glucose tolerance test (OGTT) or a **hemoglobin A1C (HbA$_{1C}$)** measurement (Table 7-2). The HbA$_{1C}$ is a form of hemoglobin that is measured to identify the average plasma glucose concentration over prolonged periods of time. It is formed in a nonenzymatic glycation pathway by hemoglobin's exposure to plasma glucose. An individual with normal levels of glucose has a normal amount of glycated hemoglobin. As the average amount of plasma glucose increases, the HbA$_{1C}$ increases in a predictable way. In the usual 120-day lifespan of the red blood cell, glucose molecules react with hemoglobin. Individuals with hyperglycemia, or poorly controlled diabetes, have a high HbA$_{1C}$. In patients with diabetes, higher levels of HbA$_{1C}$ indicate worse control of blood glucose levels, which have been associated with long-term complications of diabetes.

In the OGTT, plasma glucose is measured following an overnight fast (FPG) and 2 hours after a 75-g oral glucose load. A fasting plasma glucose $\geq$126 mg/dL or a 2-hour postglucose load $\geq$200 mg/dL confirms the diagnosis of diabetes. Symptoms of hyperglycemia together with a random plasma glucose $\geq$200 mg/dL are also diagnostic of diabetes. In 2010, the ADA adopted the HbA$_{1c}$ level to diagnose diabetes, with a threshold of $\geq$6.5%. The HbA$_{1C}$ offers several advantages over the FPG and OGTT, including greater convenience, insofar as fasting is not required and there are less day-to-day perturbations during periods of stress and illness. The HbA$_{1C}$, however, can vary with anemia, hemoglobinopathies, abnormal red cell turnover, pregnancy, and recent blood loss or transfusion. In such conditions, the diagnosis of diabetes must employ the glucose criteria during fasting or 2 hours after an OGTT.

TABLE 7-2.   Criteria for the Diagnosis of Diabetes[a]
A1C $\geq$6.5%
FPG $\geq$126 mg/dL (7.0 mmol/L). Fasting is defined as no caloric intake for at least 8 h.
2-h plasma glucose $\geq$200 mg/dL (11.1 mmol/L) during a 75 g OGTT
Plasma glucose $\geq$200 mg/dL in a patient with classic symptoms of hyperglycemia or hyperglycemic crisis.

[a]A test result diagnostic of diabetes should be repeated to rule out laboratory error, unless the diagnosis is clear on clinical grounds, such as a patient with a hyperglycemic crisis or classic symptoms of hyperglycemia and a random plasma glucose $\geq$200 mg/dL.

In general, the majority of individuals with T1D present with acute symptoms of hyperglycemia, i.e., markedly elevated blood glucose levels. Most cases are diagnosed soon after the onset of their illness based on their clinical presentation, severe hyperglycemia with or without ketosis, and the presence of positive autoimmune markers of β-cell destruction. Occasionally, the clinical classification between T1D and T2D is not clear at presentation. About 10% of patients classified as having T2D have at least one of the insulin or islet cell autoantibodies. This group is often referred to as **latent autoimmune diabetes in adults (LADA)** as they share many genetic and immunologic similarities with T1D. There are, however, differences in autoantibody clustering, T-cell reactivity, and genetic predisposition between T1D and LADA, implying important differences in the underlying disease process. Initially, most individuals with LADA are treated with oral antidiabetic agents, but with progressive β-cell destruction they require insulin treatment to maintain glycemic control.

Evidence from T1D prevention studies suggests that the measurement of insulin and islet cell autoantibodies identifies individuals at risk for developing T1D. Such testing may be appropriate in high-risk individuals, including those with prior transient hyperglycemia and who have relatives with T1D, only in the context of clinical research studies. Widespread clinical testing of asymptomatic low-risk individuals is not recommended because it would identify only a few individuals at risk. Individuals who screen positive should be counseled about their risk of developing diabetes. In patients with evidence of autoimmunity, clinical studies are currently being conducted to test various methods of preventing or reversing early T1D.

Management

Glycemic control is the cornerstone of diabetes care and is usually achieved with the administration of multiple daily injections of rapid (or short)-acting insulin with meals (bolus) combined with daily basal insulin. Some patients administer rapid-acting insulin through a continuous subcutaneous insulin infusion (CSII) pump. The goal of therapy is to achieve and maintain good glycemic control (consistent with an HbA_{1c} ≤7%) and prevent long-term complications. Recommended therapy consists of the following:

1. Use of multiple-dose insulin injections
    a. 1 to 2 basal/day,
    b. 3 to 4 prandial/day, or
    c. CSII therapy
2. Matching prandial insulin to
    a. carbohydrate intake,
    b. premeal blood glucose, and
    c. anticipated activity; and, if hypoglycemia is a significant problem
3. Use of basal and rapid-acting insulin analogs is generally preferred to the use of NPH and regular formulations.

A list of the common bolus and basal insulin preparations and their characteristics are shown in Table 7-3.

The use of CSII therapy for youths with T1D has become more widely accepted during the past two decades after rapid-acting insulin analogs were developed. Previously, diabetologists were cautious about pump use in children, particularly as a result of the threefold increase in severe hypoglycemia reported among intensively treated patients in the Diabetes Control and Complications Trial (DCCT) report, as well as the risk of DKA with pump malfunction. With advances in both insulin development and pump features,

TABLE 7-3.	Common Human Insulin Preparations			
Insulin	Onset Time	Time to Peak	Time of Duration	Dosing Schedule
Basal				
Lantus (Glargine)	1–2 h	6 h	18–26 h	Every 24 h
Levemir (Detemir)	1–3 h	8–10 h	18–26 h	Every 12–24 h
NPH	1–3 h	4–9 h	14–20 h	Every 12 h
Bolus (Premeal)[a]				
Humalog (Lispro)	10–20 min	1.5–2.5 h	4–6 h	Before eating[b]
Novolog (Aspart)	10–20 min	1.5–2.5 h	4–6 h	Before eating[b]
Regular	30–45 min	2–4 h	5–7 h	Before eating[b]
Mixtures[c]				
Humulin 70/30[d]	30–45 min	2–4 h	14–20 h	Before eating
Novolin 70/30	30–45 min	2–4 h	14–20 h	Before eating
Humalog 75/25	10–20 min	1.5–2.5 h	14–20 h	Before eating
Novolog 70/30	10–20 min	1.5–2.5 h	14–20 h	Before eating

[a]CSII uses bolus insulin only.
[b]Also used as supplement for elevated blood glucose levels.
[c]Mixtures involve combinations of NPH and Regular (Humulin and Novolin 70/30), NPH and Lispro (Humalog 75/25), and NPH and Aspart (Novolog 70/30).
[d]The first number is the percent NPH and the second number is the percent rapid- or short-acting insulin.

recent studies have shown a small but significant reduction in the frequency of hypoglycemia, ketoacidosis, and lower HbA$_{1C}$ levels in patients using insulin pumps compared to insulin injections.

The rationale for glucose control is supported by prospective and randomized studies in diabetes that correlate both the onset and progression of microvascular complications with the severity of hyperglycemia and HbA$_{1C}$ levels. Self-monitoring of blood glucose is especially important for patients treated with insulin to prevent asymptomatic hypoglycemia and extreme hyperglycemia. HbA$_{1C}$ testing is recommended at least twice a year in patients who are meeting treatment goals and who have stable glycemic control. It should be performed more frequently in those patients who are not meeting glycemic goals or whose therapy has been changed.

Because of the increased frequency of other autoimmune diseases in individuals with T1D, screening for thyroid dysfunction, vitamin B$_{12}$ deficiency, and celiac disease should be performed periodically.

Complications

There are both acute and chronic complications of diabetes. Any patient treated with insulin or a glucose-lowering agent is at risk for either acute or chronic complications. For the patient presenting with DKA, complications may occur as a result of the metabolic derangements and due to the treatment of the metabolic derangements.

Acute Complications

The acute complications are due to the immediate effects of hypoglycemia or hyperglycemia on fluid and electrolyte balance as well as cognition. Dehydration occurs in those unable to maintain sufficient water intake due to the osmotic diuresis that occurs with hyperglycemia. Excessive and prolonged hyperglycemia can lead to DKA. Individuals with diabetes are also at risk for developing hypoglycemia, which may be mild resulting in musculoskeletal weakness, or severe, resulting in seizures. These acute complications can be kept at a minimum with frequent blood glucose monitoring, maintenance of appropriate blood glucose levels, adherence to a balanced lifestyle (diet and exercise), and quarterly follow-up with a diabetes clinician.

Diabetic Ketoacidosis

DKA is characterized by a complex metabolic disturbance of carbohydrate, protein, and lipid metabolism due to lack of or ineffective insulin, with concomitant elevations of the counterregulatory hormones (glucagon, catecholamine, cortisol, and growth hormone). When insulin is deficient, hyperglycemia develops because of increased gluconeogenesis that accelerates conversion of glycogen to glucose (glycogenolysis) and inadequate use of glucose by peripheral tissues (i.e., muscle). From a quantitative standpoint, in DKA, increased hepatic glucose production represents the major pathogenic disturbance responsible for hyperglycemia. During DKA, the levels of counterregulatory hormones are increased and promote pathways that oppose insulin in the liver and peripheral tissues. Both catecholamine and glucagon inhibit insulin-mediated glucose uptake in muscles and stimulate hepatic glucose production through increased glycogenolysis and gluconeogenesis. In the absence of insulin, catecholamine, promotes triglyceride breakdown (lipolysis) to free fatty acids (FFAs) and glycerol. Fatty acids, released by fat cells, are metabolized in the liver, where ketone bodies are produced (ketogenesis). Glucagon has a central role in the pathogenesis of DKA by regulating the capacity for fatty acid oxidation in the liver that also facilitates ketone body formation. The resulting ketosis consists primarily of β-hydroxybutyrate (BOH) and acetoacetate (AA), two strong acids responsible for the acidotic state. A metabolic acidosis develops as bicarbonate is exhausted in the process of buffering the ketone bodies.

DKA is the most common hyperglycemic crisis of T1D. It is a complex disorder of fuel (glucose, fat, and to some extent protein) metabolism. Disordered metabolism is a continuum from normality to severe DKA. The triad of uncontrolled hyperglycemia, metabolic acidosis, and increased total body ketone concentration characterizes DKA. The diagnostic criteria of DKA are:

- Glucose >250 mg/dL (13.9 mmol/L)
- pH <7.30
- Serum bicarbonate <18 mEq/L
- Increased ketone bodies (BOH and AA)

These metabolic derangements result from the combination of absolute or relative insulin deficiency and increased counterregulatory hormone (glucagon, catecholamines, cortisol, and growth hormone) secretion. New onset T1D is a major cause of absolute insulin deficiency, and approximately 25% of patients newly diagnosed with T1D present with DKA. Worldwide, infection is the most common precipitating cause for DKA, occurring in 30% to 50% of cases. Urinary tract infection and pneumonia account for the majority of infections. Relative insulin deficiency, due to increased insulin requirements and elevated counterregulatory hormones, can be caused by the stress of infection, gastrointestinal bleed, myocardial infarction, burns, or trauma. Adolescents present a special problem due to behavioral changes leading to compliance problems and biologic changes leading to increased insulin requirements. Stopping insulin therapy has been described as the major precipitating cause of DKA in adult patients with T1D. In addition, psychiatric problems such as bulimia have also been reported as a significant cause of DKA in young adults.

Because the clinical presentation and management of an individual presenting with DKA clearly demonstrates the pathophysiologic mechanisms, it is discussed here. The diagnostic studies, management, and complications associated with chronic T1D follow.

Hyperglycemia

When insulin is deficient (absolute or relative), hyperglycemia results from increased gluconeogenesis, accelerated glycogenolysis, and impaired glucose utilization by peripheral tissues. Increased gluconeogenesis results from the high availability of gluconeogenic precursors (alanine, lactate, and glycerol) and from increased activity of gluconeogenic enzymes [phosphoenol pyruvate carboxykinase (PEPCK), fructose-1,6-bisphosphatase, and pyruvate carboxylase]. In addition to insulin deficiency, increased counterregulatory hormones play an important role in glucose overproduction in DKA. Elevated glucagon and catecholamine levels lead to increased gluconeogenesis and glycogenolysis. High cortisol levels stimulate protein catabolism and increased circulating amino acid concentration, providing precursors for gluconeogenesis. In addition to increased glucose production, there is impaired glucose uptake in the peripheral tissues due to a low concentration of insulin and elevated levels of counterregulatory hormones.

Ketosis

Insulin is the most important antilipolytic hormone. The association of insulin deficiency and increased concentration of catecholamines, cortisol, and growth hormone causes activation of hormone-sensitive lipase in adipose tissue. This enzyme causes endogenous triglyceride breakdown with subsequent release of large amounts of FFAs into circulation. Elevated FFAs are transported into the hepatic mitochondria where they are oxidized to ketone bodies, a process predominantly stimulated by glucagon. Glucagon lowers the level of malonyl coenzyme A (CoA), the first committed intermediate in the synthesis of long-chain fatty acids, and a potent inhibitor of fatty acid oxidation. Malonyl CoA inhibits carnitine palmitoyltransferase (CPT I), an enzyme that regulates movement of FFAs into the mitochondria. Therefore, reduction in malonyl CoA leads to stimulation of CPT I and effectively increases ketoacid production. In addition to ketoacid production, there is also evidence that decreased clearance of ketoacids also contributes to the development of DKA. The ketone bodies are relatively strong acids and produce metabolic acidosis. The large hydrogen ion load due to the accumulation of ketone bodies rapidly exceeds the buffering capacity leading to a decrease in serum bicarbonate concentration and metabolic acidosis.

Commonly available laboratory tests for "acetone" (nitroprusside reaction) primarily measure acetoacetate. In severe acidosis with altered hepatic redox status, the equilibrium between BOH and AA may lean toward BOH. With treatment and correction of the acidosis, the conversion of BOH to AA may result in an artifactual, or apparent worsening or delayed clearance of "acetone."

Kussmaul Respirations

The respiratory system attempts to compensate for the metabolic acidosis. The acidosis stimulates the central respiratory center and causes "Kussmaul" breathing (deep and rapid breathing pattern), enhancing the loss of carbon dioxide (and water loss as well). This lowers the pCO_2 and results in a loss of bicarbonate. Bicarbonate ions combine with hydronium ions, neutralizing them. The carbonic acid splits into carbon dioxide and water. The carbon dioxide can be lost through the lungs with the increased ventilation stimulated by the acidosis. The combination of acidosis, hypovolemia, and hyperosmolarity alters mental status, and patients may present confused or even comatose.

Manifestations/Consequences

High levels of glucose result in osmotic diuresis, as filtered glucose levels rise and tubular reabsorption of water is impaired because of the high concentration of glucose in the urine. With this diuresis, electrolytes including sodium, potassium, magnesium, calcium, phosphate, and bicarbonate are lost. The hydronium ions are exchanged for intracellular potassium, resulting in intracellular cation shifts with intracellular depletion of potassium, exacerbating total body potassium loss. The diuresis is noticed by the patient as increased urination (polyuria). The water loss leads to some increase in serum osmolarity, resulting in thirst and increased fluid intake (polydipsia). A failure to maintain fluid intake may be caused by anorexia or even nausea and vomiting due to acidosis/ketosis. Failure to maintain fluid intake leads to dehydration and hypovolemia. Severe hypovolemia may lead to tissue hypoperfusion, with tissue anoxia; anaerobic metabolism can lead to lactic acidosis.

Although DKA is treatable and largely preventable, DKA represents the most common cause of death in children and adolescents with T1D. Death may be the direct result of DKA, its treatment (pediatric patients), or a consequence of a comorbid condition such as multiorgan failure or, coronary artery disease combined with hypovolemia resulting in a myocardial infarction. Death may also result from a precipitating infection, trauma, or other illness. Estimates of death rates from DKA are currently under 1%.

Treatment

The therapeutic goals in the management of DKA are to: 1) improve circulatory volume and tissue perfusion, 2) decrease serum glucose, 3) clear serum ketones, and 4) correct electrolyte imbalances. Expansion of extracellular fluid with intravenous (IV) fluids results in the improvement of hyperglycemia, hypertonicity, and metabolic acidosis. These improvements are attributed to a decline in counterregulatory hormone concentration and improvement in renal perfusion, ultimately leading to increased clearance of glucose. Insulin increases peripheral glucose utilization and decreases hepatic glucose production, thereby lowering blood glucose concentration. In addition, insulin inhibits the release of FFA from adipose tissue and decreases ketogenesis, both of which lead to reversal of ketogenesis and ketoacidosis. Replacement of potassium is important because insulin administration results in a shift of potassium from the extracellular to intracellular space. It is uncommon to have to replace bicarbonate, which is generated by normal fuel metabolism. However, with very severe acidosis, certainly with pH values below 7.0, most authorities would not disagree with the administration of bicarbonate-containing fluids.

Unique to children presenting with DKA is the development of cerebral edema during or after DKA therapy. Although a number of mechanisms have been proposed, no single cause has been identified. The most likely mechanisms for the development of cerebral edema in children developing DKA during therapy are osmotic factors and brain ischemia. Clinically apparent cerebral edema occurs in approximately 1% of episodes of DKA in children and is associated with a mortality rate of 40% to 90%. Cerebral edema is responsible for 50% to 60% of diabetes-related deaths in children. Based on a number of retrospective reviews, the risk factors for cerebral edema are as follows:

- Increased serum blood urea nitrogen (BUN) level at presentation
- Severity of the acidosis
- Use of bicarbonate therapy
- Low partial pressure of arterial carbon dioxide at presentation

The management of patients suspected of cerebral edema during treatment for DKA should include:

- Raising the head of the bed to 30 degrees
- Reducing the fluid delivery rate
- Delivering mannitol (0.5 g/kg) or 3% saline (0.5 mL/kg)
- Providing mechanical ventilation
- Intracranial pressure monitoring

Chronic Complications

The chronic complications of diabetes occur when tissues freely permeable to glucose are exposed to chronic hyperglycemia. These complications are characterized as microvascular or macrovascular (Box 7-1). There is a strong association between hyperglycemia and the development and progression of diabetic microvascular complications in both T1D and T2D. In the past decade, large, long-term prospective trials involving treatment and control of hyperglycemia in diabetics have shown that microvascular-related morbidity can be significantly reduced, but not entirely prevented, through long-term glycemic control. The DCCT showed that, compared with conventional therapy, intensive therapy significantly reduced the risk of retinopathy progression and clinical neuropathy. In a long-term follow-up study to the DCCT, the likelihood that a patient would experience a cardiovascular event was also reduced in the intensive treatment group. The intensive therapy prevented one cardiovascular event for every 25 patients treated over a 10-year period in a relatively young group of patients. Intensive insulin therapy is not without risk, however, insofar as severe hypoglycemia with coma or seizure was significantly higher in the intensive therapy group.

Microvascular Complications

In microvascular complications, small arterioles and capillaries are altered by chronic hyperglycemia, leading to retinopathy, nephropathy, and neuropathy. The major pathophysiologic mechanisms underlying these microvascular diabetic complications are the polyol pathway and the diacylglycerol-stimulated protein kinase C (PKC) pathway.

Diabetes is the leading cause of blindness in the developed world. Diabetic eye disease from retinal vascular damage is categorized as follows:

- Nonproliferative retinopathy (microaneurysms and other retinal lesions)
- Proliferative retinopathy (growth of abnormal blood vessels and fibrous tissue from optic nerve head or inner retinal surface)
- Macular edema (fluid leakage from blood vessels that causes macular swelling)

Retinopathy is strongly related to the duration of diabetes and glycemic control. After 20 years, the majority of patients with T1D develop some degree of retinopathy.

BOX 7-1.	Chronic Complications of Diabetes Mellitus	
Microvascular	**Macrovascular**
Retinopathy	Coronary artery disease
Nephropathy	Cerebrovascular disease
Neuropathy	Peripheral artery disease

Randomized trials have demonstrated that lower HbA$_{1C}$ levels reduce the retinopathy risk and slow its progression.

Diabetes represents the leading cause of renal failure and transplantation nationwide insofar as 46% of patients with T1D will develop microalbuminuria, proteinuria, and end-stage renal disease (ESRD). Microalbuminuria, the earliest clinical evidence of diabetic nephropathy, is associated with a 10-fold increase in the risk of progression to overt nephropathy and eventual ESRD. The major pathogenetic factor is glomerular hyperfiltration, likely due to both an increased osmolar load and an intrarenal hypertension that results in basement membrane thickening, mesangial proliferation, and glomerulosclerosis. Angiotensin is central to the development of intrarenal hypertension. Glomerular hypertension can lead to injury to the glomerular basement membrane, causing it to leak plasma proteins into the urine. Attempts by the proximal tubules to reabsorb filtered proteins cause injury to the tubular cells, activate an inflammatory response, and produce oxidative stress. The resultant inflammatory response and renal microvascular injury result in both fibrosis and scarring of both glomerular and tubular elements of the nephron. In addition, glomerular hypertension with a reduction in glomerular filtration rate (GFR) activates growth factors and cytokines. These mediators promote an influx of monocytes and macrophages and activate pathways that result in an expansion of extracellular matrix, fibrosis, and loss of both tubular and glomerular structures. Angiotensin II (Ang-II) plays a pivotal role in the pathologic processes in hypertension that leads to renal glomerular and tubular destruction and renal failure. Acting either through signal-transducing mechanisms or directly on cells to stimulate the production or activation of mediators, Ang-II causes infiltration of inflammatory cells, increases production of mesangial and interstitial matrix, with resultant glomerular and tubular injury and destruction.

Diabetic neuropathy is a heterogeneous complication with many subtypes. The peripheral type that involves the toes, feet, legs, hands, and arms is characterized by numbness or insensitivity to pain and temperature, tingling and burning, extreme sensitivity to touch, loss of balance and coordination, and muscle weakness. The autonomic type may affect the cardiovascular, genitourinary, and digestive systems. It is characterized by postural hypotension and dizziness, lack of heart rate variability, resting tachycardia, and silent myocardial ischemia. Other symptoms of diabetic neuropathy include constipation, diarrhea, difficulty swallowing, decreased sexual response, bladder atony, urinary incontinence, and abnormal sweating.

Chronic hyperglycemia increases flux through the polyol pathway that results in increased accumulation of intracellular sorbitol, a sugar alcohol made from glucose by the aldose reductase enzyme. The aldose reductase enzyme is located in the eye and in the peripheral nerves. Sorbitol accumulation increases extracellular osmotic pressure and causes fluid retention. In the lens of the eye, increased sorbitol is followed by fluid accumulation leading to blurred vision. Vision typically improves with improved glucose; however, the long-term consequences of increased sorbitol in the lens may lead to cell ischemia or death. In the peripheral nerve, axon function is hampered due to damage of the myelin sheath that surrounds the axons. The damaged sheath affects the ability of the axons to conduct electrical impulses. Over time, the loss of function of the axons leads to a length-dependent loss of function or a "stocking glove" pattern of symmetric peripheral polyneuropathy.

Hyperglycemia stimulates de novo formation of diacylglycerol, a known activator of PKC. Activation of a specific isoform, PKC-β, by glucose, stimulates vascular endothelial growth factor, causing leaky vessels and angiogenesis. This pathway has been linked most closely to retinopathy but could also explain albuminuria and neuropathy.

Macrovascular Complications

The central pathologic mechanism in macrovascular disease is the process of atherosclerosis that leads to narrowing of arterial walls throughout the body. The macrovascular complications include coronary artery disease, cerebrovascular disease, and peripheral artery disease. The major pathophysiologic mechanism underlying macrovascular diabetic complications is the advanced glycation end products (AGE) pathway.

Atherosclerosis is thought to result from chronic inflammation and injury to the arterial wall in the peripheral or coronary vascular system. Chronic hyperglycemia may lead to endothelial injury and inflammation, enabling oxidized lipids (from LDL particles) to accumulate in the endothelial wall of arteries. Monocytes then infiltrate the arterial wall and differentiate into macrophages that accumulate oxidized lipids to form foam cells. Once formed, the foam cells stimulate macrophage proliferation and attraction of T-lymphocytes. T-lymphocytes induce smooth muscle proliferation in the arterial walls and collagen accumulation. The net result of this process is the formation of a lipid-rich atherosclerotic lesion with a fibrous cap. A rupture of this lesion can lead to an acute vascular infarction.

In addition to the atheroma formation, increased platelet adhesion and hypercoagulability may also play a role. Impaired nitric oxide generation and increased free radical formation in platelets may promote platelet aggregation. Elevated levels of plasminogen activator type 1 may also impair fibrinolysis. The combination of increased coagulability and impaired fibrinolysis likely contributes to the risk of vascular occlusion and cardiovascular events.

Patients with diabetes (T1D and T2D) develop cardiovascular problems more frequently, at an earlier age, and have a more serious course than individuals without diabetes. All of the major blood vessels are affected, and atherosclerosis also extends to the vessels in the feet. Women with diabetes do not have the protection from the development of coronary heart disease before menopause that women without diabetes do. In individuals with diabetes, thromboembolic stroke is two to three times more likely, peripheral vascular disease is four times more likely, gangrene is 15 times more likely, and amputation is two to four times more likely.

Glycation of macromolecules and its associated AGE develop naturally in tissues with slow turnover by nonenzymatic reaction in proportion to the ambient glucose. When ambient glucose levels are elevated, the number and extent of glycation increases by mass action as sugars become attached to free amino groups on proteins, lipids, and nucleic acids. Large aggregates can form and may no longer be susceptible to the normal clearance mechanisms. Some molecules may be cleared more quickly. AGE receptors on macrophages may stimulate an inflammatory response and are more susceptible to oxidation and result in oxidant damage. Advanced glycation could also explain dysfunction of neurotubules and other neural proteins as well as endothelial dysfunction.

CASE FOLLOW-UP

The young woman in the case presents to the emergency room with new onset diabetes mellitus in DKA. Based on her age and presentation, she likely has T1D. Her respiratory pattern (Kussmaul respirations) and state of poor consciousness suggest that she has metabolic acidosis due to hyperglycemia and excessive ketone production.

Due to her significant dehydration, she is treated with 1 L of intravenous normal saline. At the completion of the bolus, the laboratory studies collected at presentation are available and include the following:

(continues)

CASE FOLLOW-UP (continued)

Venous blood gas

pH: 7.13

pCO_2: 10 mmHg

Total CO_2: 5 mEq/L

Urinalysis

Large glucose and large ketones.

Laboratory studies are remarkable for metabolic acidosis with significant ketosis confirming DKA. She is aggressively treated with IV fluid and insulin. Within 5 hours of treatment, her glucose level drops below 300 mg/dL and dextrose is added to her treatment. She still requires IV insulin therapy because after 5 hours of aggressive treatment, her venous pH is only 7.21, but her pCO_2 (18) and total CO_2 (11 mEq/L) are improved.

By the following morning (14 hours after presentation), her acidosis has resolved, she is awake, alert, and well hydrated. She is switched to subcutaneous insulin injections and is ready for breakfast as well as diabetic education to learn how to monitor her blood glucose levels, take insulin, and manage her diet.

She is started on a four-injection insulin regimen that includes 1 unit of Humalog (Lispro) insulin to be taken at mealtime (breakfast, lunch, and supper) for every 10 grams of carbohydrates she eats. She will also take 25 units of the basal insulin, Lantus (glargine) at bedtime.

REFERENCES and SUGGESTED READINGS

Agus MSD, Steil GM, Wyphil D, et al. Tight glycemic control versus standard care after pediatric cardiac surgery. N Engl J Med. 2012;367(13):1208–1219.

Andresen BS, Dobrowolski SF, O'Reilly L, et al. Medium-chain acyl-CoA dehydrogenase (MCAD) mutations identified by MS/MS-based prospective screening of newborns differ from those observed in patients with clinical symptoms: identification and characterization of a new, prevalent mutation that results in mild MCAD deficiency. Am J Hum Genet. 2001;68:1408–1418.

Brent J. Fomepizole for ethylene glycol and methanol poisoning. N Engl J Med. 2009;360(21):2216–2223.

Cryer PE. Glucose counterregulation: the prevention and correction of hypoglycemia in humans. Am J Physiol. 1993;264:E149–E155.

Cryer PE, Axelrod L, Grossman AB, et al. Evaluation and management of adult hypoglycemic disorders: an Endocrine Society clinical practice guideline. J Clin Endocrinol Metab. 2009;94:709–728.

Fodor E, Hellerud, Hulting J, et al. Glycerol kinase deficiency in adult hypoglycemic academia. N Engl J Med. 2004;364:1838–1849.

Gloyn AL, Pearsen ER, Antcliff JF, et al. Activating mutations in the gene encoding the ATP-sensitive potassium-channel subunit Kir6.2 and permanent neonatal diabetes. N Engl J Med. 2011;350:1781–1782.

Guettier JM, Kam A, Chang R, et al. Localization of insulinomas to regions of the pancreas by intra-arterial calcium stimulation: the NIH experience. J Clin Endocrinol Metab. 2009;94:1074–1080.

Hermanides J, Bosman RJ, Vriesendorp TM, et al. Hypoglycemia is associated with intensive care unit mortality. Crit Care Med. 2010;38:1430–1434.

Kauhanen S, Seppänen M, Minn H, et al. Fluorine-18-L-dihydroxyphenylalanine (18F-DOPA) positron emission tomography as a tool to localize an insulinoma or beta-cell hyperplasia in adult patients. J Clin Endocrinol Metab. 2007;92:1237–1244.

Lteif, A. Hypoglycemia in infants and children. Endocrinol Metab Clin. 1999;28(3):619–646.

Murad MH, Coto-Yglesias F, Wang AT. Drug-induced hypoglycemia: a systematic review. J Clini Metb Endocrinol. 2009;94:741–745.

Noone TC, Hosey J, Firat Z, Semelka RC. Imaging and localization of islet-cell tumours of the pancreas on CT and MRI. Best Pract Res Clin Endocrinol Metab. 2005;19:195–211.

Rice G, Brazelton T, Maginot K, Srinivasan S, Hollman G, Wolff IA. Medium-chain acyl-CoA dehydrogenase deficiency in a neonate. N Engl J Med. 2007;357(17):1781.

Service FJ. Hypoglycemic disorders. N Engl J Med. 1995;332(17):1144–1152.

Service FJ. Classification of hypoglycemic disorders. Endocrinol Metab Clin. 1999;28(3):501–517.

The NICE-SUGAR Study Investigators. Intensive versus conventional glucose control in critically ill patients. N Engl J Med. 2009;360:1283–1297.

The NICE-SUGAR Study Investigators. Hypoglycemia and risk of death in critically ill patients. N Engl J Med. 2012;367(12):1108–1118.

Vaidya A, Kaiser UB, Levy BD, Loscalzo J. Lying low. N Engl J Med. 2011;364(9):871–875.

CHAPTER REVIEW QUESTIONS

1. A 14-year-old boy presents to the emergency room with new-onset diabetes mellitus. With a serum glucose level of 784 mg/dL, dry mucous membranes, and a rapid, breathing pattern he would be expected to have all of the following except:

    A. Recent history of polyuria
    B. Low serum C-peptide level
    C. Low total body potassium
    D. Hypotension
    E. Elevated pCO_2

2. A 16-year-old girl with a 3-year history of T1D forgot to take her insulin last evening and has been ill this morning. She has had three episodes of emesis, polyuria, and abdominal pain. All of the following could be consistent with her presentation except:

    A. Venous pH 7.23
    B. Serum glucose 342 mg/dL
    C. Negative serum BOH
    D. Kussmaul respirations
    E. Glycosuria

3. Which of the following serum antibodies has not been associated with development of autoimmune T1D?

    A. Insulinoma antigen 2 antibody
    B. Islet cell antibody
    C. Insulin autoantibody
    D. Antitopoisomerase antibody
    E. Glutamic acid decarboxylase antibody

4. An 8-year-old boy who was diagnosed with T1D 6 years ago, is on a four-injection insulin regimen consisting of one basal injection at bedtime and three mealtime injections. One evening, he forgets to take his bedtime basal insulin injection and by noon he feels ill, vomits twice, and becomes very dehydrated. In regard to his illness, which of the following would not be expected?

    A. Increased gluconeogenesis
    B. Increased lipolysis
    C. Increased ketosis
    D. Increased glycogen synthesis
    E. Increased amino acid oxidation

5. Which of the following is not a vascular complication of chronic hyperglycemia?

   A. Retinopathy
   B. Nephropathy
   C. Cerebrovascular disease
   D. Hypoglycemia
   E. Neuropathy

CHAPTER REVIEW ANSWERS

1. The correct answer is E. This boy has new-onset diabetes and presents in diabetic ketoacidosis (DKA). The characteristic clinical findings include a history of polyuria and polydipsia. Due to ketone production, these patients may develop a fruity (acetone) odor to their breath and body. Due to the metabolic acidosis, these patients present with hyperglycemia, ketosis, and acidosis. In an effort to improve their pH, they develop a Kussmaul respiratory pattern in which they blow off CO_2 and lower their pCO_2, rather than increase it. These patients are dehydrated, commonly hypotensive, and, because of the massive urine losses and serum acidosis, can develop a very low total body potassium level.

A recent history of polyuria (**Choice A**) would be correct because the hyperglycemia promotes excess urination. A low C-peptide level (**Choice B**) for the degree of hyperglycemia would also be correct. As glucose rises, the islet cell should be producing an excessive amount of insulin. The C-peptide is a marker for endogenous insulin production. In the case of a patient in DKA, insulin production is diminished because the islet cells are unable to produce an appropriate amount of insulin. Low total body potassium (**Choice C**) could be expected due to the acidosis (driving hydrogen into the cell and potassium out of the cell) and massive urinary loss (loss of potassium in the urine). Hypotension (**Choice D**) is correct and is due to the massive fluid losses due to the hyperglycemia.

2. The correct answer is C. This is a question regarding the findings in DKA. Due to the insulin deficiency and poor utilization of glucose, these patients generate ketones through the increase in lipolysis. If she missed an insulin injection and develops the clinical symptoms of polyuria, polydipsia, and vomiting, she could be in DKA.

A venous pH of 7.23 (**Choice A**) is an acidotic pH and consistent with her presentation. A serum glucose of 342 mg/dL (**Choice B**) is also consistent with hyperglycemia. Kussmaul respiration (**Choice D**) is the characteristic rapid and prolonged breathing pattern that patients in DKA develop in an effort to lower their pCO2, compensating for the low bicarbonate level and attempting to improve their pH. Glycosuria (**Choice E**) would also be consistent with her presentation and serum glucose level of 342 mg/dL. In general, most individuals have the presence of glucose in the urine when the blood glucose level is >180 mg/dL.

3. The correct answer is D. With the exception of the antitopoisomerase antibody, all other antibodies have been associated with autoimmune type 1 diabetes mellitus (T1D). The antitopoisomerase antibody is a type of nuclear antibody seen mainly in patients with systemic scleroderma or CREST syndrome. It is rarely seen in patients with autoimmune diabetes.

The insulinoma antigen 2 antibody (**Choice A**), islet cell antibody (**Choice B**), insulin autoantibody (**Choice C**), and glutamic acid decarboxylase antibody (**Choice E**) are all associated with T1D.

4. The correct answer is D. Glycogen synthesis involves the storage of glucose as glycogen. This process would occur in the fed state, or in the presence of insulin. It is considered an energy-storing process rather than an energy-releasing process. This boy has an insulin deficiency. All of the processes that oppose insulin should be in place because his body senses that he has poor glucose utilization and needs to generate glucose or release energy. With insulin deficiency, processes that oppose insulin increase his extracellular glucose, worsening his problem of hyperglycemia. During insulin deficiency, the body attempts to increase energy-releasing processes such as gluconeogenesis, glycogenolysis, lipolysis, ketogenesis, protein catabolism, and amino acid oxidation.

Increased gluconeogenesis (**Choice A**) would occur in this scenario because the body senses a state of starvation and a need for energy. An increase in gluconeogenesis promotes increased glucose production and increased release of energy. Increased lipolysis (**Choice B**) would also occur in this scenario because generation of fatty acids is an alternative energy source. Increased ketosis (**Choice D**) would occur because ketone products are the result of lipolysis. Increased amino acid oxidation (**Choice E**) would also occur in this scenario because oxidation of amino acids promotes release of energy.

5. The correct answer is D. Hypoglycemia is an acute complication for the management of diabetes. It is not a vascular complication of diabetes but rather a complication related to the combination of exogenous insulin therapy, carbohydrate intake, and exercise.

Retinopathy (**Choice A**) is a microvascular complication of diabetes. Nephropathy (**Choice B**) is also a microvascular complication of diabetes. Cerebrovascular disease (**Choice D**) is a macrovascular complication of diabetes. Neuropathy (**Choice E**) is also a microvascular complication of diabetes.

Type 2 Diabetes Mellitus

8

Evan T. Tiderington
Guillermo E. Umpierrez

CASE

A 37-year-old man is seen in the primary care clinic complaining of increased urinary frequency and thirst for the past month. He has had to get up twice each night for the past 2 years, but, in the past month, he has gotten up more than four times and has to leave his job to use the restroom at least four times during the day. He also reports that he drinks several glasses of liquid during the day because his mouth is dry. Other than claiming that he needs to lose weight, he states that he is healthy and is not taking any medications. His family history is remarkable for obesity—both his parents and his two brothers are extremely overweight. One of his brothers and both his parents were diagnosed with diabetes as young adults. His mother is currently taking medications for her diabetes and high blood pressure. His father died at the age of 48 from a heart attack, and he had high cholesterol and diabetes. The patient's vital signs include temperature, 98.6°F; pulse rate, 105 beats per minute; respiration rate, 14 breaths per minute; and blood pressure, 147/89 mmHg in both arms. On physical examination, he is obese (weight, 124 kg; body mass index, 35 kg/m^2) and has a dark, leathery area of skin over his axilla and abdomen.

A routine chemistry profile is significant for an elevated serum glucose level (380 mg/dL), a low serum sodium level (132 mEq/L), and an elevated HbA$_{1c}$ level (9.0%). All other biochemical parameters are normal. A urinalysis is positive for glucose and protein, and negative for ketones.

This chapter reviews the epidemiology, pathophysiology, clinical presentation, and general treatment of patients with type 2 diabetes mellitus to help the learner understand the mechanisms and treatment for this patient's hyperglycemia. We summarize the evaluation and therapeutic plan at the end of the chapter.

OBJECTIVES

1. Describe the pathogenesis of type 2 diabetes mellitus.

2. Discuss the clinical and laboratory findings in a patient with type 2 diabetes mellitus.

CHAPTER OUTLINE

Overview
  Epidemiology
  Pathophysiology
    β-Cell Dysfunction
    Mechanisms for β-Cell Failure
    Insulin Resistance
  Clinical Presentation
  Diagnostic Studies
  Management
    Metabolic Control
    Education
    Medical Nutrition Therapy
    Physical Activity
    Pharmacologic Management

(continues)

(continued)

OBJECTIVES

3. List the therapeutic options available for a patient with type 2 diabetes mellitus.

4. List the criteria for the metabolic syndrome.

OVERVIEW

Type 2 diabetes mellitus (T2D) is a heterogeneous disorder characterized by a defect in insulin secretion and increased cellular resistance to insulin action. It results in hyperglycemia and several other metabolic disturbances. The insulin deficiency is progressive and usually takes several years to progress from normal glucose tolerance to T2D. It involves intermediate stages of impaired fasting glucose (IFG) and impaired glucose tolerance (IGT), also known as **prediabetes** (Figure 8-1).

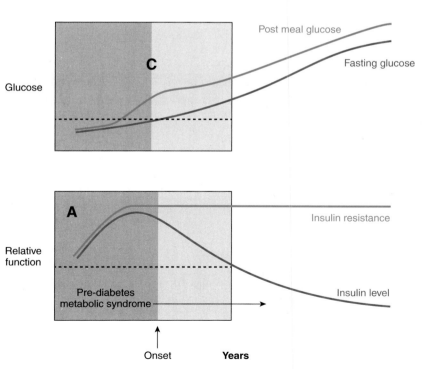

FIGURE 8-1. Fasting and postprandial glucose levels. Individuals with blood glucose levels from 140 to 199 mg/dL 2 hours after a standard amount of glucose have impaired glucose tolerance. (From McConnell TH. The Nature of Disease Pathology for the Health Professions. Philadelphia, PA: Lippincott Williams & Wilkins; 2007.)

Epidemiology

The prevalence of T2D has reached epidemic proportions in the United States and worldwide. Based on the 2010 CDC National Diabetes Database, there are 25.8 million people (8.3% of the U.S. population) with diabetes, of whom ~95% have T2D. Of those 25.8 million with diabetes, only 18.8 million have been diagnosed, leaving 7.0 million undiagnosed. Based on U.S. mortality reports, diabetes is the seventh leading cause of death. It is more common in women, especially in women with a history of gestational diabetes. Its prevalence increases after the age of 40 and is higher in all ethnic minority subgroups compared to Caucasians. It is estimated that African Americans and Hispanic Americans are twice as likely to have T2D compared to non-Hispanic Caucasians. Most patients with T2D are obese or may show an increased percentage of body fat distributed predominantly in the abdominal region. The risk factors for T2D are listed in Box 8-1.

Diabetes is the leading cause of kidney failure, adult blindness, and nontraumatic lower-limb amputations in the United States. It is also a significant cause of cardiovascular morbidity and mortality. In patients with T2D, the prevalence of heart attacks and strokes is two to four times more frequent than in nondiabetic individuals. Cardiovascular manifestations include coronary artery disease (e.g., heart attacks, angina), peripheral artery disease (e.g., leg claudication, gangrene), and carotid artery disease (e.g., strokes, dementia). Many patients with T2D have the same risk for a cardiovascular event as do nondiabetic patients who have had at least one myocardial infarction (MI). Patients with diabetes who have had a previous cardiovascular event are at 10 times the risk for a subsequent event as compared to the nondiabetic population. Management of cardiovascular risk factors plays a significant role in the care of patients with T2D.

BOX 8-1.   **Population at Risk for Type 2 Diabetes Mellitus**

Family history of diabetes
Obesity (particularly upper-body adiposity)
   Body mass index (BMI) $\geq$27 or $\geq$120% ideal body weight
Ethnic groups
   African Americans
   Hispanics
   Native Americans
   Asian Americans
Age $\geq$45 years
Previously identified impaired glucose tolerance (IGT) or impaired fasting glucose (IFG)
Hypertension ($\geq$140/90 mmHg)
Lipid abnormalities
   High-density lipoprotein (HDL) cholesterol <35 mg/dL
   Triglyceride $\geq$250 mg/dL
Women with gestational diabetes or history of having a neonate weighing >9 lb

Pathophysiology

T2D is a heterogeneous disorder, characterized by defects in insulin secretion and insulin sensitivity. Insulin resistance by itself will not result in T2D unless β-cell secretion of insulin is decreased. T2D has a progressive nature, preceded by a period of insulin resistance and IGT, or prediabetes. Endogenous insulin secretion in IGT may be increased in order to maintain the fasting blood glucose level in the normal range; however, during this time, the postprandial blood glucose is elevated because endogenous insulin secretion is decreased and ultimately leads to T2D. The conversion from IGT to T2D may take from 8 to 12 years unless there are lifestyle modifications or other therapies that may reduce this risk.

The development and rate of progression of T2D are influenced by both genetic and environmental factors, such as obesity and physical inactivity. The heritability of T2D is high (estimated at >50%), as indicated by the high concordance rates in monozygotic twins and the notably raised risk in individuals with affected first-degree relatives. Genome-wide association studies have helped to raise the number of confirmed diabetes-associated loci to more than 40. A greater number of these loci are associated with impaired β-cell function (*KCNJ11, TCF7L2, WFS1, HNF1B, SLC30A8, CDKAL1, IGF2BP2, CDKN2A, CDKN2B, NOTCH2, CAMK1D, THADA, KCNQ1, MTNR1B, GCKR, GCK, PROX1, SLC2A2, G6PC2, GLIS3, ADRA2A,* and *GIPR*) than with impaired insulin sensitivity (*PPAR-γ, IRS1, IGF1, FTO,* and *KLF14*) or obesity (*FTO*). Of these, *TCF7L2* carries the strongest susceptibility for T2D, insofar as it is associated with β-cell dysfunction. Only ~10% of the heritability of T2D can be explained by susceptibility loci that have been identified so far. The remaining heritability might be related to a large number of less common variants that are difficult to find with current approaches of genome-wide association studies, and/or epigenetic phenomena.

This chapter will focus on the patients with T2D whose β-cells are unable to overcome insulin resistance. This accounts for more than 90% of the causes of T2D. The other causes of T2D include: 1) mutations of the insulin receptor gene, 2) antibody destruction of the insulin receptor, and 3) maturity-onset diabetes of youth (**MODY**).

β-Cell Dysfunction

T2D is a progressive disease that develops slowly due to a continued decline in β-cell function. It is well accepted that for hyperglycemia to exist in T2D, β-cell dysfunction must be present. State-of-the-art diagnostic studies of insulin secretion, such as the hyperglycemic clamp, have been utilized to determine that β-cell dysfunction manifests in a number of different ways including: 1) reductions in insulin release in response to glucose and nonglucose secretagogues; 2) changes in pulsatile and oscillatory insulin secretion; 3) an abnormality in the efficiency of proinsulin to insulin conversion; and 4) reduced release of islet amyloid polypeptide (IAPP), also known as *amylin*. In addition to defective insulin secretion and action, patients with T2D also exhibit nonsuppressible glucagon secretion after a meal, resulting in increased hepatic glucose production.

Patients with T2D have impaired first- and second-phase insulin secretion. In the normal state, following intravenous (IV) glucose administration, the first-phase response peaks within 2 to 5 minutes and lasts for approximately 10 minutes (Figure 8-2). This response likely represents the release of a pool of secretory granules that is present in close proximity to the β-cell plasma membrane.

The second-phase response begins shortly after glucose administration and is more prolonged. It is maintained for the period that the glucose level is elevated. This second-phase response is believed to represent the release of secretory granules that are being mobilized within the β cell for release. It also includes many granules that contain newly synthesized insulin.

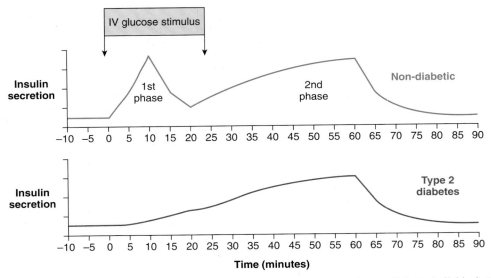

FIGURE 8-2. Biphasic insulin response to a constant glucose stimulus. In the nondiabetic individual, the peak of the first phase of insulin release occurs 2 to 5 minutes after glucose infusion; the second phase begins during the first phase and continues to increase slowly for at least 60 minutes. In the diabetic individual, both first- and second-phase responses are blunted.

For patients with T2D, both the responses are diminished. The lack of a first-phase response is an early defect and is present in all individuals with hyperglycemia. The second-phase response may appear normal at the onset in patients with T2D; however, this apparently normal response occurs at the expense of hyperglycemia. When subjects are matched for the degree of glucose elevation, it is clear that the second-phase insulin response is also reduced in patients with T2D.

Mechanisms for β-Cell Failure

The exact mechanism for the development and progression of β-cell dysfunction in T2D is not completely understood. Two hypotheses that have been proposed are as follows: 1) β-cell exhaustion due to the increased secretory demand arising from insulin resistance and 2) desensitization of the β-cell due to hyperglycemia, hyperlipidemia, and reduction in β-cell mass. The reduction in β-cell mass may also be due to amyloid deposition.

Amylin (IAPP) is a peptide hormone that is cosecreted with insulin from the β-cells. Amylin plays a role in glycemic regulation by slowing gastric emptying and promoting satiety, thereby preventing postprandial spikes in blood glucose levels. Patients with T2D are usually insulin resistant and have a greater demand for insulin production, resulting in the secretion of proinsulin and proIAPP. The enzymes that convert these precursor molecules into insulin and IAPP, respectively, however, are unable to keep up with the high levels of secretion, ultimately leading to the accumulation of proIAPP. The unprocessed proIAPP can cause IAPP to accumulate and form amyloid. The amyloid formation might be a major mediator of apoptosis in the β-cells.

Insulin resistance increases the secretory function of the β-cell. This increase in the need for insulin biosynthesis and release has led to the hypothesis that over an extended period of time, the increasing demand associated with increasing resistance will result in exhaustion of the β-cell. This exhaustion will ultimately lead to β-cell failure. Although this hypothesis is attractive, less than half of obese subjects who are insulin resistant experience β-cell failure or diabetes. Increasing evidence suggests that the failure to adequately adapt to insulin resistance may be due to a genetically programmed β-cell abnormality associated with an inability of the normal β-cell to adapt to insulin resistance and the increased secretory demand. This eventually leads to insulinopenia and hyperglycemia.

Once established, hyperglycemia has itself been shown to impair insulin secretion. Although glucose is the most potent stimulus for insulin secretion, sustained hyperglycemia affects β-cell function in a deleterious manner. This effect is known as **glucose toxicity**. In vitro and in vivo studies have confirmed that exposure to increased glucose concentrations results in dose–response reductions in insulin secretion. The increased glucose levels have been associated with a reduction in the expression of the insulin (*INS*) and *PDX-1* genes. The *PDX-1* gene is responsible for regulation of β-cell replication.

Increased dietary fat intake and/or altered fat metabolism have also been shown to have negative effects on β-cell function, a condition referred to as **lipotoxicity**. Exposure to high-fat diets is associated with reductions in insulin release in both in vitro and in vivo studies. Free fatty acids, which are critical for maintenance of β-cell function, and other factors secreted by adipose tissue such as leptin, tumor necrosis factor-α (TNF-α), resistin, and adiponectin may also have an adverse effect on insulin secretion and action.

Insulin Resistance

Insulin resistance is defined as a steady-state plasma glucose level that is higher than expected for the prevailing plasma insulin concentration. Insulin resistance is present in most patients with T2D. The term "insulin resistance" is often incorrectly used synonymously with the term "impaired insulin-stimulated glucose disposal." Insulin resistance occurs early even before the appearance of the hyperglycemia of T2D. First-degree relatives of patients with T2D are prone to having impaired insulin stimulation of muscle glycogen synthesis and suppression of lipolysis. Increased lipolysis leads to excessive production of free fatty acids and overexpression of TNF-α by adipocytes, which are important mechanisms for the development of insulin resistance in peripheral tissues and liver, as well as altered β-cell function as previously discussed.

Skeletal muscle, which makes up to 40% of the body mass of humans, is the primary tissue responsible for the peripheral disposal of glucose in response to a glucose or insulin challenge. Glucose transport into the myocyte is acutely regulated by insulin and insulin-like factors through the activation of a series of intracellular proteins. Insulin binding to the α-subunit of the insulin receptor causes an enhancement of the tyrosine kinase activity of the intracellular β-subunits. This leads to autophosphorylation of the insulin receptor and to tyrosine phosphorylation of insulin receptor substrate-1 (IRS-1). The tyrosine-phosphorylated IRS-1 molecule can then dock with the p85 regulatory subunit of phosphatidylinositol 3-kinase (PI3-kinase) that, in turn, activates the p110 catalytic subunit of this enzyme. The PI3-kinase catalyzes the production of phosphoinositide moieties, which can subsequently activate 3-phosphoinositide-dependent kinases (PDKs), including PDK1. A downstream target of PDK1 is Akt/protein kinase B (Akt/PKB), a serine/threonine kinase. The activation of these steps ultimately results in the translocation of a regulatable glucose transporter protein (GLUT-4) to the sarcolemmal membrane and the T tubules, where glucose transport takes place via a facilitative diffusion process. GLUT-4 is the only one of several isoforms in a family of facilitative glucose transporter proteins. Available evidence supports the idea that it is the magnitude of GLUT-4 translocation that dictates the capacity of a skeletal muscle to enhance glucose transport activity.

Insulin resistance in T2D is usually not associated with a decreased skeletal muscle level of the GLUT-4 protein. In patients with T2D, however, insulin stimulation fails to induce normal GLUT-4 protein translocation to the sarcolemma in skeletal muscle. Insulin-stimulated Akt/PKB kinase activity is significantly reduced in skeletal muscle from patients with insulin-resistant T2D. Apart from genetic predisposition, acquired factors that cause insulin resistance are obesity and physical inactivity. Excessive production of free fatty acids and overexpression of TNF-α by adipocytes have been proposed as mechanisms for the development of insulin resistance.

Clinical Presentation

The diagnosis of T2D is likely if an individual presents with the classic symptoms of hyperglycemia: polyuria, polydipsia, and polyphagia. Other symptoms that suggest hyperglycemia are blurred vision, lower extremity paresthesias, vaginal yeast infections (women), and acanthosis nigricans (Figure 8-3). Many patients with T2D are, however, asymptomatic, and they remain undiagnosed for years. The average patient diagnosed with T2D is likely to have had the disease for 4 to 7 years as suggested by the presence of chronic complications of retinopathy (25%), neuropathy (9%), and nephropathy (8%) at the time of diagnosis.

When the serum glucose concentration exceeds the renal threshold for glucose reabsorption (~180 mg/dL), glycosuria results, and an osmotic diuresis occurs that is manifested as polyuria. Persistent polyuria leads to hypovolemia that causes increased thirst (polydipsia). The combination of polyuria and polydipsia may actually present as nocturia.

The prevalence of T2D increases with age with one in four adults over the age of 40 having diabetes in the United States, but it should be noted that the epidemic of diabetes affects all ages. Prior to the mid-1990s, >95% of children and adolescents presenting with new onset diabetes mellitus had T1D. Over the past 15 years, however, due to the surge in obesity, up to 33% of adolescent diabetes is due to T2D.

Diagnostic Studies

There are four accepted ways to diagnose diabetes in nonpregnant adults (Box 8-2). The first two methods consist of having either a fasting plasma glucose level equal to or greater than 126 mg/dL (7 mmol/L) on two separate occasions or a random plasma glucose level greater than 200 mg/dL (11.1 mmol/L) in a subject who has symptoms of hyperglycemia (polyuria, polydipsia, or unexplained weight loss). The other method for diagnosis is to perform an oral glucose tolerance test (OGTT) in which 75 g of glucose is given by mouth and a 2-hour postprandial plasma glucose level is above 199 mg/dL. In 2010, the American Diabetes Association (ADA) recommended the use of the hemoglobin A1C (HbA$_{1C}$) test to diagnose diabetes, with a diagnostic level ≥6.5%. Recent data from

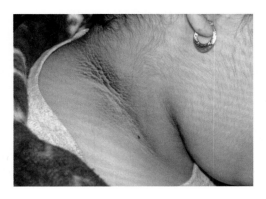

FIGURE 8-3. Acanthosis nigricans. The linear, alternating dark and light pigmentation of acanthosis nigricans becomes more apparent when the skin is stretched in this woman with type 2 diabetes (T2D). (From Goodheart HP. Goodheart's Photoguide of Common Skin Disorders, 2nd ed. Philadelphia, PA: Lippincott Williams & Wilkins; 2003.)

BOX 8-2. | Criteria for the Diagnosis of Diabetes and Prediabetes

Diabetes Mellitus

1. $HbA_{1c} \geq 6.5\%$.
2. Fasting plasma glucose (FPG) $\geq$126 mg/dL (7.0 mmol/L) on two separate occasions. Fasting is defined as no caloric intake for at least 8 hours.
3. Random BG $\geq$200 mg/dL (11.1 mmol/L) with symptoms of diabetes (polyuria, polydipsia, and unexplained weight loss). Random is defined as any time of day without regard to time since last meal.
4. 2-Hour postprandial PG $\geq$200 mg/dL (11.1 mmol/L) during an oral glucose tolerance test (OGTT). The test should be performed as described by World Health Organization using a glucose containing equivalent of 75 g anhydrous glucose in water.

Categories of Increased Risk for Diabetes (Prediabetes)

1. HbA_{1c} between 5.7% and <6.5%.
2. Impaired fasting glucose (IFG): FPG $\geq$110 mg/dL but <125 mg/dL (5.6 mmol/L).
3. Impaired glucose tolerance (IGT): 2-hour glucose $\geq$140 mg/dL (7.8 mmol/L) but <200 mg/dl (11.1 mmol/L) after a 75-g OGTT.

---

the Third National Health and Nutrition Examination Survey (NHANES III) reported a specificity of 97.4% and 99.9% for an HbA_{1c} value of 6.1% and 7% (1 and 2 standard deviations above the normal mean, respectively). The HbA_{1c} is a form of hemoglobin that is measured to identify the average plasma glucose concentration over prolonged periods of time. It is formed in a nonenzymatic glycation pathway by hemoglobin's exposure to plasma glucose. Because HbA_{1c} testing can be performed at any time of the day and without special patient preparation, it represents a convenient and highly specific method for screening and diagnosis of diabetes.

The Expert Committee recognized an intermediate group with impaired glucose homeostasis whose glucose concentration is above the normal level but below the level established for the diagnosis of diabetes. A normal fasting plasma glucose level is 100 mg/dL, and a normal 2-hour postprandial glucose level is less than 140 mg/dL. Individuals with fasting plasma glucose levels between 110 and 126 mg/dL have IFG, and those with 2-hour values after the OGTT of >140 mg/dL but <200 mg/dL have IGT. In 2010, the ADA also recommended the use of HbA_{1c} to identify people at increased risk for diabetes and proposed an HbA_{1c} range of 5.7% to 6.4%, a state that may be referred to as **prediabetes**. As with glucose measurements, the continuum of risk is curvilinear, so that as HbA_{1c} rises, the risk of diabetes rises disproportionately.

Management

Because the consequences of chronic hyperglycemia can be life-threatening, treatment of patients with T2D requires a commitment to five management principles: 1) metabolic control, 2) education, 3) nutrition, 4) physical activity, and 5) pharmacologic agents.

Metabolic Control

The rationale for glucose control is supported by prospective and randomized studies in T2D that correlate the onset and progression of microvascular complications with the severity of hyperglycemia and HbA_{1c} levels. Self-monitoring of blood glucose and measurement of $HgbA_{1c}$ has commonly been used to monitor glycemic status in patients with diabetes mellitus. A fasting and premeal glucose level between 70 and 130 mg/dL and an HbA_{1c} below or around 7% are standard goals. A more stringent glucose level or HbA_{1c} goal may be indicated for selected individual patients, as long as it can be achieved without significant hypoglycemia or other adverse effects of treatment. Patients who are appropriate candidates for intensive control include those with short duration of diabetes, long-life expectancy, and absence of significant cardiovascular disease. In addition, less-stringent HbA_{1c} goals (between 7% and 8%) are appropriate for patients with a history of severe hypoglycemia, limited life expectancy, advanced microvascular or macrovascular complications, and extensive comorbid conditions. The frequency of HbA_{1c} testing is recommended to be at least twice a year for patients who meet treatment goals and who have stable glycemic control, but it should be performed three to four times a year in patients who do not meet glycemic goals or whose therapy has been changed.

Education

Education of patients with either prediabetes or diabetes should include the following content areas: disease process, treatment options, nutritional plan, exercise plan, knowledge of diabetes medication prescribed, blood glucose monitoring, knowledge of acute and chronic complications, psychosocial issues, and individual strategies to promote health. Patients must be educated about diabetes and have a clear understanding of how to take medications and record their blood glucose. They must be instructed in what action to take during emergencies and sick days. Metabolic goals should also be discussed and emphasized.

Medical Nutrition Therapy

Medical nutrition therapy should focus on calculation of the kilocalorie requirement by multiplying the ideal body weight by 10, plus 30% to 100% added for physical activity. The diet should include 50% to 55% carbohydrate, 30% fat (of which no more than 10% should be saturated fatty acid), and 15% to 20% protein as macronutrient component of the diet, as well as fiber. It is important to remember that both the portion control in the management of diet and daily exercise play very important roles in maintaining ideal body weight.

Physical Activity

Physical activity education is of great importance as sedentary lifestyle is a powerful but modifiable risk factor for T2D. Moderate exercise is of utmost benefit in patients at risk for or who currently have T2D. Two randomized trials each found that lifestyle interventions including ~150 minutes/week of physical activity and diet-induced weight loss of 5% to 7% reduced the risk of progression from IGT to T2D by 58%. A cluster-randomized trial found that diet alone, exercise alone, and combined diet and exercise were equally effective in reducing the progression from IGT to diabetes. Therefore, there is firm and consistent evidence that programs of increased physical activity and modest weight loss reduce the incidence of T2D in individuals with IGT.

Pharmacologic Management

A large number of oral agents and insulin formulations are available for the management of T2D. Current therapeutic agents available for T2D have different mechanisms of action and include several oral agents such as insulin secretagogues, biguanides, thiazolidinediones, α-glucosidase inhibitors, dipeptidyl peptidase-IV (DPP-IV) inhibitors, bile acid sequestrants, and rapid-release bromocriptine. In addition, there are several injectable agents such as insulin, glucagon-like peptide (GLP-1) receptor agonists, and pramlintide. Most patients with newly diagnosed diabetes are treated with a single oral agent, but with progressive β-cell failure, the combination of oral agents and/or insulin is frequently needed. The classes of agents and their characteristics are listed in Table 8-1.

Biguanides

Metformin is the most commonly used antihyperglycemic agent for the treatment of T2D. It improves islet cell responsiveness to a glucose load through the correction of

TABLE 8-1. Medications Used to Treat Patients with Type 2 Diabetes Mellitus

Agent Class	Drug Effect	Route of Delivery	Examples
Biguanides	1) Enhance muscle uptake of glucose 2) Reduce hepatic gluconeogenesis 3) Suppress appetite	Oral	Metformin
Sulfonylureas	Bind to receptors on β-cells to stimulate insulin release	Oral	Glyburide, glipizide
Metiglinides	Bind to receptors on β-cells to stimulate insulin release	Oral	Repaglinide, nateglinide
Thiazolidinediones	Enhance sensitivity to insulin in peripheral tissues, primarily in muscle	Oral	Pioglitazone
α-Glucosidase inhibitors	Inhibit enzymes to reduce the rate of carbohydrate digestion and promote less absorption of glucose	Oral	Acarbose, miglitol
Incretins	1) Stimulate glucose-dependent insulin secretion 2) Inhibit glucagon production, lowering hepatic glucose output 3) Slow gastric emptying 4) Promote early satiety and reduced food intake		
Glucagon-like peptide-1 (GLP-1)	Direct incretin effect	Subcutaneous	Exenatide, liraglutide
Dipeptidyl peptidase-IV (DPP-IV) inhibitors	Inhibits degradation of GLP-1	Oral	Sitagliptin, saxagliptin
Insulin			
Bolus	Direct	Subcutaneous	Regular, lispro, aspart, glulisine
Basal	Direct	Subcutaneous	NPH (neutral protamine Hagedorn), glargine, detemir

glucose toxicity and improves peripheral glucose utilization by enhancing muscle uptake of glucose, increasing insulin receptor tyrosine kinase activity, and increasing GLUT-4 translocation and transport activity. It also reduces hepatic gluconeogenesis by inhibition of the key enzymes in this pathway and by mitochondrial depletion of the energy necessary for gluconeogenesis. Additionally, metformin has appetite-suppressive effects and inhibits leptin secretion via a mitogen-activated protein kinase signaling pathway in brown adipocytes. Metformin has been shown to reduce the fasting plasma glucose level by 50 to 70 mg/dL and the HbA$_{1c}$ by 1.4% to 2.0%. Metformin monotherapy is also associated with an increase in high-density lipoprotein (HDL) cholesterol and a reduction in triglyceride levels. It has a benign side effect profile characterized by transient gastrointestinal (GI) discomfort and nausea. Hypoglycemia is usually not a problem with metformin monotherapy. Due to the risk of lactic acidosis, which has been reported in 3 cases/100,000 patient-years, metformin should be avoided in patients with metabolic acidosis or hypoxic states, including renal failure, renal dysfunction with serum creatinine >1.5 mg/dL, liver failure, and in patients with congestive heart failure requiring pharmacologic intervention. In the Diabetes Prevention Program, metformin reduced the risk of progression from prediabetes to T2D. The ADA consensus statement advocates the use of metformin in individuals with prediabetes who are not successful with lifestyle modification.

Insulin Secretagogues

Insulin secretagogues, sulfonylureas, and glinides stimulate insulin secretion from the β-cell by interacting with the sulfonylurea receptor.

Sulfonylureas

Sulfonylureas close adenosine triphosphate (ATP)-sensitive potassium channels leading to depolarization of the β-cell membrane and increased calcium flux that stimulates insulin release. This increase in insulin secretion decreases hepatic glucose production and enhances glucose uptake in peripheral tissues, primarily muscle, leading to a reduction in plasma glucose. Approximately 25% of patients who begin therapy on sulfonylureas will achieve fasting plasma glucose <7.8 mmol/L (140 mg/dL) and are considered complete responders. About 20% have little or no reduction in plasma glucose (<1.1 mmol/L or <20 mg/dL) and are considered to have primary failure. The remaining 80% have a partial response but do not reach glycemic targets. This so-called *secondary failure of effectiveness* is common, occurring in 5% to 10% of patients per year. Hypoglycemia and weight gain are the most common side effects. Severe hypoglycemia occurs in less than 0.4 cases per 1,000 patient-treatment-years.

Meglitinides

Meglitinides, or glinides, bind to an ATP-dependent potassium channel on the cell membrane of β-cells in a similar manner to sulfonylureas but at a separate binding site. The interaction of the meglitinide with the receptor is not as "tight" as that of the sulfonylureas, translating to a much shorter duration of action. Meglitinides are roughly as effective as sulfonylureas at reducing HbA$_{1c}$ levels, causing a decrease between 1% and 2%, but they cause fewer instances of hypoglycemia. They have relatively short half-lives and must be taken less than 30 minutes prior to eating a meal. Meglitinides are safe, but do have the potential side effects of hypoglycemia and weight gain. They also interact with other drugs—particularly the cholesterol-lowering agent, gemfibrozil, which raises the blood level of meglitinide by 30- to 70-fold. Dose adjustments are also necessary in diabetic patients with moderate to severe liver dysfunction.

Thiazolidinediones

TZDs bind to peroxisome proliferator-activated receptor-γ (PPAR-γ) in muscle and fat. Their major metabolic effect is to enhance the sensitivity to insulin in peripheral tissues, primarily in muscle, although at higher doses they may also reduce hepatic glucose production. Pioglitazone is the only TZD available for clinical use. Clinical trials have shown equipotent glucose-lowering effects of approximately 30 mg/dL and a reduction of HbA_{1c} by approximately 1.3%. Overall, 20% to 30% of patients fail to respond when TZDs are used as monotherapy or added to the treatment of patients who failed sulfonylurea therapy. The most common reported side effects of TZDs include weight gain (possibly related to improvement in glycemic control), fluid retention, and expansion of plasma volume. TZDs cause fluid retention via activation of sodium channels in the distal nephron. They should not be used in patients with heart failure who are classified as class 3 or class 4 functional capacity by the New York Heart Association criteria. Several studies have linked the TZDs to osteoporosis and increased risk of fracture. Therefore, it is necessary to determine bone mineral density in patients treated with TZDs, especially in postmenopausal women who are at risk for osteoporosis.

α-Glucosidase Inhibitors

α-Glucosidase inhibitors are saccharidases that act as competitive inhibitors of enzymes needed to digest carbohydrates. The membrane-bound intestinal α-glucosidases hydrolyze oligosaccharides, trisaccharides, and disaccharides to glucose and other monosaccharides in the small intestine. Inhibition of these enzyme systems reduces the rate of digestion of carbohydrates. Less glucose is absorbed because the carbohydrates are not broken down into glucose molecules. In diabetic patients, the short-term effect of these drug therapies is to decrease current blood glucose levels; the long-term effect is a small reduction in HbA_{1c} level. α-Glucosidase inhibitors are used to establish greater glycemic control over hyperglycemia in patients with T2D, particularly with regard to postprandial hyperglycemia. They may be used as monotherapy in conjunction with an appropriate diabetic diet and exercise, or they may be used in conjunction with other antidiabetic drugs. Because α-glucosidase inhibitors are competitive inhibitors of the digestive enzymes, they must be taken at the start of meals to have maximal effect. Their effects on blood sugar levels following meals will depend on the amount of complex carbohydrates in the meal. Because α-glucosidase inhibitors prevent the degradation of complex carbohydrates into glucose, the carbohydrates will remain in the intestine. In the colon, bacteria will digest the complex carbohydrates, thereby causing GI side effects, such as flatulence and diarrhea. Since these effects are dose related, it is generally advised to start with a low dose and gradually increase the dose to the desired amount. If a patient using an α-glucosidase inhibitor suffers from an episode of hypoglycemia, the patient should eat something containing monosaccharides (e.g., glucose tablets). Because the drug will prevent the digestion of polysaccharides (or nonmonosaccharides), nonmonosaccharide foods may not effectively reverse a hypoglycemic episode in a patient taking an α-glucosidase inhibitor.

Incretins

Incretins are peptide hormones secreted by the enteroendocrine cells in the intestine that modulate glucose metabolism via their effect on pancreatic islet secretions. The gut hormones, GLP-1 and GIP, are incretins that are rapidly inactivated by the enzyme, DPP-IV, which results in a circulating half-life for GLP-1 of 2 minutes. The GLP-1 receptor analogues, exenatide and liraglutide, evade rapid clearance by DPP-IV; therefore, they have a long half-life when administered subcutaneously. The analogues stimulate glucose-dependent insulin secretion and inhibit glucagon production, thereby lowering hepatic glucose output. They also slow gastric emptying and promote early satiety and reduced food intake. Decreased food intake may be mediated locally by slowed gastric emptying and centrally by interaction with the area postrema, located in the brainstem. GLP-1 receptor agonists have also been shown to have trophic effects on the β-cell. A mechanism responsible for the expansion of β-cell mass is the inhibition of apoptosis by downregulation of caspase 3 at the mRNA level of the active protein and, upregulation of the antiapoptotic protein, Bcl-2. The GLP-1 analogues are administered subcutaneously. Exenatide and liraglutide decrease HbA_{1c} by ~1% and can be used in combination with metformin, sulfonylureas, TZDs, and insulin.

Insulin

Due to the progressive pancreatic β-cell failure, most patients with T2D will experience deficient insulin secretion leading to hyperglycemia and elevated free fatty acid levels. Although they may respond to single or combination treatment with oral agents, most patients eventually fail with oral agents and ultimately require insulin therapy to achieve and maintain adequate glycemic control because of the inexorable decline of pancreatic β-cell function. In patients with T2D, insulin therapy is indicated during sustained hyperglycemia despite maximal doses of oral agents or during intercurrent illness (e.g., infection and acute medical illness), the perioperative period, pregnancy, and severe liver or renal disease. In patients with newly diagnosed T2D who present with symptoms of hyperglycemia or weight loss, a short-term course of insulin (i.e., several weeks) to aggressively control blood glucose may induce long-lasting metabolic improvement.

Complications

There are both acute and chronic complications of diabetes. The chronic complications, both microvascular (e.g., nephropathy, retinopathy, and neuropathy) and macrovascular (e.g., coronary artery disease), have been discussed in the previous chapter insofar as the complications of T1D and T2D are similar and both develop from long-standing hyperglycemia. The life-threatening acute complications of T2D include diabetic ketoacidosis (DKA) and hyperosmolar hyperglycemia. Although most patients with T2D produce enough insulin to prevent the formation of ketone bodies and acidosis, there are a number of patients with T2D who can develop ketosis and acidosis. The clinical findings, diagnostic studies, and management strategies are similar to that of DKA, which is discussed in Chapter 7.

Hyperosmolar Hyperglycemia State

The **hyperosmolar hyperglycemic state (HHS)** is a complication of diabetes mellitus (predominantly T2D) in which high blood glucose levels cause severe dehydration, an increase in osmolarity, and a high risk for complications, such as coma and death. The diagnosis of HHS, similar to DKA in patients with T1D, is based on laboratory and clinical findings. The major difference between HHS and DKA is that patients with HHS have significantly higher serum osmolality levels and absent or minimal ketosis. Older names for HHS are *hyperosmolar nonketotic coma (HONK), nonketotic hyperosmolar coma,* and *hyperosmolar hyperglycemic nonketotic syndrome.*

 HHS is usually precipitated by an infection, myocardial infarction, stroke, or another acute illness. A relative insulin deficiency leads to a serum glucose that is usually greater than 600 mg/dL and a resulting serum osmolarity that is greater than 320 mOsm. This leads to polyuria, which, in turn, leads to volume depletion and hemoconcentration that causes a further increase in blood glucose level. Ketosis is absent because the presence of some insulin inhibits hormone-sensitive lipase (lipolysis). The increasing volume depletion may result in: 1) altered mental function (lethargy, stupor, and coma); 2) focal neurologic signs, such as sensory or motor impairments; 3) focal seizures or motor abnormalities, including flaccidity, depressed reflexes, tremors, or fasciculations; and 4) hyperviscosity and increased risk of thrombosis. Ultimately, the mortality rate in patients with HHS is between 10% and 14%.

The treatment of HHS consists of correction of the dehydration with IV fluids, reduction in the blood sugar levels with insulin, electrolyte replacement, and management of any underlying conditions that might have precipitated the illness. Treatment of HHS begins with reestablishing tissue perfusion using IV fluids. People with HHS can be dehydrated by 8 to 12 L. Attempts to correct this usually take over 24 to 48 hours with initial rates of normal saline in the range of 1 to 2 L/hour for the first few hours. Severe potassium deficits often occur. The average 70-kg person requires up to 350 mEq. This is generally replaced at a rate 10 mEq per hour as long as there is urinary output. Insulin is given to reduce blood glucose concentration; however, because it also causes the movement of potassium into cells, serum potassium levels must be sufficiently high, or dangerous hypokalemia may result. Once potassium levels have been verified to be greater than 3.3 mEq/L, an insulin infusion can be started.

METABOLIC SYNDROME

Metabolic syndrome is a combination of medical disorders that increase the risk of developing cardiovascular disease and diabetes. Some studies have shown the prevalence in the United States to be ~25% of the population, and prevalence increases with age.

Etiology

The pathophysiology of metabolic syndrome is extremely complex and has been only partially elucidated. Most patients are older, obese, and sedentary and have a degree of insulin resistance. Stress can also be a contributing factor. The most important factors are weight, genetics, endocrine disorders (such as polycystic ovary syndrome [PCOS] in women of reproductive age), aging, and sedentary lifestyle (i.e., low physical activity and excess caloric intake). There is debate regarding whether obesity or insulin resistance is the cause of the metabolic syndrome or if they are consequences of a more far-reaching metabolic derangement. A number of markers of systemic inflammation, including C-reactive protein, fibrinogen, interleukin-6, and TNF-α are often increased. Some have pointed to a variety of causes, including increased uric acid levels caused by dietary fructose.

Pathophysiology

It is common for there to have been a development of visceral fat, after which the adipocytes of the visceral fat increase plasma levels of TNF-α and alter levels of a number of other substances (e.g., adiponectin, resistin, and plasminogen activator inhibitor-1). TNF-α has been shown not only to cause the production of inflammatory cytokines but also to trigger cell signaling by interaction with a TNF-α receptor that may lead to insulin resistance. An experiment with rats fed a diet with 33% sucrose has been proposed as a model for the development of metabolic syndrome. The sucrose first elevates blood levels of triglycerides, which induce visceral fat and ultimately results in insulin resistance. The progression from visceral fat to increased TNF-α to insulin resistance has some parallels to human development of the metabolic syndrome. The increase in adipose tissue also increases the number of immune cells present within, which plays a role in inflammation. Chronic inflammation contributes to an increased risk of hypertension, atherosclerosis, and diabetes.

Clinical Findings

The symptoms and features of the metabolic syndrome include: 1) fasting hyperglycemia—T2D or IFG, IGT, or insulin resistance; 2) high blood pressure; 3) central obesity (also known as *visceral, male-pattern*, or *apple-shaped adiposity*), overweight with fat deposits mainly around the waist; 4) decreased HDL cholesterol; and 5) elevated triglycerides. The associated diseases and signs include: hyperuricemia, fatty liver progressing to nonalcoholic fatty liver disease, PCOS, and acanthosis nigricans.

Diagnostic Studies

Under current guidelines, the International Diabetes Federation consensus worldwide definition of the metabolic syndrome, revised in 2006, is shown in Box 8-3.

Therapy/Management

The first-line treatment is a change in lifestyle. Many studies have supported the value of increased physical activity and restricted caloric intake. Restricting the overall dietary carbohydrate intake is more effective in reducing the most common symptoms of metabolic syndrome than the more commonly prescribed reduction in dietary fat intake. If, after 3 to 6 months, efforts at remedying risk factors prove insufficient, then drug

---

BOX 8-3.   Criteria for the Diagnosis of Metabolic Syndrome

- Central obesity[a] [waist circumference ≥102 cm (40 in) in men or ≥88 cm (35 in) in women; if Asian American, ≥90 cm (35 in) in men or ≥80 cm (32 in) in women] and any two of the following:
  - Raised triglycerides: >150 mg/dL (1.7 mmol/L), or specific treatment for this lipid abnormality
  - Reduced high-density lipoprotein (HDL) cholesterol: <40 mg/dL (1.03 mmol/L) in males, <50 mg/dL (1.29 mmol/L) in females, or specific treatment for this lipid abnormality
  - Raised blood pressure (BP): systolic BP >130 or diastolic BP >85 mmHg, or treatment for previously diagnosed hypertension
  - Raised fasting plasma glucose (FPG)[b]: >100 mg/dL (5.6 mmol/L), or previously diagnosed type 2 diabetes (T2D)

[a]If the body mass index (BMI) is >30 kg/m², central obesity can be assumed and waist circumference does not need to be measured.
[b]If FPG is >5.6 mmol/L or 100 mg/dL, an oral glucose tolerance test is strongly recommended, but is not necessary to define presence of the syndrome.

treatment is frequently required. Generally, the individual disorders that compose the metabolic syndrome are treated separately. Diuretics and angiotensin-converting enzyme inhibitors may be used to treat hypertension. Cholesterol drugs may be used to lower LDL cholesterol and triglyceride levels, if they are elevated, and to raise HDL levels if they are low. Insulin or other antihyperglycemic agents should be used to improve blood glucose levels.

Prevention

Various strategies have been proposed to prevent the development of metabolic syndrome. These include increased physical activity and a healthy, reduced-calorie diet. Many studies support the value of a healthy lifestyle; however, these potentially beneficial measures may be effective in only a minority of people, primarily due to a lack of compliance with lifestyle and diet changes.

CASE FOLLOW-UP

This man has all of the signs, symptoms, and biochemical findings of T2D. He is also obese and has a family history of obesity, hypertension, and cardiovascular disease. The fact that he has had polyuria and polydipsia for 2 years indicates that he probably has had T2D long before he presented to the clinic.

Laboratory studies are remarkable for hyperglycemia, hyponatremia, and an elevated HbA_{1c}. The low serum sodium is due to pseudohyponatremia from the elevated serum glucose. The decreased sodium concentration does not result from a hypotonic disorder but, rather, from hyperglycemia. The hyperglycemia causes displacement of plasma water into the extracellular space, ultimately diluting the serum sodium. The elevated HbA_{1c} indicates that at least for the past 2 to 3 months, his blood glucose level has been elevated above 200 mg/dL.

Given his elevated blood glucose level and symptoms, he is started on insulin therapy. He is started on an evening dose of glargine for his basal insulin, and lispro at mealtimes. Within 24 hours, his blood glucose levels are in an acceptable range and the diabetes education team meets with him regarding management, focusing on diet, exercise, glucose monitoring, and insulin therapy.

He returns to the clinic 2 months later at which time his fasting blood glucose level is 110 mg/dL, and his HbA_{1c} is nearly normal at 6.5%. He has gained 10 lb since diagnosis. He complains of frequent episodes of hypoglycemia. Due to the weight gain and hypoglycemia, his insulin dose is significantly reduced, and metformin is added.

One month later, he reports having normal and occasionally low blood glucose levels. Insulin injections are discontinued but he continues to monitor his blood glucose levels and take metformin with breakfast and supper. He exercises between 30 and 60 minutes a day and maintains a low-calorie diet. He continues to follow up in clinic in every 6 months.

REFERENCES and SUGGESTED READINGS

American Diabetes Association. Standards of medical care in diabetes—2012. Diabetes Care. 2012;35(suppl 1):S11–S63.

Cowie CC, Rust KF, Byrd-Holt DD, et al. Prevalence of diabetes and high risk for diabetes using A1C criteria in the U.S. population in 1988–2006. Diabetes Care. 2010;33(3):562–568.

Dall TM, Mann SE, Zhang Y, et al. Distinguishing the economic costs associated with type 1 and type 2 diabetes. Popul Health Manag. 2009;12(2):103–110.

Defronzo RA. Banting Lecture. From the triumvirate to the ominous octet: a new paradigm for the treatment of type 2 diabetes mellitus. Diabetes. 2009;58(4):773–795.

Diabetes Prevention Program Research Group. Reduction in the incidence of type 2 diabetes with lifestyle intervention or metformin. N Engl J Med. 2002;346:393–403.

Hundal RS, Inzucchi SE. Metformin: new understandings, new uses. Drugs. 2003;63(18):1879–1894.

Inzucchi SE. Oral antihyperglycemic therapy for type 2 diabetes: scientific review. JAMA. 2002;287(3):360–372.

Nyenwe EA, Jerkins TW, Umpierrez GE, Kitabchi AE. Management of type 2 diabetes: evolving strategies for the treatment of patients with type 2 diabetes. Metabolism. 2011;60(1):1–23.

Pan XR, Li GW, Hu YH, et al. Effects of diet and exercise in preventing NIDDM in people with impaired glucose tolerance: the Da Qing IGT and Diabetes Study. Diabetes Care. 1997;20:537–544.

Saini V. Molecular mechanisms of insulin resistance in type 2 diabetes mellitus. World J Diabetes. 2010;1(3):68–75.

Seino S, Shibasaki T, Minami K. Dynamics of insulin secretion and the clinical implications for obesity and diabetes. J Clin Invest. 2011;121(6):2118–2125.

Stumvoll M, Fritsche A, Stefan N, Haring H. A 60 minute hyperglycemic clamp is sufficient to assess both phases of insulin secretion. Horm Metab Res. 2000;32:230–232.

Tuomilehto J, Lindstrom J, Eriksson JG, Valle TT, Hamalainen H, Ilanne-Parikka P, et al. Prevention of type 2 diabetes mellitus by changes in lifestyle among subjects with impaired glucose tolerance. N Engl J Med. 2001;344:1343–1350.

Turner R, Stratton I, Horton V, et al. UKPDS 25: autoantibodies to islet-cell cytoplasm and glutamic acid decarboxylase for prediction of insulin requirement in type 2 diabetes. UK Prospective Diabetes Study Group. Lancet. 1997;350(9087):1288–1293.

UK Prospective Diabetes Study (UKPDS) Group. Effect of intensive blood-glucose control with metformin on complications in overweight patients with type 2 diabetes (UKPDS 34). Lancet. 1998;352(9131):854–865.

Umpierrez GE, Kitabchi AE. Management of type 2 diabetes. Evolving strategies for treatment. Obstet Gynecol Clin North Am. 2001;28(2):401–419, viii.

Umpierrez GE, Smiley D, Kitabchi AE. Narrative review: ketosis-prone type 2 diabetes mellitus. Ann Intern Med. 2006;144(5):350–357.

Yki-Jarvinen H. Thiazolidinediones. N Engl J Med. 2004;351(11):1106–1118.

CHAPTER REVIEW QUESTIONS

1. A 43-year-old overweight African American man presents to the local emergency room complaining of a 3-week history of polyuria and polydipsia. He has a strong family history of diabetes. He has not eaten in almost 8 hours. Laboratory studies reveal: serum glucose, 368 mg/dL; HbA_{1c}, 8.9%; and negative urine ketones. Each of the following statements is true except:

   A. He has decreased β-cell mass.

   B. He may benefit from insulin therapy.

   C. He has increased insulin secretion compared to nondiabetic individuals with similar glucose levels.

   D. He has impaired first-phase insulin release in response to a glucose load.

   E. He has impaired second-phase insulin release in response to a glucose load.

2. A 34-year-old woman with T2D has had difficulty controlling her blood glucose level despite taking metformin and insulin. Her endocrinologist is considering adding incretin therapy. Each of the following statements is true regarding incretin therapy except:

   A. They are peptide hormones secreted by enteroendocrine cells.

   B. They can decrease HbA_{1c} by about 1%.

C. They can be used in combination with metformin, sulfonylureas, TZDs, and insulin.

D. They are only taken orally.

E. Some are inactivated by the DPP-IV enzyme.

3. A 57-year-old roofer has had T2D for 20 years. He has a family history for obesity, hypertension, and diabetes. His HbA$_{1c}$ is 10.3%. Which complication is he at the highest risk for developing?

A. Pancreatitis

B. Myocardial infarction

C. Renal failure

D. Gangrene of his foot

E. Blindness

4. A 38-year-old lawyer has a 1-week history of polyuria and polydipsia. He has also lost 4 lb in the past month. His fasting blood glucose level is 137 mg/dL and, 2 hours after drinking Glucola (75 g), his blood glucose is 276 mg/dL. His HbA$_{1c}$ is 8.7%. Each of the following is true except:

A. He would benefit from a diet with 30% of the total calories from fat.

B. He would improve his blood glucose level by increasing the amount of time he exercises.

C. He would benefit from treatment with insulin.

D. He is at risk for developing chronic complications of hyperglycemia.

E. He has islet cell antibodies.

5. A 35-year-old accountant has had diabetes for 1.5 years. She cannot tolerate metformin because of diarrhea and therefore takes pioglitazone. She has gained 20 lb in the past 3 months. She is 5 ft 3 in tall, weighs 150 lb and gets little exercise. Her HbA$_{1c}$ is 7.5%. All of the following are true except:

A. Starting insulin might result in more weight gain.

B. Her diabetes would probably get worse if she became pregnant.

C. Liraglutide would help her hyperglycemia but not her weight.

D. She might be able to stop the pioglitazone with better diet and more exercise.

E. One injection a day of long-acting insulin would lower her HbA$_{1c}$.

CHAPTER REVIEW ANSWERS

1. The correct answer is C. When individuals have the classic symptoms of diabetes in addition to a fasting blood glucose level ≥126 mg/dL, a 2-hour postglucose load ≥200 mg/dL, a random blood glucose level ≥200 mg/dL, or an HbA$_{1c}$ ≥6.5%, they are diagnosed with diabetes. This patient meets the criteria for T2D. Individuals with T2D have β-cell exhaustion and develop hyperglycemia because they are unable to secrete enough insulin to maintain a normal blood glucose level. Therefore, this patient, who has T2D, would be unable to secrete as much insulin as a nondiabetic individual faced with a similar glucose load.

This patient will have a decreased β-cell mass (**Choice A**). There are many options for pharmacologic therapy in those with T2D. This patient would benefit from insulin therapy (**Choice B**) because he is unable to secrete enough insulin to meet his body's demands. Individuals with T2D have impaired first- (**Choice D**) and second-phase (**Choice E**) insulin secretion.

2. The correct answer is D. The gut hormones GLP-1 and GIP are incretins that are only delivered subcutaneously. DPP-IV inhibitors are incretins that are delivered orally.

Incretins are peptide hormones secreted by the enteroendocrine cells in the intestine that modulate glucose metabolism via their effect on pancreatic islet secretions (**Choice A**). They have been shown to reduce HbA_{1c} by ~1% (**Choice B**). They have a different mechanism of action than that of other anti-hyperglycemic agents but do not cause drug interactions. They can be used in combination with metformin, sulfonylureas, TZDs, and insulin (**Choice D**). GLP-1 and GIP are incretins that are inactivated by the enzyme DPP-IV (**Choice E**).

3. The correct answer is B. This man has long-standing poorly controlled T2D and is at risk for long-term micro- and macrovascular complications. Patients with poorly controlled diabetes are at highest risk for MI and strokes. In patients with T2D, the prevalence of heart attacks and strokes is two to four times more frequent than in nondiabetic individuals. Many patients with T2D have the same risk for a cardiovascular event as do nondiabetic patients who have had at least one MI. Patients with diabetes who have had a previous cardiovascular event are at 10 times the risk for a subsequent event as compared to the nondiabetic population.

Pancreatitis (**Choice A**) is not a common complication of T2DM. Renal failure (**Choice C**) is a common microvascular complication of T2DM but not as common as an MI. Gangrene of an extremity is not an uncommon macrovascular complication of T2DM, but not as common as an MI (**Choice D**). Blindness (**Choice E**) is also a common microvascular complication of T2DM but not as common as an MI.

4. The correct answer is E. Management of patients with T2D includes five principles: 1) metabolic control, 2) education, 3) nutrition, 4) physical activity, and 5) pharmacologic agents. Patients with T2D would be unlikely to have islet cell antibodies, as these are typically found in patients with T1D.

He would benefit from a diet with 30% of the total calories from fat (**Choice A**). He should also have 10% or less of fat as saturated. He would improve his blood glucose level by increasing the amount of time he exercises (**Choice B**). He would benefit from insulin therapy (**Choice C**) as well as other antihyperglycemic agents. The diagnosis of diabetes places patients at risk for developing long-term complications (**Choice E**).

5. The correct answer is C. Liraglutide is a long-acting incretin that affects blood glucose by a number of mechanisms. The analogs stimulate glucose-dependent insulin secretion and inhibit glucagon production, thus lowering hepatic glucose output. They also slow gastric emptying and promote early satiety and reduced food intake. Decreased food intake may be mediated locally by slowed gastric emptying and centrally by interaction with the area postrema. Therefore, liraglutide would reduce her blood glucose and should result in weight loss, rather than weight gain.

Insulin therapy may improve glycemic control, but may also cause an increase in weight (**Choice A**). This is due to the improvement in glucose and calorie utilization. Gestation places an increased stress on glucose homeostasis. Without a change in hyperglycemic therapy, her diabetes would probably get worse if she became pregnant (**Choice B**). If she improves her diet and exercise, she will increase her insulin sensitivity and likely not require TZD therapy (**Choice D**). Adding just one injection a day of insulin should improve her glycemic control, thereby lowering her HbA_{1c} (**Choice E**).

Obesity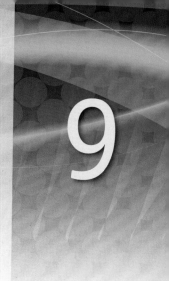

9

Adva Eisenberg
Jason Zhu
Andrew B. Muir

CASE

A 43-year-old Hispanic woman presents to her primary care physician for a new employee physical examination. She is unemployed, lacks health insurance, and has therefore not been to a doctor in more than 5 years. She describes mild pain without swelling or erythema in both of her knees, daytime fatigue, and postprandial abdominal discomfort. On physical exam, her blood pressure is 140/90 mmHg. She is 5 ft 6 in (1.68 m) tall, weighs 220 lbs (100 kg), and has a body mass index (BMI) of 35.5 kg/m². She has mild lower extremity edema and velvety hyperpigmentation in her neck and axillae consistent with acanthosis nigricans. The remainder of her physical exam is normal. Social history reveals that she does not smoke, and she drinks alcohol socially. She does not "watch her diet" and she exercises "on and off." Family history reveals that her father died of a heart attack at age 71 years. Her mother is alive and has hypertension and type 2 diabetes mellitus (T2D).

Initial laboratory evaluation reveals normal serum electrolytes and a fasting glucose of 118 mg/dL. A serum fasting lipid panel reveals a total cholesterol of 241 mg/dL, LDL cholesterol of 165 mg/dL, HDL cholesterol of 40 mg/dL, and triglycerides of 180 mg/dL. Her serum thyroid-stimulating hormone (TSH) level is 2.5 µIU/L.

This chapter reviews the physiology and pathophysiology of obesity and the gut hormones to help the learner classify this woman's obesity, determine her risk for complications of obesity, decide what further evaluation is necessary, and understand the treatment options. At the end of the chapter, we summarize the work-up along with proper counseling options to give the learner a better understanding of the care of obese patients.

Because the etiology and consequences of obesity are complex and multifaceted, this chapter enumerates how gut hormones and other endocrinologic factors are involved. This chapter has been organized to: 1) present the basic physiology

(continues)

(*continued*)

of energy homeostasis; 2) introduce the relevant gut hormones; 3) establish the concept that adipose tissue is an endocrine organ; 4) summarize the genetic contributors to obesity and its secondary causes; 5) review the pathophysiologic complications of obesity on genetic, metabolic, and endocrinologic levels; and 6) address the treatment options for obesity including lifestyle, pharmacotherapeutic, and surgical options.

OBJECTIVES

1. Describe the major gut hormones and their role in appetite control and weight regulation.

2. Differentiate primary from secondary causes of obesity.

3. Describe the metabolic syndrome.

4. Describe the evaluation and management of an overweight, obese, or morbidly obese individual.

EPIDEMIOLOGY

Obesity is the top cause of preventable death across the United States and worldwide. It is projected to affect 40% of the population by the year 2020. The estimated decrease in life expectancy for obese individuals is 8 years. This is a consequence not of obesity per se but, rather, of the metabolic derangements that result from its complications. Fat distribution that is primarily upper body and associated with an increase in visceral fat is linked to an abnormal metabolic profile. The complications of obesity include endothelial dysfunction, hepatic steatosis, premature puberty, hypogonadism, obstructive sleep apnea, restrictive lung disease, bone and joint disease, cholelithiasis, and pseudotumor cerebri. Mortality ratios are significantly higher among overweight and obese individuals for cardiovascular disease, stroke, cancer, and digestive disease. Consequently, determining the mechanisms behind the causes of obesity has tremendous public health implications.

Although national surveys tracking population prevalence of obesity showed minimal change between 1960 and 1980, in the 1988 to 1994 survey, the population prevalence of obesity increased almost 8%, with a similar increase in the 1999 to 2000 survey. However, similar prevalence in the 2003 to 2008 and 2009 to 2010 surveys provide hope that a ceiling may soon be reached. In 2009 to 2010, the prevalence of obesity among 8,397 adult men and women was 36% with no intersex difference.

CLASSIFICATION

The majority of obesity research uses BMI as the unit of reference, which is calculated by dividing an individual's weight (in kilograms) by the square of his or her height (in meters squared). The BMI-based classifications of weight diagnoses have been established in adults and children (Table 9-1). The BMI is an invaluable tool that provides a standardized definition of obesity for clinical and epidemiologic research and can guide decisions made in clinical practice. Among National Health and Nutrition Examination Surveys (NHANES), the BMI has been highly correlated with the percentage of body fat. Nevertheless, BMI is an imperfect unit because it distinguishes neither fat from lean mass, nor visceral fat from subcutaneous fat. Although subcutaneous fat contributes to mechanical complications of obesity (e.g., pulmonary and orthopedic problems), visceral fat contributes more significantly to excess mortality from metabolic complications (e.g., cardiovascular disease).

PHYSIOLOGY

Energy homeostasis is the steady state in which energy balance and body fat mass remain constant in a constant environment. Obesity is due to a positive imbalance of caloric intake and caloric expenditure over time. There are many central and peripheral factors that play a role in energy homeostasis.

Energy Homeostasis

In the body's system of energy homeostasis, the brain is the decision maker with many "advisors" (central homeostasis).

In addition to the numerous brain nuclei that communicate among themselves, human energy management systems are linked to the gastrointestinal tract, adipose tissue, and pancreas (peripheral homeostasis).

Central Homeostasis

Within the arcuate nucleus of the hypothalamus there are two primary pairs of neuronal networks that regulate appetite; these networks have opposing actions.

TABLE 9-1.	Clinical Classification of Adiposity by Body Mass Index (BMI)	
Classification	**BMI in Children**	**BMI in Adults (mg/m²)**
Underweight	<5th percentile for age	<18.5
Healthy/normal	5th–84th percentile for age	18.5–24.9
Overweight	≥85th–94th percentile	25.0–29.9
Obese	≥95th percentile	30.0–39.9
Morbidly obese	Not Used	≥40.0

The first pair of neuronal networks synthesizes **neuropeptide Y (NPY)** and **agouti-related protein (AGRP)** as orexigenic neurotransmitters that increase appetite while decreasing metabolism and energy expenditure. The axonal release of both AGRP and NPY from these neurons inhibits the actions of α-melanocyte-stimulating hormone (α-MSH) on neurons in the ventromedial hypothalamus that express the **melanocortin 4 receptor (MC4R)**. This disrupts the normal anorexigenic actions of MC4R. NPY also causes increased caloric intake by increasing the synthesis of the orexigenic melanin-concentrating hormone, a neuropeptide that is synthesized in the lateral hypothalamus.

The second pair of neuropeptides releases **proopiomelanocortin (POMC)** and **cocaine/amphetamine-regulated transcript (CART)** and has an anorexigenic effect by promoting MC4R activation and suppressing appetite. Inactivating mutations within the POMC gene, the proconvertase gene (prevents cleavage of melanocortin from POMC) and the MC4R gene, result in early-onset obesity. CART requires several mechanisms for its anorexigenic effects, including decreasing the rate of gastric emptying and increasing the postprandial satiety effects of **cholecystokinin (CCK)**.

In addition to the hypothalamic network, a third system has been implicated in the regulation of appetite, the **endocannabinoid system**. Cannabinoid receptors are present throughout the central and peripheral nervous systems. When activated, they increase food intake, promote weight gain, and decrease muscle glucose uptake. These receptor antagonists suppress appetite, promote weight loss, and improve dyslipidemia, hypertension, and glucose uptake. **Rimonabant**, a pharmacologic cannabinoid receptor antagonist, showed promise in decreasing body weight in randomized controlled trials with obese human patients but has been excluded from the US market because of its associated risk of serious psychiatric disorders, especially depression.

In addition to the hypothalamus, studies of experimental animal models suggest that the caudal brainstem and telencephalon both contribute to an individual's eating behavior. Although it normally receives neural inputs from both the hypothalamus and telencephalon, the caudal brainstem may act independently to allow for meal initiation and meal termination, a finding that has been documented in studies with decerebrate rats. The caudal brainstem contains the nucleus of the solitary tract (NTS), with its receptors for leptin, ghrelin, insulin, and glucose-sensing neurons. The NTS is able to modulate eating behavior based on plasma glucose and the individual's preferences or aversions for specific foods. The NTS receives input from the hypothalamus that is regulated by leptin, a hormone critical to long-term energy homeostasis. Rats that lack the leptin receptor have a diminished response in the NTS and are less sensitive to the satiating effect of CCK.

The telencephalon, which contains the nucleus accumbens, the amygdala, and various areas of the limbic, orbitofrontal, and cingulate areas, helps regulate the cognitive, emotional, and social aspects of eating. Two broad categories of neurotransmitters have been reported to interact between the telencephalon and hypothalamus: those that are released because one "likes" to eat a food and those that are released because one "wants" to eat a food. Dopamine, which is released from the nucleus accumbens and is part of the brain's reward system, is in the "wanting" category, whereas γ-aminobutyric acid (commonly known as *GABA*) is released when there is an emotional impetus (i.e., "liking" a food).

Peripheral Homeostasis

Peripheral human energy management systems (i.e., linked to the stomach, adipose tissue, and pancreas) are divided into short-term and long-term energy homeostasis.

Short-term Energy Homeostasis

Once an individual begins to eat, several factors impact satiation and the perception of fullness, ultimately leading to meal termination. They guide the individual to stop eating before gastric capacity is exceeded and allow an appropriate time interval to pass before the next meal. These factors are a response to the combined effects of gastric distention and the release of peptide signals from the enteroendocrine cells that line the gastrointestinal (GI) tract.

The mechanoreceptor neurons in the stomach are responsible for sensing gastric distension and, via vagal afferent and spinal sensory nerves, notify the hindbrain. Satiation-inducing gut peptides also communicate with the hindbrain via vagal afferent fibers, and directly through circulation. Anorexigenic peptides including CCK, **glucagon-like peptide-1 (GLP-1)**, oxyntomodulin, peptide YY (PYY3–36), apolipoprotein A-IV, and enterostatin are released by intestinal enteroendocrine cells. The pancreas also secretes anorexigenic peptides including pancreatic polypeptide, glucagon, and amylin. The most important anorexigenic peptides are discussed here. GLP-1 is a glucose-dependent insulin secretagogue produced by intestinal L cells after an individual consumes a meal containing carbohydrates and fat. GLP-1 and **gastric inhibitory peptide (GIP)** are both incretins (i.e., hormones that potentiate insulin secretion after an oral rather than an intravenous glucose challenge). This incretin effect accounts for approximately 50% to 70% of the total amount of insulin secreted after an oral glucose load, making these hormones significant contributors to the body's glucoregulatory mechanisms. In addition to increasing postprandial insulin levels, GLP-1 inhibits glucagon secretion, decreases hepatic gluconeogenesis, decreases insulin resistance, and increases postmeal satiety. An obesity-related reduction of the GLP-1 response to an oral carbohydrate challenge can be reversed by surgically induced weight loss.

CCK, released by neuroendocrine I-cells in the duodenum and ileum, is both a gut peptide hormone and a central nervous system neurotransmitter. CCK is secreted during and after meals in response to high gut concentrations of protein and long-chain fatty acids. It helps stimulate gut motility, gallbladder contraction, gastric emptying, and acid secretion. It is one of the principle hormones involved in satiation by its actions on upper abdominal vagal afferent fibers. CCK also communicates with the hypothalamus through the CCK1 receptor, which informs the brain that fat and proteins are being processed.

Ghrelin is an acylated peptide secreted from the gastric mucosa that promotes meal initiation. It peaks before meals and falls immediately after eating, thus representing the only gut peptide whose blood levels rise when fasting and fall when eating. Ghrelin activates the orexigenic NPY and AGRP neurons. The metabolic effects of ghrelin include enhanced use of carbohydrates, reduced fat utilization, and increased gastric motility and acid secretion. Ghrelin's effect on glucose homeostasis is derived from its ability to increase hepatic glucose production and glucose conservation in muscles and adipose tissue. During states of caloric restriction, ghrelin increases serum glucose levels, thereby preventing hypoglycemia. In obese individuals, however, ghrelin may induce a diabetic phenotype by promoting hyperglycemia.

In addition to stimulating feeding, ghrelin acts on the pituitary to increase growth hormone (GH) secretion, in concert with growth hormone-releasing hormone. Furthermore, it has been reported that fasting plasma ghrelin levels are reduced in obese individuals and increased in individuals with anorexia nervosa. These data indicate that humans may downregulate ghrelin as a result of excessive energy production.

Long-term Energy Homeostasis

Leptin, secreted by adipocytes, is the key hormone in the management of long-term energy homeostasis. Leptin receptors have been found in a variety of peripheral tissues, including liver, skeletal muscle, and pancreas. Centrally, leptin receptors are concentrated in the hypothalamus and brainstem, where they regulate satiety, energy expenditure, and neuroendocrine function. The anorexigenic neuropeptides, α-MSH and POMC, directly increase in response to activation of leptin-sensitive neurons that are located in the arcuate nucleus. Leptin deficiency promotes the urge for food intake that results in fat accumulation. By reducing thermogenesis, it creates a chronic positive energy balance. Obese individuals typically have elevated serum leptin levels, which reflects the leptin resistance commonly found in these individuals. Inactivating genetic mutations of the leptin gene are rarely found in obese individuals. Replacement of leptin has been shown to nearly normalize metabolic dysfunction in affected individuals. Unfortunately, its therapeutic use in obese individuals with intact leptin signaling has not been successful, most likely due to the acquired leptin resistance. Leptin plays a role in several other important processes including angiogenesis, inflammation, and insulin secretion.

Adipose Tissue: An Endocrine Organ

A growing body of evidence has shown that adipose tissue is an active endocrine organ and not simply a passive storage depot for lipids. Adipose cells are comprised of adipocytes, preadipocytes, vascular cells, and macrophages. They produce and secrete a variety of biologically active molecules collectively known as **adipokines**. Many of these adipokines act locally in an autocrine or paracrine fashion, whereas others circulate systemically to regulate function in the liver, skeletal muscle, and vascular endothelium. A large number of these substances play key roles in maintaining the body's energy balance and regulating insulin sensitivity, blood pressure, lipid metabolism, hemostasis, and immune responses.

Noninflammatory Mediators

In addition to **leptin**, the most essential adipokines, or **noninflammatory mediators of adipose tissue**, include **adiponectin, resistin, visfatin, glucocorticoids**, and **free fatty acids (FFAs)**.

Adiponectin

Adiponectin plays a role in both whole-body metabolism and glucose and lipid homeostasis. It has a strong association with cardiovascular health and, unlike the majority of other adipokines, an *inverse* association with vascular inflammatory markers such as **C-reactive protein (CRP)** and fibrinogen. The level of adiponectin has an inverse relationship with several components of the metabolic syndrome including hypertension, BMI, insulin resistance, and dyslipidemia. In addition, hypoadiponectinemia is linked to fatty liver disease as well as endothelial dysfunction and ischemic heart disease.

Human case-control studies have demonstrated that elevated serum adiponectin levels have a protective effect against myocardial infarction. This effect persists even when controlling for family history, BMI, alcohol intake, history of T2D, hypertension, and levels of hemoglobin A1c (HbA1c), CRP, and lipoproteins. The principal mechanism responsible for this protective effect is its antiinflammatory properties. There are therapeutic agents including the thiazolidinediones, renin-angiotensin system (RAS) blocking agents, and antagonists of type 1 cannabinoid receptors (rimonabant) that increase the serum concentration of adiponectin.

Resistin

Resistin, in contrast to adiponectin, is proinflammatory. It targets the liver, adipose tissue, and skeletal muscle. Resistin upregulates hepatic gluconeogenesis and downregulates uptake and metabolism of fatty acids in skeletal muscle.

Visfatin

Visfatin is a recently discovered pre–B-cell colony-enhancing factor. It is found in high concentrations in the visceral fat of both humans and mice. Its circulating levels rise with the development of obesity. Visfatin displays insulin-mimetic effects on the liver, adipose tissue, and skeletal muscle.

Glucocorticoids

Glucocorticoids play an integral role in adipose tissue metabolism. As addressed later in the chapter, obesity is linked to the metabolic syndrome. The metabolic syndrome closely resembles Cushing syndrome with central obesity, insulin resistance, T2D, and dyslipidemia. However, in the common forms of obesity, circulating glucocorticoid levels are not elevated. This seeming contradiction may be explained by the fact that adipocytes, particularly those comprising visceral fat deposits, express **11β-hydroxysteroid dehydrogenase (11β-HSD)** at high levels. This enzyme converts circulating inactive cortisone to active cortisol, leading to *locally* elevated intracellular glucocorticoid concentrations. A phenotype similar to the metabolic syndrome has been reported in mice that overexpress 11β-HSD in their adipose tissue. In contrast, 11β-HSD knockout mice had decreased visceral fat accumulation and less metabolic dysfunction.

Free (Nonesterified) Fatty Acids

FFAs are elevated in the plasma of obese individuals; their main source is visceral adipose tissue. FFA concentrations are primarily regulated by catecholamines, which promote lipolysis, and insulin, which promotes lipogenesis. Acute, postprandial increases in FFAs contribute to hyperinsulinemia, whereas more chronic elevations lead to lipotoxicity and β-cell apoptosis. Studies that use recombinant genetic models to increase the release of FFAs to the heart are similar to diabetic cardiomyopathy, which suggests an association between insulin resistance and cardiovascular risk. The proposed mechanism for the pathologic effects of FFAs is linked to individuals with both oxidative stress and to elevations in proinflammatory cytokines.

Inflammatory Mediators

It is well recognized that excess visceral fat (e.g., intraabdominal, omental, perirenal) is associated with a higher risk of metabolic disease than is excess subcutaneous fat. The cause of this effect has not been clearly determined, but current proposals suggest that interacting genetic, developmental, and environmental factors determine the capacity and distribution of stored triglyceride in these two adipose depots. Subcutaneous sites appear to be the storage sites of first choice. When these metabolically "inactive" sites approach their capacity, demand arises for new fat deposition sites. Individual variations in the differentiation of adipocytes from preadipocytes may determine the capacity of subcutaneous fat storage, and the extent to which excess energy is stored as triglycerides in new fat cells (hyperplasia) or in enlarging existing cells (hypertrophy). In central storage sites, adipocyte hypertrophy induces intracellular stress causing release of FFAs, proinflammatory adipokines, and cytokines, resulting in tissue invasion by macrophages. The chronic systemic inflammation created by this environment promotes local and systemic insulin resistance; endothelial cell dysfunction; a prothrombotic state; and, ultimately, T2D, hypertension, and atherosclerosis. FFAs released from dysfunctional, hypertrophied adipocytes exacerbate metabolic disease because they are taken up by muscle, liver, and pancreatic islets. Here, intracellular toxic lipid metabolites (e.g., ceramides) accumulate and induce organ dysfunction that further promotes insulin resistance, insulinopenia, and dyslipidemia. Several of the inflammatory mediators involved with obesity are discussed in more detail below.

Tumor Necrosis Factor-α

TNF-α is a proinflammatory cytokine that stimulates other inflammatory factors, including leptin and interleukin-6, while reducing the expression of the antiinflammatory adiponectin. High levels of TNF-α are associated with insulin resistance and elevated systolic blood pressure. Treatment with the 3-hydroxy-3-methylglutaryl-coenzyme A (HMG-CoA) reductase inhibitor simvastatin will lower the levels of both TNF-α and CRP. Although weight loss and physical activity reduce the serum level of TNF-α, the administration of TNF-α inhibitors (i.e., etanercept, infliximab, and adalimumab) does not affect insulin resistance in obese individuals with T2D.

Interleukin-6

Interleukin-6 (IL-6) increases proportionally with body mass. Approximately 30% of it is derived from the stromal/vascular adipose tissue. Increased adipose and serum levels of IL-6 are associated with obesity, insulin resistance, and cardiovascular disease. In fact, serum IL-6 concentrations are three times higher in patients with obesity and T2D than in normal-weight individuals.

C-reactive Protein

CRP is synthesized in the liver (not in adipose tissue) and is an available, sensitive, and objective indicator of inflammation. It is also an independent predictor of cardiovascular disease and early arterial change. The relationship between adipose tissue and circulating CRP concentration is determined by the production of the immune mediators IL-6 and TNF-α from adipose tissue. Population-based studies have shown that overweight individuals have a higher serum CRP concentration than normal-weight individuals. The magnitude of the serum CRP increase has been correlated to BMI, waist circumference, and serum leptin concentrations.

Plasminogen Activator Inhibitor-1

Plasminogen activator inhibitor type 1 (PAI-1) is a serine-protease inhibitor. It inhibits the production of plasmin in the coagulation cascade, thereby preventing fibrinolysis. Like other proinflammatory adipokines, its circulating level correlates with both the degree of visceral obesity and with other constituents of the metabolic syndrome, including hyperinsulinemia, hypertension, hypertriglyceridemia, increased FFA concentration, increased low-density lipoprotein (LDL) cholesterol, and decreased high-density lipoprotein (HDL) cholesterol concentration. PAI-1 levels can be reduced with weight reduction and physical activity.

The inhibition of fibrinolysis by PAI-1 in combination with obesity-related increases in clotting factors and platelet activation produces a hypercoagulable state that predisposes to thrombosis, atherogenesis, and cardiovascular risk. In individuals with T2D, serum levels of PAI-1 are three times higher than in those without diabetes. Angiotensin-converting enzyme (ACE) inhibitors and angiotensin-receptor blockers have been shown to decrease PAI-1 levels, whereas metformin and thiazolidinediones have been shown to increase PAI-1 activity.

Angiotensinogen

Angiotensinogen and other agents in the RAS, including renin, ACE, angiotensin II (Ang-II), and AT-1 and AT-2 receptors, can be produced and released from visceral adipose tissue deposits. The RAS affects both fluid and electrolyte balance and vascular tone, which, in turn, affects the cardiovascular system. High serum concentrations of angiotensinogen and Ang-II are present in obese individuals and are associated with hypertension, vascular inflammation, angiogenesis, and atheromatous changes. In addition, Ang-II promotes lipogenesis and preadipocyte differentiation, which illustrates the relationship between the RAS and the metabolic syndrome.

CAUSES OF OBESITY

The prevalence of obesity was initially recognized in adults in developed countries. Recently this occurrence has extended to developing countries and to children and adolescents. Most of the obesity seen today is due to a combination of environmental factors and a genetic predisposition. This type is referred to as *primary obesity*. In less than 5% of obese individuals, a specific genetic or secondary cause can be identified.

Primary Causes: Environmental

The startling rise in the prevalence of obesity in the United States in the last two decades has been termed an *epidemic*. This rapid rise in a short period of time points to environmental factors as the major culprit. The expansion of the global food system and its marketing forces has increased the affordability, availability, and accessibility of calorically-dense food. Furthermore, the rise in technology has led to decreased reliance on human labor and activity in food production. Changes in the family structure and school physical education programs during the last three to four decades are among the societal factors that have aggravated the obesity epidemic.

A negative association between socioeconomic status (SES) and education has been noted in many obesity studies. As SES and education decline, obesity rises. This relationship is explained by both exposure to high calorie-dense, palatable, and inexpensive foods (i.e., fast-food restaurants) and an elevated consumption of these foods. Race and ethnicity have also contributed to the obesity epidemic, with African American and Hispanic populations having disproportionately higher obesity rates than non-Hispanic Caucasians. Although often difficult to separate from education and SES, biologic determinants have also been proposed to account for this epidemic. For example, Asian subjects have a higher total body fat mass than Caucasians of equal BMI, which might explain their greater susceptibility to obesity-related T2D.

In addition to physiologic explanations correlating ethnicity and obesity, cultural differences in conceptions of ideal body image exist between non-Hispanic Caucasians, Hispanics, and African Americans, with some cultures valuing overweight or obesity as a sign of health or attractiveness. Studies using standardized quantitative surveys found that African American women had a heavier ideal body image compared to Caucasian women. Clinically overweight African American women were more likely than Caucasian women to perceive themselves as being of normal weight. Those who considered themselves overweight reported less body dissatisfaction compared to Caucasian women. Almost identical results were found among a cohort of Puerto Rican women.

Finally, "social facilitation" describes the "contagious" association of social networks and obesity. Christakis et al. reported that, in Americans, the risk of becoming obese increased by 57% among those who had a friend who became obese during the observation period. In this study the development of obesity was associated with a 40% greater risk of obesity developing in a subject's sibling.

Primary Causes: Genetic

Although lifestyle factors have played a prominent role in the development of obesity, its effect is most significant in individuals who have a permissive genetic profile. Family and twin studies have shown that 40% to 70% of the interindividual variation in obesity susceptibility can be ascribed to genetic differences in the population.

Obesity provides no known survival benefits; to the contrary, an increased proportion of body fat is associated with higher mortality. In the context of modern society, in which food is generally abundant and advances in technology have made life increasingly sedentary, it appears that there is no biologic advantage to being predisposed to obesity. Yet, during periods of hunger and famine endured by our "hunter-gatherer" ancestors, efficient energy storage might have provided a survival advantage. This is the **"thrifty gene hypothesis"** by geneticist James V. Neel. Although Neel originally applied the concept to insulin resistance as an evolutionary response to glucose conservation by the brain, his theory has been extended to include obesity as well.

An alternative explanation to the thrifty gene hypothesis is the **"thrifty phenotype"** hypothesis, first introduced by Hales and Barker. It is based on their clinical observations that poor intrauterine and postnatal nutrition are linked to an increased risk for obesity and T2D later in life. Their theory alleges that fetal malnutrition leads to an enduring modification of metabolic processes that facilitates conservation of energy. The persistence of these modifications into a postnatal environment in which nutrition is ample then promotes obesity and diabetes. In contrast to the slow evolution central to the thrifty gene hypothesis, the thrifty phenotype hypothesis supports the idea of *epigenetic* gene expression as a rapid, real-time adaptation to the fetal environment. Such alterations favor early life survival but result in metabolic dysfunction later in life.

Genome-wide Association Study Loci

Human obesity has genetic components, but they are seldom monogenic. Genome-wide association studies (GWAS) have completely transformed the search for genes that underlie genetically complex traits and diseases, including obesity and its complications. At least 52 genetic loci have been identified through GWAS as having a direct association with obesity-related traits including BMI, body fat percentage, and waist circumference. While promising to expand our understanding of adipose tissue physiology, these loci nevertheless have very minor individual effects and together account for only a small percentage of the total variance of obesity susceptibility. Furthermore, their ability to predict obesity suffers in comparison to that of traditional risk factors, such as parental obesity and childhood obesity. Nonetheless, these loci provide potential insights into the permissive physiologic pathways and gene-environment interactions that underlie obesity susceptibility.

There have been four waves of large-scale high-density GWAS for loci linked specifically to BMI, and altogether 32 loci have been located that reached genome-wide significance. One locus that has consistently been found to be associated with BMI, body fat percentage, and waist circumference is the first intron of the fat mass and obesity-associated gene (**FTO**), which promotes obesity and overeating. It was originally discovered in white European adults, but has recently been associated with obesity-related traits in children and adolescents. In addition, FTO effects were observed in individuals of African, East Asian, and Indian Asian descent. The genotypic effect of FTO, however, manifests more strongly in inactive individuals than in active ones. Individuals who meet daily physical activity recommendations may stave off FTO effects on obesity-related traits, such as T2D, hypertension, and the metabolic syndrome.

Another locus associated with BMI is near the MC4R, the gene that is also implicated in the most common monogenic form of extreme childhood obesity. The **near-MC4R** locus has also been identified in South Asians, East Asians, and African Americans, including children and adolescents. Since it was found downstream of MC4R, it is still unclear whether its association with BMI is connected to the MC4R's role in monogenic obesity or whether it plays a separate role in controlling body mass.

Despite their clear-cut associations, the contributions of these loci must be considered in light of their absolute effect on obesity susceptibility. For example, each FTO risk allele, one of the most prevalent loci and the one with the highest known effect, increases BMI by an average of 0.39 kilograms, with an increase in obesity risk of 1.20 times. Therefore, the FTO locus explains a mere 0.34% of the interindividual variation in BMI. Altogether, the 32 loci identified for BMI represent only 1.45% of the interindividual variation in BMI. In contrast, studies have found that having one obese parent increases an individual's risk of obesity by 2.2 to 3.2 times and having two obese parents increases the odds ratio between 5 and 15.3 times. Furthermore, although obesity during infancy does not increase the risk of adulthood obesity, obesity during the ages of 10 to 14 years increases the risk of adulthood obesity by over 20 times.

The imperfect association between BMI and body fat composition suggests that application of GWAS to a more accurate measure of adiposity (i.e., body fat percentage) might uncover new genetic associations. One locus identified in such studies was near **SPRY2**, which is part of the RAS/mitogen-activated protein kinase pathway and has been implicated in the pathogenesis of T2D in East Asians. An additional locus was found near **IRS1**, which was identified in past GWAS for T2D, cardiovascular disease, and dyslipidemias. Surprisingly, the fat percentage *decreasing* allele of the near-IRS1 gene was associated with an increased risk of T2D, low HDL cholesterol, and cardiovascular disease. On further examination, this allele decreases subcutaneous fat but not the more dangerous visceral fat, implying that it may play a role in fat distribution. Also notable is that although all of the loci that were identified for waist circumference had already been identified for BMI, 14 loci reached genome-wide significance for waist–hip circumference ratio (WHR) when adjusted for BMI, indicating that WHR possibly affects predominantly abdominal obesity rather than overall obesity.

The underlying physiologic pathways represented by the obesity-related loci have yet to be completely elucidated. Most individuals likely carry a large combination of these and many additional unidentified variants. Further research is needed before therapeutic interventions targeted toward specific steps in these pathways can be developed.

Monogenic and Syndromic Obesity

Although rare, and comprising less than 5% of the overall prevalence of obesity, there are certain monogenic forms of severe, early-onset obesity that are due to a single gene mutation (Table 9-2). Genetic syndromes that include obesity can also be caused by a single gene mutation, in which affected individuals have dysmorphic and functional features that are clinically recognizable (Table 9-3). These syndromes, while uncommon, have significant implications for treatment and genetic counseling.

Secondary Causes

The vast majority of obese patients have no identifiable pathological cause. Less than 5% of obese patients have an endocrinopathy contributing to secondary obesity. Usually, a careful history and physical examination provides enough information to determine this pathologic cause of obesity, but there is no one specific finding with ideal predictive value. Children with an endocrine disease that causes them to be overweight or obese are associated with linear growth failure. Modest centripetal obesity is most typical of endocrine conditions compared to the diffuse adiposity of the limbs and trunk seen in patients with primary obesity. Many conditions that suggest an underlying endocrine cause of obesity are also complications of common obesity. For example, hyperglycemia and hypertension are characteristic features of Cushing syndrome, but they also occur in individuals with primary obesity. Individuals with non-specific clinical findings of secondary obesity may require a more detailed investigation to search for a pathologic cause of obesity. Dietary and family histories as well as specific physical findings are helpful in differentiating between primary and secondary causes of obesity (Table 9-4).

TABLE 9-2.	Monogenic Obesity
Gene	**Description**
Leptin	• Deficiency leads to severe, early-onset obesity with uncontrolled hyperphagia • Linear growth normal in childhood • Puberty often delayed secondary to hypogonadotropic hypogonadism • Abnormalities in T-cell number and function
Leptin receptor	• Deficiency leads to severe, early-onset obesity with uncontrolled hyperphagia • Puberty is often delayed secondary to hypogonadotropic hypogonadism
Melanocortin-4 receptor (MCR4)	• Both heterozygous and homozygous mutations • Deficiency leads to early-onset obesity in the setting of hyperphagia • Increases in both fat and lean body mass • Increases in bone mineral density • Accelerated linear growth in childhood • Hyperinsulinemia
Proopiomelanocortin (POMC)	• Incomplete deficiency in early life: adrenal insufficiency, pale skin, and red hair • After glucocorticoid therapy, develop hyperphagia and obesity
Prohormone covertase-1 (PC1)	• Severe early-onset obesity • Hypocortisolemia • Hypogonadotropic hypogonadism • Postprandial (reactive) hypoglycemia

Cushing Syndrome

Cushing syndrome resembles the metabolic syndrome. The high level of circulating glucocorticoids causes insulin resistance in muscle, liver, and adipocytes. Between 20% and 50% of individuals have diabetes, and more than 70% have hypertension. Nearly all individuals with Cushing syndrome are either overweight or obese, and a key finding is abdominal visceral adiposity. Glucocorticoids increase appetite and enhance adipocyte differentiation and lipoprotein lipase activity, more so in visceral than in subcutaneous adipocytes. Effective treatment of hypercortisolism improves all five components of the metabolic syndrome but does not eliminate them completely, especially cardiovascular risk. Therefore, close management of comorbidities such as hypertension, dyslipidemia, and diabetes is imperative in patients with Cushing syndrome, regardless of the cause.

Hypothyroidism

Thyroid hormones increase basal metabolic rate, whereas a decrease in circulating thyroid hormones has a negative effect. Individuals with overt hypothyroidism often present with weight gain, but overt obesity is uncommon. The correlation between thyroid status and obesity is bidirectional, with hypothyroidism influencing an individual's weight and

TABLE 9-3.   Syndromic Obesity

Syndrome	Description
Albright hereditary osteodystrophy (pseudohypoparathyroidism)	• Short stature • Round facies • Subcutaneous ossifications • Brachydactyly and skeletal anomalies • PTH and multiple hormone resistance (types 1A and 1C)
Alström	• Short stature • Blindness • Sensorineural hearing loss • Type 2 diabetes mellitus • Dilated cardiomyopathy (~70%) • Renal, pulmonary, hepatic, and urologic dysfunction • Systemic fibrosis develops over time
Bardet-Biedl	• Late childhood obesity • Retinitis pigmentosa • Polydactyly • Intellectual disability • Hypogonadism • Renal cysts and failure
Börjeson-Forssman-Lehmann	• Severe intellectual disability • Epilepsy • Hypogonadism • Swelling of subcutaneous tissue of face • Narrow palpebral fissures • Large ears
Beckwith-Wiedemann	• Neonatal macrosomia • Postnatal overgrowth and organomegaly • Hyperinsulinemic hypoglycemia • Abdominal wall defects • Macroglossia • Midface hypoplasia • Hemihypertrophy • Increased risk of embryonal tumors
Carpenter	• Craniosynostosis • Polysyndactyly • Cardiac defects
Fragile X	• Prominent lower jaw • Large protruding ears • Macroorchidism • Intellectual disability • Joint hyperextensibility
Prader-Willi	• Short stature • Hyperphagia • Hypotonia • Intellectual disability • Hypogonadotropic hypogonadism • Small hands and feet

(continues)

TABLE 9-3.	Syndromic Obesity *(continued)*
Syndrome	**Description**
Rapid-onset obesity, hypothalamic dysfunction, hypoventilation, autonomic dysregulation (ROHHAD)	• Rapid onset of obesity in first few years of life • Pituitary hormone deficiencies • Prone to death from hypoventilation
Rubinstein-Taybi	• Short stature • Characteristic facial features • Broad thumbs and first toes • Moderate to severe intellectual disability • Eye abnormalities • Heart and kidney defects
WAGR	• **W**ilms tumor • **A**niridia • **G**enitourinary anomalies • Mental **r**etardation

TABLE 9-4.	Distinguishing Primary from Secondary Obesity	
	Primary (Common)	**Secondary**
History	Longstanding problem	Cushing syndrome: past or current steroid use, proximal muscle weakness, rapid onset of centripetal fat distribution, neurologic symptoms (e.g., nocturnal headache, visual field defects), new-onset hypertension or hyperglycemia
	Unhealthy food choices*	Hypothyroidism: cold intolerance, fatigue, constipation, muscle cramps, dysmenorrhea, galactorrhea
	Sedentary*	Polycystic ovary syndrome: oligomenorrhea/amenorrhea, infertility, premature adrenarche
	Family history of obesity	Growth hormone deficiency Children: delayed physical maturation and slow growth velocity Adults: history of brain tumor or radiation, memory loss, fatigue
	Short-term success with weight control efforts in the past	Hypogonadism: delayed or absent puberty, infertility, fatigue, depression/anxiety, dysmenorrhea/amenorrhea, erectile dysfunction
		Hypothalamic obesity: history of central nervous system tumor, radiation, trauma or surgery, hyperphagia, central diabetes insipidus

(continues)

TABLE 9-4.	**Distinguishing Primary from Secondary Obesity (*continued*)**	
	Primary (Common)	**Secondary**
Physical Exam	Normal stature	Cushing syndrome: central obesity, muscle wasting, buffalo hump, moon facies, extensive, wide purple striae at atypical sites, hypertension, virilization
		Hypothyroidism: bradycardia, hypotonia, dry skin, thinning of outer 1/3 of eyebrows, slow relaxation of tendon reflexes
	BMI >30	Polycystic ovary syndrome: central obesity, acne, hirsutism
		Growth hormone deficiency **Children:** short stature, cherubic face, modest central obesity, midline facial anomalies **Adults:** central obesity, reduced muscle mass/strength, baldness in men
	Limbs and trunk affected	Hypogonadism: modest central/visceral obesity, eunuchoid body habitus, dry skin, lack of facial, axillary, and pubic hair, muscle atrophy, gynecomastia, anosmia (Kallman syndrome)
	Thin, pink, or pale striae on abdomen, loins, buttocks, thighs	Hypothalamic obesity: central/visceral obesity, effects of central nervous system injury (cranial nerves, optic discs, mentation)

*Initial history often underestimates caloric intake and overestimates activity

adiposity in addition to obesity directly affecting thyroid function. Studies have also shown that obese individuals have elevated serum TSH levels in the setting of normal free thyroxine (T_4) and normal or elevated free triiodothyronine (T_3) levels. What remains unclear is whether these high TSH levels are a response to increased weight or whether they represent subclinical hypothyroidism and actually contribute to lipid and/ or glucose dysregulation.

Although the mechanism behind the increased TSH and T_3 levels in obese individuals is not completely clear, leptin is definitely a contributing factor, insofar as it enhances gene expression of thyrotropin-releasing hormone from the paraventricular nucleus of the hypothalamus, which eventually stimulates TSH release. Leptin may also promote T_4 to T_3 conversion by deiodinase enzymes in a tissue-specific fashion. Unfortunately, in patients with clinical hypothyroidism who are treated with levothyroxine therapy, the degree of TSH suppression does not have a significant impact on body weight. Many clinicians believe that any weight loss with levothyroxine is principally due to a loss of excess body water.

Polycystic Ovary Syndrome

PCOS also has a striking similarity with the metabolic syndrome, and the extensive overlap between the two entities has led many to speculate that dysregulation of adipose tissue function is the underlying process behind both. Approximately 40% of women with PCOS are obese. Furthermore, women with PCOS are prone to a visceral pattern of fat distribution.

There are no studies that have shown a difference in leptin levels among women with PCOS compared with normal women after controlling for obesity. However, a recent systematic review and metaanalysis showed that women with PCOS had lower levels of adiponectin, which are associated with insulin resistance, and this was regardless of obesity status. Oral contraceptives are the first-line treatment for women with PCOS who are not trying to become pregnant. Metformin provides moderate improvements in metabolic dysfunction when used as adjunct therapy in these women, although the response is variable and may depend on the presence or absence of insulin resistance.

Growth Hormone Deficiency

Adults with GH deficiency have an increased proportion of fat mass, specifically abdominal fat, in addition to disturbances in lipid metabolism, bone mineral density, and increased cardiovascular risk. Isolated GH deficiency rarely leads to severe obesity, but GH replacement in patients who are deficient decreases abdominal fat mass and increases lean tissue mass. This redistribution may have a more significant effect on morbidity and mortality than pure weight loss. Children with GH deficiency present with short stature and also have higher proportions of fat mass, which is distributed more prominently on the trunk than on the limbs. Affected children treated with GH replacement have a return of body fat to normal within several months. The targeted effects of GH replacement on abdominal and visceral obesity to reduce weight in adults with primary obesity have been disappointing.

Hypogonadism

Hypogonadotropic hypogonadism is associated with an increased proportion of abdominal fat and should be included in the differential diagnosis for any adolescent with modest abdominal obesity and pubertal delay. In adults and adolescents, testosterone decreases fat tissue by inhibiting lipoprotein lipase-mediated triglyceride uptake. A deficiency of testosterone leads to triglyceride accumulation in fat tissue.

Female sex hormones also contribute to fat mass distribution and metabolism. This is exemplified by the increase in visceral fat and the associated metabolic disturbances that are seen following menopause, when female sex hormone levels drop precipitously. Estrogen replacement in postmenopausal women leads to a lower WHR as well as improved insulin sensitivity in women with T2D.

As with other forms of secondary obesity, there appears to be a bidirectional relationship between obesity and a form of hypogonadotropic hypogonadism. Males with morbid obesity display a decrease in free testosterone that is believed to be the result of decreased luteinizing hormone (LH) compared to nonobese males of a similar age. One possible explanation for this decrease is that the enhanced conversion of testosterone to estrogen by the enzyme aromatase in excess fat stores leads to an estrogen-driven inhibition of LH via a negative feedback mechanism. An excess of circulating leptin has also been reported to be an LH-inhibiting mechanism in obese males.

Hypothalamic Obesity

Hypothalamic obesity can result from any process that damages the hypothalamus, including head trauma, tumors, radiation, neurosurgery, anoxic brain injury, meningitis, and encephalitis. It can also be due to genetic defects of the melanocortin system and to medications (especially antipsychotic drugs) that interrupt the normal function of the hypothalamic center for energy regulation. Interrupted leptin and insulin actions on the POMC and AGRP/NPY neurons in the arcuate nucleus or disinhibition of vagus nerve control of insulin (via the ventromedial hypothalamus) may be the pathophysiologic mechanism for the higher fasting circulating insulin levels in individuals with hypothalamic obesity compared to individuals with primary obesity.

Severe hyperphagia is a common finding in individuals with hypothalamic obesity, yet obesity can occur even in the absence of hyperphagia. The typical pattern of weight gain is rapid onset that immediately follows hypothalamic injury. This suggests that this initial postinjury phase might be a critical time for intervention. Hypothalamic obesity can be extremely resistant to the typical therapeutic measures of caloric restriction and increased exercise, which may be explained by a defect, not only in appetite control, but also in energy expenditure. Nevertheless, a healthy diet and physical activity should be advocated because animal data suggest that increased exercise may help offset the dysregulated sympathoadrenal activation seen in individuals with hypothalamic obesity.

ENDOCRINOLOGIC COMPLICATIONS OF OBESITY

There are a number of endocrine- and nonendocrine-associated complications that occur as a result of obesity. Because there are an extensive number of nonendocrine-associated complications, this section only reviews the most important endocrine-associated complications including metabolic syndrome, T2D, and dyslipidemia.

Metabolic Syndrome

The metabolic syndrome is a constellation of cardiovascular and endocrinologic comorbidities. Central obesity, defined by waist circumference and ethnicity-specific values, is a mandatory criterion, in addition to at least two of the following laboratory abnormalities: elevated serum triglycerides, reduced serum HDL cholesterol, elevated blood pressure, and elevated fasting plasma glucose. It is estimated that a quarter of the world's adult population has the metabolic syndrome. Individuals with the metabolic syndrome have more than triple the risk of stroke and heart attack compared to those without it. Metabolic syndrome is no longer an adult-only disease; these biochemical disturbances exist in more than 25% of obese adolescents. Formal criteria for establishing the diagnosis of the metabolic syndrome in children have not been established.

Insulin resistance appears to be the primary pathogenic process underlying the metabolic syndrome. It is defined as the inability to suppress hepatic glucose output and stimulate glucose uptake in muscle and adipocytes that leads to glucose intolerance and T2D in predisposed individuals. The exact etiology of insulin resistance has yet to be determined, but obesity and its associated adipokine profile are implicated in its pathogenesis. The inflammatory cytokines, such as TNF-α and IL-6, are both increased in obesity and interfere with the insulin-receptor signaling pathway. The overabundance of macrophages in adipose tissue produces an excess of the proinflammatory mediators TNF-α, IL-1, and resistin. These mediators affect multiple transcription factors that interfere with normal insulin action, which results in insulin resistance. In addition, adiponectin, an insulin sensitizer, is abnormally low in obese individuals.

It is critical that physicians monitor obese individuals for the abnormal laboratory components of the metabolic syndrome and carefully control the blood pressure, blood glucose, and lipid profile abnormalities.

Type 2 Diabetes Mellitus

Obesity increases the risk of T2D in predisposed individuals by increasing insulin resistance and reducing pancreatic β-cell function. Insulin resistance is a reversible process, but it has a complex etiology. The most important pathophysiologic components are altered production of adipokines, FFAs, and inflammatory mediators by adipose tissue. Excess adiposity itself, however, does not cause insulin resistance. For instance, individuals with obesity secondary to Prader-Willi syndrome are more insulin sensitive than are BMI-matched individuals with primary obesity. This conclusion is based on insulin and glucose levels measured in the fasting state and using the euglycemic blood glucose clamp procedures. Although subcutaneous fat predominates over visceral fat, it is not certain that this accounts entirely for the preservation of insulin action in peripheral tissues (i.e., muscle, adipose tissue, and liver).

To compensate for systemic insulin resistance, obese individuals who are euglycemic develop increased β-cell mass and function. The β-cells of these obese individuals may increase in volume by 50% and release up to five times more insulin, compared to the β-cells of nonobese individuals. FFAs, released by adipose tissue, are elevated in those with obesity and T2D. Chronic exposure to FFAs has been associated with decreased insulin synthesis as well as glucose-stimulated insulin release. Therefore, FFAs may be the link between insulin resistance and β-cell dysfunction.

Dyslipidemia

Obesity is associated with several lipid abnormalities, including hypertriglyceridemia, increased LDL, and reduced HDL. These metabolic disturbances are most prevalent in individuals who have a predominantly central fat distribution. The average triglyceride concentration of an obese individual (BMI >30) is more than 60 mg/dL greater than individuals with a BMI less than 21 mg/dL. For every one-unit increase in BMI, there is an associated decrease of 1.1 mg/dL in HDL in men and 0.6 mg/dL in women. Taken together, these dyslipidemias are atherogenic and increase risk for serious cardiovascular disease. Exercise and even moderate weight loss may improve the lipid profile and reduce cardiovascular disease risk.

NONENDOCRINOLOGIC COMPLICATIONS OF OBESITY

An exhaustive discussion of the nonendocrinologic complications of obesity is beyond the scope of this chapter. Serious complications that affect almost every organ system may affect an obese individual's quality of life and mortality. See Table 9-5 for many of the endocrine and nonendocrine complications of obesity.

ASSESSMENT OF OBESITY

The U.S. Preventive Services Task Force (USPSTF) recommended that all adults be screened for obesity, and that all patients with a BMI of 30 or more should receive intensive, multicomponent behavioral interventions.

TABLE 9-5.	**Complications of Obesity**
Cardiovascular/ Cerebrovascular	*Hypertension* • Every 10% increase in body weight is associated with a 6.5 mmHg increase in systolic blood pressure. *Coronary Heart Disease* • The proinflammatory state of obesity is an independent risk factor for coronary disease, independent of age, smoking status, hypercholesterolemia, and diabetes. *Cerebrovascular Disease* • Men and women in the third or fourth quartiles of waist–hip circumference ratio have twice as high risk of stroke as those in the bottom quartile.
Pulmonary	*Obstructive Sleep Apnea (OSA)* • Approximately 60–90% of OSA patients are obese. *Obesity Hypoventilation Syndrome* • Leptin is implicated as a neurohumoral modulator impacting CO_2 chemosensitivity and increased minute ventilation.
Musculoskeletal	*Knee Osteoarthritis* • Leptin is implicated in the direct proinflammatory and catabolic role of cartilage metabolism, whereas adiponectin appears to be protective. *Gout* • Obesity more than triples the risk of developing gout, not only by increasing uric acid production but also by decreasing renal excretion.
Gastrointestinal	*Gallstones* • Obesity is a risk factor for gallstones due to the increased saturation of bile with cholesterol. *Pancreatitis* • Obesity is a risk factor for exacerbating and increasing the complications of acute pancreatitis and the severity and susceptibility to acute pancreatitis have been linked to adipokines including adiponectin, leptin, visfatin, and resistin. *Liver Disease* • The increased metabolism and release of free fatty acids by visceral fat into the portal circulation decreases the clearance of insulin by the liver and increases hepatic secretion of glucose and very low-density lipoprotein.
Cancer	• It is estimated that obesity accounts for 1 in 7 cancer deaths in men and 1 in 5 in women. Obesity is a preventable risk factor for cancers of the colon, female breast, endometrium, kidney, and esophagus.
Psychiatric	• Obesity has been implicated as both a cause and effect of low self-esteem, mood disorders, impaired social interactions, and eating disorders.

Screening

After examining intensive behavioral interventions, the USPSTF found that weight loss improved glucose tolerance and other cardiovascular risk factors. Height, weight, and BMI of all children should be plotted on standardized growth charts. Those with a BMI in the overweight or obese category (see Table 9-1) require special attention and treatment. Children with a normal BMI but an obese first-degree relative (especially mothers) should also be considered at risk for obesity.

Clinical Evaluation

A complete evaluation of an obese individual should focus on both the cause and its complications. Patients and/or clinicians may be uncomfortable initiating a discussion about an overweight or obesity problem. A health-care provider may prevent this uneasiness by commenting on an objective observation (e.g., BMI) and then asking the patient for permission to discuss this abnormality. Motivational interviewing is a technique of directing a patient-provider encounter toward specific problems emphasizing those that the patient feels are most important. Although this approach is a departure from the traditional patient-provider encounter, it encourages a trusting relationship that is an essential element when discussing obesity. A thorough weight history, including maximum body weight, history of weight gain, patterns of food consumption (including meal omission, binge eating, private eating, food hoarding), and physical activity (type, frequency, duration, and intensity) are required. Insight is often gained by asking a patient to link adiposity changes to major life milestones (e.g., college, bereavement, employment, illness). The assessment should also include risk factors and medications, especially corticosteroids, thiazolidinediones, and antipsychotics.

A complete physical examination should focus on the individual's affect, height, weight, BMI, heart rate, and blood pressure. Cutaneous manifestations of insulin resistance are extremely important to discern and include acanthosis nigricans (Figure 9-1), skin tags, monilia, abscess formation, or violaceous striae. These may help clinicians make the appropriate diagnosis and also provide concrete evidence for the patient's treatment. Hepatomegaly, cardiomegaly, and respiratory problems are additional physical signs that suggest obesity complications. A determination of a patient's willingness to make changes in order to lose weight is a vital part of the discussion and evaluation, because it is predictive of a successful outcome.

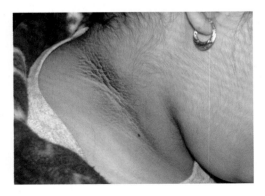

FIGURE 9-1. Acanthosis nigricans. Linear, alternating dark and light pigmentation becomes more apparent when the skin is stretched. (From Goodheart HP. Goodheart's Photoguide of Common Skin Disorders. 2nd ed. Philadelphia, PA: Lippincott Williams & Wilkins; 2003.)

The initial laboratory evaluations should be directed by the history and physical examination findings. Occult complications can be uncovered by measuring fasting blood glucose, lipids, and liver function tests (e.g., transaminases and γ-glutamyl transferase). More extensive evaluations for high-risk individuals should include a chest X-ray, electrocardiogram, echocardiogram, and serum levels of 25-hydroxy vitamin D_3 and CRP. An oral glucose tolerance test is required, and is superior to serum insulin levels, for identifying individuals who have or are at risk for developing T2D.

MANAGEMENT OF OBESITY

Management or treatment of obese individuals involves a number of factors and options. The most important factor in the management of obesity is lifestyle modification in which obese individuals must make changes to their behavior, diet, and exercise. For obese individuals who are unable to improve their weight with lifestyle modification and/or who are at risk for complications from obesity, pharmacologic agents and surgical procedures are options.

Lifestyle Modifications

The National Heart, Lung, and Blood Institute recommend diet, physical activity, and behavioral therapy for all patients with a BMI >25. Although there are many different diets, losing weight ultimately requires consumption of fewer calories than is expended throughout the day. In the absence of physical activity, a sustained daily decrease of 500 kilocalories/day will generate a weight loss of 1 lb/week. Common dietary strategies include eating a nourishing breakfast, increasing the amount of dietary fiber consumed, eating several smaller meals throughout the day, and using commercial meal replacement plans. Of those strategies, only meal replacements have proved successful in randomized controlled trials. In the primary care setting, the involvement of a dietician has been shown to improve weight reduction.

Diet

There are currently four major diet subtypes: low-fat diet, low-carbohydrate diet, low glycemic index (GI) diet, and high-protein diet. The low-fat diet relies on restricting dietary fats to less than 30% of the total caloric intake. The Lifestyle Heart Trial, a clinical trial involving dietary counseling, moderate exercise, and a low-fat diet (only 7% of all calories came from fat) resulted in a weight loss of 24 lbs after 1 year and a reduction of coronary heart disease at 5 years. Unfortunately, low-fat diets are difficult to maintain on a long-term basis.

The low-carbohydrate diet has been studied extensively and is now commercialized into the *Atkins* and *South Beach* diets. These plans typically start with less than 20 grams of carbohydrates per day. Randomized trials found that diets low in carbohydrates benefited patients with hyperglycemia by decreasing fasting glucose levels as well as lowering plasma triglycerides and increasing HDL cholesterol levels. Unfortunately, this diet also led to increased LDL cholesterol levels.

The low glycemic index diet is based on limiting the consumption of foods that raise postprandial blood glucose levels. According to the glycemic index scale, consuming pure glucose has a rating of 100, whereas consuming oatmeal has a glycemic index of 42. Items with a rating less than 55 have a low glycemic index. In randomized trials, the low glycemic index diet did not promote weight loss beyond the mechanism of caloric restriction. Plasma insulin levels were reduced with this diet, but it is not known whether or not this translates into beneficial clinical outcomes.

High-protein diets increase satiety and meal-induced thermogenesis. In randomized trials, protein was substituted for carbohydrates in calorie-restricted diets. Individuals who consumed more protein had greater weight loss. High-protein diets also appeared to provide better long-term maintenance of reduced intraabdominal fat stores compared with low-protein diets.

Exercise

Even without diet modification, increased physical activity may reduce visceral adipose tissue and improve insulin resistance. However, absolute weight loss associated with exercise alone is minimal. A synergistic relationship exists between diet and exercise, with greater reductions in triglyceride levels and blood pressure among cohorts who do both, compared with those who only do one. It is recommended that all overweight and obese patients who exercise also follow a calorie-restricted diet for optimal weight loss and improvement in their metabolic profile.

Behavioral Therapy

The basis of behavioral therapy relies on an increased self-awareness of weight, physical activity, goal setting, and stimulus control (e.g., identifying and limiting exposure to situations that may encourage incidental eating). Cognitive restructuring (i.e., changing self-defeating thoughts and feelings that undermine weight-loss efforts) and a strong social support system are critical. In most studies, behavioral treatment may help individuals lose up to 10% of body weight in 6 months.

Pharmacologic Management

For some patients, pharmacologic therapy is an appropriate addition to diet and exercise. Current guidelines recommend the use of pharmacologic weight-loss agents in patients with a BMI more than 30 or in patients with a BMI more than 27 who have a comorbid condition such as diabetes, hypertension, and/or hypercholesterolemia. It is important to educate patients about the role pharmacotherapy plays in the weight-loss program. The role of the medication is to help an individual stay on a diet and exercise plan, not to replace it. In the United States, there are currently five Food and Drug Administration (FDA)-approved medications for weight reduction: phentermine, diethylpropion, Qsymia™, lorcaserin, and orlistat. These medications may be divided into two classes: satiety increasers, or appetite suppressants (the first four) and nutrient-absorption inhibitors (orlistat).

Metformin is an antihyperglycemic agent used in the treatment of T2D. Although it is not approved for use as an adjuvant therapy in weight-loss programs, empiric observations suggest BMI may be reduced by metformin treatment, especially in adults.

Appetite Suppressants

Phentermine and **diethylpropion** decrease appetite by increasing the pre-synaptic release of norepinephrine. In randomized controlled trials, weight reduction was 4% greater in the experimental group compared to those receiving a placebo. Due to their sympathomimetic mechanism of action, blood pressure must be closely monitored in prehypertensive or hypertensive patients on medical therapy. Although these drugs have only been approved for short-term use (less than 12 weeks), some studies suggest that these medications may be effective for up to 10 years.

In 2012, the FDA approved two new weight-loss drugs, Qsymia™ (phentermine and topiramate), an appetite suppressant and anticonvulsant medication, and lorcaserin. The precise mechanism of action is unknown, but, in clinical trials, there was an additional 10% weight loss compared with placebo. **Lorcaserin** is a serotonin 2C-receptor agonist. In randomized, placebo-controlled trials, 48% of patients receiving lorcaserin had lost greater than 5% of their body weight (i.e., more than twice the amount of patients on placebo). Over the 12 months of the clinical trial, patients had significant improvements in serum lipid, insulin, and fasting blood glucose levels. Although past serotonin agonists increased the risk of mitral and aortic valvulopathies, the serotonin 2B receptor present on heart valves is not triggered by lorcaserin. No risk of heart disease has been reported to date. The makers of both lorcaserin and Qsymia™ are sponsoring extensive postmarketing trials to further establish the safety of these medications.

Nutrient Absorption Inhibitor

Orlistat is a triacylglycerol lipase inhibitor that reduces dietary fat absorption by up to 30% in the intestinal lumen. Combined with lifestyle changes, orlistat reduced body weight 3% more than lifestyle modification alone. In the Prevention of Diabetes in Obese Subjects trial, orlistat also reduced the incidence of diabetes, with a risk reduction of 37%. Its use is often limited by the adverse GI effects caused by fat malabsorption.

Metformin

Metformin suppresses hepatic gluconeogenesis and enhances insulin sensitivity by activating hepatic adenosine monophosphate kinase. It causes significant GI distress, an effect that partially contributes to drug-induced weight loss. Patients receiving metformin often lose weight without any change in energy expenditure, indicating that the weight loss may result from decreased food intake. Typical weight loss of 2 to 6 lbs is published with a maximum of 22 lbs reported in one study. Other popular "off-label" applications of metformin have exploited its ability to reduce androgen production in women with PCOS and to potentially delay the onset of T2D in people with abnormal glucose tolerance. However, repeated and consistent reports of benefit are lacking. Although metformin may be a safe pharmacologic therapy for weight loss, it is probably best reserved for patients with T2D who may simultaneously derive benefit from drug-induced weight loss.

Surgical Treatment

A 1991 National Institutes of Health consensus conference recommended that surgery be considered only for motivated obese patients who meet BMI eligibility criteria, who have a good understanding of the risks, and, in whom the benefits of surgery outweigh the risks. Patients with a BMI >40 or >35 with serious comorbidities such as obstructive sleep apnea and other cardiopulmonary diseases were recommended as potential candidates. These eligibility criteria are subject to revision, however, as the balance between risk and benefit changes with time. With increasing experience, surgical complications have become less frequent. This reduction in complication rate may be due to less stringent criteria (i.e., lower presurgical BMI). Such bias in case selection is suggested by the exponential increase in the use of surgical therapies. The number of bariatric surgeries per year has increased from 13,386 in 1998 to over 220,000 in 2008.

Although there are numerous forms of bariatric surgery, the two most common operations are the Roux-en-Y gastric bypass and the adjustable gastric band (Figure 9-2). Sleeve gastrectomy is a recent innovation that is rapidly gaining popularity, but it has not

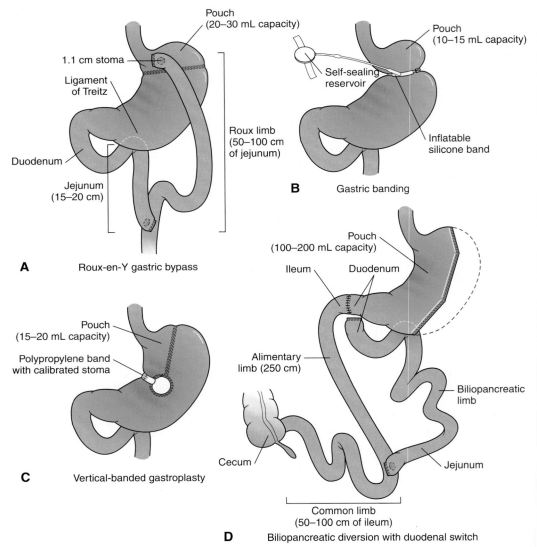

FIGURE 9-2. Surgical procedures for morbid obesity. **(A)** Roux-en-Y gastric bypass. A horizontal row of staples across the fundus of the stomach creates a pouch with a capacity of 20 to 30 mL. The jejunum is divided distal to the ligament of Trietz and the distal end is anastomosed to the new pouch. The proximal segment is anastomosed to the jejunum. **(B)** Gastric banding. A prosthetic device is used to restrict oral intake by creating a small pouch of 10 to 15 mL that empties through the narrow outlet into the remainder of the stomach. **(C)** Vertical-banded gastroplasty. A vertical row of staples along the lesser curvature of the stomach creates a new, smaller stomach pouch of 10 to 15 mL. **(D)** Biliopancreatic diversion with duodenal switch. Half of the stomach is removed, leaving a small area that holds about 60 mL. The entire jejunum is excluded from the rest of the GI tract. The duodenum is disconnected and sealed off. The ileum is divided above the ileocecal junction and the distal end of the jejunum is anastomosed to the first portion of the duodenum. The distal end of the biliopancreatic limb is anastomosed to the ileum.

yet been subjected to long-term scrutiny. All of these procedures anatomically modify the GI tract to decrease gastric food capacity. The gastric bypass operation decreases the stomach to 30 cc, or the size of a golf ball, and then connects the new stomach to a point in the proximal jejunum, about 30 cm below the ligament of Treitz. The adjustable gastric band is a small bracelet placed around the stomach to create a small proximal compartment. Both of these procedures are associated with postoperative vomiting, nutritional deficiencies, and **dumping syndrome**, in which ingested foods bypass the stomach and enter the small intestine mostly undigested. Both gastric bypass and gastric banding induce significant weight loss. Though gastric bypass typically results in more weight loss than the banding procedure, it is associated with a higher risk of complications. In a study of 1,035 patients who underwent bariatric surgery in the Swedish Obese Subjects trial, the mean BMI decreased from 50 to 33 in 2 years, and overall mortality decreased by more than 30% compared with the control group, which received conventional lifestyle modification therapy.

In a large meta-analysis of over 22,000 subjects, Buchwald et al. reported that 76.8% of the patients who had T2D underwent remission after surgery. The remission percentage varied based on the procedure, from 48% of all patients who had undergone adjustable gastric banding to 99% who had a biliopancreatic bypass. Unfortunately, recurrence of diabetes occurred in almost 25% of patients after the gastric bypass procedure, especially those who had a lower preoperative BMI and those who regained a greater percentage of their weight. The mechanism of improved glycemic control appears to involve improvements in insulin sensitivity through increased release of the incretins GLP-1 and GIP.

CASE FOLLOW-UP

Mild fatigue and postprandial abdominal pain in a severely obese individual requires further investigation. Although this woman's obesity may be secondary to diet and lack of exercise, it is important to rule out treatable causes such as hypothyroidism. A serum TSH level is a sufficient screening test, although 10% to 15% of obese individuals have obesity-induced hyperthyrotropinemia that will require further evaluation including measurement of free T_4 and autoantibodies against thyroid peroxidase and thyroglobulin. Postprandial abdominal pain has many causes, but this patient is at particular risk for gastroesophageal reflux, esophagitis, constipation, and diabetic autonomic neuropathy that causes gastroparesis and cholelithiasis. Her ethnicity, age, and gender make gallbladder disease a likely cause of her symptoms.

The laboratory report shows a normal serum TSH with an elevated fasting blood glucose level. An abdominal ultrasound reveals a 0.4-cm gallstone near the neck of the gallbladder. On her return visit, her blood pressure measurement is elevated with the lowest of three automated blood pressure measurements at her pharmacy being 135/90 mmHg. Her current problem list now includes obesity, stage 1 hypertension, dyslipidemia, impaired fasting glucose, and cholelithiasis. Almost all of these conditions may improve with weight loss, with the exception of cholelithiasis, which may worsen during rapid weight loss. At her clinic visit she is educated about the importance of losing weight and setting up a weight-loss strategy. Before attempting pharmacologic treatment or bariatric surgery, it is imperative that the patient make a concerted attempt to lose weight through lifestyle modification. Setting up an appointment with a dietician is essential. If she will be considered for pharmacotherapy or bariatric

(continues)

> **CASE FOLLOW-UP** (*continued*)
>
> surgery, an exercise physiologist and a behavioral therapist should be consulted. Cardiovascular and orthopedic evaluations are also necessary to determine the intensity of activity this patient can tolerate.
>
> It is also important to address her hypercholesterolemia and hypertension. Although her calculated Framingham risk score is less than 5%, her LDL cholesterol is above the threshold of 160 mg/dL. Treatment with a statin medication is indicated at this time. Her hypertension should be treated with a single antihypertensive agent, such as a thiazide diuretic. A smoking history and family history of premature cardiovascular disease may be decisive factors in determining the risk/benefit ratio of more intensive therapies.
>
> The last issue that must be addressed concerns her cholelithiasis. The indication for a cholecystectomy is based on her symptoms, and a referral to a general surgeon is warranted. Despite the benefit of combining a cholecystectomy with a bariatric surgical procedure and the advantages of a single anesthetic, a cholecystectomy should not be accompanied by a bariatric procedure in the short term, because months of obesity management are still required. She will undergo the cholecystectomy and, shortly thereafter, will begin a lifestyle behavior-modification program to lose weight.

REFERENCES and SUGGESTED READINGS

Baggio LL, Drucker DJ. Biology of incretins: GLP-1 and GIP. Gastroenterology. 2007;132(6):2131–2157.

Barness LA, Opitz JM, Gilbert-Barness E. Obesity: genetic, molecular, and environmental aspects. Am J Med Gen Part A. 2007;143A(24):3016–3034.

Chanson P, Salenave S. Metabolic syndrome in Cushing's syndrome. Neuroendocrinology. 2010;92 (suppl 1):96–101.

Chung WK. An overview of mongenic and syndromic obesities in humans. Pediatr Blood Cancer. 2012;58(1):122–128.

Clifton PM. Bariatric surgery: effects on the metabolic complications of obesity. Curr Atheroscler Rep. 2012;14(2):95–100.

Eckel RH. Clinical practice. Nonsurgical management of obesity in adults. N Engl J Med. 2008;358(18): 1941–1950.

Farooqi IS, et al. Clinical and molecular genetic spectrum of congenital deficiency of the leptin receptor. N Engl J Med. 2007;356(3):237–247.

Flegal KM, et al. Prevalence and trends in obesity among US adults, 1999–2010. JAMA. 2012; 307(5):491–497.

Gale SM, Castracane VD, Mantzoros CS. Energy homeostasis, obesity and eating disorders: recent advances in endocrinology. J Nutr. 2004;134(2):295–298.

Gnacinska M, et al. Role of adipokines in complications related to obesity: a review. Adv Med Sci. 2009;54(2):150–157.

Guyenet SJ, Schwartz MW. Regulation of food intake, energy balance, and body fat mass: implications for the pathogenesis and treatment of obesity. J Clin Endocrinol Metab. 2012;97(3):745–755.

Hagan S, Niswender KD. Neuroendocrine regulation of food intake. Pediatr Blood Cancer. 2012;58(1):149–153.

Hutley L, Prins JB. Fat as an endocrine organ: relationship to the metabolic syndrome. Am J Med Sci. 2005;330(6):280–289.

Kahn SE, Hull RL, Utzschneider KM. Mechanisms linking obesity to insulin resistance and type 2 diabetes. Nature. 2006;444(7121):840–846.

Lazar MA. How obesity causes diabetes: not a tall tale. Science. 2005;307(5708):373–375.

Lee M, Korner J. Review of physiology, clinical manifestations, and management of hypothalamic obesity in humans. Pituitary. 2009;12(2):87–95.

Loos RJF. Genetic determinants of common obesity and their value in prediction. Best Pract Res Clin Endocrinol Metab. 2012;26(2):211–226.

Pacifico L, et al. Thyroid function in childhood obesity and metabolic comorbidity. Clin Chim Acta. 2012;413(3–4):396–405.

Rasmussen MH. Obesity, growth hormone and weight loss. Mol Cell Endocrinol. 2010;316(2):147–153.

Sabin MA, Werther GA, Kiess W. Genetics of obesity and overgrowth syndromes. Best Pract Res Clin Endocrinol Metab. 2011;25(1):207–220.

Villa J, Pratley R. Adipose tissue dysfunction in polycystic ovary syndrome. Curr Diabetes Rep. 2011;11(3):179–184.

CHAPTER REVIEW QUESTIONS

1. Obesity is associated with an elevated level of all of the following molecules, *except*:

A. Leptin
B. Adiponectin
C. Interleukin-6
D. Insulin
E. Free fatty acids

2. Taken together, the monogenic causes of obesity established to date account for approximately what percentage of severe obesity?

A. 0.1%
B. 1.0%
C. 5.0%
D. 10%
E. 15%

3. The criteria necessary for diagnosis of the metabolic syndrome include which of the following?

A. Elevated BMI, reduced HDL cholesterol, elevated LDL cholesterol, elevated blood pressure, and elevated fasting plasma glucose
B. Elevated BMI, elevated triglycerides, elevated LDL cholesterol, elevated blood pressure, and elevated fasting plasma glucose
C. Central obesity, elevated LDL cholesterol, reduced HDL cholesterol, elevated blood pressure, and elevated fasting plasma glucose
D. Central obesity, elevated triglycerides, reduced HDL cholesterol, elevated blood pressure, and elevated fasting plasma insulin
E. Central obesity, elevated triglycerides, reduced HDL cholesterol, elevated blood pressure, and elevated fasting plasma glucose

4. All of the following medications help patients lose weight via an increase in norepinephrine or serotonin, thus increasing satiety and suppressing appetite except:

A. Diethylpropion
B. Orlistat
C. Phentermine
D. Qsymia™
E. Lorcaserin

5. A 47-year-old Caucasian female presents to your office for an annual physical exam. She is 5 ft 2 in tall and weighs 240 lbs (BMI = 43.9). Her past medical history includes hypertension, osteoarthritis, T2D, hypercholesterolemia, and obstructive sleep apnea. Current medications include lisinopril, metoprolol, atorvastatin, and metformin. She uses a bilevel positive airway pressure machine at night (BIPAP). She recently quit her job, as the pain from her osteoarthritis made getting out of bed unbearable, and has been feeling more fatigued than usual. She is embarrassed about her weight and has developed agoraphobia over the past few years. She has been working with your dietician to lose weight for the past 3 years but this has been unsuccessful despite caloric restriction and exercise. She has attempted pharmacologic therapy with phentermine and orlistat without success. The next best step in management is:

A. Increase her BIPAP settings because her current pressures may be insufficient.

B. Check TSH for possible hypothyroidism.

C. Increase her antihypertensive medications.

D. Implement a trial of Qsymia™ in addition to caloric restriction and exercise.

E. Refer her to a bariatric surgery specialist.

CHAPTER REVIEW ANSWERS

1. The correct answer is B. Obesity has been found in association with elevated serum levels of leptin (**Choice A**), IL-6 (**Choice C**), insulin (**Choice D**), and free fatty acids (**Choice E**) but an inverse relationship exists between obesity and adiponectin levels.

2. The correct answer is C. Monogenic forms of obesity are rare and comprise only a small fraction of the overall prevalence of obesity. Monogenic causes of obesity account for less than 5% of severe obesity. These include mutations in the gene for leptin, the leptin receptor, the melanocortin-4 receptor (MCR4), proopiomelanocortin (POMC), and prohormone covertase-1 (PC1).

3. The correct answer is E. Central obesity, defined by waist circumference and ethnicity-specific values, is a mandatory criterion for establishing a diagnosis of metabolic syndrome. This reflects the metabolically adverse effects of increased visceral obesity, which are not fully accounted for by BMI alone (**Choices A and B**). In addition to central obesity, at least two of the following four factors must also be present: elevated triglycerides, reduced HDL cholesterol, elevated blood pressure, and elevated fasting plasma glucose, not insulin (**Choice D**). Elevated LDL cholesterol (**Choices A, B, and C**) is NOT one of the criterion for diagnosing metabolic syndrome.

4. The correct answer is B. As of August 2012, there are only five medications approved for weight reduction: diethylpropion, orlistat, phentermine, Qsymia™, and lorcaserin. Of these, orlistat is the only one that is not an appetite suppressant. Its primary mechanism of action works at reducing the absorption of fats from the human intestine by inhibiting pancreatic lipases. In clinical trials, patients taking orlistat achieved on average a 5% decrease in body mass.

5. The correct answer is E. The patient is morbidly obese with numerous comorbidities such as hypertension, obstructive sleep apnea, T2D, and hypercholesterolemia. Obesity has impacted her physical, social, and psychological well-being. After unsuccessfully working with a dietician on caloric restriction, exercise, and pharmacologic intervention, the next step is to assess her as a candidate for bariatric surgery.

Adrenal Gland Disorders

Josh A. Hammel
Guillermo E. Umpierrez

CASE

A 44-year-old woman presents to the trauma center at a local hospital following a car accident. On arrival, she is conscious but drowsy, tachycardic (120 beats/minute), and hypotensive (70/40 mmHg). She has several rib fractures and complains of severe back pain. There is no major external bleeding. After a rapid infusion of 2 L of normal saline, her blood pressure remains low (80/50 mmHg).

This chapter begins with a review of adrenal gland physiology and proceeds to the etiology, evaluation, and treatment of disorders of adrenal insufficiency and adrenal excess to help readers develop hypotheses for the etiology of this woman's hypotension, hyponatremia, and hyperkalemia. We provide a summary of the work-up and a therapeutic plan at the end of the chapter to give the learner a better understanding of this entity.

OBJECTIVES

1. List the etiology of hypofunction and hyperfunction of the adrenal gland.

2. Recognize the clinical and laboratory findings in patients with abnormal adrenal gland function.

3. Describe the evaluation and management of patients with abnormal adrenal gland function.

CHAPTER OUTLINE

(continues)

PHYSIOLOGY

The adrenal gland is made up of two separate organs, the **adrenal medulla** and the **adrenal cortex**. The adrenal medulla produces the catecholamines—epinephrine, norepinephrine, and dopamine. These hormones activate the sympathetic nervous system (SNS) during periods of stress. The adrenal cortex produces steroid hormones that regulate metabolism, electrolyte/fluid balance, and gonadal function.

Adrenal Medulla

The adrenal medulla resides in the innermost portion of the adrenal gland and houses granule-containing cells responsible for the production of catecholamines. The medulla is a collection of postsynaptic cells in the SNS that release hormones into the bloodstream rather than synapsing on a target tissue. Approximately 90% of the cells in the adrenal medulla produce epinephrine, with the remainder responsible for norepinephrine and dopamine production. Norepinephrine is a derivative of tyrosine, and epinephrine is formed by methylation of norepinephrine.

The adrenal medulla secretes catecholamines under control of the SNS. Basal secretion of catecholamines is very low; however, under periods of stress, sympathetic activity results in release of catecholamines into the bloodstream in preparation for a "fight or flight" response. Epinephrine and norepinephrine act on multiple α- and β-adrenergic receptors to elicit various effects in target tissues. Vasoconstrictive and vasodilatory effects are prominent in different tissues, as are positive chronotropic and inotropic effects on the heart. Epinephrine and norepinephrine increase the metabolic rate; stimulate glycogenolysis; and raise blood glucose, free fatty acids, and lactate levels. Epinephrine and norepinephrine also increase alertness.

Adrenal Cortex

The adrenal cortex is composed of three zones based on structure and function: 1) zona glomerulosa, 2) zona fasciculata, and 3) zona reticularis (Figure 10-1). The outermost

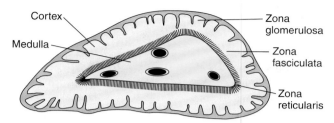

FIGURE 10-1. Adrenal cortex. The adrenal gland, showing the medulla (site of epinephrine and norepinephrine synthesis) and the three layers of the cortex. The zona glomerulosa is the outer layer of the cortex and is primarily responsible for mineralocorticoid production. The middle layer, the zona fasciculata, and the inner layer, the zona reticularis, produce the glucocorticoids and the adrenal sex hormones, respectively. (From Porth CM. Pathophysiology Concepts of Altered Health States. 7th ed. Philadelphia, PA: Lippincott Williams & Wilkins; 2005.)

zona glomerulosa is responsible for production of the mineralocorticoids that maintain sodium, potassium, and fluid balance. The middle zona fasciculata is the largest zone and makes up 80% of the cortex. It produces glucocorticoids that affect metabolism of glucose and proteins. The innermost zona reticularis secretes androgens.

Cholesterol forms the backbone of all of the products of the adrenal cortex. Cholesterol derivatives are classified by the number of carbon atoms in their backbone. The human adrenal cortex produces mostly C_{19} and C_{21} steroids. C_{19} steroids are androgens, whereas C_{21} steroids have varying degrees of glucocorticoid and mineralocorticoid activity.

Cortisol (hydrocortisone) is the main glucocorticoid produced in the adrenal cortex. It drives many metabolic reactions that involve all three macronutrients as well as maintenance of blood pressure. Cortisol has counterregulatory action to insulin, so it increases blood glucose by increasing hepatic glucose production (gluconeogenesis) and decreasing glucose uptake in peripheral tissues. Circulating levels of cortisol are increased during hypoglycemia (insulin-counterregulatory effect). In the absence of cortisol, hypoglycemia may occur due to the inability to sustain gluconeogenesis. In addition, without cortisol, individuals may develop hypotension caused by the inability of the vascular system to respond to the pressor effects of catecholamines.

Cortisol production is controlled by adrenocorticotropic hormone (ACTH) secretion from the anterior pituitary. ACTH secretion is stimulated by the hypothalamic secretion of corticotropin-releasing hormone (CRH). Through its negative feedback effect, elevated levels of cortisol can inhibit production of both ACTH and CRH, a system that is known as *the hypothalamic–pituitary–adrenal (HPA) axis* (Figure 10-2).

Aldosterone is the main mineralocorticoid, governing retention and excretion of sodium and potassium, thereby indirectly affecting the water balance of the entire body. Aldosterone functions to retain sodium; it acts on the collecting ducts in the kidney to cause increased exchange of sodium for potassium and hydrogen ions, resulting in a loss of potassium and acidification of the urine.

Three factors control secretion of aldosterone: the renin-angiotensin system (RAS), ACTH from the HPA axis, and the plasma concentration of potassium. Angiotensin II, the terminal signal of the RAS that is secreted during hypovolemic states, stimulates secretion of aldosterone. Aldosterone, in turn, acts on the kidney causing it to retain sodium and water, to conserve volume and maintain blood pressure. Increased levels of ACTH also increase aldosterone secretion, but only temporarily (i.e., 1 to 2 days). Finally, increases in plasma potassium concentrations cause aldosterone secretion to promote potassium diuresis and maintain a normokalemic state.

Androstenedione and dehydroepiandrosterone (DHEA), both 1-carbon steroid hormones, are the two major androgens produced in the adrenal cortex. Androstenedione is

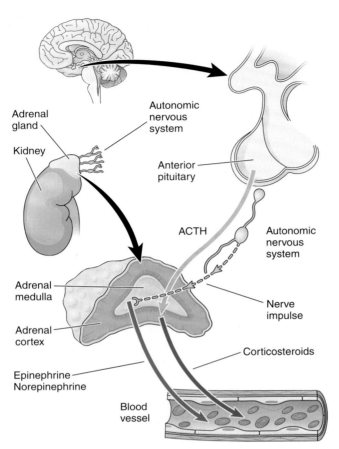

FIGURE 10-2. Hypothalamic–pituitary–adrenal (HPA) axis. Normal adrenal gland. The cortex and the medulla secrete hormones directly into blood—the cortex under command of pituitary ACTH, the medulla under command of autonomic nerve impulse. (From McConnell TH. The Nature of Disease Pathology for the Health Professions. Philadelphia, PA: Lippincott Williams & Wilkins; 2007.)

produced in the adrenal glands and the gonads as a precursor of the sex hormones, testosterone in men and estrogen in women. DHEA, the most abundant circulating steroid in humans, is produced in the adrenal glands and the gonads. It functions predominantly as a metabolic intermediate in the biosynthesis of the androgen and estrogen sex steroids. Both androstenedione and DHEA potentiate protein anabolism and virilization but are only about one-fifth as potent as testosterone. Unlike testosterone secretion, which is mediated by the gonadotropin luteinizing hormone (LH), androstenedione and DHEA secretion is mediated by ACTH.

ADRENAL INSUFFICIENCY

Adrenal insufficiency is a condition characterized by the inability to produce adequate amounts of steroid hormones, primarily cortisol, but may also include impaired aldosterone production.

Etiology

There are two major types of adrenal insufficiency: *primary*, due to impairment of the adrenal glands and *central*, caused by impairment of the pituitary gland or hypothalamus. Adrenal insufficiency can also be classified as congenital or acquired. The causes of adrenal insufficiency are listed in Table 10-1.

TABLE 10-1.	Causes of Adrenal Insufficiency	
Condition	**Cause**	**Treatment**
Primary (Congenital)		
CAH	Steroid biosynthesis enzyme deficiency	GC ± MC
AHC	Mutation of *DAX1*	GC + MC
Wolman disease	Deficiency of lysosomal lipase enzyme	GC + MC
ALD	Elevated long-chain fatty acids	GC + MC
FGD	ACTH-receptor gene defect	GC only
AAA	ACTH resistance	GC + MC
Primary (Acquired)		
Autoimmune	Antibodies against adrenal tissue	GC + MC
Infectious	Direct damage to adrenal gland	GC + MC
Trauma	Direct damage to adrenal gland	GC + MC
Pharmacologic agents	See Table 10-3	GC ± MC
Central (Congenital)		
Hypopituitarism	Defect in hypothalamus or pituitary	GC only
Central (Acquired)		
Tumor	Direct damage to HT and/or pituitary	GC only
Chronic glucocorticoid therapy	Zona fasciculata atrophy	GC only
Brain irradiation	Direct damage to HT and/or pituitary	GC only
Pharmacologic agents	See Table 10-3	GC only
Aldosterone Deficiency		
Pseudohypoaldosteronism	Mineralocorticoid receptor defect	MC only

Notes: CAH, congenital adrenal hyperplasia; AHC, adrenal hypoplasia congenita; ALD, adrenoleukodystrophy; FGD, familial glucocorticoid deficiency; AAA, Allgrove syndrome; GC, glucocorticoid; MC, mineralocorticoid.

Clinical Findings

The clinical findings of chronic glucocorticoid and mineralocorticoid insufficiency include poor weight gain (in the growing child) or weight loss, dehydration, hypotension, weakness, fatigue, anorexia, nausea, vomiting, diarrhea, salt craving, frequent illnesses, and vague gastrointestinal complaints. Hyperpigmentation of the skin and mucosa is observed in patients with primary (but not with secondary) adrenal insufficiency due to increased CRH and ACTH levels, which causes excess stimulation of propiomelano-cortin and melanocyte-stimulating hormone (MSH). Laboratory findings include hypo-glycemia, hyponatremia, and hyperkalemia. Hyperkalemia occurs frequently in patients with primary adrenal insufficiency due to lack of mineralocorticoid (aldosterone) secretion and is not seen in patients with central adrenal insufficiency because ACTH plays only a minor role in secretion of aldosterone. These individuals have a small heart on chest radiograph and low-voltage on the electrocardiogram. In addition, individuals with chronic glucocorticoid deficiency but preserved aldosterone secretion do not crave salt and rarely experience significant dehydration and hypotension. These individuals do, however, have hyponatremia because the inhibitory effect that normal cortisol secretion has on anti-diuretic hormone (ADH) is absent.

In addition to the symptoms of chronic adrenal insufficiency, individuals with acute adrenal insufficiency may experience fever, abdominal pain, and confusion.

Diagnostic Studies

The diagnosis of primary adrenal insufficiency is based on clinical signs, symptoms, and laboratory confirmation of a low early-morning serum cortisol level, elevated plasma ACTH level, and lack of response to ACTH (Cortrosyn®) stimulation. Because the range for serum cortisol levels is wide, and cortisol secretion is diurnal, confirmatory biochemical dynamic testing is performed with agents such as Cortrosyn or insulin. Stimulation testing is discussed in detail in Chapter 19.

A low early-morning serum cortisol level, a low or normal plasma ACTH level, and impaired response to Cortrosyn or to insulin-induced hypoglycemia provides biochemical evidence of central adrenal insufficiency. Similar to the testing for individuals suspected of having primary adrenal insufficiency, dynamic testing is the preferred method for confirming the diagnosis.

Treatment

Treatment is directed toward deficient hormone replacement therapy. Individuals with both glucocorticoid and mineralocorticoid deficiency will require replacement of both, whereas those with only glucocorticoid deficiency will only need glucocorticoid replacement. Individuals with primary adrenal insufficiency require hydrocortisone (8 to 12 mg/m^2/day) and fludrocortisone (0.05 to 0.2 mg/day). Children usually require higher glucocorticoid and mineralocorticoid doses than do adults; infants may require 20 to 30 mg/m^2/day and children 12 to 15 mg/m^2/day of hydrocortisone. Infants and children require between 0.1 to 0.2 mg/day of fludrocortisone, whereas teenagers and adults usually need 0.05 to 0.1 mg/day. For most individuals with central adrenal insufficiency, fludrocortisone is not needed, and the dose of hydrocortisone is lower (6 to 10 mg/m^2/day) than for those with primary adrenal insufficiency. The doses given are available in standard guidelines, but the clinician should adjust the dose of the medication based on the individual's symptoms, vital signs, linear growth, weight gain, and biochemical results. Chronic glucocorticoid overdosing should be avoided insofar as cortisol excess has serious medical consequences including osteoporosis, hyperglycemia, diabetes, and weight gain (see section on Cushing Syndrome later in this chapter).

During periods of stress, such as infection, general anesthesia, or injury, individuals with adrenal insufficiency are unable to produce the necessary rise in cortisol secretion and, therefore, require a higher dose of glucocorticoid therapy during these episodes. Individuals with primary adrenal insufficiency should be instructed to increase their dose of glucocorticoid therapy to provide 60 to 100 mg/m^2/day of hydrocortisone for at

TABLE 10-2.	Potencies of Glucocorticoids Relative to Hydrocortisone			
Preparation	**Glucocorticoid Potency**	**Mineralocorticoid Potency**	**Plasma Half-life (min)**	**Duration of Action (h)**
Cortisol (Hydrocortisone)	20 mg	20 mg	90	8–12
Cortisone	25 mg	16 mg	30	8–12
Prednisone	5 mg	16 mg	60	12–36
Prednisolone	5 mg	16 mg	200	12–36
Triamcinalone	4 mg	0	300	12–36
Methylprednisolone	4 mg	10 mg	180	12–36
Dexamethasone	0.75 mg	0	200	36–54
Betamethasone	0.60 mg	0	300	36–54
Fludrocortisone	0	3,000 mg	240	24–36
Aldosterone	0	8,000 mg	20	-----

least 48 hours and then return to the maintenance dose. Fludrocortisone is not increased during periods of stress.

In order to treat individuals with adrenal insufficiency appropriately, the clinician must recognize the various potencies of synthetic glucocorticoid and mineralocorticoid preparations compared to hydrocortisone (Table 10-2).

PRIMARY ADRENAL GLAND INSUFFICIENCY (CONGENITAL)

The most common cause of congenital adrenal insufficiency is congenital adrenal hyperplasia (CAH). In addition to CAH, other causes include adrenal hypoplasia congenita (AHC), adrenoleukodystrophy, Wolman disease, familial glucocorticoid resistance, and Allgrove syndrome.

Congenital Adrenal Hyperplasia

CAH is a group of autosomal-recessive disorders that is the result of a deficiency of one of the five enzymes required for cortisol synthesis from the adrenal cortex (Figure 10-3).

Etiology

The most common cause is 21-hydroxylase deficiency, accounting for more than 90% of cases. A large spectrum of phenotypes is possible. A severe form, with a concurrent defect in aldosterone biosynthesis (salt-wasting form), and a form with apparently normal aldosterone biosynthesis (simple virilizing type) are grouped together and termed *classic 21-hydroxylase (21-OHase) deficiency*. There is also a mild, nonclassic form that may be either asymptomatic or associated with signs of postnatal androgen excess.

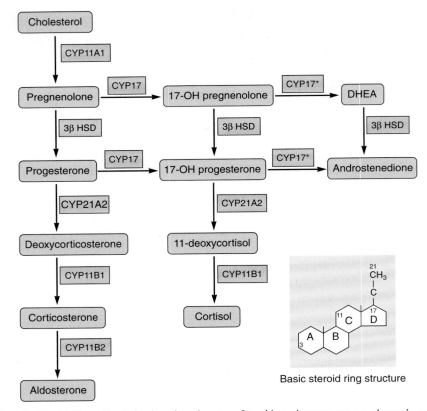

FIGURE 10-3. Steroid biosynthesis in the adrenal cortex. Steroids and precursors are shown in square boxes. Enzymes are shown in stippled boxes. Enzyme gene symbol designations are *CYP11A1*, desmolase; *CYP17*, 17α hydroxylase (±17,20 lyase*); 3β HSD, 3-β-hydroxysteroid dehydrogenase; *CYP21A2*, 21 hydroxylase; *CYP11B1*, 11β hydroxylase; *CYP11B2*, aldosterone synthase. Inset: Basic steroid ring structure. The four basic carbon rings are designated A, B, C, and D. Individual carbons at sites of steroidegonic enzyme activity are designated numerically. (From Mulholland MW, Maier RV, et al. Greenfield's Surgery Scientific Principles and Practice. 4th ed. Philadelphia, PA: Lippincott Williams & Wilkins; 2006.)

Pathology

For any cause of CAH, in which CRH and ACTH are overstimulated due to a lack of cortisol production, the gross pathology demonstrates adrenal gland hyperplasia (Figure 10-4).

Pathophysiology

The most common cause is 21-OHase deficiency, accounting for more than 90% of cases and caused by mutations in *CYP21A2*. The spectrum of phenotypes is large. Steroid 21-OHase (a cytochrome P450 enzyme) converts 17-hydroxyprogesterone (17-OHP) to 11-deoxycortisol and progesterone to 11-deoxycorticosterone (11-DOC) (see Figure 10-3). Because 11-deoxycortisol and 11-DOC are precursors for cortisol and aldosterone, respectively, complete loss of 21-OHase activity results in deficiencies of both of these vital corticosteroids.

Clinical Findings

The clinical phenotype is categorized as *classic salt-losing*, *classic nonsalt-losing* (or *simple virilizing*), or *nonclassic* forms. Females with classic CAH usually present at birth

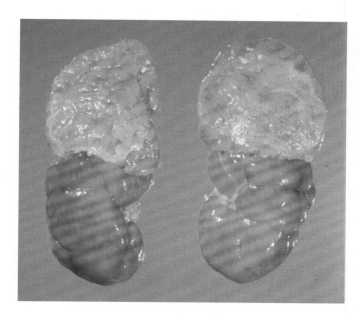

FIGURE 10-4. Adrenal gland hyperplasia. Congenital adrenal hyperplasia (CAH). A 7-week-old male died of severe salt-wasting CAH. At autopsy, both adrenal glands were markedly enlarged. (From Rubin E, Farber JL. Pathology. 3rd ed. Philadelphia, PA: Lippincott Williams & Wilkins; 1999.)

with ambiguous genitalia due to in utero exposure to excess fetal adrenal androgens. In fact, CAH is the most common cause of ambiguous genitalia. Males with classic CAH do not have phenotypic abnormalities at birth. The diagnostic features in boys vary according to the severity of 21-OHase impairment and the extent of aldosterone deficiency.

Nonclassic CAH is a mild form of the disease. Although the same gene, *CYP21A2*, is involved in both the severe and mild forms, genetic mutations typically associated with nonclassic CAH only partially impair 21-OHase activity. Therefore, individuals with nonclassic CAH do not have cortisol deficiency but, instead, have manifestations of hyperandrogenism later in childhood or in early adulthood. Females are born with normal genitalia, and some individuals with nonclassic CAH have no apparent clinical symptoms at all. Treatment with hydrocortisone is beneficial for females with signs of virilization and for children who have early onset of the disease and rapid skeletal age progression.

Diagnostic Studies

In the United States and most other developed countries, neonatal screening for CAH is performed at birth. Neonatal screening reduces morbidity and mortality, particularly among boys, by identifying infants with the severe, salt-wasting form before they develop adrenal crises. Initial testing usually consists of an immunoassay for 17-OHP levels; this assay has a low positive predictive value (approximately 1%), which results in many follow-up evaluations that have negative results. Infants with markedly elevated levels should have immediate determination of their serum glucose, sodium, potassium, and 17-OHP levels at baseline and after ACTH stimulation to confirm the diagnosis.

If the diagnosis is still in question after biochemical testing, molecular testing can be performed to determine if a *CYP21A2* mutation exits. The *CYP21A2* mutation can be detected in DNA samples extracted from the same dried blood spots used for hormonal screening. The positive predictive value of this strategy depends on the carrier rate for classic CAH in the general population.

CAH after infancy is diagnosed by measuring an early-morning baseline serum 17-OHP in symptomatic individuals. The severity of the hormonal abnormality depends on the degree of the enzymatic impairment, which, in turn, depends on the genotype.

Treatment

The goal of therapy for patients with CAH is to reduce excessive androgen secretion by replacing the deficient hormones. Proper treatment with glucocorticoid therapy prevents adrenal crisis and virilization and allows for normal growth and development. During childhood, the preferred glucocorticoid is hydrocortisone because its short half-life minimizes the adverse side effects (i.e., growth suppression) of the more potent longer-acting agents (e.g., dexamethasone).

In addition to glucocorticoid therapy, infants with salt-wasting 21-OHase deficiency require mineralocorticoid replacement and, possibly, supplemental sodium chloride. Although the aldosterone biosynthetic defect is clinically apparent only in the salt-wasting form, subclinical aldosterone deficiency is present in all forms of 21-OHase deficiency. It is best evaluated by the plasma renin activity (PRA)/plasma aldosterone ratio. Individuals with an elevated PRA level or PRA/aldosterone ratio benefit from fludrocortisone therapy and adequate dietary sodium.

Individuals with severe forms of 21-OHase deficiency are unable to produce a sufficient cortisol response to physical stress (e.g., febrile illness, gastroenteritis with dehydration, surgery, or trauma) and require increased glucocorticoid therapy during these episodes. Hydrocortisone (glucocorticoid) and fludrocortisone (mineralocorticoid) supplementation are the mainstays of therapy. During periods of stress, the glucocorticoid dose should be significantly increased (60 to 100 mg/m^2/day of a cortisol equivalent) for at least 48 hours or until complete recovery has occurred. Failure to provide stress-dose levels of cortisol in these circumstances can lead to shock and death.

Adrenal Hypoplasia Congenita

AHC is an inherited disorder of the adrenal cortex caused by mutations of the *DAX-1* (dosage-sensitive sex reversal-AHC critical region on the X chromosome gene 1) gene. This gene encodes a nuclear transcription factor that participates at various steps in the differentiation of adrenal and gonadal tissues as well as in gonadotropin expression. In this disorder, the definitive zone of the fetal adrenal gland does not develop, resulting in glucocorticoid and mineralocorticoid deficiencies in the neonate. In addition to the glucocorticoid and mineralocorticoid deficiencies, individuals may not enter puberty due to combined failure of hypothalamic gonadotropin-releasing hormone (GnRH) release and a pituitary defect in gonadotropin production. AHC is a lethal disease if untreated because of the glucocorticoid and mineralocorticoid deficiencies. Prognosis is very good for those receiving replacement therapy in the neonatal period.

Adrenoleukodystrophy

Adrenoleukodystrophy (ALD) is an X-linked congenital disease characterized by progressive brain damage followed by adrenocortical deficiency. It is characterized by high ratios of C_{26} to C_{22} very-long-chain fatty acids in plasma and tissues. Symptoms develop in mid-childhood, but a variant of the disorder, adrenomyeloneuropthy (AMN), presents in early adulthood. Both disorders are caused by mutations in the *ALDP* gene on the X chromosome. The earliest clinical findings are associated with central nervous system leukodystrophy and include behavioral changes, poor school performance, and dysarthria that progresses to severe dementia. Symptoms of adrenal insufficiency usually appear after symptoms of white matter disease. In contrast to ALD, AMN begins with adrenal insufficiency in childhood, and neurologic disease follows 10 to 15 years later. Treatment with replacement doses of glucocorticoid and mineralocorticoid is effective for adrenal function, but no therapy has proven effective for the neurologic disease.

Wolman Disease

Wolman disease is caused by a deficiency of lysosomal acid lipase, the enzyme necessary for mobilizing cholesterol esters from adrenal lipid droplets. This disease affects all cells, not just steroidogenic cells, because every cell must store and utilize cholesterol. Wolman disease is inherited in an autosomal-recessive pattern. The diagnosis should be suspected in newborns with feeding difficulties, diarrhea, hepatomegaly, splenomegaly, failure to grow, and adrenal gland calcification. The diagnosis is established by bone marrow aspiration yielding foam cells containing large lysosomal vacuoles engorged with cholesterol esters and is confirmed by finding absent cholesterol esterase activity in fibroblasts, leukocytes, or marrow cells. The complications of Wolman disease progress over time, eventually leading to the life-threatening problems of anemia and liver failure. Very few infants survive beyond the first year of life.

Familial Glucocorticoid Deficiency

Familial glucocorticoid deficiency (FGD) is a rare autosomal-recessive condition. Individuals with FGD have marked atrophy of both the zona fasciculata and zona reticularis of the adrenal cortex. Individuals have clinical manifestations of both glucocorticoid deficiency and ACTH excess. The biochemical findings include low serum cortisol levels and markedly increased ACTH levels. The zona glomerulosa is well preserved, and mineralocorticoid production is normal, insofar as it is dependent on the unaffected RAS. The most common causes of FGD are molecular defects of the ACTH receptor gene and mutations in the MC2 receptor accessory protein (*MRAP*). The other causes of FGD have unknown mutations that may affect ACTH signal transduction, expression of the ACTH receptor, or differentiation of the adrenal cortex.

Allgrove Syndrome (Triple A Syndrome)

Triple A syndrome is a rare autosomal-dominant disorder consisting of a clinical triad of: 1) ACTH-resistant adrenal (glucocorticoid) insufficiency, 2) achalasia (failure of the lower esophageal sphincter to relax, delaying food into the stomach, and causing dilation of the thoracic esophagus), and 3) alacrima (absence of tear secretion). This disorder resembles ACTH resistance, but mutations in the ACTH receptor have been excluded. Many individuals have progressive neurologic symptoms including intellectual impairment, sensorineural deafness, peripheral neuropathies, and autonomic dysfunction.

PRIMARY ADRENAL GLAND INSUFFICIENCY (ACQUIRED)

The most common cause of acquired adrenal gland insufficiency is Addison disease. Other causes are pharmacologic agents, infection, hemorrhage, metastases, and surgical removal of the adrenal glands.

Addison Disease

The most common cause of primary adrenal failure is an autoimmune destruction of the gland called **Addison disease**, or *autoimmune adrenalitis*, which accounts for up to 80% of all cases.

Etiology

Autoimmune adrenalitis may be part of autoimmune polyglandular syndrome type 2 (APS2), which will be discussed in detail in Chapter 16. Other causes of acquired primary adrenal failure include granulomatous infiltration, tuberculosis, fungal infections, hemochromatosis, metastatic tumors, and pharmacologic agents.

Pathology

Regardless of the etiology, the gross pathology shows adrenal gland atrophy, and the histopathology reveals atypical nuclei secondary to prolonged ACTH stimulation. Most histopathologic features are dependent on the etiology of the adrenal insufficiency. For autoimmune destruction, the adrenal cortex contains lymphocytes (Figure 10-5). In infiltrative cases, amyloid (amyloidosis) or iron (hemochromatosis) deposition is present. In granulomatous conditions such as tuberculosis and fungal infections, calcifications are present in both the gross and histopathology specimens. The Waterhouse-Friderichsen syndrome (Figure 10-6), most commonly seen in individuals with meningococcemia, involves bilateral adrenal hemorrhage, resulting in a syndrome of adrenocortical deficiency, disseminated intravascular coagulation, hypotensive shock, and, possibly, death.

Pathophysiology

In Addison disease, both glucocorticoid and mineralocorticoid hormones are deficient. Without cortisol, the vascular system is unable to respond to catecholamines, and hypotension and shock ensue. Glucocorticoid deficiency also inhibits many anabolic metabolic reactions and results in weight loss and hypoglycemia. Mineralocorticoid deficiency leads to an inability of the renal tubules to retain sodium and excrete potassium, resulting in hyponatremia and hyperkalemia. The loss of sodium further exacerbates the hypotension resulting from glucocorticoid deficiency, eventually leading to shock if treatment is not provided.

Clinical Findings

Early symptoms of Addison disease may be fairly nonspecific, such as fatigue, weight loss, anorexia, irritability, myalgias, arthralgias, nausea, vomiting, and fever. Individuals may appear diffusely hyperpigmented as a result of elevated CRH and ACTH levels

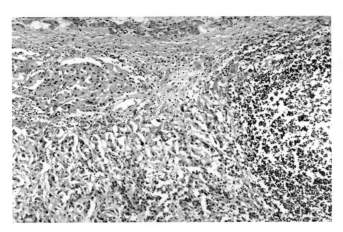

FIGURE 10-5. Autoimmune adrenalitis. A section of the adrenal gland from a patient with Addison disease demonstrates chronic inflammation and fibrosis in the cortex, an island of residual atrophic cortical cells, and an intact medulla. (From Rubin E, Farber JL. Pathology. 3rd ed. Philadelphia, PA: Lippincott Williams & Wilkins; 1999.)

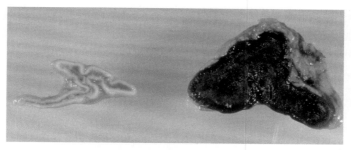

FIGURE 10-6. Waterhouse-Friderichsen syndrome. A normal adrenal gland (*left*) is contrasted with an adrenal gland enlarged by extensive hemorrhage obtained from a patient who died of meningococcemic shock. (From Rubin E, Farber JL. Pathology. 3rd ed. Philadelphia, PA: Lippincott Williams & Wilkins; 1999.)

(due to reduced feedback inhibition of cortisol), which causes excess stimulation of propiomelanocortin and MSH. MSH and ACTH share the same precursor molecule. As adrenal cortical function continues to decline, those with Addison disease will experience hypotension and hypoglycemia. If treatment is not quickly initiated, individuals will develop hypotensive shock and death.

Diagnostic Studies

Adrenal insufficiency is diagnosed biochemically by measuring the serum cortisol level before the administration of 250 mcg of synthetic ACTH, and 30 and 60 minutes afterward. Any basal or stimulated value ≥18 mg/dL defines a normal response. Serum baseline levels <3 mg/dL in the presence of stress are highly suggestive of adrenal insufficiency; however, basal (nonstimulated) serum cortisol lacks diagnostic accuracy. For individuals with chronic Addison disease, serum sodium is low and commonly serum potassium elevated. Individuals may also have hypoglycemia.

Treatment

Definitive treatment consists of replacing the deficient hormones with daily supplementation. Hydrocortisone (glucocorticoid) and fludrocortisone (mineralocorticoid) supplementation are the mainstays of therapy. For the majority of those with Addison disease, a dose of 8 to 12 mg/m^2/day of hydrocortisone will provide enough cortisol to meet the body's physiologic needs. During periods of stress, the glucocorticoid dose should be significantly increased (60 to 100 mg/m^2/day of a cortisol equivalent) for at least 48 hours or until complete recovery has occurred. Failure to provide stress-dose levels of cortisol in these circumstances can lead to shock and death.

Prognosis

Individuals with Addison disease have relatively normal life expectancy provided that they are compliant with their replacement therapy. Some studies show that there might be a slight increase in all-cause mortality. When these individuals complain of chronic fatigue, it may be the result of inadequate supplementation.

Other Causes of Acquired Primary Adrenal Insufficiency

Pharmacologic agents, infection, hemorrhage, metastases, and surgical removal of the adrenal glands are other causes of primary adrenal insufficiency. With the exception of

TABLE 10-3.	Pharmacologic Agents Causing Adrenal Insufficiency
Condition and Mechanism of Action	**Pharmacologic Agents**
Primary Adrenal Insufficiency	
Hemorrhage	Heparin, warfarin, tyrosine kinase inhibitors (sunitinib)
Inhibition of cortisol-synthesis enzyme	Aminoglutethimide, trilostane, ketoconazole, fluconazole, etomidate
Activation of cortisol metabolism	Phenobarbital, phenytoin, rifampin, troglitazone
Central Adrenal Insufficiency	
HPA axis suppression	Glucocorticoids, megestrol acetate, medroxyprogesterone, ketorolac tromethamine, opiate drugs
Peripheral resistance to glucocorticoids	Mifepristone, antipsychotic drugs (chlorpromazine), antidepressant drugs (imipramine)

complete removal of both adrenal glands, these other causes may spare some adrenal tissue leaving compromised adrenal gland function, rather than complete absence of adrenal function. The most common infections that cause adrenal insufficiency are tuberculosis, fungemia, diphtheria, and streptococcemia. Pharmacologic agents can cause both primary and central adrenal insufficiency (Table 10-3).

CENTRAL ADRENAL GLAND INSUFFICIENCY (CONGENITAL)

Central adrenal insufficiency is caused by impairment of the pituitary gland or hypothalamus. Congenital causes of insufficient stimulation of the adrenal gland involve defects in development of the hypothalamus, pituitary gland, and cells that secrete GnRH and ACTH. Nearly all individuals with central adrenal gland insufficiency have normal mineralocorticoid production because aldosterone is primarily governed by the RAS and serum potassium concentration. One congenital cause of aldosterone hypofunction is due to the rare condition of pseudohypoaldosteronism (PHA).

Hypopituitarism

Congenital isolated CRH or ACTH deficiency is rare, and a number of transcription factors have been implicated in inherited hypothalamic and pituitary hormone deficiencies. Usually these individuals are identified shortly after birth with genital abnormalities, small size, and hypoglycemia. Individuals born with midline brain defects such as a cleft lip, cleft-lip-palate, and septo-optic dysplasia may also have defects in hypothalamic and pituitary gland development. In these infants, who are usually easy to identify at birth, it is important to exclude pituitary hormone deficiencies as soon as possible.

Pseudohypoaldosteronism

Aldosterone secretion is unaffected by CRH or ACTH deficiency because its secretion is dependent on the RAS. Pseudohypoaldosteronism type 1 (PHA1) is a rare inherited condition that is characterized by renal insensitivity to the action of mineralocorticoids. At least two forms of PHA1, autosomal dominant and recessive, have been identified. Individuals with autosomal-dominant PHA1 generally have much milder symptoms than those with the autosomal-recessive type. The autosomal-recessive type of PHA1 has multiple target organ unresponsiveness to mineralocorticoids including the sweat and salivary glands, the colon, and the kidney. Mutations in the mineralocorticoid receptor (MR) gene leads to autosomal-dominant renal PHA1, whereas mutations in the epithelial sodium channel (ENaC) α, β, and γ subunit genes lead to autosomal recessive severe systemic PHA1. The biochemical findings in individuals with PHA1 are similar to the findings in individuals with aldosterone deficiency and include hyponatremia and hyperkalemia. However, individuals with PHA1 have an elevated aldosterone level, consistent with a receptor defect.

Individuals with autosomal-dominant renal PHA1 generally require oral salt supplementation but typically show a gradual clinical improvement in renal salt loss during childhood. Some individuals are clinically asymptomatic but may have elevated PRA and aldosterone levels.

CENTRAL ADRENAL GLAND INSUFFICIENCY (ACQUIRED)

The most common cause of acquired central adrenal insufficiency is the result of chronic use of exogenous steroids. Exogenous administration of supraphysiologic doses of corticosteroids not only can result in Cushing syndrome (discussed under "Adrenal Gland Excess," later in this chapter), but also, while on therapy and after abrupt discontinuation, results in suppression of CRH and ACTH release, leading to atrophy of the adrenal cortex. Acute discontinuation of exogenous steroid administration or the inability of the adrenal gland to increase endogenous cortisol production in situations of stress results in acute adrenal insufficiency or crisis. In addition to long-term glucocorticoid therapy, other pharmacologic agents as well as pituitary and hypothalamic defects such as tumors, infiltration, infarction, and surgery are associated with acquired adrenal insufficiency. The pituitary gland and hypothalamic defects are discussed in more detail in Chapter 2.

Hypothalamic/Pituitary Tumors

Approximately 25% of individuals with pituitary tumors develop ACTH and, ultimately, cortisol deficiency. Adrenal insufficiency is rarely the presenting complaint but may contribute to the clinical picture. After surgery and/or radiation therapy, many individuals will develop ACTH deficiency as part of their surgical or radiation-induced pituitary damage. Therefore, all individuals should receive glucocorticoid therapy during treatment, irrespective of the status of the HPA axis at the time the tumor is identified. Because cortisol is required to inhibit ADH, treatment with glucocorticoids may unmask a previously unapparent deficiency of ADH and, thus, precipitate diabetes insipidus.

Iatrogenic Causes

Long-term glucocorticoid therapy can suppress the synthesis and storage of CRH and ACTH. Recovery of the HPA axis from long-term glucocorticoid therapy entails recovery of multiple components in a sequential cascade and, therefore, typically requires considerable time. Depending on the preparation, dose, frequency, and duration of treatment, individuals on high doses (>12 mg/m^2/day of an equivalent dose of hydrocortisone) for more than 10 days may need to wean off of therapy slowly. Some studies have reported a failure of HPA axis recovery up to several months to 1 year in individuals on high-dose glucocorticoid therapy. Caution must be taken when weaning these individuals. Until it can be biochemically proven that those individuals who are on high doses for a long time have normal adrenal function, it must be assumed that they are adrenally insufficient, and they should receive stress dosing for any possible stressful encounter. As discussed in acquired primary adrenal insufficiency, pharmacologic agents can also cause central adrenal insufficiency (see Table 10-3).

ACUTE ADRENAL CRISIS

An adrenal crisis occurs most commonly in an individual with undiagnosed chronic adrenal insufficiency who is subjected to a severe stress, such as a major illness, trauma, or surgery. Treatment initially consists of fluid and electrolyte administration, glucocorticoid and mineralocorticoid replacement therapy, and treatment of the precipitating illness.

ADRENAL GLAND EXCESS

The most common condition in which excess hormone is secreted from the adrenal gland is Cushing syndrome, in which cortisol is excessively produced. Most of this section is devoted to Cushing syndrome; hyperaldosteronism is discussed in detail in Chapter 11, and excess adrenal androgen production is discussed earlier in this chapter as well as in Chapter 15 with CAH.

Cushing Syndrome

Chronic cortisol excess is known as *Cushing syndrome* and is divided into excess exogenous administration and excess endogenous production by the adrenal gland. With millions of individuals using pharmacologic doses of glucocorticoids for a variety of illnesses, the most common cause of Cushing syndrome is iatrogenic. The pathogenic mechanisms of endogenous Cushing syndrome can be divided into two forms: ACTH-dependent (i.e., elevated ACTH level produced by the pituitary or by ectopic tissues) and ACTH-independent (i.e., suppressed or normal ACTH level due to excessive production of cortisol by the adrenal gland).

Etiology

For individuals aged 7 years and older, the most common form of endogenous Cushing syndrome is ACTH-dependent. The most commonly reported form, with an incidence of 5 to 25 per million, is due to an ACTH-secreting pituitary adenoma. This form of Cushing syndrome is termed *Cushing disease*. Ectopic ACTH secretion, from benign and malignant tumors, is common but is often not diagnosed considering that about 1% of patients with small cell lung cancer have ectopic ACTH syndrome. The most common causes of ACTH-independent Cushing syndrome are adrenocortical tumors, either benign or malignant types, and bilateral primary micronodular and macronodular adrenocortical hyperplasia. In infants and children aged 7 years and younger, adrenal tumors are the most common cause.

Clinical Findings

The clinical manifestations of Cushing syndrome are characterized by central obesity, weight gain, moon facies, supraclavicular fat accumulation, a cervical fat pad (buffalo hump), thinned skin, easy bruising, purple striae, proximal muscle weakness, fatigue, hypertension, impaired glucose tolerance, diabetes, acne, hirsutism, and menstrual irregularities. Osteoporosis, fractures, and neuropsychologic disturbances (depression, emotional irritability, sleep disturbances) may also occur. In addition to exhibiting poor linear growth, growing children have similar symptoms as adults with Cushing syndrome. Two women with clinical features of Cushing syndrome are shown in Figure 10-7.

Buffalo hump fat

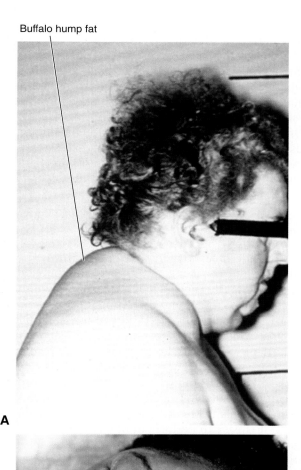

A

B

FIGURE 10-7. Cushing syndrome. **(A)** Cushingoid obesity, including "buffalo hump" of dorsal fat. **(B)** Cushingoid moon facies. (From McConnell TH. The Nature of Disease Pathology for the Health Professions. Philadelphia, PA: Lippincott Williams & Wilkins; 2007.)

Pathophysiology

The pathophysiology of Cushing syndrome is due to an excessive production (endogenous) or intake (exogenous) of cortisol. Cushing disease is a primary pituitary abnormality. The excessive cortisol depresses the immune system, creating an increased susceptibility to infection and a catabolic metabolism. These derangements of metabolism cause muscle breakdown, increased deposition of central fat, and the classic cushingoid appearance. For ACTH-dependent Cushing syndrome due to ectopic ACTH secretion, the high levels of ACTH may have a mineralocorticoid effect by stimulating production of DOC from the zona glomerulosa. Elevated cortisol causes hypertension by overwhelming the enzyme, 11-β-hydroxysteroid dehydrogenase (HSD) type 2 that converts cortisol to its inactive metabolite, cortisone. The excess cortisol then binds to the mineralocorticoid receptor, leading to hypertension.

Excess cortisol prevents linear growth likely through its inhibition of insulin-like growth factor (IGF)-1 secretion and effect at the growth plate. Excess cortisol interferes with the growth hormone–IGF-1 axis at the hypothalamic, pituitary, and target organ levels, affecting hormone release, receptor abundance, signal transduction, gene transcription, pre-mRNA splicing, and mRNA translation. Direct effects at the growth plate include the suppression of multiple gene expression, chondrocyte proliferation and matrix proteoglycan synthesis, sulfation, release, and mineralization, as well as the augmentation of hypertrophic cell apoptosis. At the tissues adjacent to the growth plate, excess cortisol enhances osteoclast and suppresses osteoblast recruitment and function. Excess cortisol also reduces muscle strength and disrupts the normal control of vascular invasion at the cartilage-bone interface.

Diagnostic Studies

The critical screening laboratory tests include measurements of 24-hour urinary free cortisol (UFC), late-night salivary cortisol, and the 1-mg (30 mcg/kg for individuals <34 kg) overnight dexamethasone suppression test. The diagnosis of Cushing syndrome is based on documentation of excess cortisol secretion and impairment of physiologic feedback of the HPA axis. The 24-hour UFC gives an integrated value of cortisol production during the entire day and is the most widely used screening test for establishing the diagnosis of Cushing syndrome. The 1-mg overnight dexamethasone test results in suppression of endogenous production of cortisol in normal individuals. Individuals with Cushing syndrome will not suppress cortisol production; their morning cortisol level is >5 mcg/dL. The late-night salivary cortisol determination has also been shown to be a useful screening test for hypercortisolism. Measurement of cortisol in saliva has some advantages over 24-hour UFC: it is easy to perform at home, is noninvasive, and, by collecting late at night, it can be used to determine the presence or absence of appropriate cortisol diurnal variation. Two measurements of UFC and/or nighttime salivary cortisol are recommended to screen patients with suspected hypercortisolism. The UFC and salivary cortisol tests, however, have low sensitivity and specificity in patients with poorly controlled diabetes, obesity, or depression or in individuals with inconsistent bedtimes (night-shift workers), licorice ingestion, cigarette smoking, and tobacco chewing. These individuals have been recognized as having pseudo-Cushing syndrome insofar as they have the phenotypic appearance, elevated 24-hour UFC, and random serum cortisol levels. However, they usually maintain low salivary cortisol levels in the middle of the night and suppress their cortisol production after low- or high-dose dexamethasone suppression testing.

Once the diagnosis has been established, it is important to determine the source of the excessive endogenous cortisol by measuring the serum ACTH. Low levels of ACTH suggest that the etiology is ACTH independent (such as an adrenal tumor or exogenous source), whereas increased levels of ACTH suggest ACTH-dependent causes, such as Cushing disease or ectopic ACTH.

When ACTH levels are low and excess exogenous cortisol administration has been excluded as a possible cause, a computed tomography (CT) scan or MRI of the abdomen and pelvis is needed to locate a probable adrenal tumor. When ACTH and cortisol levels are high, several laboratory procedures can be used to determine if the increased ACTH production is due to Cushing disease or ectopic ACTH. Magnetic resonance imaging (MRI) of the pituitary gland reveals an adenoma in 50% of ACTH-dependant Cushing syndromes, which establishes the diagnosis of Cushing disease. When the MRI is equivocal or negative, bilateral inferior petrosal sinus sampling of ACTH is required and may localize ACTH production to the pituitary gland. If Cushing disease is ruled out with the above two procedures, an ectopic source of ACTH should be undertaken. A CT scan of the chest and abdomen is performed first to look for benign or malignant lesion(s) that may explain the ectopic source of ACTH. An algorithm for the work-up and determination of the etiology of Cushing syndrome is shown in Figure 10-8.

The high-dose dexamethasone suppression test can be used to differentiate Cushing disease from ectopic ACTH production because pituitary adenomas retain CRH receptors and suppress with very high levels of cortisol. Ectopic ACTH production, on the other hand, does not suppress. Dexamethasone suppression testing is discussed in more detail in Chapter 19.

Treatment

Cushing syndrome has many etiologies, and successful treatment is dependent on determining the correct one. For example, iatrogenic Cushing syndrome is treated by reduction and careful tapering of exogenous glucocorticoid administration. Cushing syndrome due to an adrenal adenoma is treated with resection of the neoplasm. Cushing disease is treated with resection of the pituitary adenoma (transsphenoidal approach). After resection of a pituitary tumor or an adrenal adenoma, individuals must be maintained

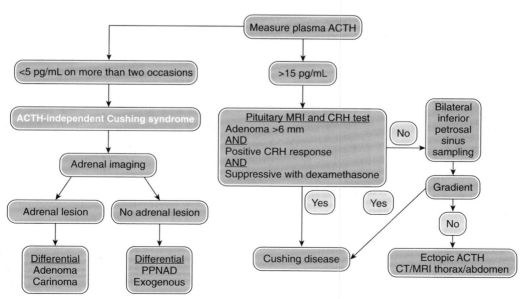

FIGURE 10-8. Algorithm for determining the etiology of Cushing syndrome.
Notes: PPNAD, primary pigmented nodular adrenocortical disease.

on hydrocortisone supplementation to prevent short-term adrenocortical insufficiency. Individuals with ectopic ACTH secretion must be treated with resection of the responsible neoplasm. If resection is not possible, a bilateral adrenalectomy and subsequent hydrocortisone replacement therapy is a reasonable alternative.

Prognosis

Prognosis depends on the etiology. For example, iatrogenic Cushing syndrome is dependent on the reason for the need for glucocorticoid therapy. Prognosis for an adrenal adenoma is excellent, with a 10-year survival of 90%. Cushing disease also has an excellent prognosis if tumor resection is complete. Prognosis is obviously worse for patients with a recurrence of the tumor. An ACTH-secreting tumor of unknown etiology has a 10-year survival of only 55%.

Carney Complex

A rare cause of excess cortisol production is a multiple neoplasia syndrome known as *the Carney complex*. It is inherited in an autosomal-dominant manner and is characterized mostly by benign skin tumors and pigmented lesions, myxomas, schwannomas, and various endocrine tumors. The most common endocrine tumor is primary pigmented nodular adrenocortical disease (PPNAD).

Inactivating mutations of the *PRKAR1A* gene coding for the regulatory type I-α (RIα) subunit of protein kinase A (PKA) are responsible for the disease in most patients. The overall penetrance among *PRKAR1A* mutation carriers is near 98%. It is genetically and clinically heterogeneous, with specific mutations providing some genotype–phenotype correlation. Phosphodiesterase-11A (the *PDE11A* gene) and phosphodiesterase-8B (the *PDE8B* gene) mutations have been found in patients with isolated adrenal hyperplasia and Cushing syndrome as well as in patients with PPNAD. Dysregulation of the cyclic adenosine monophosphate/PKA pathway can modulate other signaling pathways and contributes to adrenocortical tumorigenesis.

CASE FOLLOW-UP

Our patient sustained severe injuries in a motor vehicle collision. Her hypotension and unresponsiveness to fluid therapy suggest internal bleeding or a metabolic process. The severe back pain could be due to an aortic transection or renal damage. Because of her drowsy condition, in addition to a complete blood count, a metabolic panel is collected when the intravenous line is placed. Her blood count is reported as normal, indicating that anemia and thrombocytopenia are not present. Her metabolic panel, on the other hand, is remarkable for a serum glucose of 55 mg/dL, a serum sodium of 127 mEq/L, and a serum potassium of 7.2 mEq/L. Her electrocardiogram is normal.

Her drowsy state may be due to hypoglycemia, or to a closed head injury. The presence of hyponatremia and hyperkalemia with systemic hypotension that is unresponsive to fluid is highly suggestive of adrenal insufficiency. Her simultaneous plasma ACTH, serum cortisol, and serum aldosterone levels are shown below and confirm primary adrenal insufficiency.

(continues)

CASE FOLLOW-UP (*continued*)

Hormone	Level	Normal Range
ACTH (pg/mL)	345	10–60
Cortisol (mcg/dL)	2	8–22
Aldosterone (ng/dL)	2	7–30

In preparing for a chest and abdominal CT scan to determine if she has an aortic rupture or any other cause for bleeding, she receives both a stress dose of IV hydrocortisone (200 mg, ~100 mg/m²) and IV dextrose.

Within 30 minutes, her blood pressure and serum glucose improve. The CT scan reveals fractured ribs and bilateral adrenal hemorrhage, the latter having caused her to develop primary adrenal insufficiency.

She is admitted to the hospital and started on daily hydrocortisone at 200 mg/day over the next 48 hours. As she improves, the hydrocortisone is decreased to a maintenance dose (~12 mg/m²/day), and fludrocortisone (0.1 mg/day) is added. Within 5 days, her electrolytes and glucose levels are all within normal limits.

Over the next 2 months, she improves significantly, and an abdominal CT scan shows no evidence of adrenal hemorrhage. She is slowly weaned off of her hydrocortisone and fludrocortisone over 6 weeks. Four weeks later, a high-dose ACTH stimulation test is performed at 8 a.m. After collection of a plasma ACTH and serum cortisol, 250 mcg of Cortrosyn is infused intravenously, and serum cortisol levels are collected 30 minutes and 60 minutes later. The results are shown in the table below, confirming that her adrenal glands produce an adequate amount of cortisol and aldosterone:

Hormone	Baseline (T = 0)	T = 30 min	T = 60 min
ACTH (pg/mL)	35	—	—
Cortisol (mcg/dL)	15	35	45
Aldosterone (ng/dL)	12	25	33

REFERENCES and SUGGESTED READINGS

Almeida MQ, Stratakis CA. Carney complex and other conditions associated with micronodular adrenal hyperplasias. Best Pract Res Clin Endocrinol Metab. 2010;24(6):907–914.

Arlt W, Allolio B. Adrenal insufficiency. Lancet. 2003;361:1881–1893.

Bornstein SR. Predisposing factors for adrenal insufficiency. N Engl J Med. 2009;360(22):2328–2339.

Carol T, Raff H, Findling JW. Late-night salivary cortisol measurement in the diagnosis of Cushing's syndrome. Nat Clin Pract Endocrinol Metab. 2008;4(6):344–350.

Chakera A, Vaidya B. Addison disease in adults: diagnosis and management. Am J Med. 2010;123(5):409–413.

Chrousos GP, Detera-Wadleigh SD, Karl M. Syndromes of glucocorticoid resistance. Ann Intern Med. 1993;119(11):1113–1124.

Erickson D, Natt N, Nippoldt T, Young WF Jr, Carpenter PC, Peterson T, et al. Dexamethasone suppressed corticotropin-releasing hormone stimulation test for diagnosis of mild hypercortisolism. J Clin Endocrinol Metab. 2007;92(8):2972–2976.

Felner EI, Thompson MT, Ratliffe AF, White PC, Dickson BA. Recovery of adrenal function in children treated for leukemia. J Peds. 2000;137:21–24.

Felner EI. Reducing the risk for adrenal insufficiency in those treated for ALL: Tapering glucocorticoids prior to abrupt discontinuation. J Ped Heme Oncol. 2011;33(6):406–408.

Habiby RL, Boepple P, Nachtigall L, Sluss PM, Crowley WF Jr, Jameson JL. Adrenal hypoplasia congenital with hypogonadotropic hypogonadism: evidence that DAX-1 mutations lead to combined hypothalamic and pituitary defects in gonadotropin production. J Clin Invest. 1996;98:1055–1062.

Hittle K, Hsieh S, Sheeran P. Acute adrenal crisis masquerading as septic shock in a healthy young woman. J Pediatr Health Care. 2010;24(1):48–52.

Hochberg, Z. Mechanisms of steroid impairment of growth. Horm Res. 2002;58(suppl 1):33–38.

Kempna P, Fluck CE. Adrenal gland development and defects. Best Pract Res Clin Endocrinol Metab. 2008;22:77–93.

Kidambi S, Raff H, Findling JW. Limitations of nocturnal salivary cortisol and urine free cortisol in the diagnosis of mild Cushing's syndrome. Eur J Endocrinol. 2007;157(6):725–731.

Lehmann SG, Lalli E, Sassone-Corsi P. X-linked adrenal hypoplasia congenital is caused by abnormal nuclear localization of the DAX-1 protein. PNAS. 2002;99(12):8225–8230.

Newell-Price J. Diagnosis/differential diagnosis of Cushing's syndrome: a review of best practice. Best Pract Res Clin Endocrinol Metab. 2009;23(supp 1):S5–S14.

Nieman LK, Biller BM, Findling JW, Newell-Price J, Savage MO, Stewart PM, et al. The diagnosis of Cushing syndrome: an Endocrine Society Clinical Practice Guideline. J Clin Endocrinol Metab. 2008;93:1526–1540.

Oelkers W. Adrenal insufficiency. N Engl J Med. 1996;335:1206–1212.

Raff H, Findling J. A physiologic approach to the diagnosis of the Cushing syndrome. Ann Intern Med. 2003;138(12):980–991.

Riepe FG. Clinical and molecular features of type pseudohypoaldosteronism. Horm Res. 2009;72(1):1–9.

Speiser PW, White PC. Congenital adrenal hyperplasia. N Engl J Med. 2003;349(8):776–788.

CHAPTER REVIEW QUESTIONS

1. A 46-year-old Caucasian woman presents to your office complaining of fatigue, back pain, intermittent nausea, and vomiting of insidious onset over the past several months. Her blood pressure is 97/69 mmHg, heart rate 86 beats per minute, and temperature 37.2°F. Physical exam shows diffuse hyperpigmentation on both sun-exposed and non–sun-exposed skin. What will a basic metabolic profile most likely show?

   A. Sodium 140, potassium 4.5
   B. Sodium 140, potassium 5.6
   C. Sodium 145, potassium 3.5
   D. Sodium 128, potassium 5.3
   E. Sodium 115, potassium 3.2

2. A 56-year-old man with no previous medical problems presents to your office complaining of weakness, fatigue, weight gain, polydipsia, and polyuria. His blood pressure is 156/100 mmHg, heart rate 65 beats per minute, and temperature 37.8°F. Physical exam reveals central obesity, thin extremities, and purple striae across his abdomen. A random blood glucose is 96 mg/dL. His only medication is occasional ibuprofen for back pain. Which of the following tests should be ordered first?

   A. CT scan abdomen/pelvis
   B. 24-hour urine free cortisol
   C. Head MRI
   D. High-dose dexamethasone suppression test
   E. Inferior petrosal sinus sampling

3. A 36-year-old female requires long-term dexamethasone therapy. After taking the dexamethasone for 3 months, what would her plasma ACTH and serum cortisol levels be?

A. ACTH high, cortisol high
B. ACTH normal, cortisol normal
C. ACTH low, cortisol high
D. ACTH low, cortisol low
E. ACTH high, cortisol low

4. A 28-year-old woman presents with weight gain and amenorrhea. She has facial hirsutism and states that she has been under stress lately. Physical exam reveals purple striae, central obesity, and hypertension (160/110 mmHg). Which of the following biochemical findings would you expect her to have?

A. Suppression of plasma cortisol with overnight (1 mg) dexamethasone
B. Elevated urine free cortisol excretion
C. Hyponatremia
D. Hyperkalemia
E. Hypoglycemia

5. A 35-year-old woman presents with a recent weight gain of 20 lbs and new-onset depression. On physical examination she has a blood pressure of 135/82 mmHg, pulse of 76 beats per minute, and generalized obesity. She does not have facial plethora, and her proximal muscle strength is good. Laboratory data show 24-hour urine free cortisol excretion, 120 mcg (normal, 20 to 90 mcg). The most appropriate next test would be:

A. Nighttime salivary cortisol measurement
B. CT scan of the adrenal glands
C. MRI of the pituitary gland
D. Bilateral inferior petrosal sinus sampling
E. CRH stimulation test

CHAPTER REVIEW ANSWERS

1. The correct answer is D. This woman's presentation is consistent with Addison disease secondary to bilateral autoimmune destruction of the adrenal cortex. Such patients are deficient in both glucocorticoid and mineralocorticoid production. As a result of the lack of aldosterone's action on the kidneys, this woman will waste sodium and retain potassium, resulting in low serum sodium levels and elevated serum potassium levels.

The serum values in **Choice A** are normal. If a patient's blood sample is hemolyzed, the sodium level (and all other blood levels) may be normal and the potassium spuriously high (**Choice B**). Patients with high sodium and low potassium (**Choice C**) may have an endocrine disorder such as hyperaldosteronism (Conn syndrome), whereby aldosterone is oversecreted, leading to potassium wasting and sodium retention. These patients would also be hypertensive instead of mildly hypotensive. A patient presenting with a severely low sodium and borderline low potassium (**Choice E**) may be suffering from any number of conditions leading to hypervolemia, such as heart failure or the syndrome of inappropriate ADH secretion (SIADH).

2. The correct answer is B. This patient's presentation is consistent with Cushing syndrome. The first-line testing modalities for ruling out Cushing syndrome are the overnight dexamethasone suppression test, a 24-hour urine free cortisol measurement, or late-night salivary cortisol measurement.

A CT scan of the abdomen/pelvis (**Choice A**) may be useful to look for an adrenal adenoma once the diagnosis of Cushing syndrome has been established but not as an initial test. A head MRI (**Choice C**) would also be useful if he was experiencing neurologic symptoms or if one of the initial screening tests was consistent with Cushing syndrome. Inferior petrosal sinus sampling (**Choice E**) should also be performed after screening studies suggest Cushing syndrome. The high-dose dexamethasone suppression test (**Choice D**) is used to differentiate ACTH-dependent from ACTH-independent causes of Cushing syndrome, but would also not be performed until one of the screening tests were positive.

3. The correct answer is D. In a patient undergoing long-term steroid supplementation, the HPA axis will be depressed, and both ACTH production from the pituitary and cortisol production from the adrenal cortex will be low as a result of feedback inhibition. Unlike prednisone, measurement of dexamethasone does not cross-react with hydrocortisone. If the patient were taking prednisone, however, the woman's serum cortisol level would likely be elevated.

Both ACTH and cortisol will be high (**Choice A**) in ACTH-dependent Cushing syndrome. Possible causes include Cushing disease or ectopic ACTH production. In either case the excess ACTH drives increased production of cortisol from the adrenal cortex. An individual with a normal functioning HPA axis will have normal ACTH and cortisol levels (**Choice B**). ACTH would be low and cortisol high (**Choice C**) in an individual with a cortisol-producing adrenal adenoma or taking hydrocortisone or prednisone. The excess cortisol production would inhibit ACTH production from the pituitary, resulting in a low ACTH level. In an individual with primary adrenal insufficiency, the plasma ACTH level would be high and cortisol low (**Choice E**).

4. The correct answer is B. This woman has features of hypercortisolism (striae, central obesity) and virilization (hair on face). She may also have a component of excess aldosterone (hypertension), although she could be hypertensive from the excess cortisol. Therefore, she likely has adrenal-mediated Cushing syndrome. Cushing syndrome results in elevated urinary free cortisol levels.

She would not be expected to suppress her early-morning cortisol level with a nighttime dose of dexamethasone (**Choice A**). With increased cortisol, and possibly aldosterone, she would not have hyponatremia (**Choice C**), hyperkalemia (**Choice D**), or hypoglycemia (**Choice E**). With excess cortisol, individuals are more likely to have hyperglycemia. In those with excess aldosterone, hypernatremia and hypokalemia are present.

5. The correct answer is A. With just a mild elevation in urinary free cortisol along with depression and weight gain, it is more likely that this woman has pseudo-Cushing syndrome and not true Cushing syndrome. It is therefore, more appropriate to perform the least invasive test to rule it out. In normal individuals, ACTH and cortisol levels would be low at night, but individuals with Cushing syndrome lose this diurnal variation. If her nighttime cortisol levels are low it is unlikely that she has Cushing syndrome.

The other choices are not screening tests and should only be ordered after the diagnosis of Cushing syndrome is suggested by elevated cortisol levels on a screening test. In addition, a CT scan of the adrenal glands (**Choice B**), an MRI of the pituitary gland (**Choice C**), bilateral inferior petrosal sinus sampling (**Choice D**), and CRH stimulation testing (**Choice E**) are tests that should be used to identify the etiology of Cushing syndrome.

Endocrine Hypertension 11

Mark H. Adelman
Eric I. Felner

CASE

A 38-year-old woman presents for follow-up with her primary care physician with a history of poorly controlled hypertension despite the use of multiple antihypertensive medications. Her major complaints are headache and fatigue. In the physician's office, her blood pressure is 160/100 mmHg in both arms. The remainder of the physical examination is normal. Social history reveals that she does not drink or smoke. She also denies eating licorice or chewing tobacco. Family history reveals that her father died of lung cancer. There is no family history of hypertension, cardiovascular disease, or strokes.

Initial laboratory evaluation reveals elevated serum levels of sodium (149 mEq/L), chloride (113 mEq/L), and bicarbonate (22 mEq/L) along with a low level of potassium (2.9 mEq/L).

This chapter reviews adrenal gland physiology and the endocrine causes of hypertension to help the learner develop hypotheses conveying the etiology of this woman's hypertension. We summarize the work-up and provide a therapeutic plan at the end of the chapter to give the learner a better understanding of the diagnosis. Although there are several causes of hypertension due to endocrine disorders, this chapter emphasizes the adrenal causes of hypertension. This chapter is organized to: 1) review the basic physiology of hypertension involving the renal and endocrine systems and 2) review the causes of hypertension due to adrenal gland, catecholamine, and mineralocorticoid pathology.

OBJECTIVES

1. List the endocrine causes of hypertension.

2. Recognize clinical and laboratory findings in a patient with an endocrine cause of hypertension.

PHYSIOLOGY

An understanding of renal physiology as it relates to endocrine causes of hypertension requires a review of blood pressure physiology, and the basics of the renal system, mineralocorticoids, glucocorticoids, and catecholamines.

Blood Pressure Physiology and the Endocrine System

The endocrine system plays an important role in the regulation of blood pressure through direct and indirect effects on blood volume, venous capacitance, vascular resistance, heart rate, and cardiac contractility. These effects are most apparent in states of hormonal excess or deficiency. Although endocrine causes of hypertension are relatively uncommon, several endocrine pathologies result in hypertension including states of excess production of adrenocortical steroids and catecholamines, growth hormone excess, hypercortisolism, and hyperthyroidism.

Primary or essential hypertension is idiopathic and accounts for more than 95% of cases of hypertension. When there is a specific cause for an increased blood pressure, the hypertension is considered secondary. Other than an elevated blood pressure, most hypertensive patients, regardless of the cause, are asymptomatic and have normal biochemical studies. Early detection and effective treatment are the top priorities in managing patients with hypertension in order to reduce long-term complications such as cardiovascular disease, stroke, and chronic renal disease. In patients with resistant hypertension (defined as persistently elevated blood pressure >140/90 mmHg despite the use of multiple antihypertensive agents), a family history of multiple endocrine neoplasia (MEN) syndrome, or in the presence of hypokalemia, an endocrine cause should be considered.

Of the 5% of hypertensive individuals with a secondary cause, most (40% to 60%) have a renal or renovascular disturbance. Endocrine abnormalities are much less common, accounting for only 10% to 15% of all causes of secondary hypertension.

A brief discussion of the hormones and enzymes involving mineralocorticoid physiology facilitates the understanding of the role of endocrine pathophysiology.

Renal and Mineralocorticoid Physiology

The renal system lies retroperitoneal in the upper area of the abdomen and consists of the pair of kidneys, ureters, bladder, and urethra. The functions of the renal system are performed by the kidneys and include the

- regulation of water and inorganic ion balance,
- removal of metabolic waste products and foreign chemicals from the blood and excretion in urine,
- production of erythropoietin, and
- production of glucose through stimulation of gluconeogenesis.

The endocrine system relies on the renal system for the production of two hormones: renin and 1,25-dihydroxyvitamin D. 1,25-dihydroxyvitamin D, or calcitriol, is converted from 25-hydroxyvitamin D by the 1α-hydroxylase enzyme in the kidney where it promotes calcium and phosphate reabsorption from the small intestine. Calcium homeostatsis is discussed in detail in Chapters 4 and 5. The secretion of renin, from the juxtaglomerular apparatus, ultimately leads to secretion of aldosterone, the most potent mineralocorticoid, from the glomerulosa of the adrenal cortex.

The juxtaglomerular apparatus is the principal site of regulation of angiotensin II (Ang-II) production. The synthesis of prorennin, its conversion to renin, and its systemic secretion are stimulated by blood volume contraction detected by stretch receptors, β-adrenergic stimulation of the sympathetic nervous system, and prostaglandins I_2 and E_2. The synthesis and secretion of these prostaglandins and the normal function of the stretch receptors are dependent upon intracellular ionized calcium concentration. Renal prostaglandin secretion is stimulated by catecholamines and Ang-II. These processes are inhibited by volume expansion and atrial natriuretic peptide (ANP). Renin converts angiotensinogen, a proenzyme synthesized in the liver, into angiotensin I, which is then converted in the lungs into Ang-II, by angiotensin-converting enzyme. Ang-II is both a stimulator of aldosterone secretion and a potent vasopressor. Ang-II is metabolized to angiotensin III, also a stimulator of aldosterone secretion (Figure 11-1).

Aldosterone is a steroid hormone produced exclusively in the zona glomerulosa of the adrenal cortex. It is the major circulating mineralocorticoid in humans. The principal regulators of its synthesis and secretion are the renin–angiotensin system (RAS) and K^+ concentration. Minor regulators include adrenocorticotropic hormone (ACTH) from the pituitary, ANP from the heart, and local adrenal secretion of dopamine. Numerous aldosterone precursors, including deoxycorticosterone (DOC) and 18-hydroxycorticosterone, have mineralocorticoid activity and may produce or exacerbate features typical of mineralocorticoid hypertension when present in excessive amounts in various pathologic states. The principal site of action of aldosterone is the distal nephron, although several other sites of aldosterone-sensitive Na+ regulation are noted, including the sweat glands and gastrointestinal (GI) tract.

The mechanisms regulating aldosterone secretion are complex and involve the zona glomerulosa of the adrenal cortex, the juxtaglomerular apparatus in the kidneys, the cardiovascular system, the autonomic nervous system, the lungs, and the liver. Aldosterone

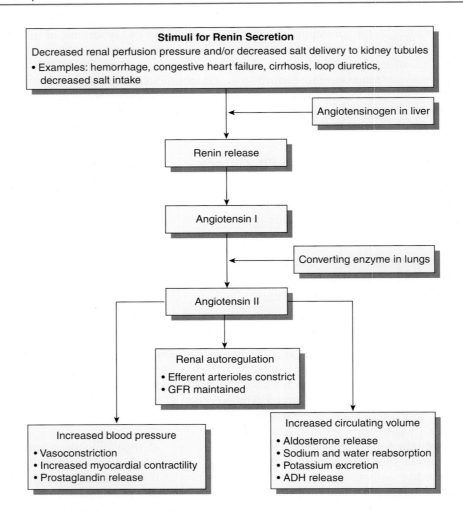

*GFR, glomerular filtration rate; ADH, antidiuretic hormone.

FIGURE 11-1. Renin–angiotensin system. (From Smeltzer SC, Bare BG. Textbook of Medical-Surgical Nursing. 9th ed. Philadelphia, PA: Lippincott Williams & Wilkins; 2000.)

secretion is stimulated by depletion in blood volume detected by stretch receptors and by an increase in serum K^+ concentration. Conversely, aldosterone secretion is suppressed by hypervolemia and hypokalemia.

ACTH stimulates aldosterone secretion in an acute and transient fashion but does not affect chronic regulation of mineralocorticoid secretion. Individuals with an inability to appropriately secrete ACTH, due to hypothalamic or pituitary dysfunction, are unable to secrete cortisol. These individuals, however, despite the loss of the ability to secrete ACTH, will still be able to secrete aldosterone because aldosterone is primarily controlled by the RAS.

The complex regulation of aldosterone synthesis and secretion provides several points where a disturbance in aldosterone secretion may occur. Aldosterone is synthesized from cholesterol in a series of six biosynthetic steps (see Chapter 10). Only the last two steps are specific to aldosterone synthesis. The first four are common to cortisol synthesis in the zona fasciculata. Consequently, a defect in one of the specific aldosterone synthetic enzymes does not lead to hypercortisolism and secondary ACTH-mediated adrenal hyperplasia. The enzyme aldosterone synthase is encoded by the gene *CYP11B2* and has

11-β-hydroxylase, 18-hydroxylase, and 18-hydroxydehydrogenase activity. This gene is located on human chromosome arm 8q24.3, close to the gene *CYP11B1* that encodes 11-β-hydroxylase, the enzyme that catalyzes the final step of cortisol synthesis. Mutations in these genes can result in a number of disorders of aldosterone synthesis.

Aldosterone action on target tissues (e.g., distal renal tubule, sweat glands, salivary glands, and large intestinal epithelium) is mediated via a specific mineralocorticoid receptor. Mineralocorticoid receptors exhibit equal affinity for mineralocorticoids and cortisol, yet the aldosterone receptors in the distal tubule and elsewhere are protected from the activation by cortisol by 11-β-hydroxysteroid dehydrogenase (11β HSD) type 2, which locally converts cortisol to inactive cortisone.

Aldosterone's major effect on electrolytes is to increase Na^+ reabsorption and increase K^+ excretion from the kidney. Aldosterone stimulates sodium transport in the renal collecting duct by activating the epithelial sodium channel (ENaC). The ENaC is a membrane-bound ion-channel that is permeable to lithium ions, protons, and sodium ions (Figure 11-2). The

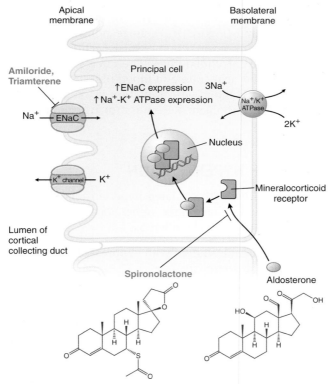

FIGURE 11-2. Cortical collecting duct principal cell. Cortical collecting duct principal cells absorb Na^+ via an apical membrane Na^+ channel (ENaC). Cytoplasmic Na^+ is then transported across the basolateral membrane via the Na^+-K^+ ATPase. In addition, collecting duct cells express apical membrane K^+ channels that allow K^+ to exit into the urinary space. ENaC expression and apical surface localization is modulated by aldosterone. Aldosterone binds to the mineralocorticoid receptor, which then increases transcription of the gene encoding ENaC as well as genes encoding other proteins involved in Na^+ reabsorption (such as Na^+-K^+ ATPase). The collecting duct principal cell is the site of action of the two classes of potassium-sparing diuretics. Mineralocorticoid receptor antagonists such as spironolactone competitively inhibit the interaction of aldosterone with the mineralocorticoid receptor, and thereby decrease expression of ENaC. Direct inhibitors of ENaC, such as amiloride and triamterene, inhibit Na^+ influx through the ENaC channel. (From Golan DE, Tashjian AH, Armstrong EJ. Principles of Pharmacology: The Pathophysiologic Basis of Drug Therapy. 2nd ed. Baltimore, MD: Wolters Kluwer Health; 2008.)

apical membrane of many tight epithelia contains sodium channels that are primarily characterized by their high affinity to the diuretic blocker amiloride. These Na^+ channels mediate the first step of active Na^+ reabsorption. This is essential for maintenance of body salt and water homeostasis. Together with the Na^+-K^+ ATPase, these channels permit reabsorption of Na^+ in the kidney, colon, lungs, and sweat glands. Aldosterone increases the function of the Na^+-K^+ ATPase and activity of the epithelial Na^+ channels in the kidney. In the kidney, the Na^+ channels can be blocked by diuretics, such as amiloride or triamterene, or inhibited by ANP, resulting in natriuresis and diuresis.

ADRENAL CORTEX AND MEDULLA

Catecholamines, cortisol, and aldosterone have profound effects on blood pressure. Excessive levels can cause hypertension, whereas insufficient levels can cause hypotension.

The adrenal medulla is both an endocrine organ and a highly specialized part of the sympathetic nervous system. It is composed mainly of hormone-producing chromaffin cells, where the amino acid tyrosine is converted to the catecholamines epinephrine, norepinephrine, and dopamine (Figure 11-3). In response to stressors (i.e., exercise, danger, or other deviations from normal homeostasis), chromaffin cells are stimulated by nerve impulses to release catecholamines. The effects of epinephrine and norepinephrine include: 1) increased heart rate and blood pressure, 2) blood vessel constriction in the skin and GI tract, 3) blood vessel dilation in skeletal muscle, 4) bronchiole dilation, and 5) decreased metabolism. Receptors for catecholamines are widely distributed throughout the body.

ENDOCRINE STATES OF HYPERTENSION

The most common causes of endocrine-related hypertension are due to elevated levels of mineralocorticoids, hormones that mimic mineralocorticoids, or adrenal medullary hormones. The causes can further be classified as:

- elevated levels of plasma aldosterone with suppressed plasma renin activity (PRA) (primary hyperaldosteronism),
- elevated levels of aldosterone with elevated PRA (secondary hyperaldosteronism),
- elevated levels of catecholamines (adrenal medullary hormones), and
- biochemical and clinical effects mimicking elevated aldosterone but with normal or low levels of plasma aldosterone (pseudohyperaldosteronism).

Secondary hyperaldosteronism is not considered an endocrine-related cause of hypertension and therefore will not be discussed in this chapter. The causes of secondary hyperaldosteronism include: 1) liver cirrhosis, 2) heart failure, 3) nephrotic syndrome, 4) renal artery stenosis, 5) a renin-producing tumor, 6) or a juxtaglomerular tumor. These conditions should be reviewed in other pathophysiology texts.

ADRENAL CORTEX MINERALOCORTICOID HORMONES

Primary hyperaldosteronism and excess DOC are two conditions representing causes of hypertension due to excess production of mineralocorticoid hormones from the adrenal cortex. Pseudohyperaldosteronism is a condition that mimics hyperaldosteronism.

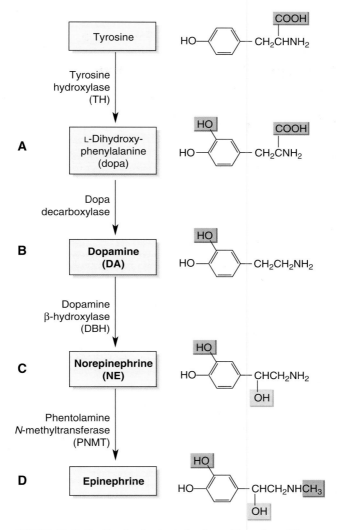

FIGURE 11-3. Synthesis of catecholamines. (From Bear MF, Connors BW, Parasido, MA. Neuroscience: Exploring the Brain. 2nd ed. Philadelphia, PA: Lippincott Williams & Wilkins; 2001.)

Primary Hyperaldosteronism

Primary hyperaldosteronism (PH) most commonly occurs as a result of adrenal hyperplasia, accounting for almost 60% of all causes, with aldosterone-producing adenomas (APAs) accounting for the remaining 40%. Adrenal carcinomas that are purely aldosterone-secreting occur in less than 1% of patients with PH. The majority of PH due to hyperplasia is bilateral (70%), whereas the majority of APAs are unilateral (85%). For solitary nodules, the left adrenal gland is most often affected.

Etiology

The most common cause of adrenal-mediated hypertension is primary PH. Although adrenal hyperplasia and adrenal carcinoma also cause primary PH, when the hyperaldosteronism is due to a solitary adrenal adenoma, it is known as **Conn syndrome**.

TABLE 11-1. Biochemical Findings, Tests, and Treatment for Endocrine Causes of Hypertension

Serum Aldosterone	Plasma ACTH	Serum Cortisol	Serum K$^+$	Confirmatory Tests	Treatment
Elevated					
Hyperaldosteronism	N	N	↓	SLT, AVS, imaging	Surgery
Normal					
DOC-secreting tumor	N/↓	N/↑	↓	↑DOC levels and Imaging	Surgery
DSH	N	N	↓	Gene analysis	Dexamethasone
Cushing syndrome	↑/↓	↑	↓	CRH stim, DST, imaging	Surgery
11-OHase deficiency	↑/↓	L	↓	Cortrosyn test and gene analysis	Hydrocortisone
Pheochromocytoma	N	N	N	↑HVA, VMA levels	Phenoxybenzamine, surgery
Low					
17-OHase deficiency	↑	↓	↓	Cortrosyn test and gene analysis	Hydrocortisone
Glucocorticoid resistance	N/↓	N/↑	↓	DST and gene analysis	Dexamethasone
AME	N/↓	N	↓	↑Cortisol/cortisone	Dexamethasone
Licorice ingestion	N	N	↓	History and ↑Cortisol/cortisone	Stop licorice
MR mutation	N	N	↓	Gene analysis	Decrease progesterone
Liddle syndrome	N	N	↓	Gene analysis	Amiloride/triamterene
Gordon syndrome	N	N	↑	Gene analysis	Thiazide diuretic

Notes: K$^+$, serum potassium level; ↑, high; ↓, low; N, normal; MR, mineralocorticoid receptor; DSH, dexamethasone-suppressible hyperaldosteronism; SLT, salt-loading test; AVS, adrenal vein sampling; DST, dexamethasone-suppression test; HVA, homovanilic acid; VMA, vanillylmandelic acid; DOC, deoxycorticosterone; ACTH, adrenocorticotropic hormone; AME, apparent mineralocorticoid excess; CRH, corticotropin-releasing hormone.

TABLE 11-2.	Pharmacologic Agents Used in the Treatment for Endocrine Causes of Hypertension	
Agent	**Mechanism of Action**	**Effects**
Hydrocortisone	Binds to glucocorticoid and mineralocorticoid receptors	Suppresses CRH and ACTH secretion
Dexamethasone	Binds to glucocorticoid but not mineralocorticoid receptor	Suppresses CRH and ACTH secretion
Phenoxybenzamine	Binds to and inhibits $\alpha1$ and $\alpha2$ receptors	Muscle relaxation and dilatation of blood vessels
Amiloride	Binds to amiloride-sensitive Na^+ channels	Promotes Na^+ and water loss from the kidneys but spares K^+
Triamterene	Binds to and inhibits the epithelial sodium channels on principal cells in the late distal convoluted tubule and collecting tubule	Inhibits Na^+ reabsorption and K^+ excretion
Spironolactone	Competitive antagonist of the aldosterone-dependent Na^+/K^+ exchange site in the distal convoluted tubule	Promotes excretion of Na^+ and water but spares K^+
Thiazide	Inhibits the Na^+/Cl^- cotransporter in the distal convoluted tubule	Inhibits water reabsorption

Pathology

PH is principally a disease of adulthood, with its peak incidence in the fourth to sixth decades of life. APAs are usually benign encapsulated adenomas that are <2 cm in diameter. Most cases are solitary, although in as many as one-third of cases, evidence exists of nodularity in the same adrenal, suggesting that it has arisen in a previously hyperplastic gland.

Pathophysiology

In the renal tubules, elevated aldosterone promotes excessive Na^+ reabsorption as well as K^+ excretion. Na^+ retention results in water retention, expansion of the extracellular volume, arterial hypertension, and suppression of PRA production. Excessive K^+ and H^+ loss results in hypokalemic alkalosis that may be associated with various complications that are described below.

Clinical Findings

Primary hyperaldosteronism is characterized by moderate-to-severe hypertension. If hypokalemic alkalosis occurs, muscle weakness, polydipsia, polyuria, nocturia, paresthesia, tetany, headaches, and abnormal electrocardiographic features (i.e., low voltage or inverted T waves) may develop. Other clinical manifestations include subarachnoid hemorrhage, postural hypotension, and bradycardia. In rare cases, high Na^+ levels may cause edema. A neonatal form of idiopathic hyperaldosteronism has been described in which neonates present with constipation, hypokalemia, and hypertension.

Diagnostic Studies

The diagnosis of PH is based on elevated aldosterone levels, suppressed PRA, an elevated aldosterone/PRA ratio, and lack of aldosterone suppression with endocrine suppression tests. The classic finding is the presence of high aldosterone and low PRA. A PRA <1 ng/dL/hour is not only common to virtually all patients with PH but also occurs in 20% to 25% of patients with essential hypertension. The ratio of aldosterone (ng/dL) to PRA (ng/mL/hour) is a better screening study than either aldosterone or PRA alone. Ratios <20 make the diagnosis of PH less likely, whereas ratios of 20 to 40 suggest PH. Ratios >65 are highly suggestive of PH. The plasma aldosterone/PRA ratio is the best screening test, but aldosterone suppression testing is required to confirm the diagnosis. Several tests are used to demonstrate the autonomous production of aldosterone. These tests are discussed in detail in Chapter 19.

The work-up in patients in whom primary PH is suspected starts with appropriate biochemical analysis and, when the diagnosis is confirmed, is followed by a computed tomography (CT) scan or magnetic resonance image (MRI) of the abdomen, including the adrenal glands. High-resolution CT scans and MRIs are equally effective in differentiating between an APA and adrenal hyperplasia, and APAs >5 mm in size can be detected with either imaging modality. If the diagnosis is still not established, and especially if no adrenal mass is seen, several nuclear scans are available to determine the physiologic function of an APA or adrenal hyperplasia, but all have limited reliability.

Treatment

In 75% to 90% of patients with a solitary aldosterone-producing tumor, surgical adrenalectomy corrects the hypertension and hypokalemia. In the other patients with idiopathic hyperaldosteronism associated with bilateral adrenal hyperplasia, surgery rarely cures the hypertension. Restriction of salt in the diet (<100 mEq/day) and use of a nonselective, mineralocorticoid receptor antagonist (i.e., spironolactone) may be necessary. Additional agents may be necessary in some patients who do not achieve target blood pressure. Although K^+ supplementation may be needed to improve serum K^+ levels, it is typically of little benefit in controlling blood pressure. Maintaining a healthy weight, exercising regularly, and avoiding tobacco may also be helpful. Surgical intervention should be entertained in those patients with confirmed PH in whom imaging studies suggest an adenoma. Radiation therapy should be reserved for those who are not surgical candidates and do not respond to medical therapy.

Prognosis

In cases of APAs, the prognosis is excellent with early diagnosis and treatment. Surgical removal of an adrenal tumor results in complete resolution of symptoms and normalization of the blood pressure in about 70% of cases. Blood pressure, however, does not return to normal immediately following surgery, but rather normalizes gradually over 1 to 4 months. Individuals whose blood pressure does not normalize within 4 months after tumor removal likely have essential hypertension. If a tumor is responsible for the disease but cannot be removed surgically, or if both adrenals are involved, the prognosis still remains excellent with medical therapy. The majority of patients with PH will have a complete recovery if the diagnosis is made early and the symptoms treated promptly. If, on the other hand, PH is untreated or if treatment is delayed, irreversible damage to the heart and/or kidneys may occur.

Excess Deoxycorticosterone

Excess levels of deoxycorticosterone (DOC) are due to either an enzyme deficiency in the steroid biosynthesis pathway or to a DOC-producing adrenal tumor. The enzyme-deficiency causes are discussed in detail in the discussion of congenital adrenal hyperplasia in Chapter 10. The DOC-producing tumors are rare and usually malignant. Due to the relatively weak mineralocorticoid activity of DOC, these tumors do not always result in symptoms of mineralocorticoid excess.

Clinical manifestations resembling hyperaldosteronism result from DOC excess. Although a relatively weak mineralocorticoid, DOC, when secreted in excessive amounts, causes excess Na^+ retention and K^+ wasting. Na^+ retention promotes water retention, expansion of the extracellular volume, hypertension, and suppression of renin production. K^+ wasting results in hypokalemic alkalosis. The clinical findings are similar to those found in PH.

The diagnosis is based on the same biochemical findings seen with PH with the exception that the DOC level is significantly elevated, and the aldosterone level is low to normal. The demonstration of suppressed PRA and elevated DOC is vital to the diagnosis. A NaCl suppression test can be used to demonstrate the inability to suppress DOC secretion. This test is described in detail in Chapter 19.

In addition to secreting DOC, these tumors commonly secrete other adrenal hormones, behaving similarly to an adrenal cortical carcinoma. The staging system for these tumors depends upon tumor size, nodal involvement, invasion of adjacent organs, and presence of distant metastases. Only stages I and II are curable by surgery. Most patients, however, have either stage III or IV disease at the time of diagnosis. Despite surgical correction, the 5-year survival is only 30% and 20% for stage III and stage IV disease, respectively.

Pseudohyperaldosteronism

Pseudohyperaldosteronism is a condition that mimics hyperaldosteronism. Like hyper-aldosteronism, individuals with pseudohyperaldosteronism present with hypertension, hypokalemia, metabolic alkalosis, and low plasma renin activity. Unlike hyperaldosteronism, aldosterone levels in individuals with pseudohyperaldosteronism are normal or low. The most common causes of pseudohyperaldosteronism are genetic and include 11β HSD-2 deficiency, Liddle syndrome, Gordon syndrome, and mutations of the mineralocorticoid receptor. Licorice ingestion, the only dietary cause, inhibits the 11β HSD-2 enzyme, thereby overwhelming the mineralocorticoid receptor by cortisol. Cushing syndrome also causes pseudohyperaldosteronism by overwhelming the mineralocorticoid receptor and is discussed in detail in Chapter 10. Pseudohyperaldosteronism and its causes for hypertension are discussed as adrenal cortex glucocorticoid hormones, ACTH-dependent disorders, sodium reabsorption disorders, and mutations of the mineralocorticoid receptor.

ADRENAL CORTEX GLUCOCORTICOID HORMONES

11β HSD-2 deficiency and hypercortisolism are causes of pseudohyperaldosteronism due to adrenal cortex glucocorticoid hormones.

11-β-Hydroxysteroid Dehydrogenase Deficiency

Apparent mineralocorticoid excess (AME) is a rare autosomal recessive disorder characterized by hypertension, hypokalemia, and hypernatremia. It results from mutations in the *HSD11B2* gene, which encodes the kidney isozyme 11-β-hydroxysteroid dehydrogenase (11β HSD) type 2. In unaffected individuals, the isozyme inactivates circulating cortisol to the less-active metabolite, cortisone. Those with an inactivating mutation have elevated renal concentrations of cortisol. At high concentrations, cortisol cross-reacts and activates the mineralocorticoid receptor, leading to aldosterone-like effects in the kidney such as hypokalemia, hypernatremia, and hypertension.

The initial presentation is usually in childhood. There is a history of severe hypertension, low birth weight, failure to thrive, and short stature. The biochemical findings include hypokalemia, hypernatremia, metabolic alkalosis, low serum aldosterone, and low PRA level. If the K^+ level is severely low, additional clinical findings include muscle weakness, tetany, and decreased tendon reflexes. The condition can be differentiated from other causes of pseudohyperaldosteronism through the measurement of urinary metabolites of cortisol (tetrahydrocortisol) and cortisone (tetrahydrocortisone). In the unaffected individual, the ratio of tetrahydrocortisol to tetrahydrocortisone is 1, whereas in those with apparent mineralocorticoid excess (AME), it is between 6 and 70.

Treatment involves the delivery of a synthetic glucocorticoid, such as dexamethasone, which results in minimal endogenous production of cortisol. As this only corrects 60% of cases, other treatment options include spironolactone, a reduction in dietary sodium with supplementation of potassium, or even a renal transplant. Spironolactone, a mineralocorticoid receptor antagonist, binds competitively to the mineralocorticoid receptor and protects receptors against any mineralocorticoid excess.

Hypercortisolism

As discussed previously, states of hypercortisolism cause hypertension by activation of the mineralocorticoid receptor or by overwhelming the 11β HSD-2 enzyme. Cushing syndrome and Cushing disease, the most common causes of endogenous hypercortisolism, are discussed in detail in Chapter 10.

ADRENOCORTICOTROPIC HORMONE–DEPENDENT DISORDERS

Aldosterone regulation is primarily under the control of the RAS. Adrenocorticotropic hormone (ACTH), however, can affect the release of aldosterone through its stimulation of steroid biosynthesis. As discussed in Chapter 10, excessive ACTH secretion that results in hypercortisolism causes hypertension by overwhelming the 11β HSD-2 enzyme. The excess cortisol, after saturating the glucocorticoid receptor, binds to and activates the mineralocorticoid receptor. Excessive ACTH secretion may also occur when specific enzymes of steroid biosynthesis (such as 21-hydroxylase and 11-hydroxylase) are deficient, resulting in cortisol deficiency. Cortisol deficiency may further stimulate ACTH secretion and overwhelm the mineralocorticoid pathway, resulting in hypertension. These conditions are discussed in depth in Chapter 15 with disorders of sexual reproduction and ambiguous genitalia.

Hypertension due to excess ACTH secretion without hypercortisolism may be seen in familial glucocorticoid resistance. Another ACTH-dependent disorder, dexamethasone-suppressible hyperaldosteronism (DSH), involves the stimulation of aldosterone by ACTH due to a mutation involving the fusion of the gene for the promoter region of an enzyme necessary for cortisol production with the gene for the coding sequences of an enzyme necessary for aldosterone production.

Familial Glucocorticoid Resistance

Glucocorticoid resistance results from the partial inability of glucocorticoids to exert its effects on target tissues. This condition is associated with compensatory increases in circulating ACTH and cortisol, with the former causing excess secretion of both adrenal mineralocorticoids and androgens. The manifestations of glucocorticoid resistance include chronic fatigue (possibly due to central nervous system glucocorticoid deficiency), various degrees of hypertension, and hyperandrogenism. The familial forms of glucocorticoid resistance are due to molecular defects that alter the functional characteristics or concentrations of the intracellular glucocorticoid receptor. Therefore, in an effort to produce a sufficient amount of glucocorticoid in those with a receptor defect, excess glucocorticoid is stimulated by a compensatory increase in corticotropin-releasing hormone (CRH) and ACTH secretion. At high sustained levels, ACTH not only increases glucocorticoid production but also mineralocorticoid and androgen production. The variability in the manifestations of familial glucocorticoid resistance can be explained by the overall degree of glucocorticoid resistance—that is, different sensitivity of target tissues to mineralocorticoids or androgens, or both, as well as different biochemical defects of the glucocorticoid receptor, and maintaining selective resistance of certain glucocorticoid responses in specific tissues. There are four keys to making this diagnosis:

1. Lack of phenotypic evidence for hypercortisolism,
2. Elevated levels of 24-hour urinary free cortisol,
3. Elevated levels of cortisol after dexamethasone-suppression testing (DST), and
4. Intact hypothalamic–pituitary–adrenal axis with normal circadian rhythmicity.

This syndrome should be diagnosed by the biochemical features listed above in conjunction with the absence of the typical clinical findings seen in other states of hypercortisolism.

The gene encoding the glucocorticoid receptor on chromosome 5 is very complex and contains 10 exons. A number of point mutations and gene microdeletions have been discovered in families with this condition. Mutations have resulted in a decreased number, affinity, and DNA binding of the glucocorticoid receptor.

Treatment of this condition involves the use of a synthetic glucocorticoid with minimal intrinsic mineralocorticoid activity. Dexamethasone, with no mineralocorticoid activity, will reduce ACTH stimulation and, ultimately, reduce excess mineralocorticoid and androgen secretion.

Dexamethasone-Suppressible Hyperaldosteronism

Dexamethasone-suppressible hyperaldosteronism (DSH) is a rare autosomal dominant disorder characterized by hypertension and hypokalemia but may not come to attention until profound hypokalemia occurs after treatment with a thiazide diuretic. It results from a mutation in which the promoter region for the gene (CYP11B1) encoding 11-hydroxylase (enzyme catalyzing the conversion of deoxycortisol to cortisol) in the zona fasciculata fuses with the coding sequences for the gene (CYP11B2) encoding aldosterone synthetase (enzyme catalyzing the conversion of DOC to corticosterone and corticosterone to aldosterone) in the zona glomerulosa. This results in ACTH-dependent activation of the aldosterone synthase effect on cortisol, deoxycortisol, corticosterone, 18-oxocortisol, 18-hydroxycortisol, and aldosterone. The hyperaldosteronism results in suppression of PRA.

The most common presentation of this condition is severe hypertension that occurs in infancy or early adulthood. A strong family history of hypertension, often with early death of affected family members due to cerebrovascular accidents, is common. An important distinction between this condition and other causes of hyperaldosteronism is the age of onset of hypertension. In DSH, the diagnosis is usually made in the first two decades of life, whereas in the other causes of hyperaldosteronism, diagnosis is usually made in the third to sixth decades of life. The biochemical findings include hypokalemia, low PRA, and elevated aldosterone levels. If hypokalemia occurs, the clinical findings may include muscle weakness, tetany, and decreased tendon reflexes.

Genetic testing for the chimeric gene is 100% specific and sensitive for making the diagnosis. Biochemically, the condition can be differentiated from other causes of hyperaldosteronism by the presence of elevated levels of 18-oxocortisol and 18-hydroxycortisol. The simplest test to perform is the DST in which serum aldosterone levels are measured before and 8 hours after dexamethasone administration. Elevated levels of aldosterone prior to dexamethasone administration fall to near undetectable levels in those with DSH. It is not, however, as specific a test as genetic testing, and an appropriate response to dexamethasone usually requires genetic testing for the chimeric gene.

Treatment involves the delivery of a synthetic glucocorticoid such as dexamethasone, which inhibits ACTH, resulting in reduction of excessive aldosterone stimulation.

SODIUM-REABSORPTION DISORDERS

Although extremely rare, Liddle syndrome and Gordon syndrome are two Na^+-reabsorption disorders that cause hypertension and result in biochemical findings consistent with pseudohyperaldosteronism.

Liddle Syndrome

Liddle syndrome (pseudohyperaldosteronism I) is an autosomal dominant renal disorder characterized by hypertension, hypokalemia, and inappropriate kaliuresis. Liddle syndrome is caused by mutations in the β- or γ-subunit of the amiloride-sensitive ENaC. During normal physiologic conditions, in an effort to prevent excess Na^+ reabsorption, the E3 ligase (Nedd4) presents the ENaC to the cellular proteasome for ENaC degradation. Liddle syndrome is caused by dysregulation of the ENaC due to a genetic mutation at the 16p13-p12 locus. This mutation changes a domain in the channel so it can no longer be degraded properly by the ubiquitin proteasome system. Therefore, there is increased activity of this channel, leading to increased Na^+ reabsorption, leading to an increase in extracellular volume, and, in turn, ultimately leading to hypertension.

The biochemical findings include hypokalemia, hypernatremia, metabolic alkalosis, low plasma aldosterone, and low PRA. If the K^+ level is severely low, in addition to hypertension, the clinical findings may include muscle weakness, tetany, and decreased tendon reflexes. Genetic testing for the mutation is available.

Treatment includes a low-salt diet and a K^+-sparing diuretic that directly blocks the ENaC such as amiloride or triamterene. These agents are very effective in treating the hypertension and hypokalemia; however, spironolactone, a K^+-sparring diuretic, is ineffective because it acts by blocking aldosterone secretion. Liddle syndrome can be distinguished from apparent mineralocorticoid excess (AME) based on the clinical response to amiloride and triamterene and the lack of response to spironolactone.

Gordon Syndrome

Gordon syndrome (pseudohyperaldosteronism II) is an autosomal dominant disorder characterized by early, and frequently severe, hypertension. It involves abnormal kidney function, combining volume-dependent salt-sensitive hypertension, hyperkalemia, hyperchloremia, metabolic acidosis, and a normal glomerular filtration rate. During normal physiologic conditions, and in an effort to prevent excess Na^+ loss, the thiazide-sensitive NaCl cotransporter (NCCT) in the distal convoluted tubule is inhibited by a protein kinase (WNK-4). Gordon syndrome is caused by the loss of function of WNK-4 that results in increased NCCT activity and decreased Na$^+$ reaching the collecting duct and ultimately leads to lower electrogenic Na$^+$ reabsorption, with reduced tubular electronegativity. This drives K$^+$ and H$^+$ secretion causing hyperkalemia and a metabolic acidosis. In addition, the inactivation of WNK-4 reduces the activity of the renal outer medullary K$^+$ channel in the collecting duct.

The biochemical findings include hyperkalemia, hyperchloremia, metabolic acidosis, hypoaldosteronism, and low PRA. The key difference in this condition, as compared to Liddle syndrome, is that these patients are hyperkalemic, rather than hypokalemic. Treatment includes a low-salt diet and a thiazide diuretic.

MUTATIONS OF THE MINERALOCORTICOID RECEPTOR

Although extremely rare, gain-of-function mutations of the mineralocorticoid receptor can produce similar symptoms, electrolyte disturbances, and blood pressure elevations as seen in hyperaldosterone or excess-DOC states. A mutation that encodes the gene for the mineralocorticoid receptor has been reported. This autosomal dominant, missense mutation activates the mineralocorticoid receptor despite low PRA and aldosterone. This results in a change in the ligand-binding domain, leading to similarities between the mineralocorticoid receptor and progesterone. Therefore, hypertension and hypokalemia occur in individuals affected with this mutation who encounter elevated progesterone states such as pregnancy. Interestingly, spironolactone, the model compound for antagonizing aldosterone action, acts as an agonist for this abnormal receptor. The only known treatment for this condition is to minimize progesterone excess. Although pregnancies should not necessarily be aborted, delivery of the fetus usually results in an improvement in blood pressure.

ADRENAL MEDULLARY HORMONES

Pheochromocytoma is the one adrenal medullary hormone cause for hypertension.

Pheochromocytoma

In adults, 85% of pheochromocytomas are found in the adrenal glands, with 80% of those being unilateral and solitary tumors. The other 15% are extra-adrenal. In children, however, 25% are bilateral and 25% are extra-adrenal.

Etiology

A pheochromocytoma is a neuroendocrine tumor that usually arises in the adrenal medulla from chromaffin cells or is extra-adrenal from chromaffin tissue that failed to involute after birth. These tumors secrete excessive amounts of catecholamines (epinephrine, norepinephrine, and their metabolites). In the United States, the prevalence is approximately 5 per 1,000,000, with an incidence of 1,000 cases per year. It is seen mostly in young or middle-aged adults. Most occur sporadically, but at least 25% are due to genetic mutations. A number of gene mutations are associated with familial pheochromocytoma. The pheochromocytoma is also a tumor of the MEN syndrome (type 2A or 2B). Mutations in the autosomal *RET* proto-oncogene account for MEN 2A and 2B (Box 11-1). The MEN syndromes are discussed in detail in Chapter 17.

Pathology

The tumors are made up of large, polyhedral, pleomorphic chromaffin cells. Malignancy is indicated by local invasion of surrounding tissues or by distant metastases. Less than

BOX 11-1.	Features of Multiple Endocrine Neoplasia Syndromes 2A and 2B

MEN 2A

- Medullary carcinoma of the thyroid gland
- Pheochromocytoma
- Parathyroid tumors
- Nonendocrine findings
  - Pruritic cutaneous lichen amyloidosis
  - Hirschsprung disease

MEN 2B

- Medullary carcinoma of the thyroid gland
- Pheochromocytoma
- Nonendocrine findings
  - Marfanoid habitus
  - Mucosal neuromas
  - Ganglioneuromas

Notes: MEN, multiple endocrine neoplasia.

10% are malignant. A pheochromocytoma is classified in one of four stages: localized and benign, regional, metastatic, or recurrent.

Pathophysiology

The effects of catecholamine excess produce the clinical findings. Understanding the biochemistry of catecholamine production is the key to understanding the pathophysiology of pheochromocytoma. In the adrenal medulla, tyrosine is converted to dihydroxyphenylalanine, which is converted to dopamine. Dopamine is then converted to epinephrine and norepinephrine, which are ultimately metabolized to homovanillic acid (HVA) and vanillylmandelic acid (VMA). The principal catecholamines produced by a pheochromocytoma are epinephrine, norepinephrine, HVA, and VMA. These catecholamines activate $\alpha1$, $\alpha2$, $\beta1$, and $\beta2$ receptors. Norepinephrine, the catecholamine principally produced by extra-adrenal pheochromocytomas, has $\alpha1$, $\alpha2$, and $\beta1$ effects. Activation of the α and β receptors causes the following effects:

- $\alpha1$—smooth muscle contraction
- $\alpha2$—smooth muscle constriction
- $\beta1$—heart muscle contraction
- $\beta2$—smooth muscle relaxation.

Clinical Findings

Virtually all patients have moderate-to-severe hypertension. The most common symptoms include headache, sweating, and increased heart rate. These symptoms may occur suddenly but usually subside in less than an hour. Other symptoms include orthostasis, palpitations, anxiety, pallor, weight loss, and hyperglycemia. A pheochromocytoma may cause resistant hypertension and may be fatal if it results in malignant hypertension. The classic symptoms of pheochromocytoma include paroxysms of the "5 Ps": palpitations, perspiration, pallor, pain, and pressure.

Diagnostic Studies

First, the diagnosis of a catecholamine-producing tumor must be suspected and then confirmed biochemically by increased concentrations of fractionated metanephrines and catecholamines in the urine or plasma. The diagnosis can be established by measuring fractionated cathecholamines (dopamine, norepinephrine, and epinephrine) and metanephrines (metanephrine and normetanephrine) in plasma or in a 24-hour urine test. The most accurate case-finding method for identifying catecholamine-secreting tumors is measuring fractionated metanephrines and catecholamines in a 24-hour urine collection (sensitivity 98%, specificity 98%).

Although rarely necessary, suppression testing with clonidine may be considered if the diagnosis is still uncertain after initial testing. Clonidine is a centrally acting α-agonist that mimics catecholamines in the brain. It causes reduced activity of the sympathetic nerves controlling the adrenal medulla. A normal adrenal medulla will respond to clonidine with lower catecholamine levels, whereas a pheochromocytoma will prevent the catecholamine levels from dropping.

Once the diagnosis of a pheochromocytoma is confirmed by biochemical testing, the next step is to localize the tumor(s) to help guide the potential surgical approach. Computer-assisted adrenal and abdominal imaging (with MRI or CT) is the first localization test (Figure 11-4A,B). Most pheochromocytomas (98%) are located in the abdomen and pelvis, of which almost 90% are in the adrenal glands. If the findings on abdominal

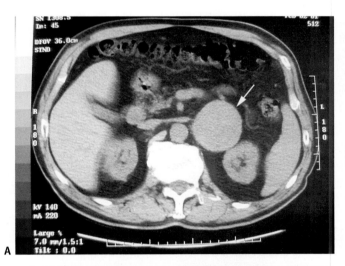

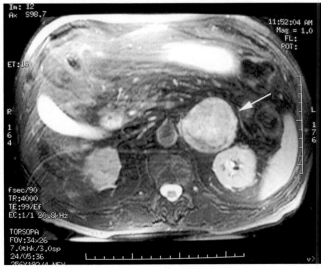

FIGURE 11-4. Pheochromocytoma. **(A)** Computed tomography (CT) scan shows a well-circumscribed left adrenal mass (*arrow*). **(B)** The T2-weighted magnetic resonance imaging (MRI) shows the mass to be heterogeneously bright (*arrow*). (From Mulholland MW, Lillemoe KD, Doherty GM, et al. Greenfield's Surgery: Scientific Principles and Practice. 4th ed. Philadelphia, PA: Lippincott Williams & Wilkins; 2006.)

imaging are negative, scintigraphic localization with [123-I]-metaiodobenzylguanidine may help localize the tumor.

Treatment

The treatment of choice for a pheochromocytoma is surgical resection. Most of the tumors are benign and can be excised. To ensure a successful surgical outcome, the chronic and acute effects of excess circulating catecholamines should be reversed preoperatively. Combined α- and β-adrenergic blockade is required preoperactively to control blood pressure and prevent intraoperative hypertensive crises. α-Adrenergic blockade should be initiated 7 to 10 days preoperatively to allow expansion of the contracted blood volume.

Laparoscopic adrenalectomy is the procedure of choice for patients with solitary intra-adrenal pheochromocytomas. Hypotension may occur after surgical resection, and it should be treated with fluids and small, intermittent doses of intravenous pressor agents as needed. Postoperative hypotension is less frequent in patients who have had adequate preoperative α-adrenergic blockade and volume expansion.

Prognosis

The prognosis depends on the stage of the pheochromocytoma and the patient's age and general health. Blood pressure usually normalizes within a week, but some patients may

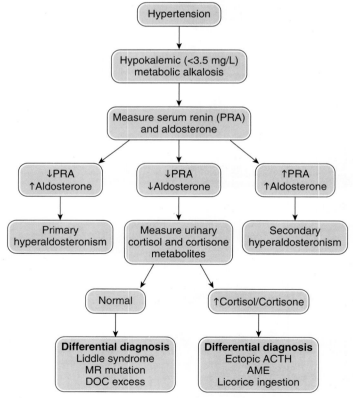

FIGURE 11-5. Algorithm for determining the etiology of hypertension in a patient with hypokalemia.
Note: PRA, plasma renin activity; MR, mineralocorticoid receptor; DOC, deoxycorticosterone; ACTH, adrenocorticotropic hormone; AME, apparent mineralocorticoid excess

remain hypertensive for several weeks after surgery. About 1 to 2 weeks after surgery, 24-hour urinary fractionated metanephrines and catecholamines should be measured. If the levels are normal, the resection of the pheochromocytoma is considered complete. Increased levels, however, indicate residual tumor, which could be the result of a second primary lesion or occult metastases. Annual biochemical testing allows for the assessment of metastatic disease, tumor recurrence, or delayed appearance of multiple primary tumors. Recurrence rates are highest for those with familial disease or a paraganglioma. A follow-up CT scan or MRI is not needed unless the fractionated metanephrines and/or catecholamine levels are elevated, or the original tumor was nonfunctioning. A localized and regional tumor stage has the most favorable prognosis, whereas metastatic and recurrent stages are less favorable.

In evaluating a patient with hypertension and hypokalemia, an algorithm can be followed based on the serum aldosterone and PRA levels (Figure 11-5).

CASE FOLLOW-UP

With a history of poorly controlled hypertension, despite multiple antihypertensive medications, and hypokalemia, further laboratory testing is indicated. Her plasma aldosterone level (30 ng/dL) is elevated, and her PRA (0.3 ng/mL/hour) is low. The ratio of plasma aldosterone to PRA (100) is significantly elevated and highly suggestive of primary hyperaldosteronism (PH).

A saline suppression test is performed in which plasma aldosterone levels are collected before, during, and after she receives 2 L of normal saline for 4 hours.

The results of the saline suppression test confirm suppressed PRA levels without suppression of plasma aldosterone levels (Table 11-3). The significantly elevated ratio of plasma aldosterone/PRA is highly suggestive of PH. Imaging with abdominal CT reveals normal appearing adrenal glands. Bilateral adrenal vein sampling is performed in an effort to help localize the elevated aldosterone secretion. Results of adrenal vein sampling reveal an elevated aldosterone level in the left adrenal vein (Table 11-4).

Our patient is taken to surgery, and the left adrenal gland is removed laporoscopically revealing an aldosterone-secreting tumor. One month after surgery, the patient maintains a normal blood pressure without the use of any medications.

TABLE 11-3.   Saline Suppression Test Results

Parameter	Baseline	2 h	4 h
Serum sodium (mEq/L)	147	146	146
Serum potassium (mEq/L)	3.3	3.2	3.2
Plasma aldosterone (ng/dL)	30	31	32
PRA (ng/mL/h)	0.3	0.2	0.2
Aldosterone/PRA	100	155	160

(continues)

CASE FOLLOW-UP (*continued*)

TABLE 11-4.   Adrenal Vein Sampling Results

Parameter	Right Adrenal Vein	Left Adrenal Vein
Plasma aldosterone (ng/dL)	800	8,300
Serum cortisol (mcg/dL)	1,200	1,300
Plasma aldosterone/serum cortisol ratio	0.67	6.4

The work-up for this patient (Figure 11-5) focused on conditions that did not suppress aldosterone in the presence of suppressed PRA, virtually ruling out secondary causes of hyperaldosteronism. The only logical conclusion for this patient's hypertension is primary hyperaldosteronism. Other conditions that should have been considered include causes of pseudohyperaldosteronism, such as Liddle syndrome, apparent mineralocorticoid excess (AME), and mutations of the mineralocorticoid receptor. Because these conditions are associated with aldosterone suppression, they were less likely.

REFERENCES and SUGGESTED READINGS

Charmandari E, Kino T, Ichijo T, Chrousos GP. Generalized glucocorticoid resistance: clinical aspects, molecular mechanisms, and implications of a rare genetic disorder. J Clin Endocrinol Metab. 2008;93:1563–1572.

Dluhy RG, Williams GH. Aldosterone–villain or bystander? N Engl J Med. 2004;351(1):8–10.

Eisenhofer G, et al. Biochemical diagnosis of pheochromocytoma: how to distinguish true from false-positive test results. J Clin Endocrinol Metab. 2003;88:2656–2666.

Felner EI, Taweevisit M, Gow K. Hyperaldosteronism in an adolescent with Gardner's syndrome. J Pediatr Surg. 2009;44:e21–e23.

Furuhasi M, et al. Liddle's syndrome caused by a novel mutation in the proline-rich PY motif of the epithelial sodium channel β-subunit. J Clin Endocrinol Metab. 2005;90:340–344.

Geller DS, et al. Activating mineralocorticoid receptor mutation in hypertension exacerbated by pregnancy. Science. 2000;289(5476):119–123.

Guerrero MA, Schreinmakers JM, Vriens MR, et al. Clinical spectrum of pheochromocytoma. J Am Coll Surg. 2009;209:727–732.

McKenzie TJ, Lillegard JB, Young WF Jr, Thompson GB. Aldosteronomas–state of the art. Surg Clin North Am. 2009;89:1241–1253.

Neary NM, King KS, Pacak K. Drugs and pheochromocytoma–don't be fooled by every elevated metanephrine. N Engl J Med. 2011;364(23):2268–2270.

Pacak K. Preoperative management of the pheochromocytoma patient. J Clin Endocrinol Metab. 2007;92:4069–4079.

Palmer BF, Alpern RJ. Liddle's syndrome. Am J Med. 1998;104:301–309.

Vasan RS, Evans JC, Larson MG, et al. Serum aldosterone and the incidence of hypertension in nonhypertensive persons. N Engl J Med. 2004;351(1):33–41.

Scholten A, Cisco RM, Vriens MR, et al. Pheochromocytoma crisis is not a surgical emergency. J Clin Endocrinol Metab. 2013;98(2):581–91.

Speiser PW, Martin KO, Kao-Lo G, New MI. Excess mineralocorticoid receptor activity in patients with dexamethasone-suppressible hyperaldosteronism is under adrenocoticotropic control. J Clin Endocrinol Metab. 1985;61:297–302.

Trebble P, Matthews L, Blaikley J, Wayte AWO, Black GCM, Wilton A, et al. Familial glucocorticoid resistance caused by a novel frameshift glucocorticoid receptor mutation. J Clin Endocrinol Metab. 2010;95:E490–E499.

White PC. Disorders of aldosterone biosynthesis and action. N Engl J Med. 1994;331:250–258.

White PC, Mune T, Agarwal AK. 11β-Hydroxysteroid dehydrogenase and the syndrome of apparent mineralocorticoid excess. Endocr Rev. 1997;18:135–156.

Yamamoto A, et al. Deoxycorticosterone-secreting adrenocortical carcinoma. Endocr Pathol. 1993;4(3):165–168.

CHAPTER REVIEW QUESTIONS

1. A 46-year-old man presents to your office with hypertension that is refractory to the most common antihypertensive agents. He is not overweight, but does have a strong family history for strokes. You prescribe a trial of dexamethasone and his blood pressure normalizes by his next visit with you. The most likely cause of this man's hypertension is

   A. Secondary hyperaldosteronism
   B. Glucocorticoid-remediable hyperaldosteronism
   C. Congenital adrenal hypoplasia
   D. Addison disease
   E. Liddle syndrome

2. A 48-year-old woman has blood pressure (BP) readings of 177/123, 194/129, and 182/118 mmHg on three consecutive days. On the fourth day, her BP is 189/121 mmHg, serum Na$^+$ level is 154 mEq/L, and serum K$^+$ level is 2.1 mEq/L. Regarding her diagnosis, which of the following statements is most likely *true*?

   A. Her aldosterone level is low.
   B. Her aldosterone/renin ratio is low.
   C. She has Kimmelstiel-Wilson syndrome.
   D. She has Conn syndrome.
   E. She has Nelson syndrome.

3. A 52-year-old male presents with hypertension. A serum K$^+$ level of 1.9 mEq/L (normal 3.5 to 5.0) leads to a more formal work-up including the measurement of serum aldosterone and PRA levels. Both aldosterone and PRA levels are low. All of the following should be considered as possible causes of his hypertension *except*:

   A. Apparent mineralocorticoid excess
   B. Liddle syndrome
   C. Excess licorice ingestion
   D. Gordon syndrome
   E. Deoxycorticosterone excess

4. A 57-year-old man is referred by his primary care provider for a 9-month history of episodic palpitations, sweating, and headaches that typically last an hour. Prior blood pressure readings while on maximal doses of four antihypertensive medications are as follows: 184/108, 146/86, 192/98, 176/90, and 136/78 mmHg. Physical examination reveals no abnormal findings. His serum Na$^+$ level is 142 mEq/L and serum K$^+$ level is 4.1 mEq/L. The most likely biochemical abnormality is

   A. Elevated urine free cortisol
   B. Elevated ratio of plasma aldosterone to PRA
   C. Elevated urine total metanephrines
   D. Elevated serum 17-hydroxyprogesterone
   E. Increase in serum cortisol of 10 mcg/dL 60 minutes after cortrosyn-stimulation test

5. A 21-year-old woman is brought to the emergency department by her boyfriend because she was too weak to get out of bed. Family history includes a brother with hypertension, and father who died of a stroke at 48 years of age. Physical examination is notable for generalized weakness and hypoactive deep tendon reflexes. Blood

pressure is 164/92 mmHg. Serum Na^+ level is 158 mEq/L and serum K^+ level is 2.8 mEq/L. Plasma aldosterone and PRA levels are both low. Which of the following medications would be the most appropriate treatment for her hypertension?

A. Hydrochlorothiazide
B. Amlodipine
C. Metoprolol
D. Amiloride
E. Spironolactone

CHAPTER REVIEW ANSWERS

1. The correct answer is B. The hypertension in those individuals with this condition, as its name implies, responds to dexamethasone. There is commonly a family history of strokes or cardiovascular disease related to early-onset hypertension. All of the other choices are incorrect.

In secondary hyperaldosteronism (**Choice A**), nonendocrine causes of hypertension such as heart failure, liver cirrhosis, renal tumors, and renal artery stenosis are the most common causes. Dexamethasone would not improve his blood pressure. In congenital adrenal hypoplasia (**Choice C**), the adrenal gland fails to completely develop and those affected produce insufficient amounts of glucocorticoids and mineralocorticoids. They usually present shortly after birth with hyponatremia, hyperkalemia, hypoglycemia, and hypotension. The condition is caused by a mutation in the *DAX1* gene on the X chromosome. Addison disease (**Choice D**) is most commonly caused by an autoimmune destruction of the adrenal cortex resulting in insufficient production of glucocorticoids and mineralocorticoids. These patients usually present with hyponatremia, hyperkalemia, hypoglycemia, and hypotension. Liddle syndrome (**Choice E**) is an autosomal dominant disorder characterized by early, and frequently severe, hypertension. It involves abnormal kidney function, with excess resorption of Na^+ and loss of K^+ from the renal tubule. The biochemical findings include hypokalemia, hypernatremia, metabolic alkalosis, hypoaldosteronism, and low PRA. Treatment includes a low-salt diet and a K^+-sparing diuretic that directly blocks the epithelial Na^+ channel, such as amiloride or triamterene. The hypertension does not improve with dexamethasone.

2. The correct answer is D. These findings are characteristic of Conn syndrome (primary hyperaldosteronism) in which increased aldosterone secretion causes Na^+ retention, increased total plasma volume, increased renal artery pressure, and inhibition of PRA. All of the other choices are incorrect.

The patient would have an elevated, not a low, aldosterone level (**Choice A**). Because the patient's aldosterone level is high and PRA level should be appropriately suppressed, her aldosterone/PRA ratio should be very high, not low (**Choice B**). Kimmelstiel-Wilson syndrome (**Choice C**) is a late complication of diabetes mellitus in which intercapillary glomerulosclerosis, hypertension, and edema occurs, accompanied by proteinuria. The syndrome develops approximately 20 years after the onset of diabetes. Nelson syndrome (**Choice E**) is the rapid enlargement of a pituitary adenoma after removal of both adrenal glands. The clinical manifestations include weakness (from glucocorticoid deficiency) and hyperpigmentation (from excess melanocyte-stimulating hormone).

3. The correct answer is D. All of the other choices can present with hypertension, hypernatremia, and hypokalemia. Gordon syndrome is an autosomal dominant disorder characterized by early, and frequently severe, hypertension. The biochemical findings include hyperkalemia, hyperchloremia, metabolic acidosis, hypoaldosteronism, and low PRA. The key difference in this condition, as compared to Liddle syndrome, is that these patients are hyperkalemic, rather than hypokalemic. Treatment includes a low-salt diet and a thiazide diuretic.

Apparent mineralocorticoid excess (**Choice A**) is a rare autosomal recessive disorder characterized by hypertension, hypokalemia, and hypernatremia resulting from mutations in the *HSD11B2* gene. Mutations in this gene inhibit the conversion of cortisol to cortisone. The cortisol then binds to and activates the mineralocorticoid receptor. Liddle syndrome (**Choice B**) is an autosomal dominant disorder characterized by early, and frequently severe, hypertension. It involves abnormal kidney function, with excess resorption of Na^+ and loss of K^+ from the renal tubule. The biochemical findings include hypokalemia, hypernatremia, metabolic alkalosis, hypoaldosteronism, and low PRA. Treatment includes a low-salt diet and a K^+-sparing diuretic that directly blocks the epithelial Na^+ channel, such as amiloride or triamterene. The hypertension does not improve with dexamethasone. Excess licorice ingestion (**Choice C**), which contains glycyrrhizin, an inhibitor of the enzyme 11β HSD type 2, impairs conversion of cortisol to cortisone. This is similar to the condition of apparent mineralocorticoid excess (AME). Deoxycorticosterone (DOC) (**Choice E**), although a relatively weak mineralocorticoid, when secreted in excessive amounts, causes excess Na^+ retention at the expense of K^+ wasting. Na^+ retention promotes water retention, expansion of the extracellular volume, hypertension, and suppression of renin production. K^+ wasting results in hypokalemic alkalosis. The clinical findings are similar to those found in primary hyperaldosteronism.

---

4. The correct answer is C. The patient's history is consistent with pheochromocytoma. His complaint of paroxysmal headache, palpitations, and diaphoresis can be explained by episodic release of catecholamines from a tumor of the adrenal medulla. Note also that some, but not all, of his blood pressure readings were severely elevated for the same reason. Pheochromocytoma may occur sporadically or in association with the multiple endocrine neoplasia (MEN) syndrome (type 2A or 2B). Elevated levels of catecholamines in the blood result in increased urinary excretion of catecholamines as well as their breakdown products including metanephrines, homovanillic acid, and vanillylmandelic acid.

Patients suffering from hypercortisolism would be expected to have an elevated level of urinary free cortisol (**Choice A**), due to the increased secretion of cortisol from the adrenal glands. This may occur in an adrenocorticotropic hormone (ACTH)–dependent manner, as in Cushing disease or syndrome, or in an ACTH-independent manner, as in adrenocortical adenoma or carcinoma. An elevated ratio of plasma aldosterone to PRA (**Choice B**) is characteristic of Conn syndrome (primary hyperaldosteronism) in which increased aldosterone secretion causes Na^+ retention, increased total plasma volume, increased renal artery pressure, and inhibition of renin secretion. An elevated serum 17-hydroxyprogesterone level (**Choice D**) is seen in patients with congenital adrenal hyperplasia (CAH). 21-Hydroxylase deficiency is the most common form of CAH and typically results in virilization of female newborns. As intermediates in the biosynthesis of mineralocorticoids and glucocorticoids build up, they are shunted into the androgen pathway, an intermediate of which is 17-hydroxyprogesterone. Lack of an appropriate cortisol response to the ACTH-stimulation test (**Choice E**) is diagnostic of adrenal insufficiency, which may be either primary or secondary in nature. The etiology of adrenal insufficiency may be further determined by measuring plasma levels of ACTH (high in primary, low in secondary). Patients with adrenal insufficiency are more likely to have hypotension and not hypertension.

5. The correct answer is D. This patient's generalized weakness is due to severe hypokalemia. Her relatively young age and a strong family history suggest a genetic basis for her hypertension and metabolic abnormalities. Note that her plasma aldosterone level is low. Taken together, these findings suggest a diagnosis of Liddle syndrome, an autosomal dominant mutation causing overactivity of the epithelial Na^+ channel in the renal tubules with resultant Na^+ retention and K^+ wasting. Appropriate treatment of this condition includes a medication that blocks the activity of epithelial sodium channel (ENaC), such as amiloride or triamterene.

Hydrochlorothiazide (**Choice A**) is a thiazide diuretic that inhibits Na^+ reabsorption in the renal distal convoluted tubule. Although commonly used in the treatment of essential hypertension, thiazide diuretics do not directly act on ENaCs and so would not be the most appropriate choice of medication for a patient with Liddle syndrome. Amlodipine (**Choice B**) is a dihydropyridine calcium-channel antagonist, which achieves its antihypertensive effect by direct vasodilation. Because its mechanism of action is independent of the underlying defect in Liddle syndrome, amlodipine would not be the best choice of medication for this patient. Metoprolol (**Choice C**) is a $\beta1$-selective adrenergic receptor antagonist, although the exact mechanisms by which it reduces blood pressure in hypertensive patients are not fully understood. Spironolactone (**Choice E**) is a K^+-sparing diuretic that blocks aldosterone secretion. It does not act on the ENaC and therefore would not be an appropriate choice of medication for a patient with Liddle syndrome.

Female Reproductive Disorders

12

Steven A. Gay
Mary S. Dolan

CASE

A 16-year-old girl presents to her primary care physician with a concern that she has not yet experienced a menstrual period. Her past medical, surgical, and family history is unremarkable. A review of systems indicates breast development at age 10 years and pubic hair development at age 11 years. Over the past 5 years, she has maintained consistent linear growth and weight gain. Breast and pubic hair have progressed appropriately. She does not drink or smoke. She is not sexually active and does not take any medications. Family history reveals that her grandmother died of colon cancer. There is no family history of short stature, abnormal age of menarche, or delayed puberty. On physical examination, she has Tanner V breast development, pubic, and axillary hair. She has no signs of virilization. The pelvic examination is not performed.

This chapter reviews the embryology and physiology of the female reproductive system, followed by the etiology, pathophysiology, and management of female reproductive disorders to allow the reader to develop hypotheses for the etiology of this girl's amenorrhea. At the end of the chapter, a summary of the work-up and treatment will be presented to provide the reader a better understanding of the diagnosis. There are several causes of menstrual irregularities that are caused by endocrine disorders. This chapter will emphasize the hypothalamic, pituitary, ovarian, and adrenal causes of abnormal menarche and reproduction with brief descriptions of other less common etiologies.

OBJECTIVES

1. Describe the physiologic processes that occur during the menstrual cycle.

2. List the causes of female hypogonadism.

(*continued*)

OBJECTIVES

3. Describe the clinical findings and laboratory abnormalities in a patient with irregular menses.

4. Develop a differential diagnosis for a female with irregular menses.

5. Describe the evaluation and management of a female with irregular menses.

6. Classify the major female reproductive disorders.

CHAPTER OUTLINE

Female Hypogonadism
  Hypogonadotropic Hypogonadism
    Disorders of Hypothalamic Function
    Disorders of Pituitary Origin
  Hypergonadotropic Hypogonadism
    Turner Syndrome
    Gonadal Dysgenesis
    Miscellaneous Genetic Causes
    Autoimmunity
    Radiation and Chemotherapy
Congenital Outflow Tract Abnormalities
  Imperforate Hymen
  Transverse Vaginal Septum and Cervical Atresia
  Müllerian Agenesis
Acquired Outflow Tract Abnormalities
  Leiomyomas
  Endometriosis
  Asherman Syndrome
  Cervical Stenosis
Ovarian Disorders
  Polycystic Ovary Syndrome
  Ovarian Stromal Hyperthecosis
  Theca Lutein Cysts
  Luteomas
  Neoplasias
Adrenal Gland Disorders
  Virilizing Disorders
    Idiopathic Hirsutism
    Idiopathic Hyperandrogenism
  Evaluation and Management

ANATOMY

The ovaries, fallopian tubes, and uterus together with the cervical outflow tract, vagina, and vulva form the female reproductive system. This system creates an ideal intrauterine environment to support the implantation of an embryo and the development of a fetus until the end of pregnancy.

The ovaries are the reproductive gonads and the main site of sex hormone synthesis in women. They are bilateral organs located in the pelvis adjacent to the fallopian tubes with their own arterial supply directly from the abdominal aorta along with collateral supply from the uterine artery. At infancy, the ovaries contain all the female gametes that will be produced. The gametes are surrounded by a supportive layer called the *granulosa cells*. Together they form the follicles, several hundred of which are contained within the ovarian stroma and its overlying epithelium. These follicles are in a primordial state until activated by the autocrine and paracrine signals. Ten to 20 primordial cells are recruited and undergo a process of selective atresia until a dominant follicle is selected. This dominant follicle enters into the full ovarian cycle that culminates in ovulation.

The fallopian tubes, ampulla, and fimbriae form the passageway for the oocyte to enter the uterus. The fimbriae, a component of the distal fallopian tubes, partially surround each ovary and capture the oocyte from the follicle. The rhythmically beating cilia that line the fallopian tubes facilitate movement of the oocyte into the uterine cavity. Fertilization usually occurs in the fallopian tubes or its most distal portion, the ampulla.

The uterus is the organ that supports the embryo during implantation and pregnancy. It has three layers: the outer serosal layer, the middle myometrium, and the inner endometrium. The myometrium contains smooth muscle, which increases during pregnancy to help push the infant through the birth canal in the final stage of pregnancy. The endometrium serves as the site of implantation and undergoes the monthly cycle of proliferation and shedding known as the *menstrual period*.

The outflow tract is composed of the muscular cervix, the vagina, and the vulva. Together they form the birth canal through which the infant passes or through which the endometrium is shed as menstrual blood.

EMBRYOLOGY

The internal female reproductive system is derived from the Müllerian ducts (paramesonephric ducts) and the primordial gonads. The Müllerian ducts are a pair of mesoderm-derived ducts that give rise to the fallopian tubes, uterus, cervix, and upper two-thirds of the vagina. Initially induced by the development of the Wolffian ducts, the Müllerian ducts persist in a female embryo. In the absence of male testes producing anti-Müllerian hormone (AMH), the Müllerian ducts elongate laterally to form the fallopian tubes and fuse centrally to form the urogenital sinus. The urogenital sinus then differentiates into the uterus, cervix, and upper portion of the vagina.

The ovary arises from the urogenital ridge and the yolk sac, which is derived from germ cells. The urogenital ridge begins as a thickening of the abdominal peritoneum and later becomes populated by primordial germ cells, which migrate from the endodermal yolk sac. These primordial germ cells undergo an expansive mitosis into oogonia and then undergo meiotic division arresting as primary oocytes at the termination of meiosis I. This is a depletion process, beginning with 5 to 6 million oogonia that are reduced to 1 million at birth, followed by further reduction until the start of puberty.

PHYSIOLOGY

The differentiation of the gonad into an ovary and the production and secretion of estrogen from the ovary via the hypothalamic–pituitary–ovarian (HPO) axis are the major physiologic mechanisms in female development as well as in reproduction.

Female Gonadal Differentiation

The differentiation of the bipotential gonad into an ovary requires less critical factors and events than differentiation of the gonad into a male testis. In the absence of the sex determining region on the Y-chromosome (SRY), the undifferentiated gonad will develop into an ovary. In the absence of AMH, the female internal genitalia will develop. In the absence of testosterone and dihydrotestosterone (DHT), female external genitalia will develop.

Hypothalamic–Pituitary–Gonadal Axis

In women, the hypothalamic–pituitary–gonadal (HPG) axis drives estrogen secretion from the ovary. Gonadotropin-releasing hormone (GnRH), released by the hypothalamus, stimulates the pituitary release of both follicle-stimulating hormone (FSH) and luteinizing hormone (LH). FSH stimulates the release of inhibin, whereas LH stimulates release of testosterone and progesterone (Figure 12-1). The HPG axis also drives the development of the secondary sex characteristics associated with puberty. GnRH-producing cells are located primarily in the paraventricular nucleus of the hypothalamus. These neurons receive modulatory input from other sites within the central nervous system (CNS), although the complete regulatory pathways have not been determined. Estrogen and inhibin from the ovaries provide negative feedback on the hypothalamus.

A key feature of the HPG axis is that for the gonadal secretion of hormones to occur properly, both GnRH and the gonadotropins must be secreted in a pulsatile fashion (Figure 12-2). These pulses must be secreted every 90 to 120 minutes. Women lacking either the normal pulse frequency or amplitude may be hypogonadal or infertile.

Although the hypothalamic–pituitary–adrenal (HPA) axis is best known for the production of glucocorticoids from the zona fasciculata and mineralocorticoids from the zona glomerulosa, it also plays a vital role in female puberty by initiating production of androgens from the zona reticularis.

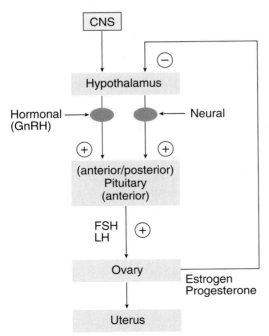

FIGURE 12-1. Hypothalamic–pituitary–gonadal axis in females. The hypothalamus secretes gonadotropin-releasing hormone (GnRH) into the hypothalamic–pituitary portal system in a pulsatile pattern. GnRH stimulates gonadotroph cells in the anterior pituitary gland to synthesize and release luteinizing hormone (LH) and follicle-stimulating hormone (FSH). These two hormones, referred to as gonadotropins, promote ovarian synthesis of estrogen. Estrogen inhibits release of GnRH, LH, and FSH. Depending on the time in the menstrual cycle, the concentration of estrogen in the plasma, and the rate at which estrogen concentration increases in the plasma, estrogen can also stimulate pituitary gonadotropin release (e.g., at ovulation). The ovaries secrete inhibin, which selectively inhibits FSH secretion, and activin, which selectively promotes FSH secretion. (Beckmann CRB, Ling FW, Smith RP, et al. Obstetrics and Gynecology. 5th ed. Philadelphia, PA: Lippincott Williams & Wilkins; 2006.)

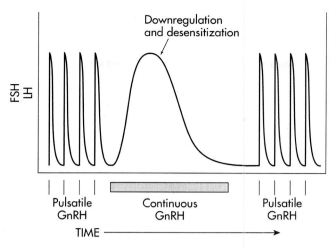

FIGURE 12-2. Gonadotropin-releasing hormone pulsatility. Schematic representation of the intermittent release of follicle-stimulating hormone (FSH) and luteinizing hormone (LH) in response to sporadic GnRH. Constant GnRH produces a reversible decrease in both gonadotropins after 7 to 10 days. Return of intermittent release produces a normal FSH and LH response. (Baggish MS, Valle RF, Guedj H. Hysteroscopy: Visual Perspectives of Uterine Anatomy, Physiology and Pathology. Philadelphia, PA: Lippincott Williams & Wilkins; 2007.)

Female Reproductive Hormones

The most important hormones involved in female reproduction include estrogen, progesterone, androgens, activin, inhibin (A and B), and follistatin.

Estrogen

Estrogens exert a wide range of effects throughout the body beyond the obvious role of feminization. Estradiol, estrone, and estriol are the three estrogens found in circulation. Estradiol, the most potent estrogen, is produced primarily in the ovaries by the granulosa cells from androgen substrate. It is formed by theca cells under FSH and LH stimulation. 17-β Estradiol is the primary circulating estrogen in premenopausal women. Estrone, a metabolite of estradiol and androstenedione, is formed by aromatase activity in peripheral adipose tissues. Estriol, the weakest estrogen and a metabolite of dehydroepiandrosterone (DHEA), is formed by aromatase activity in peripheral adipose tissues and by the fetoplacental unit from the conversion of maternal cholesterol during pregnancy.

Because estrogens are not water soluble, they require a transport mechanism to enter the systemic circulation. Estrogen itself induces increased production of sex hormone–binding globulin (SHBG). This globulin, along with albumin, is bound to most estrogens in the circulation. However, only free circulating estrogens, which account for just 2% to 3% of total estrogen, have biological action.

The effects of estrogen on reproductive tissues are wide ranging. On a cellular level, estrogens bind to several subclasses of estrogen receptors (mainly α and β), which then form homo- or heterodimers within the nuclear space. These receptors are differentially expressed by the amount and tissue type that determines the agonist and antagonist properties of many selective estrogen receptor–modulator drugs (SERMs). In the uterus, estrogen stimulates endometrial proliferation through basal mitotic stimulation and angiogenesis, sensitizes smooth muscle to oxytocin, and decreases mucus viscosity. In the ovary, it increases mitosis of the granulosa layer. In breast tissue, it promotes the growth and stimulation of ductal cells and connective tissues.

The estrogen effects on nonreproductive tissues are also wide ranging and are critical to health considerations with advancing age. Estrogen has direct effects on bone, CNS, and liver function and an indirect effect on cardiovascular health. Estrogen decreases bone resorption and promotes maturation and closure of epiphyseal plates in young women. It has neuroprotective effects on cognition and memory. In the liver, it increases lipoprotein receptor production, leading to decreased circulating cholesterol and low-density lipoprotein (LDL) and increased high-density lipoprotein (HDL) levels. It also affects the production of procoagulant and fibrinolytic enzymes and increases production of the thyroxine (T_4) transport protein and transcortin. These roles are especially relevant because estrogen wanes in menopause, leading to bone density loss, acceleration of age-dependent memory loss, and increased cardiovascular problems including myocardial infarction.

Progesterone

Progesterone is synthesized from the theca and granulosa cells in the ovary. Most of its production occurs during the luteal phase due to action of the corpus luteum. During pregnancy, the placenta is also able to synthesize progesterone from maternal cholesterol.

Progesterone is transported primarily bound to albumin. Its main function is to prepare the reproductive tract for the potential and maintenance of pregnancy. Progesterone stimulates oocyte maturation, facilitates implantation of the embryo by increasing endometrial proteins that lyse the zona pellucida, maintains the endometrial lining, and promotes secretory functioning. In nonendometrial tissue, progesterone induces cell proliferation and differentiation as pregnancy progresses, inhibits myometrial contractility by raising resting membrane potential, decreases electrical coupling and prostaglandin synthesis, and blocks α-adrenergic receptors. It also induces lobular development of the breast in preparation for lactation.

The cellular effects of progesterone are closely tied to estrogen. It opposes estrogen induction of many of the estrogen-responsive genes, especially those that impact uterine function. Estrogen and progesterone increase progesterone receptor expression. Progesterone also affects GnRH pulsatility, increases hypothalamic opioid activity, decreases LH secretion, and increases FSH secretion.

Androgens

Androgens play a role as a substrate for other ovarian hormones. In excess, they may result in virilization (development of male features) and hirsutism (increase in terminal hair in a male pattern).

Androgens include dehydroepiandrosterone (DHEA), DHEA sulfate (DHEAS), androstenedione, testosterone, and dihydrotestosterone (DHT). DHEA, DHEAS, and androstenedione are prehormones that have little or no intrinsic andronergic activity; they require conversion to testosterone or DHT to exert their androgenic effects. Androstenedione, made in equal amounts by the adrenal glands and ovaries, is the substrate for most testosterone production by peripheral conversion of 17-hydroxylase (17-OHase) in adipose tissue. Testosterone is usually produced by conversion of androstenedione, but up to a third of testosterone is from direct ovarian synthesis.

Women should have an adequate amount of androgen for strength and energy. Most androgens are converted to estrogens by the aromatase enzyme. The surge in aromatase activity occurs with ingestion of simple carbohydrates. For women with diets high in simple carbohydrates, a surge in aromatase activity occurs, converting more androgen into estrogen. Excess estrogen in women is associated with a number of pathologic conditions, such as premenstrual syndrome, fibroids, mood swings, decreased libido, and a lack of energy.

Transport of androgens is similar to that of estrogens; however, the high expression of sex hormone binding globulin (SHBG) from estrogen in women results in very little testosterone being available in the free form. Therefore, there is very little substrate available for peripheral conversion into DHT, the more potent androgen. The testosterone that is available is usually aromatized within adipose tissue into estrogen.

Androgens contribute to the female sexual drive; however, at pathologic levels, androgens reduce SHBG concentrations and promote peripheral conversion of increased free androgens and estrogens into DHT and testosterone. This may result in virilization with a deepened voice, clitoromegaly, frontal balding, increased muscle mass, and a male habitus.

Ovarian Peptide Hormones

The ovary produces several peptide hormones including activin, inhibins A and B, and follistatin. They are important in folliculogenesis, aiding granulosa formation, and augmenting gonadotropin regulation at the level of the hypothalamus and pituitary gland. The preantral follicle exclusively secretes inhibin B, which provides negative feedback on the pituitary for FSH production. Inhibin A, a marker of corpus luteal functioning, decreases late in the menstrual cycle, thereby aiding in the repletion of FSH for the next cycle. Activin, produced by the granulosa cell during folliculogenesis, promotes granulosa proliferation, upregulates FSH receptors, and modulates steroidogenesis in the follicle. Follistatin is also produced in the follicle and binds to and neutralizes activin.

Menstrual Cycle

Menstrual cycle is the term for the physiologic changes that occur in fertile women for sexual reproduction. The menstrual cycle is commonly divided into three phases: the follicular phase, ovulation, and the luteal phase. The menstrual cycle is centrally regulated by the hypothalamus and anterior pituitary gland.

Central Regulation

Pulsatile release of GnRH from the arcuate nucleus of the hypothalamus travels through the portal system in the pituitary stalk to the anterior pituitary and stimulates LH and FSH secretion. LH and FSH bind G protein-coupled receptors on the ovary that increase cyclic adenosine monophosphate and protein kinase A activity. This results in an increase in the side-chain cleavage (P450 scc) enzyme expression and activity, and converts cholesterol into pregnenolone, which is the rate-limiting step in steroidogenesis. This forms the substrate for later conversion to androgens and estrogens and provides feedback for central regulation. The frequency and amplitude of the GnRH pulse generator is an important factor in gonadotropin release and regulation of the ovarian cycle. A slower frequency release favors FSH repletion and LH depletion. Fast pulses result in the reverse.

The ovarian cycle comprises a follicular phase and a luteal phase. Together, they further the development of the dominant follicle; the ovulation of the oocyte; and the maintenance of the follicular remnants, referred to as the *corpus luteum*. These correspond with the endometrial proliferative and secretory phases, respectively. Ovulation defines the transition between these two phases. During the follicular phase, gonadotroph cells of the anterior pituitary gland secrete LH and FSH in response to pulsatile GnRH stimulation. Circulating LH and FSH promote growth and maturation of ovarian follicles. Developing follicles secrete increasing amounts of estrogen. At first, the estrogen has an inhibitory effect on gonadotropin release; however, just before the midpoint in the menstrual cycle, estrogen exerts a brief positive feedback effect on LH and FSH release. This is followed by follicular rupture and release of an egg into the fallopian tube. During the second half of the cycle, the corpus luteum secretes both estrogen and progesterone. Progesterone induces a change in the endometrium from a proliferative to a secretory type. If fertilization and implantation of a blastocyst does not occur within 14 days after ovulation, the corpus luteum involutes, secretion of estrogen and progesterone declines, menses occurs, and a new cycle begins.

Follicular Phase

The initial cohort of preselected primordial follicles is under FSH stimulation. The FSH stimulates the granulosa layer to proliferate and induces the development of both the granulosa and the theca layers. The theca cells contain the enzymes necessary to convert cholesterol to androstenedione, but lack the enzymes needed to convert it to estrogen and progesterone. The granulosa cells convert the steroid product of the theca cells, androstenedione, to estrogen and progesterone. Simultaneous with the development of the theca and granulosa layers, FSH promotes steroidogenesis and upregulation of LH receptors. These LH receptors act as an FSH receptor surrogate after the FSH levels decrease, due to rising estrogen levels. During this follicular stage, estrogen exerts negative feedback on FSH and positive feedback on LH. As a result, only the follicle that maintains LH stimulation and FSH inhibition becomes the dominant follicle. The remaining follicles, which are under partial FSH stimulation and do not meet the necessary self-sustaining threshold, degenerate.

At the optimal threshold, the theca and granulosa layers continue to make steroid products, which enter the systemic circulation and drive the endometrial proliferative phase. The dominant follicle is selected from the cohort of primordial follicles via FSH stimulation to become the primary follicle. This primary follicle develops, enlarges, and forms a central cavity surrounding the oocyte that is known as the *antrum*.

A fully developed follicle, known as a *Graafian follicle*, is now ready to ovulate. The increased estrogen production positively feeds back on the hypothalamus and pituitary gland to increase GnRH production, secretion, and receptor expression. This further increases LH release, ovarian stimulation, and estradiol production. The result is an LH spike that causes the smooth muscle surrounding the follicle to contract, thereby thrusting the oocyte into the extraovarian space. From here, the oocyte continues its path down the fallopian tubes and into the endometrium. This completes the follicular phase of the menstrual cycle.

Luteal Phase

The luteal phase of the ovarian cycle is named after the follicular remnants, called the *corpus luteum*. It exerts its effects on the HPO axis and the endometrium. Once ovulation occurs, the follicular remnants persist and continue to produce estradiol and progesterone by the action of LH. Together, estradiol and progesterone maintain the endometrial lining and promote implantation of a fertilized ovum in the very short timeframe (20 to 24 days) known as the *implantation window*. Progesterone also acts centrally, antagonizing LH production and changing GnRH pulsatility to favor FSH repletion. Without continued hormonal support from LH and lacking human chorionic gonadotropin (which acts as an LH analogue) from an implanted embryo, the corpus luteum regresses, as does its production of progesterone and estradiol. Without these hormone actions, the endometrium loses its support and is shed. This shedding process is known as *menstruation* (Figure 12-3).

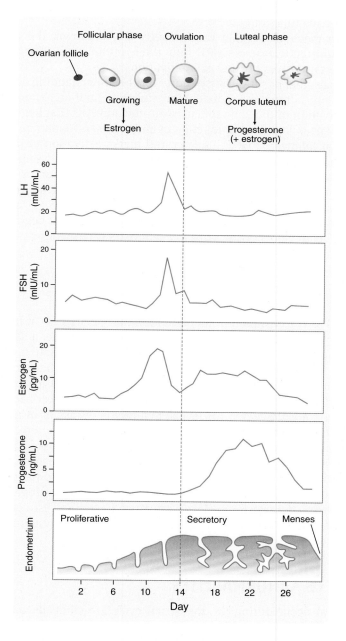

FIGURE 12-3. The menstrual cycle: Changes of the ovary, uterus, and hormones. (Adapted with permission from Thorneycroft IH, Mishell DR Jr, Stone SC, et al. The relation of serum 17-hydroxyprogesterone and estradiol-17β levels during the human menstrual cycle. Am J Obstet Gynecol 1971;111(7): 947–951.)

Puberty

Puberty is the process of biological and sexual maturation. It is defined as the development of secondary sexual characteristics and important cognitive and psychosocial changes as well as the ability to reproduce. The female secondary sexual characteristics are breast and pubic hair development, which are indicators of underlying estrogen potential and reproductive function.

Although the exact mechanisms that start puberty are unknown, the earliest signs are a change in the pulsatile release of GnRH from the hypothalamus. This GnRH "pulse generator" is an important driver of HPO axis activation.

There are five changes that occur during puberty for the understanding and/or staging of puberty's progression: adrenarche, gonadarche, thelarche, pubarche, and menarche. Adrenarche is the activation of the zona reticularis in the adrenals that begins about age 6 years. It marks the start of low-level production of androgens. Gonadarche is the activation of the ovaries that follows 2 to 3 years later and marks activation of the HPO axis, which drives the growth spurt, thelarche (breast development), and pubarche (pubic hair development). In general, thelarche precedes pubarche in Caucasians (average age 10.0 and 10.5 years, respectively), but racial differences exist. African American girls generally reach both stages simultaneously (average age 8.8 and 8.9 years, respectively). Menarche, the final stage of female puberty, is the start of menses that begins at an average age of 12 years. Thelarche occurring prior to age 7 years is termed *precocious puberty* and may require further evaluation to determine the etiology.

Menopause

Menopause is defined as the cessation of menstruation that persists for at least a year. It is due to the loss of ovarian activity. It is preceded by perimenopause, a state of irregular menstrual bleeding that occurs 1 to 2 years before complete cessation of menstrual activity. There is marked variability in FSH, LH, and estradiol in the perimenopausal period. Once in the fully menopausal state, estradiol and inhibin B levels stabilize as low or undetectable. This, in turn, results in loss of central negative feedback, leading to elevated FSH and moderately elevated LH levels. Symptoms of loss of ovarian function include hot flashes, flushing, night sweats, vaginal dryness, painful intercourse (dyspareunia), loss of neuronal protection, decreased bone mass, and decreased libido. In addition, the loss of the estrogen's protective effects on LDL and vascular tone results in an increased risk for cardiovascular diseases. Furthermore, peripheral aromatase activity in adipose tissue is reduced and causes minimal levels of extragonadal estrogen production from androgen precursors. If progesterone levels are much lower than estrogen levels, the unopposed estrogen can lead to endometrial hyperplasia, anovulatory uterine bleeding, and endometrial cancer.

MENSTRUAL CYCLE ABNORMALITIES

The abnormalities that occur during the menstrual cycle are clinically evident with a lack of or excess of blood flow, irregularity of bleeding, and pain during the cycle. The menstrual cycle is centrally regulated by the hypothalamus and anterior pituitary gland. Abnormalities in the menstrual cycle may be due to a hormonal abnormality or a structural abnormality of the outflow tract. Insofar as these disorders can effect pubertal development and reproduction, they will be presented as menstrual cycle irregularities, hypogonadism, and congenital and acquired outflow obstructions.

Amenorrhea

Primary amenorrhea is defined by either absence of menses by age 14 years in the absence of growth or secondary sexual characteristics or absence of menses by age 16 years regardless of pattern of growth or secondary sexual characteristics. *Secondary amenorrhea* includes women who have menstruated previously but have not had menses in at least three previous cycles or 6 months. The most common cause of secondary amenorrhea is pregnancy which, should be ruled out prior to initiating an extensive workup.

For normal menstruation to occur, functional hormonal signals must travel from the hypothalamus to the anterior pituitary and to a functional ovary. The functional ovary must then influence the uterine endometrium to shed its lining, which must pass through the cervix and vagina. Disorders of amenorrhea can be classified by the level at which the disturbance occurs. Diagnostic tests are aimed at determining the functional capacity of each level. After ruling out pregnancy, algorithms for evaluating the cause of amenorrhea and chronic anovulation are shown in Figures 12-4 and 12-5, respectively.

Dysmenorrhea

Dysmenorrhea is pain and cramping during menses that interferes with normal daily activity. *Primary dysmenorrhea* is pain and cramping that results from myometrial contractions without a known cause. *Secondary dysmenorrhea* results from a known cause such as endometriosis, uterine fibroids, or adenomyosis. The causes of secondary dysmenorrhea can be excluded by imaging or surgical evaluation. The diagnosis and treatment of secondary dysmenorrhea is beyond the scope of this chapter.

Dysmenorrhea is prevalent in adolescent females who have achieved ovulatory cycles. Moderate to severe dysmenorrhea is estimated to occur in 60% of U.S. adolescent females with 15% regularly missing school. Risk factors include a body mass index (BMI) less than 20, menarche prior to age 12 years, irregular or heavy menses, longer duration of cycles, premenstrual symptoms, smoking, and history of sexual assault. Protective factors include exercise, oral contraceptive use, higher number of pregnancies, and stable partner relationships.

The pathophysiology of primary dysmenorrhea is most likely due to myometrial ischemia from prolonged contractions. The secretory endometrium contains multiple prostaglandin products of arachidonic acid breakdown. Prostaglandins $F_{2\alpha}$ and E_2 within the endometrium have been shown to correlate with disease severity.

Primary dysmenorrhea begins just prior to or at the start of the menstrual cycle. It gradually declines over a 72-hour period. The pain is described as variable in timing and intensity and is usually located in the suprapubic area. This contrasts with secondary dysmenorrhea, which is dependent on the underlying cause. Endometriosis usually causes pain the week prior to or in the middle of the cycle. It is associated with deep pain in the lower back, legs, lower abdomen, and upon defecation. Uterine fibroids usually cause pain that correlates with increased menstrual flow, intermenstrual spotting, or increased size of the fibroids. The diagnosis is based on clinical symptoms after other causes of secondary amenorrhea have been excluded either by clinical history, imaging, or diagnostic laparoscopy. The first-line treatment for primary dysmenorrhea is nonsteroidal anti-inflammatory drugs. These medications decrease myometrial contractions by decreasing prostaglandin synthesis. Oral contraceptives or other hormone contraceptives (ring, patch, or implant) are also effective. Women who fail to experience any symptomatic relief should consider undergoing diagnostic laparoscopy.

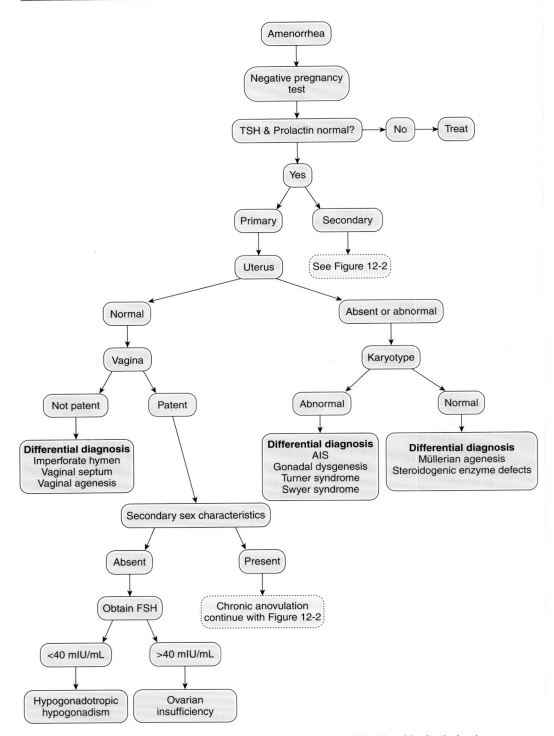

FIGURE 12-4. Algorithm for evaluating a female with amenorrhea. TSH, thyroid-stimulating hormone; FSH, follicle-stimulating hormone; AIS, androgen insensitivity syndrome.

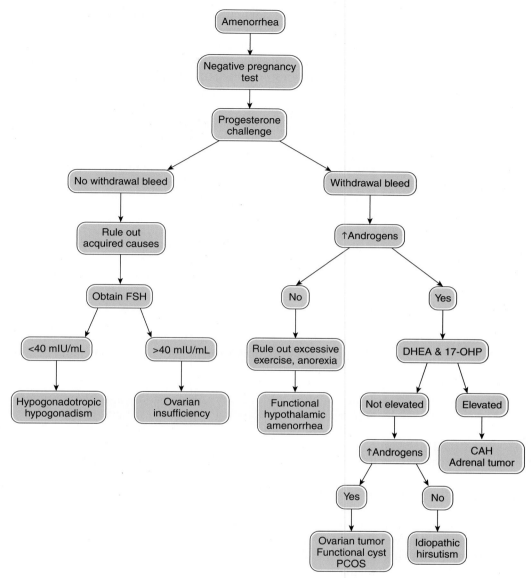

FIGURE 12-5. Algorithm for evaluating a female with chronic anovulation. FSH, follicle-stimulating hormone; DHEA, dehydroepiandrosterone; 17-OHP, 17α-hydroxyprogesterone; CAH, congenital adrenal hyperplasia; PCOS, polycystic ovary syndrome.

Abnormal Uterine Bleeding

Abnormal uterine bleeding includes abnormalities in cycle length, days of menses, or amount of menstrual flow. The normal length of a cycle is 21 to 35 days with normal menses lasting 3 to 5 days and average blood loss of 30 to 80 mL. Deviations from these provide valuable clues to the underlying disorder. For example, an irregular cycle length between menses suggests an anovulatory condition, in which the functional ovarian cycle and ovulation are abnormal.

Menorrhagia is defined as a regular cycle length that is excessive in either days of menses (>7 days) or amount of blood lost (>80 mL). A finding of menorrhagia may suggest an area of endometrial tissue that is poorly supported or perfused as a result of a uterine fibroid, endometrial polyp, or adenomyosis. Less commonly, endometrial hyperplasia or cancer is associated with menorrhagia. Adolescent females presenting with clinically significant menorrhagia need evaluation for a bleeding or clotting disorder, such as von Willebrand disease, thrombocytopenia, or malignancy. In women older than 35 years with menorrhagia, underlying endometrial hyperplasia or cancer should be excluded with an endometrial biopsy.

Hypomenorrhea is defined as regular timed cycles that are unusually light in flow volume. This is suggestive of a failure of the endometrial lining to proliferate. This may be due to a failure of hormonal stimulation as in hypogonadotropic hypogonadism, ovarian insufficiency as in hypergonadtropic hypogonadism, or an acquired disorder that prevents proliferation as in the development of intrauterine adhesions such as occurs in Asherman syndrome (discussed later in this chapter). Contraceptives increase progesterone levels, which may antagonize endometrial proliferation and result in low-volume menses.

Oligomenorrhea is defined as cycles exceeding 35 days. This is usually the result of anovulation that may be caused by polycystic ovary syndrome (PCOS), thyroid disease, or other causes of chronic anovulation. Pregnancy should always be ruled out before any other work-up is undertaken. This diagnosis exists on a spectrum with amenorrhea because secondary amenorrhea is defined as the absence of menses for at least three previous cycles or 6 months.

Polymenorrhea is defined as cycles lasting less than 21 days and, like oligomenorrhea, is usually the result of anovulation. It is usually caused by thyroid dysfunction.

Metrorrhagia is defined as bleeding that occurs between regular periods. When it is associated with excessive flow, the term **menometrorrhagia** is used, indicating heavy, irregular cycles. The etiology of these disorders is similar to menorrhagia and includes fibroids, adenomyosis, polyps, and endometrial hyperplasia.

These disorders are evaluated on the basis of history, examination, and laboratory testing. The physical examination should exclude bleeding from a source other than the uterus, such as the cervix, vagina, urethra, or rectum. Disorders for thyroid function, PCOS, and bleeding should be investigated. The pelvic examination may reveal fibroids, adenomyosis, or cancer. In patients with hypomenorrhea, laboratory tests should include a pregnancy test and measurement of thyroid-stimulating hormone (TSH), prolactin, and FSH levels to determine if the patient has hormonal dysregulation or ovarian insufficiency. In patients with excessive or prolonged menses associated with frequent cycles, a pregnancy test and measurement of TSH, complete blood count, prothrombin time/partial thromboplastin time, factor VIII, and von Willebrand antigen and activity levels should be ordered. Biopsy or endometrial sampling is recommended in women over age 35 years with intermenstrual bleeding or heavy periods. Finally, imaging studies such as a sonohysterogram (SHG) or pelvic ultrasound may reveal an underlying uterine abnormality.

Treatment should be aimed at the underlying disorder, and any desired future fertility must be considered. Menstrual regulation with hormonal contraceptives may be curative in some women, whereas more definitive treatment, such as endometrial ablation or hysterectomy may be necessary in others.

FEMALE HYPOGONADISM

In females with **hypogonadism**, the ovaries do not produce enough estrogen to meet the body's needs. The level at which this deficiency occurs helps distinguish the etiology of hypogonadism. *Primary hypogonadism*, or *hypergonadotropic hypogonadism*, involves failure of the ovaries to respond to FSH and LH. When primary hypogonadism affects estrogen production, the lack of estrogen fails to inhibit production of FSH and LH; thus, FSH and LH are elevated. *Central hypogonadism*, or *hypogondatropic hypogonadism*, is a failure of the hypothalamus or pituitary gland to produce adequate pulses of GnRH, FSH, and/or LH.

Hypogonadotropic Hypogonadism

Hypogonadotropic hypogonadism is the state of decreased gonadotropin (LH and FSH) secretion that usually results from a loss of GnRH pulsatility. This lack of pulsatility abolishes the ovarian cycle and results in amenorrhea. The biochemical findings include decreased FSH and estradiol levels. If loss of estrogen production is suspected, a progesterone challenge test is warranted. In this test, exogenous progesterone is given for 5 to 7 days and then discontinued. If the patient has menstrual bleeding, then the patient has sufficient estrogen to proliferate the endometrium. If the patient does not experience menstrual bleeding, her ovaries unlikely produce sufficient estrogen.

These disorders are the result of decreased or absent gonadotropins due to hypothalamic or pituitary dysfunction.

Disorders of Hypothalamic Function

Hypothalamic disorders that result in hypogonadotropic hypogonadism (decreased gonadotropins and ovarian hormones) may be due to overt suppression of all ovarian function, or it may be limited to poor luteal functioning from decreased LH stimulation. In this section, the common forms of functional hypothalamic amenorrhea (FHA) and hypothalamic amenorrhea due to anorexia nervosa and exercise will be discussed. The rare forms of amenorrhea due to hypothalamic dysfunction, such as infiltrative diseases (lymphoma, sarcoidosis, Langerhans cell histiocytosis) and Kallman syndrome (congenital GnRH deficiency), are not discussed in this chapter.

Functional Hypothalamic Amenorrhea

Functional hypothalamic amenorrhea (FHA) is a diagnosis of exclusion based on clinical findings alone. It is due to stress, which inactivates the HPO axis. The pathophysiology is suggested by studies of nonhuman primates showing environmental stressors induce secretion of corticotropin-releasing hormone (CRH). In addition to its stimulatory effects on adrenocorticotropic hormone (ACTH) and cortisol, CRH increases GnRH-inhibitory endorphins and directly inhibits GnRH pulsatility. This lack of proper GnRH pulsatility abolishes regular menses and ovulation. The characteristic features in most patients include proneness to anxiety and underlying metabolic, endocrine, or other psychological characteristics. Patients tend to be underweight. Laboratory findings revealing decreased gonadotropins together with menstrual abnormalities suggestive of anovulation (amenorrhea or oligomenorrhea) are diagnostic after exclusion of other causes. Many patients lack a classic stressor. Biochemical investigation of GnRH pulsatility is seldom necessary to diagnosis of FHA after other causes of amenorrhea have been excluded. Approximately 80% to 90% will have a decreased GnRH, decreased frequency of GnRH pulses, or decreased amplitude of pulses. Treatment is aimed at alleviating the stressor and improving BMI to appropriate levels. Even without treatment, spontaneous recovery occurs in 70% of patients after 6 to 8 years. Those prone to spontaneous recovery are those with normal BMIs, lower cortisol levels, and an identifiable stressor.

Anorexia Nervosa

Anorexia nervosa is a disorder that is associated with amenorrhea or oligomenorrhea. The etiology of the menstrual abnormalities is similar to FHA and likely includes abnormal leptin and insulin-like growth factor (IGF)-1 levels, known modulators of hypothalamic function. Findings in these patients include refusal to reach a normal weight (≤85% of ideal body weight), fear of gaining weight or becoming fat, and distorted body image. Additional findings include cycles of binging and self-induced vomiting as well as laxative or diuretic abuse.

The clinical findings reflect a dysfunctional hypothalamus, a decrease in adipose tissue, hypotension, bradycardia, hypothermia, soft fine body hair (lanugo), and dry skin. Women may complain of nausea, fatigue, early satiety, or bloating. These abnormalities may be severe and life threatening given that regulation of appetite, thirst, autonomic balance, and endocrine functioning can be severely impaired.

The laboratory findings include decreased serum levels of FSH, LH, estradiol, IGF-1, and leptin. Serum cortisol levels are increased. Serum levels of TSH and T_4 are usually normal but triiodothyronine (T_3) may be decreased and reverse T_3 (rT_3) increased.

Treatment is aimed at correcting body weight to normal levels. The treatment is complex, requiring mental health professionals; dieticians; and, commonly, hospitalization. To prevent the effects of estrogen deficiency, oral contraceptives may be used.

The prognosis depends on the degree of malnutrition that has occurred. Approximately half will have a good outcome with return of normal body weight and menses. However, 25% will have relapses; in another 25%, outcomes are poor. Osteopenia and osteoporosis are common from the combined nutritional and estrogen deficiencies.

Exercise

Extreme exercise, such as intense running or vigorous gymnastics, even with its many health benefits, can cause amenorrhea in women of reproductive age. The exact mechanism remains to be determined, but higher energy demand, lean body weight, and endogenous opioids released after exercise act synergistically to limit menses and ovulation. Women with <22% body fat have lower leptin levels. This, in turn, may abolish GnRH pulsatility and lead to anovulation and amenorrhea. The primary health concerns arise from estrogen depletion secondary to the resultant anovulatory state. Because these athletes are especially prone to osteopenia and osteoporosis, it is important to obtain baseline bone density measurements in women presenting with amenorrhea who exercise excessively. For women who do not reduce their exercise intensity, estrogen should be supplemented in the form of a contraceptive, which provide both estrogen and progesterone. Calcium and vitamin D supplements may also help fortify bone density.

Disorders of Pituitary Origin

Pituitary disorders that result in hypogonadotropic hypogonadism are discussed in Chapter 2. These disorders include adenomas; empty sella syndrome; Sheehan syndrome; and infiltrative diseases, such as hemochromatosis and lymphocytic hypophysitis. Hyperprolactinemia, which may be associated with hypo- or hypergonadotropic hypogonadism, is also discussed in detail in Chapter 2.

Hypergonadotropic Hypogonadism

Hypergonadotropic hypogonadism is defined as gonadotropin (LH and FSH) elevation due to a loss of negative feedback. This is also traditionally referred to as *ovarian insufficiency* or *premature menopause* if it occurs before age 40 years. It is usually due to a genetic or autoimmune condition, infectious disease, or the result of radiation/chemotherapy. Many of the disorders that present as secondary amenorrhea can also present as primary amenorrhea if they occur before the age of menarche. Patients with ovarian insufficiency may present with dyspareunia (pain during intercourse) or hot flashes as a result of diminished ovarian function associated with increased levels of FSH and inhibin B. On physical examination, signs of estrogen depletion, such as breast and vulvar atrophy, may be found. Biochemical findings include elevated FSH and decreased estradiol levels. Women who present with ovarian insufficiency, especially those who present before age 30 years, need a karyotype analysis to exclude a Y chromosome genotype or X chromosome abnormalities. Additional screening for gene mutations and adrenal or thyroid autoimmune diseases is also indicated.

Turner Syndrome

Turner syndrome (TS) is characterized by short stature and absence of sexual development. The incidence is approximately 1 in 2,000 to 5,000 live births. The classic karyotype is 45,XO, but approximately 50% are mosaics, resulting from chimerism in which some cells retain a complete or partial 46,XX karyotype. Other variations include structural abnormalities of the X chromosome, such as partial deletions and ring structures. This is important insofar as TS mosaics have less severe phenotypes than those with complete 45,XO. Approximately 15% of females with TS begin, but do not finish puberty, and about 5% actually complete puberty. This is a result of gonadal dysgenesis because the absent X usually results in defective formation of the ovaries.

Only one-third of females with TS will have ovaries detected on pelvic ultrasound. The remaining patients have limited follicles or a high number of follicles in atresia that depend on the severity and degree of X chromosome loss. This results in a predominance of ovarian stroma, known as a **streak gonad**. The majority of females with TS have elevated levels of FSH and LH due to the ovarian insufficiency.

The pathophysiology of TS depends on the degree of X chromosome loss. In 45,XO individuals, loss of homeobox-containing genes (*SHOX*) is located at the terminal end of the X chromosome and results in short stature. Other genes lost result in wide-ranging effects that vary between individuals.

In addition to the signs listed above, the classical phenotype of TS includes a webbed neck, micrognathia, widely spaced nipples, low-set ears, and posteriorly shifted hairline (Figure 12-6). At birth, many have lymphedema. Renal abnormalities (e.g., horseshoe kidney) affect 30% to 50% and predispose them to hydronephrosis. Cardiac manifestations include a biscupid aortic valve (20% to 30%), coarctation of the aorta (5% to 10%), aortic root elongation (50%), persistent left superior vena cava, and anomalous pulmonary venous return. Osteoporosis is common and is a result of the low estrogen produced from ovarian insufficiency. Other findings may include hypothyroidism, ocular abnormalities such as red–green color blindness, hearing loss, liver function abnormalities, and celiac disease. These later findings are related to the absence of the gene on the deleted portion of the X chromosome.

Treatment requires management of the multitude of anomalies including the short stature. These females require cardiac and renal ultrasonography to look for any congenital abnormalities. Periodic biochemical monitoring should include thyroid, renal, and liver function. Screening for celiac disease and audiometry tests should be performed and repeated at least every 10 years if normal. Monitoring of linear growth is important because females with TS may benefit from growth hormone (GH) therapy. Finally, estrogen therapy should be started between ages of 12 and 15 years. Within 6 to 12 months of starting estrogen therapy, progesterone should be added, and 6 to 12 months later, linear growth should be completed.

The prognosis for females with TS varies depending on the severity of the phenotype. Intelligence is normal, but there is an increased prevalence of attention deficit/hyperactive disorder. Overall mortality is increased threefold and is due to a combination of cardiovascular disease, diabetes, renal impairment, and liver disease. The overall cancer risk is not increased, but the risk for endometrial, bladder, and CNS neoplasms is. With the administration of human GH, most females with TS will achieve a height of 10 to 15 cm greater than the average height of 150 cm.

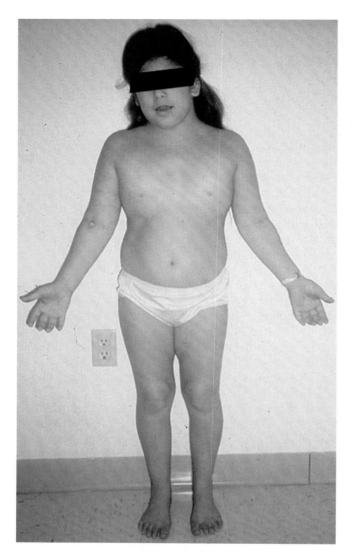

FIGURE 12-6. Turner syndrome. Short stature, stocky build, crest chest, lack of breast development, and cubitus valgus are evident in this 13-year-old girl. (From Shulman D, Beru B. Atlas of Clinical Endocrinology: Neuroendocrinology and Pituitary Disease. Philadelphia, PA: Current Medicine Inc.; 2000.)

Gonadal Dysgenesis

Gonadal dysgenesis is the incomplete or defective formation of the gonads. It results from disturbances in either germ cell migration or formation of the urogenital ridge. The most common cause of gonadal dysgenesis is TS, but different chromosomal abnormalities and gene mutations may also be causal. Dysgenesis may occur in a complete form with full cessation of gonad function or in an incomplete (mixed) form with some residual gonad functioning.

In the rare Swyer syndrome, females have complete gonadal agenesis. These females usually present for medical attention because of delayed puberty and primary amenorrhea. Despite a 46,XY karyotype, female internal and external genitalia develop because the completely dysgenic gonad fails to produce anti-mullerian hormone (AMH) or androgens. Because adrenal glands are not affected, adrenarche with the presence of pubic hair usually occurs at the appropriate age. The diagnosis is made by karyotype. Once the diagnosis is confirmed, prompt gonadectomy is recommended because 20% to 30% of gonads undergo malignant transformation before age 20 years. Sex hormone therapy should be implemented between ages of 12 and 15 years to ensure a smooth transition into puberty.

Miscellaneous Genetic Causes

Several gene mutations increase the risk of ovarian insufficiency. The most important of these is the **fragile X syndrome**. The X-linked *FMR1* gene with CGG sequence expansions characterize this syndrome. It occurs in 1 in 4,000 to 8,000 births. As an X-linked disorder, females are partially protected, but 70% have a borderline or low IQ and experience menopause 5 years earlier than expected. A second group of gene mutations includes those that impair follicular development but do not cause ovarian insufficiency. They include steroidogenic enzyme defects, defects in gonadotropins or their receptors (e.g., Savage syndrome), and disorders of paracrine regulation of the ovary. Treatment typically involves exogenous administration of sex steroids.

Autoimmunity

Autoimmune causes of ovarian insufficiency account for approximately 4% of cases. Autoimmunity can be directed at the adrenals, ovaries, and thyroid gland. A strong association exists between adrenal autoimmunity and ovarian failure, which justifies screening for antiadrenal or anti-21-hydroxylase antibodies. Screens for antithyroglobulin and antithyroperoxidase antibodies have demonstrated that approximately 15% to 25% are prevalent in females with ovarian insufficiency. Autoimmune disorders are discussed in greater detail in Chapter 16.

Radiation and Chemotherapy

Radiation exposure that results in ovarian insufficiency is dependent on the patient's age of exposure, radiation dose, and the radiation field. Radiation that does not include the pelvis has minimal, if any, effect. Radiation dosages of approximately 600 rad will cause complete ovarian failure in women over age 40 years. In those who are younger, however, pregnancies have occurred with a dose of 600 rad. The radiosensitivity of oocytes is estimated at 200 rad, suggesting that half will not survive each exposure.

Females treated for neoplasms with chemotherapy are also at risk for developing ovarian insufficiency. Oocytes are extremely sensitive to cytotoxic agents, and the oocyte depletion from these agents occurs in a drug- and dose-dependent manner. The most toxic drugs are the alkylating agents such as cyclophosphamide. Less toxic agents include those that impair cellular metabolism (e.g., methotrexate and 5-fluorouracil). Treatment with a long-acting GnRH agonist prior to chemotherapy may confer some protection from cytotoxic agents by inducing a hypogonadal state in which ovarian cells are minimally active. This approach is controversial. Other approaches include oocyte collection prior to chemotherapy.

CONGENITAL OUTFLOW TRACT ABNORMALITIES

There are a number of congenital causes of outflow tract abnormalities including imperforate hymen, transverse vaginal septum, cervical atresia, and Müllerian agenesis.

Imperforate Hymen

The hymen is formed by the invagination of the urogenital sinus and usually ruptures in the perinatal period. Failure to rupture is referred to as an **imperforate hymen** (Figure 12-7). Most cases occur sporadically. During menarche, females with an imperforate hymen develop pelvic and abdominal pain due to the buildup of trapped menses. Findings on physical examination include a bulging membrane, often with blue coloration due to retained menses referred to as **hematocolpos**. The treatment involves surgery to create a perforation.

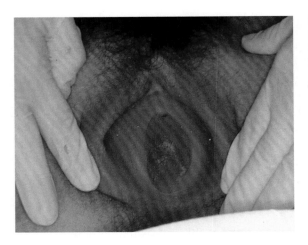

FIGURE 12-7. Imperforate hymen. (From Fleisher GR, Ludwig S, Baskin MN. Atlas of Pediatric Emergency Medicine. Philadelphia, PA: Lippincott Williams & Wilkins; 2004.)

Transverse Vaginal Septum and Cervical Atresia

When the vaginal plate in embryogenesis fails to canalize, an obstructing septum or poorly formed cervix results. Females with this abnormality have similar symptoms as those with an imperforate hymen. The abdominal and pelvic pain is due to increased retrograde menstrual flow. These females are at risk for endometriosis. In addition to poor visualization of the cervix and hematocolpos, other developmental anomalies, such as fallopian tube atresia, may be detected on physical examination. Secondary sexual characteristics are unaffected because the ovaries usually develop normally.

Müllerian Agenesis

Müllerian agenesis, also known as *Mayer-Rokitanksy-Küster-Hauser* (*MRKH*) *syndrome*, occurs in 1 in 5,000 newborn females. These females usually come to attention because they have primary amenorrhea but normal thelarche and adrenarche. The MRKH syndrome is defined by failure of complete formation and fusion of Müllerian-derived structures, that is, the uterus, fallopian tubes, and cervix. Two general types (A and B) have been described. Females with type A have a symmetric, muscular, and rudimentary uterus with normally developed fallopian tubes. Females with type B have an asymmetric rudimentary uterus with absent or underdeveloped fallopian tubes. It is also associated with unilateral renal agenesis; urological malformation; and, occasionally, skeletal abnormalities of the spine. The diagnosis is usually made by taking a careful history and performing a pelvic examination. A pelvic ultrasound and diagnostic laparoscopy may be useful for diagnosis. The treatment involves the use of dilating devices to enlarge the vaginal opening or the surgical creation of a functional vagina.

ACQUIRED OUTFLOW TRACT ABNORMALITIES

The acquired causes of outflow tract abnormalities include leiomyomas, endometriosis, Asherman syndrome, and cervical stenosis.

Leiomyomas

Leiomyomas, or *uterine fibroids*, are benign smooth muscle proliferations within the uterus. They can be subserosal (along the exterior portion of the uterus), intramural (within the myometrium of the uterus), or submucosal (within the uterine cavity). **Leiomyosarcomas** are a malignant proliferation of uterine smooth muscle cells.

Fibroid tumors affect nearly 30% of all women in the United States by age 40 years. African American women are especially prone, with 50% affected by the fifth decade. Fibroid tumors are rarely of concern but may cause pain, bleeding, or infertility in some women. The pain occurs as a result of degenerative changes within the fibroid as it outgrows its blood supply. Menorrhagia and/or metrorrhagia occur commonly because the fibroids alter the support of the overlying endometrial tissue. If the bleeding is excessive, affected women are at risk for anemia due to iron deficiency.

Fibroids develop from the proliferation of a single smooth muscle cell. This proliferation of cells is hormonally responsive to estrogen and commonly enlarges during pregnancy, when estrogen levels are elevated.

The diagnosis of fibroid tumors is usually made with imaging studies, such as a pelvic ultrasound or sonohysterogram (SHG). Fibroids should be surgically removed if they cause significant symptoms, grow rapidly, or are suspected of causing infertility. For women who do not desire future pregnancies, a uterine artery embolization can be performed. This procedure destroys the blood supply to the fibroid, causing it to degenerate. To definitively remove the fibroids and eliminate any chance of recurrence, a hysterectomy should be performed.

Endometriosis

Endometriosis is the presence of endometrial tissue outside the uterine cavity (Figure 12-8). Women with endometriosis have pain, may develop adhesions, and may become infertile. Approximately 20% of women with chronic pelvic pain have endometriosis. Up to 40% of female infertility is due to endometriosis. It can occur anywhere within the body, but it is mostly commonly found within the pelvic peritoneum and on the ovaries. There are reports of endometrial tissue within the lungs that resulted in hemoptysis. The pathophysiologic mechanism of endometriosis is likely due to a combination of retrograde flow, ectopic distribution during early embryogenesis, lymphatic transport, and metaplastic transformation into endometrial tissue. Endometriosis clinically presents as cyclic pelvic and lower back pain that occurs the week prior to the onset

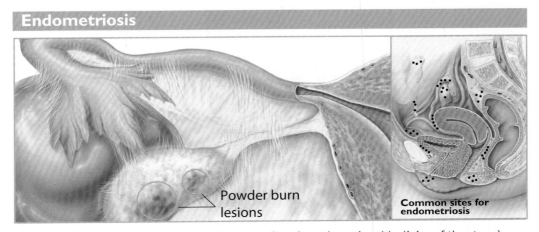

Endometriosis

Powder burn lesions

Common sites for endometriosis

FIGURE 12-8. Endometriosis. Endometriosis occurs when the endometrium (the lining of the uterus) grows outside of the uterus. Pain symptoms can occur before and during periods and during or after intercourse.

of menses. This form of dysmenorrhea is a result of cyclic proliferation and shedding of endometrial tissue within contained cystic formation. Scarring may occur and distort the pelvic anatomy, which may exacerbate the dysmenorrhea and cause infertility. Depending on the site of implantation, endometriosis can also cause dyspareunia or even pain with defecation.

The diagnosis is made histologically after biopsy of the affected area. The pelvic examination is remarkable for dense adhesions, nodularity, and/or a fixed retroverted uterus. On laparoscopy, "powder burn" lesions are characteristic of endometriosis (Figures 12-8 and 12-9). The initial treatment is the administration of hormonal contraceptives that suppress the cyclical proliferation of the ectopic endometrial tissue. In women who do not get relief and seek a pregnancy, a conservative surgical thermal or laser ablation of the visualized lesions can be effective. Definitive treatment may be necessary for those without adequate relief and involves the removal of all of the affected tissue. Usually, a complete hysterectomy with removal of the fallopian tubes and ovaries is ultimately necessary.

Asherman Syndrome

Asherman syndrome is an acquired anatomical defect of the uterus due to adhesions that develop as a result of extensive surgical procedures, inflammation, or retained products of conception. Females with Asherman syndrome usually present with amenorrhea. A progesterone challenge test results in no withdrawal bleeding. Ultrasonographic studies, such as SHG or hysterosalpingography, can demonstrate adhesions within the uterus. The treatment involves surgical lysis of the adhesions. Hysteroscopic dissection is usually necessary to remove uterine adhesions.

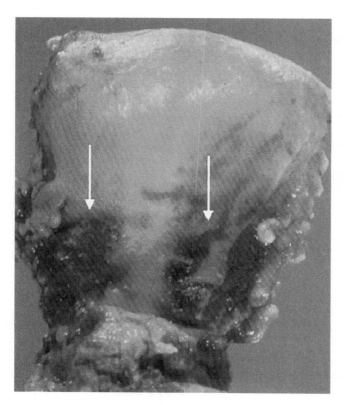

FIGURE 12-9. "Burned-out" endometriosis. This hysterectomy specimen shows dark red to gray serosal discoloration (*white arrows*) characteristic of the gunpowder burn appearance of "burned-out" endometriosis. (From Baggish MS, Valle RF, Guedj H. Hysteroscopy: Visual Perspectives of Uterine Anatomy, Physiology and Pathology. Philadelphia, PA: Lippincott Williams & Wilkins; 2007.)

Cervical Stenosis

Cervical stenosis is an acquired condition that occurs as a result of extensive surgical manipulation of the cervix, multiple vaginal births, or infection. The diagnosis is made by physical and pelvic examination. The treatment for cervical stenosis is gradual dilation of the cervix with ultrasound guidance.

OVARIAN DISORDERS

The ovarian disorders that affect female reproduction include PCOS, ovarian stromal hyperthecosis, theca lutein cysts, luteomas, and neoplasia.

Polycystic Ovary Syndrome

Polycystic ovary syndrome (PCOS) is an acquired disorder characterized by hyperandrogenism; menstrual irregularities; and enlarged, cystic ovaries. The etiology is controversial, but it is believed that an abnormally elevated LH/FSH ratio leads to aberrant ovulation (i.e., anovulation) and ovarian cyst formation. PCOS is a complex interaction of genetic, metabolic, and environmental derangements that cause prolonged anovulation, resulting in a polycystic ovary.

The pathophysiology of PCOS is due to the effects of a hyperestrogenic state that results from the anovulatory polycystic ovaries. Androgens are elevated because of the increased peripheral conversion of estrogen by the aromatase enzyme and from direct ovarian synthesis by sustained LH levels. The estrogen and androgen levels remain elevated, and, because they do not rise and fall in a cyclical pattern, menstrual irregularities, such as oligomenorrhea or amenorrhea, occur. These persistently high androgen levels are responsible for most of the clinical findings in PCOS including impaired glucose tolerance, type 2 diabetes, hirsutism, virilization, and increased adipose deposition. The resultant obesity worsens the situation and increases the risk for insulin resistance, dyslipidemia, hypertension, and cardiovascular disease. The elevated androgens also decrease SHBG, which causes an increase in the proportion of unbound biologically active androgens. As a result, PCOS leads to a self-reinforcing cycle of hormone and metabolic derangements. The ultimate effect of chronic exposure to unopposed estrogen that occurs in these anovulatory women places them at a high risk for endometrial hyperplasia and carcinoma.

After other androgen excess disorders have been excluded, the diagnosis of PCOS is confirmed if a female has two of the following three criteria: (1) oligomenorrhea and/or anovulation, (2) biochemical or clinical evidence of hyperandrogenism, and (3) polycystic ovaries on imaging studies. The treatment for PCOS requires restoration of gonadotropin, estrogen, and androgen levels to normal and the evaluation and management of the sequelae of PCOS. To restore normal hormone levels, females with PCOS are treated with contraceptive agents that contain estrogen and progesterone. This not only decreases androgen levels but also increases progesterone levels. Progesterone opposes the hyperestrogenic state, decreasing the risk of endometrial hyperplasia. Metformin, an agent used to treat individuals with type 2 diabetes, reduces androgen levels; decreases hepatic glucose production; reduces weight; and, ultimately, improves the gonadotropin and sex hormone levels in many females with PCOS.

The sequelae of PCOS include insulin resistance, diabetes, dyslipidemia, obesity, hypertension, and infertility. For effective treatment, these conditions must be recognized early and clinical intervention started immediately. Defects in insulin actions or insulin signaling pathways are central to the pathogenesis of PCOS. Most women with PCOS are insulin resistant due to a combination of genetic predisposition and obesity.

Ovarian Stromal Hyperthecosis

Ovarian hyperthecosis is a histologic diagnosis based on stromal hyperplasia. Females with ovarian hyperthecosis have similar yet extremely advanced clinical features as those with PCOS. These women have severe insulin resistance, elevated serum testosterone levels, severe hirsutism, and virilization, and most of them have acanthosis nigricans. The treatment is similar to that for PCOS but may require a surgical intervention to remove the hyperthecosis.

Theca Lutein Cysts

Theca lutein cysts are hyperfunctioning theca cells. They produce an abnormally increased amount of androgen that overwhelms the normal aromatization process, resulting in elevated estrone and estradiol levels. The elevated androgen level results in virilization. Theca lutein cysts are most commonly found in pregnant females with multiple pregnancies, molar or trophoblastic disease, or diabetes. The diagnosis is confirmed histologically by ovarian biopsy.

Luteomas

Ovarian luteomas are pregnancy-associated hyperplastic masses of luteinized ovarian tissue that usually secrete little or no androgen. However, in some cases, luteomas can secrete elevated levels of androstenedione, testosterone, and DHT that results in rapid virilization and hirsutism. Most luteomas are 6 to 10 cm in length, and nearly half occur bilaterally. After pregnancy, luteomas usually spontaneously regress and seldom require removal. Newborn females exposed to elevated androgen levels in utero may appear virilized at birth.

Neoplasias

Tumors usually of sex cord–stroma include granulosa-theca cell tumors, Sertoli-Leydig tumors, and fibromas. They originate from the stroma or the layers near the oocyte and cause hyperandrogenism. These tumors are undifferentiated cell types capable of forming either ovarian or testicular cells. They can present in women of any age but are usually discovered in the fifth to seventh decades of life. Sex cord–stroma tumors are usually unilateral and low grade, and account for 5% to 10% of all ovarian tumors. The diagnosis is made by biopsy following positive imaging studies. However, if suspicion remains after a negative imaging study, ovarian venous sampling may help detect an androgen gradient suggestive of a unilateral neoplasm. Findings depend on the sex cord–stromal tumor type. Histologically, Call-Exner bodies are "coffee-bean" in configuration and are pathognomonic for granulosa-theca cell tumors. Fibromas may be present as a Meigs syndrome with associated ascites and a right hydrothorax. The treatment depends on the extent of the lesion. In women with low-grade growth tumors, a unilateral salpingo-oophorectomy of the fallopian tube and ovary may be sufficient. If childbearing is complete, removal of the ovaries, fallopian tubes, and uterus is recommended because of the distinct possibility of a late recurrence. Radiation and chemotherapy are seldom required for sex cord–stroma cell tumors.

ADRENAL GLAND DISORDERS

In women, androgens are produced within the adrenal glands and ovaries. In the adrenal glands, ACTH stimulates cholesterol conversion into pregnenolone, which is then converted to 17α-hydroxypregnenolone. This becomes the substrate for the weak adrenal androgens DHEA, DHEAS, and androstenedione. In the ovaries, LH stimulates the theca cells to produce androstenedione and testosterone, which may either enter systemic circulation bound to SHBG or be aromatized to estrone and estradiol, respectively.

Therefore, in women, androgen excess disorders may result from either a primary increase in androgen synthesis, secondary to increased stimulation, or to ectopic androgens that are derived from another source, such as a tumor or medication. Because a decrease in SHBG will result in an increase in unbound free testosterone, an excess of androgens will decrease SHBG levels, thereby exacerbating the increase in free testosterone.

The majority (~80%) of women presenting with hyperandrogenism have PCOS. The remaining 20% are due to androgen-secreting neoplasms, congenital adrenal hyperplasia (CAH), idiopathic hyperandrogenism, or idiopathic hirsutism. As PCOS has been discussed earlier in this section and CAH in Chapter 15, the following discussion will be limited to hyperandrogenism, hirsutism, and the evaluation of women with states of possible androgen excess.

Virilizing Disorders

Virilizing disorders are classified as hirsutism or hyperandrogenism and may develop as an inherited or an acquired condition. Hirsutism is defined as excessive growth of facial and body hair in females who do not have elevated androgen levels. Hyperandrogenism, also known as *virilization*, is defined as having both the clinical (e.g., excess growth of facial and body hair) and laboratory features of elevated serum androgen levels.

Idiopathic Hirsutism

Idiopathic hirsutism is a diagnosis of exclusion. It typically affects middle-aged women traditionally of Mediterranean or Middle Eastern descent. These women usually have mild to moderate hirsutism despite a normal or mildly elevated testosterone level and normal menstrual history. One explanation for the cause of idiopathic hirsutism is upregulated 5α-reductase activity at the hair follicle that causes higher local levels of DHT. A helpful diagnostic test is to evaluate the serum level of 3α-androstanediol glucuronide, a DHT metabolite. Medications that lower 5α-reductase activity (e.g., finasteride) are effective but must be used in conjunction with effective birth control because of the potential birth defects that may occur in male fetuses during pregnancy. Estrogen–progesterone contraceptives may also be beneficial because they increase androgen binding and decrease androgen synthesis.

Idiopathic Hyperandrogenism

Idiopathic hyperandrogenism is also a diagnosis of exclusion. Females present with excess facial and body hair and elevated serum levels of androgens but usually ovulate normally. The management is similar to that for idiopathic hirsutism with antiandrogen and oral contraceptive administration. The same pregnancy precautions and use of a highly effective birth control should be employed when antiandrogens are utilized.

Evaluation and Management

Women who present with signs of virilization should be tested for free testosterone, 17α-hydroxyprogesterone (17-OHP), TSH, prolactin, and DHEAS insofar as these hormones confirm the diagnosis and guide the management. An elevation in 17-OHP suggests

CAH, due to the congenital deficiency of the 21α-hydroxylase enzyme. DHEAS elevation with increased free testosterone strongly indicates an adrenal origin for virilization and necessitates an imaging evaluation such as an abdominal computed tomography scan. TSH and prolactin levels should also be obtained because a large proportion of anovulatory women, with or without androgen excess, have thyroid or prolactin abnormalities. This may alert the clinician to another etiology for the anovulatory cycles.

The rate of progression of virilization is an important clinical finding. Rapidly progressive disorders may indicate an underlying neoplasm, whereas an indolent process suggests PCOS, idiopathic hyperandrogenism, or idiopathic hirsutism.

Adrenal disorders that result in androgen excess include both neoplastic and non-neoplastic lesions. Most adrenal tumors that secrete androgens (DHEA, DHEAS, testosterone) are carcinomas. Nonneoplastic lesions include classical and nonclassical CAH, Cushing syndrome, and glucocorticoid resistance. A more in-depth discussion of these disorders and their management is given in Chapter 10.

CASE FOLLOW-UP

A pelvic examination is necessary to evaluate her genitalia. The patient has to wait a week before the gynecologist can see her. The primary care physician orders several laboratory tests with the following results: FSH (4.2 mIU/L), LH (2.4 mIU/L), and a comprehensive metabolic panel is within the normal range. Her karyotype reveals a 46,XX genotype.

A week later, the gynecologist performs a pelvic examination. According to the gynecologist's examination, our patient has normal external female genitalia, including labia minora, labia majora, and a clitoris. Her vagina is shallow with a blind pouch. Her cervix could not be visualized.

Based on suspicion for Müllerian agenesis, an ultrasound is performed, but a uterus is not clearly identified. On diagnostic laparoscopy, an asymmetric rudimentary uterus and absent fallopian tubes are noted. Unilateral renal agenesis is noted as well. The patient is referred for surgical evaluation for creation of a functional vagina. Her final diagnosis is MRKH syndrome type B.

REFERENCES and SUGGESTED READINGS

Azziz R. The evaluation and management of hirsutism. Obstet Gynecol. 2003;101(5 Pt 1):995–1007.

Baptiste CG, Battista MC, Trottier A, Baillargeon JP. Insulin and hyperandrogenism in women with polycystic ovary syndrome. J Steroid Biochem Mol Biol. 2010;122(1–3):42–52.

Bianco SD, Kaiser UB. The genetic and molecular basis of idiopathic hypogonadotropic hypogonadism. Nat Rev Endocrinol. 2009;5:569–576.

Bouligand J, Ghervan C, Tello JA, et al. Isolated familial hypogonadotropic hypogonadism and a GNRH1 mutation. N Engl J Med. 2009;360:2742–2748.

Caronia LM, Martin C, Welt CK, et al. A genetic basis for functional hypothalamic amenorrhea. N Engl J Med. 2011;364(3):215–225.

Davenport ML. Approach to the patient with Turner syndrome. J Clin Endocrinol Metab. 2010;95(4):1487–1495.

De Vos M, Devroey P, Fauser BC. Primary ovarian insufficiency. Lancet. 2010;376(9744):911–921.

Ehrmann DA. Polycystic ovary syndrome. N Engl J Med. 2005;352(12):1223–1236.

Fritz M, Speroff L. Clinical Gynecologic Endocrinology and Infertility. 8th ed. Philadelphia, PA: Lippincott Williams and Wilkins, 2011.

Gupta J, Kai J, Middleton L, Pattison H, Gray R, Daniels J. Levonorgestrel intrauterine system versus medical therapy for menorrhagia. N Engl J Med. 2013;368:128–137.

Guzick DS. Polycystic ovary syndrome. Obstet Gynecol. 2004;103(1):181–193.

Jensen JT, Lefebvre P, Laliberté F, et al. Cost burden and treatment patterns associated with management of heavy menstrual bleeding. J Womens Health (Larchmt). 2012;21:539–547.

Kaunitz AM, Inki P. The levonorgestrel-releasing intrauterine system in heavy menstrual bleeding: a benefit-risk review. Drugs. 2012;72:193–215.

Melmed S, Casanueva FF, Hoffman AR, Kleinberg DL, Montori VM, Schlechte JA, et al. Diagnosis and treatment of hyperprolactinemia: an Endocrine Society clinical practice guideline. J Clin Endocrinol Metab. 2011;96(2):273–288.

Plant TM. Hypothalamic control of the pituitary-gonadal axis in higher primates: key advances over the last two decades. J Neuroendocrinol. 2008;20: 719–726.

Santoro N. Update in hyper- and hypogonadotropic amenorrhea. J Clin Endocrinol Metab. 2011;96(11):3281–3288.

Sweet MG, Schmidt-Dalton TA, Weiss PM, Madsen KP. Evaluation and management of abnormal uterine bleeding in premenopausal women. Am Fam Physician. 2012;85(1):35–43.

Viswanathan V, Eugster EA. Etiology and treatment of hypogonadism in adolescents. Pediatr Clin North Am. 2011;58(5):1181–1200.

CHAPTER REVIEW QUESTIONS

1. An 18-year-old ballerina presents with a chief complaint of absent menses. She states that she is in good health, but has never achieved menarche and her breast development occurred much later than most of her girlfriends. Visual inspection reveals Tanner stage V breasts and pubic hair. On pelvic examination, her cervical os is visualized and appears normal. She has a normal bimanual pelvic examination and a normal transvaginal ultrasound. She denies any associated symptoms. The most likely etiology of her delayed menarche is:

   A. Anorexia nervosa
   B. Prolactin-secreting adenoma
   C. Polycystic ovarian syndrome
   D. Androgen insensitivity syndrome
   E. Functional hypothalamic amenorrhea

2. A 36-year-old female presents to clinic with the complaint of failure to conceive. She describes wanting to have a child with her husband of 3 years and they have had intercourse without any form of contraception for 18 months. Apart from a brief period of depression in college, her medical history is not significant. She denies any hot flashes, dyspareunia, vaginal dryness, excessive stress, or exercise. She has had constipation for 10 months. Her partner has a child from a previous relationship. She does not take any medication. Her vital signs and physical examination are normal with Tanner stage V breasts and pubic hair as well as a normal bimanual pelvic examination. She describes irregular menstrual cycles lasting 40 to 45 days. Transvaginal ultrasound performed in the clinic is normal. Laboratory findings are consistent with

   A. An elevated 17α-hydroxyprogesterone (17-OHP) and decreased serum potassium (CAH)
   B. An elevated androstenedione level and positive glucose tolerance test (PCOS)
   C. Elevated FSH and inhibin B levels with a low antral follicle count (POF)
   D. An elevated TSH and prolactin (hyperprolactinemia/hypothyroidism)
   E. Low FSH and LH with decreased estradiol and progesterone (hypogonadism)

3. A 53-year-old obese female presents to clinic with complaints of vaginal spotting for 3 days. She believes this is very unusual since she has been in menopause for 4 years and has not had any vaginal bleeding. Further work-up and an endometrial biopsy confirm a diagnosis of endometrial hyperplasia, a precursor for endometrial cancer. The pathophysiology of this condition is the result of:

   A. Elevated FSH with loss of negative feedback at the hypothalamus and anterior pituitary
   B. Loss of estrogen negative feedback on the endometrium secondary to menopause

C. Peripheral estrogen production by adipose tissue without progesterone opposition

D. Failure of the patient to take estrogen supplements as phytoestrogens from tofu

E. Peripheral androgens that were converted from circulating C19 steroids

4. A 21-year-old college student presents to the Student Health Clinic complaining of irregular menses. She states she has never had a regular period and that her periods are often heavy and lasting 8 to 9 days. Additional questioning reveals that she developed breasts and pubic hair at approximately age 10 and menarche at 11 years. Her vitals are HR 66, BP 110/75, RR 14, and she is afebrile. On physical examination, she is slightly obese (BMI 30.5) and has moderate acne. Biochemical and imaging work-up reveals multiple ovarian cysts. This condition most likely results from:

A. Anovulatory follicles with subsequent excess estrogen production and peripheral aromatization

B. Excess androstenedione production due to adrenal hyperplasia

C. Low insulin-like growth factor (IGF)-1 expression in the ovaries with subsequent insulin resistance

D. Ovulatory cycles with insufficient progesterone production

E. Negative feedback on the arcuate nucleus with subsequent gonadotropin inhibition

5. A 31-year-old female presents to clinic for the evaluation of primary infertility. She has attempted to conceive with her male partner for 2 years without any success. She describes having less interest in sex lately but desires to have a large family with her husband. She admits to using an over-the-counter ovulation predictor kit to help conceive, but has yet to have a positive result. Her menses she describes were "like clockwork" in college but are now irregular, sometimes months between cycles, and her last period ended 45 days ago. She denies any cramping, dyspareunia, or pain with defecation. There is no history of sexually-transmitted infections or pelvic inflammatory disease. On examination, she is a well-appearing female without any abnormal findings. Her breasts and pubic hair are both Tanner stage V and her speculum and bimanual pelvic examinations are unremarkable. Her husband's semen analysis was normal and her uterine ultrasound was also normal. Her biochemical tests reveal an elevated FSH and LH and a decreased estradiol. This patient is most likely suffering from

A. Idiopathic adrenal hyperplasia

B. Functional pituitary adenoma

C. Ovarian insufficiency

D. Hypogonadotropic hypogonadism

E. Müllerian agenesis

CHAPTER REVIEW ANSWERS

1. The correct answer is E. This patient has primary amenorrhea resulting from hypogonadotropic hypogonadism that is most commonly functional hypothalamic amenorrhea (FHA). This disorder is the result of absent GnRH pulsatility that is due to the inhibitory effects of intense exercise and stress from her profession as a ballerina.

Although an important disorder to consider in young women presenting with amenorrhea, her overall clinical picture of good health is not consistent with anorexia nervosa (**Choice A**). A prolactin-secreting adenoma (**Choice B**), a type of pituitary adenoma, is much less common than FHA and is associated with galactorrhea and neurological findings such as visual changes and headache. Polycystic ovarian syndrome (**Choice C**), though a common disorder, usually includes signs of hyperandrogenism and acne. Individuals with androgen insensitivity syndrome (**Choice D**) have an XY karyotype. Due to a dysfunctional androgen receptor, they cannot adequately respond to androgens. In the complete AIS form, patients have fully formed breasts, no pubic hair, and lack a fully formed vagina or uterus. This is due to the inhibitory effects of Müllerian inhibitory hormone, which is secreted by the XY testes.

2. The correct answer is D. These findings are characteristic of hypothyroidism with an elevated TSH, with or without elevated prolactin levels. Elevations in thyrotropin-releasing hormone (TRH) have cross-stimulatory properties for prolactin, which in turn inhibits GnRH pulsatility and cyclical gonadotropin release. Although hyperprolactinemia is classically associated with galactorrhea, less than half of patients have galactorrhea.

An elevated serum 17α-hydroxyprogesterone (17-OHP) level with an elevated serum potassium level is characteristic of congenital adrenal hyperplasia (CAH). CAH includes several adrenal steroidogenic enzyme defects, which often lead to accumulation of androgens (**Choice A**). Elevations in the androgen, androstenedione, are suggestive of polycystic ovarian syndrome (PCOS), CAH, or another condition that results in elevated androgens such as a functional tumor. Hyperandrogenism would either be demonstrated biochemically or clinically if this were present (**Choice B**). A high FSH/inhibin B and low antral follicle count would suggest an estrogen-depleted state [hypergonadotropic hypogonadism or premature ovarian failure (POF)] (**Choice C**). These states are associated with hot flashes, dyspareunia, and vaginal atrophy, all of which are absent in this patient. Low gonadotropins and low ovarian hormones (**Choice E**) characterize hypogonadotropic hypogonadism. This patient lacks the characteristic neurological symptoms, the positive partum history, and exercise stress that make an anatomic or acquired defect in hypothalamic or pituitary function unlikely.

3. The correct answer is C. Estrogen is the steroid hormone responsible for endometrial proliferation. Progesterone halts this proliferative process and promotes the secretory functioning of the endometrium. In the postmenopausal state, circulating C19 steroids are converted by aromatase contained in adipose tissue into estrogen, which, in the absence of progesterone, leads to a state of chronic endometrial proliferation. Obese individuals are especially at risk because of their large amount of adipose tissue. Treatment depends on the staging and includes progesterone-containing medications, dilation and curettage, or hysterectomy.

Low estrogen levels due to menopause causes a loss of negative feedback and elevated FSH and inhibin B levels (**Choice A**) that drives the symptoms of perimenopause (i.e., hot flashes, night sweats, etc.). Estrogen is a direct stimulator of endometrial proliferation and provides negative feedback to the hypothalamus and pituitary gland, but not the endometrium (**Choice B**). There is evidence that suggests that natural estrogen supplements, such as tofu, alleviate perimenopausal symptoms (**Choice D**). However, these levels are insufficient to support endometrial growth and would not cause significant hyperplasia. Most androgens found in menopausal women are converted from the estrogens aromatized from circulating C19 steroids (**Choice E**). These androgens, however, may exacerbate hyperlipidemia and signs of virilization.

4. The correct answer is A. Polycystic ovarian syndrome (PCOS), a diagnosis of exclusion, is a very common endocrine disorder in reproductive-aged women with a prevalence of 10% in the United States. The pathophysiology of PCOS is not fully understood, but many of the clinical sequelae stem from an estrogen excess state with concomitant aromatization into androgens. The excess estrogen arises from the large number of anovulatory follicles, which produce high amounts of estrogen.

Hyperandrogenism is a major criterion for the diagnosis of PCOS. Congenital adrenal hyperplasia (CAH), with elevated androgen production from the adrenal glands, must be excluded before making a diagnosis of PCOS (**Choice B**). Insulin resistance is an important abnormality in PCOS, and is often present at the time of diagnosis. However, insulin resistance is not the primary cause of PCOS. An elevated insulin-like growth factor (IGF)-1 is expected in an insulin-resistant state secondary to elevated insulin levels (**Choice C**). PCOS has anovulatory cycles, which cause the failure of the corpus luteum to develop. The subsequent loss of cyclical progesterone is an important clinical component of endometrial hyperplasia risk in patients with PCOS (**Choice D**). Many aspects of PCOS pathology are driven by excess gonadotropin production in part by a loss of negative feedback from cyclical hormone production and not, insufficient gonadotropin secretion (**Choice E**).

---

5. The correct answer is C. The increased gonadotropins and decreased estradiol levels are characteristic of hypergonadotropic hypogonadism or premature ovarian insufficiency. The clinical picture supports this diagnosis, and in the presence of an unremarkable history and physical examination, the other options are less likely.

A patient with idiopathic adrenal hyperplasia (**Choice A**) has clinical or biochemical evidence of hyperandrogenism. A patient with a functional pituitary adenoma (**Choice B**), usually a prolactinoma, has either bilateral hemianopsia or galactorrhea. In the case of a prolactinoma, excess levels of gonadotropins would not be seen. Hypogonadotropic hypogonadism (**Choice D**) is associated with low FSH and LH levels, and ovarian hormone production, which is not consistent with the biochemical findings in this patient. Functional hypothalamic amenorrhea (FHA) is the most common cause of hypogonadotropic hypogonadism. Another potential cause that is seen in women with obstetrical complications is pituitary necrosis, known as *Sheehans syndrome*. Müllerian agenesis (**Choice E**), in which the Müllerian-derived structures (fallopian tubes, uterus, cervix, and upper vagina) are malformed, is much less likely because her bimanual pelvic examination is normal, as was the uterine ultrasound.

Male Reproductive Disorders

13

David Kappa
Eric I. Felner

CASE

A 15-year-old male presents to his primary care physician with a concern that his penis and testes are small. The young man is self-conscious around his peers when he is changing in the locker room for physical education class at school. He has no other complaints. His past medical, surgical, and family history are unremarkable. A review of his systems indicates that he developed pubic hair at age 12 years. His vital signs are within normal limits. On physical examination, he has thin pubic and axillary hair. He does not have gynecomastia. Examination of his genitalia shows that the length of his penis is 5 cm. His testes are prepubertal, soft, and small, measuring only 2 cm^3 in volume. His visual fields are intact.

With the exception of precocious puberty, which is discussed in detail in Chapter 15, this chapter reviews the etiology and pathophysiology of male reproductive disorders to help the learner develop hypotheses to better understand this young man's genital disorder. This chapter is organized to facilitate a review of the: 1) hormone effects resulting in the development and maintenance of normal male genitalia, 2) clinical characteristics in males with reproductive disorders, 3) etiology of male reproductive disorders, and 4) evaluation and treatment of male reproductive disorders.

OBJECTIVES

1. List the causes of primary and central hypogonadism in males.

2. Recognize the clinical and laboratory findings in males with hypogonadism.

3. Develop a differential diagnosis for male reproductive disorders.

4. Describe the evaluation and management of a male with a reproductive system disorder.

CHAPTER OUTLINE

Physiology
  Male Gonadal Differentiation
  Hypothalamic–Pituitary–Gonadal
    Axis
  Androgen Functions
Hypogonadism
  Etiology
  Clinical Findings
  Diagnostic Studies
  Treatment
Primary Hypogonadism
(Congenital)
  Klinefelter Syndrome
  Anorchia
  Cryptorchidism
  Leydig Cell Aplasia
  Gonadotropin-Receptor Mutation
  Defects in Testicular Biosynthesis
  Androgen-Receptor Defects
Primary Hypogonadism (Acquired)
  Infection
  Trauma
  Autoimmune Destruction

(continues)

PHYSIOLOGY

The development of the male reproductive tract is due to gonadal androgen hormone production and action. These hormones are primarily synthesized in the testes but also in the zona reticularis of the adrenal cortex. At various stages of development, androgens produce the male phenotype including the male internal genitalia, penis, scrotum, testes, male-pattern hair, muscle mass, vocal cord elongation, and bone mass. The critical function of the male gonadal system is the androgen contribution to fertility and conception. Testosterone, produced from the testes, is directly responsible for the development of normal male internal gonadal structures. Testosterone, through its conversion to dihydrotestosterone (DHT) by the 5α-reductase (5α-R) enzyme, is essential for the development of male external gonadal structures.

Male Gonadal Differentiation

For the differentiation of the normal testis, a number of critical factors and a sequence of events must occur. For the undifferentiated gonad to develop into a testis, the Y chromosome must have a functional sex-determining region Y (*SRY*) gene. In order for testosterone action to occur, the testes must produce a sufficient amount of testosterone, and the target tissues must have the appropriate receptors and enzymes to mediate its actions. Testosterone must be capable of converting to DHT by the 5α-R enzyme for the development of male external genitalia. The testes must also produce Müllerian-inhibiting hormone (MIH) during development to inhibit the formation of internal female reproductive structures. In addition, the testes must respond to follicle-stimulating hormone (FSH) and luteinizing hormone (LH).

Hypothalamic–Pituitary–Gonadal Axis

In males, the hypothalamic–pituitary–gonadal (HPG) axis drives testosterone secretion from the testes. Gonadotropin-releasing hormone (GnRH), released from the hypothalamus, stimulates the pituitary to release the gonadotropins FSH and LH. FSH and LH both stimulate the testes. FSH stimulates the release of inhibin and sperm production, and LH stimulates the release of testosterone. The HPG axis also drives the development of the secondary sex characteristics associated with puberty in both males and females (Figure 13-1). Within the hypothalamus, GnRH-producing cells are located primarily in the paraventricular nucleus. These neurons receive modulatory input from other sites within the central nervous system, although the complete regulatory pathways have not as of yet been determined. Negative feedback on the hypothalamus is provided by testosterone and inhibin from the testes.

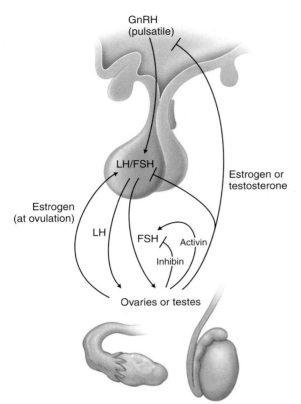

FIGURE 13-1. Hypothalamic–pituitary–gonadal axis in males. The hypothalamus secretes gonadotropin-releasing hormone (GnRH) into the hypothalamic–pituitary portal system in a pulsatile pattern. GnRH stimulates gonadotroph cells in the anterior pituitary gland to synthesize and release luteinizing hormone (LH) and follicle-stimulating hormone (FSH). These two hormones, referred to as gonadotropins, promote testicular synthesis of testosterone. Testosterone inhibits release of GnRH, LH, and FSH. The testes secrete inhibin, which selectively inhibits FSH secretion, and activin, which selectively promotes FSH secretion. (From Golan DE, Tashjian AH, Armstrong EJ. Principles of Pharmacology: The Pathophysiologic Basis of Drug Therapy. 2nd ed. Baltimore, MD: Wolters Kluwer Health; 2008.)

A key feature of the HPG axis is that for gonadal secretion of hormones to occur properly, both GnRH and the gonadotropins must be secreted in a pulsatile fashion (Figure 13-2). Pulses are secreted every 90 to 120 minutes. Men lacking normal pulse frequency or amplitude may be hypogonadal or infertile.

Although the hypothalamic–pituitary–adrenal (HPA) axis is best known for the production of glucocorticoids from the zona fasiculata and mineralocorticoids from the zona glomerulosa (see Chapter 10), it also plays a role in puberty for both males and females by initiating the production of androgens from the zona reticularis.

Androgen Functions

The principal effects produced by the male reproductive axis result from the production and action of androgens, which are classic steroid hormones. They are synthesized primarily in the testes (adrenals contribute only a small fraction in men) and travel in the circulation bound to carrier proteins (Figure 13-3). The major androgen produced by the testes is testosterone. Testosterone is converted to the more active DHT in target tissues and estradiol in adipose tissues. Approximately 60% of testosterone in the circulation is bound to sex hormone–binding globulin (SHBG), and approximately 38% is bound to albumin. The remaining 2% is unbound, or free, testosterone and can enter target cells and bind to the cytoplasmic receptor. Men secrete about eight times more testosterone than women, but women are more sensitive to it. The anabolic effects include enhancement of muscle mass, strength, and bone density. The androgen effects include sex organ maturation; voice deepening; and facial, chest, and axillary hair development.

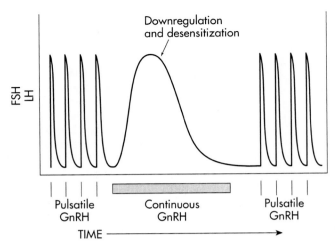

FIGURE 13-2. Gonadotropin-releasing hormone pulsatility. Schematic representation of the intermittent release of follicle-stimulating hormone (FSH) and luteinizing hormone (LH) in response to sporadic gonadotropin-releasing hormone (GnRH). Constant GnRH produces a reversible decrease in both gonadotropins after 7 to 10 days. Return of intermittent release produces a normal FSH and LH response. (From Baggish MS, Valle RF, Guedj H. Hysteroscopy: Visual Perspectives of Uterine Anatomy, Physiology and Pathology. Philadelphia, PA: Lippincott Williams & Wilkins; 2007.)

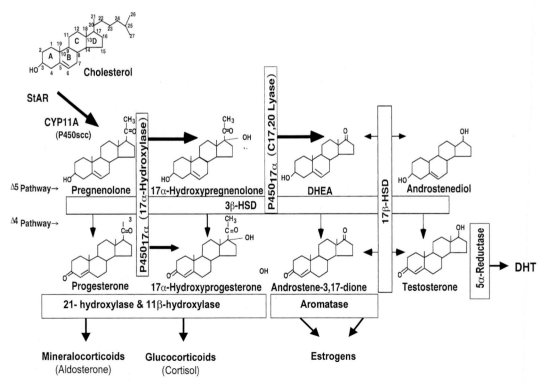

FIGURE 13-3. Steroid biosynthesis pathway. The ovary, the testis, and the adrenal gland produce six common core steroids. The core D5 steroids are pregnenolone, 17-hydroxypregnenolone, and dehydroepiandrosterone. The core D4 steroids are progesterone, 17-hydroxyprogesterone, and androstenedione (androstene-3,17-dione). The core steroids are important precursors for the production of sex steroids, glucocorticoids, and mineralocorticoids.

In males, testosterone exerts its effect at three major developmental milestones: 1) in the fetus for promotion of internal and external genitalia; 2) at puberty for maturation of genitalia, secondary sex characteristics, growth spurt, and epiphyseal closure; and 3) in adults for maintenance of libido, fertility, strength, and bone mass.

Once androgenization has occurred, the male phenotype tends to persist even if androgen levels decrease. However, prolonged hypoandrogenization decreases male pattern body hair and muscle mass and may reduce the efficiency of erection, libido, and other sexual behaviors. The male fat pattern also changes to a more female pattern with fat deposition in the hips and thighs.

Impotence is another manifestation of androgen deficiency. Impotence is defined as the inability to achieve an erection adequate for successful intercourse. Male penile erection is a complex biological event that is dependent on adequate arterial dilatation for blood flow into the corpora cavernosa. These events require normal neurologic, vascular, and hormonal inputs to the penis and are affected by a number of disorders that affect these systems. Hypogonadism is a prominent cause of impotence, although most impotent men are not hypogonadal, and not all hypogonadal men are impotent. Impotent men should be evaluated for testosterone deficiency as well as for thyroid disorders, hyperprolactinemia, and diabetes mellitus. Because most cases of impotence are multifactorial, it will not be discussed in this chapter.

Disorders of male reproduction are most commonly related to states of hypogonadism and testosterone deficiency, although excess testosterone production and infertility occur. In this chapter, the major focus will be on hypogonadism and conditions involving testosterone deficiency. Disorders of ambiguous genitalia will be discussed in detail in Chapter 15.

HYPOGONADISM

In males with **hypogonadism**, the testes do not produce enough testosterone. The level at which this deficiency occurs helps distinguish the etiology of hypogonadism.

Etiology

Testosterone deficiency may occur because of **primary** or **central hypogonadism**. *Primary hypogonadism* involves failure of the testes to respond to FSH and LH. When primary hypogonadism affects testosterone production, testosterone is insufficient to inhibit production of FSH and LH; hence, FSH and LH are elevated. *Central hypogonadism* is a failure of the hypothalamus or pituitary gland to produce adequate pulses of GnRH, FSH, and/or LH. As in primary hypogonadism, serum testosterone levels are low, but FSH and LH levels are low or inappropriately normal.

Clinical Findings

The clinical findings of hypogonadism, and subsequently, testosterone deficiency, depend on the age when the deficiency occurs. If the deficiency occurs during fetal development, there is likely to be impaired male sex organ development. Depending on when the deficiency occurred, the male child may have female-appearing genitalia (first trimester) or ambiguous genitalia (second or third trimester). Defects in sexual differentiation and ambiguous genitalia are discussed in detail in Chapter 15.

Testosterone deficiency that occurs in the child has few consequences but usually goes unrecognized until puberty is delayed. Affected boys will not develop muscle mass, a deeper voice, pubic hair, or enlargement of the penis and testes, and they will have slow growth at a time (pubertal growth spurt) when growth should be accelerated. If they are able to produce estrogen, from conversion of testosterone through the aromatase enzyme in adipose tissue, they will likely develop gynecomastia. If they produce little or no estrogen, they will develop a eunuchoid-like body because of delayed fusion of the epiphyses and continued long bone growth.

Hypogonadism in the adult male who previously reached puberty and developed secondary sexual characteristics causes variable manifestations depending on the degree and duration of the deficiency. Men with adult-onset testosterone deficiency may have decreased lean body mass, increased visceral fat, decreased testicular volume, osteopenia, gynecomastia, sparse body hair, decreased libido, erectile dysfunction, impaired cognitive skills, sleep disturbances, and mood changes.

Diagnostic Studies

The diagnosis of hypogonadism in the adult who has experienced puberty and normal development is based on clinical signs, symptoms, and laboratory confirmation of low morning testosterone levels on two different occasions. The normal range for serum testosterone is 300 to 1,000 ng/dL. For the adolescent who has not experienced signs of puberty or who has clinical signs of androgen deficiency, biochemical studies are useful only if the gonadotropin levels (FSH and LH) are extremely elevated and the bone age is older than age of 14 years. For boys with younger bone ages or who have serum gonadotropins in the prepubertal range without formal stimulation testing, hypogonadism may be difficult to differentiate from constitutional delay. Formal testing involves the use of GnRH and/or human chorionic gonadotropin (hCG) stimulation. These tests are discussed in detail in Chapter 19.

Because there are many causes of primary hypogonadism, establishing a differential diagnosis may seem daunting. The first and most important step after taking a thorough history and performing a physical examination is establishing whether the defect is a primary gonadal one, or if it is a central problem, affecting the hypothalamus or pituitary gland. The diagnosis of primary hypogonadism is established with a low serum testosterone level in the presence of an elevated serum LH level. More sophisticated genetic and biochemical tests may be required to further classify this condition if a congenital cause is likely.

The diagnosis of central hypogonadism, like that of primary hypogonadism, depends on identifying the site of the defect. First determine the relative levels of gonadotropins and testosterone. If serum LH, FSH, and testosterone levels are all low, then the site of origin is most likely the hypothalamus or pituitary gland. An imaging study, such as a magnetic resonance image (MRI) of the brain with a focus on the hypothalamus and pituitary gland, is necessary for identifying structural or mass effects.

Treatment

Treatment is directed toward providing adequate androgen replacement. Although patients with primary hypogonadism will not become fertile with any endocrine therapy, patients with central hypogonadism may become fertile with gonadotropin therapy.

For adolescent males with testosterone deficiency, monthly intramuscular (IM) injections of testosterone cypionate or enanthate (50 mg) should be initiated for 4 to 8 months. For the adolescent males who have a constitutional delay of growth, usually within 6 months of initiation, secondary sex characteristics and testicular volume will progress normally, and therapy will no longer be necessary. For those adolescents with true, permanent hypogonadism, after 4 to 8 months of the monthly therapy, the dose should

TABLE 13-1.	Treatment of Adult Male Hypogonadism
Treatment	**Dose**
Intramuscular testosterone (cypionate, enanthate)	100 mg/7 d or 200 mg/14 d
Testosterone gel (1%)	5–10 g/d (delivers 5–10 mg/d)
Testosterone transdermal patch	5–10 mg/d

be maintained at 50 mg/m^2 every 14 days for the next 18 to 24 months. Thereafter, testosterone replacement should be maintained at 100 mg/m^2 every 14 days. Although transdermal gels and patches are available, they are expensive, can be transferred to others during close contact, and pose dosing difficulties in adolescents, and therefore, only older adolescents should use them if they desire.

Adults with testosterone deficiency can utilize the same preparations as described above. Dosing for adults with testosterone deficiency is shown in Table 13-1.

Adolescent and adult men who developed hypogonadism prior to puberty are unlikely to develop complications from therapy unless an excessive dose is administered. For those who developed hypogonadism after completing puberty and likely may still produce some endogenous testosterone, there are risks to therapy. Potential adverse effects of testosterone therapy and its analogs include erythrocytosis, acne, gynecomastia, and enlargement of the prostate. Treatment may enhance growth of an existing prostate carcinoma and theoretically may awaken a dormant prostate cancer. These men should have their hematocrit and prostate-specific antigen (PSA) checked every 6 to 12 months. Significant increases in either should prompt referral to a specialist.

PRIMARY HYPOGONADISM (CONGENITAL)

The most common cause of congenital primary hypogonadism is Klinefelter syndrome (KS), an inherited chromosomal abnormality characterized by two or more X chromosomes with a single Y chromosome. The 47,XXY karyotype is the most common. In addition to other genetic syndromes, other causes of congenital primary hypogonadism may include defects in testicular function, testosterone biosynthesis, Leydig cell function, and gonadotropin receptors.

Klinefelter Syndrome

Individuals with Klinefelter syndrome (KS) most commonly have an extra X chromosome (47,XXY) as a result of meiotic nondisjunction of the sex chromosomes. Despite the frequency, only 25% of individuals with KS are diagnosed correctly, and only 10% are diagnosed as children.

The primary clinical features of KS include small testicles, infertility, testosterone deficiency, and tall stature. The most consistent features are the small, firm, atrophic testicles, which result from progressive hyalinization of the seminiferous tubules (Figure 13-4). These pathologic changes result in primary gonadal failure and azoospermia. The dysfunctional testes produce deficient testosterone, which becomes apparent as puberty progresses. Although these boys ultimately become testosterone deficient, they may progress through puberty appropriately prior to developing atrophic testes. They usually have azoospermia due to the hyalinization of the seminiferous tubules and obliteration

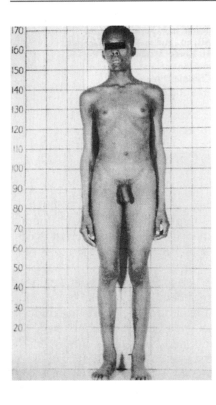

FIGURE 13-4. Klinefelter syndrome. A patient with Klinefelter syndrome (KS) showing normal phallus development but gynecomastia. (Reprinted with permission from McKusick VA. Klinfelter and Turner's syndromes. J Chronic Dis. 1960;12:52.)

of the passage of sperm to the ejaculatory ducts, but 50% of individuals with KS produce sperm.

The cognitive function of individuals with KS usually includes some degree of language acquisition or reading impairment. Neuropsychologic testing often reveals deficits in executive functions, although these deficits can often be successfully ameliorated through early intervention. There may also be delays in motor development that can be addressed through occupational therapy.

The diagnosis of KS is elusive as evidenced by the high rate of undiagnosed patients. These individuals typically present to medical attention with infertility or gynecomastia. Biochemical studies show elevated serum FSH and LH levels in association with low serum testosterone levels. The definitive diagnosis is made with a karyotype that reveals the presence of a Y chromosome and at least one extra X chromosome. Testicular biopsies are not needed for confirmation of the diagnosis but show diffuse hyalinization.

Management is focused on the problem of infertility and testosterone supplementation. Due to the progressive testicular failure, it is important to attempt to recover sperm as early as possible. Early in puberty, ejaculated sperm may be collected for cryopreservation. If azoospermia is present, then testicular sperm extraction is possible in 50% of KS patients that can be used for in vitro fertilization. Testosterone supplementation will enhance libido, virilization, bone density, and muscle mass. If testosterone replacement therapy is administered, the prognosis is excellent.

Anorchia

Anorchia, also referred to as the *vanishing testes syndrome*, results when the testes are absent at birth. If the testes fail to develop, the individual will be internally and externally female. If the testes fail to develop or function by 8 to 10 weeks gestation, the baby will have ambiguous genitalia. If, however, the testes develop, but are compromised after 14 weeks, the baby will have normal-appearing male genitalia, including penis and scrotum. The scrotum, however, will be empty and the gonads absent. The most likely cause of anorchia is due to an interruption in blood flow to the testes, similar to what occurs during a testicular torsion, ultimately resulting in a nonfunctional gonad.

Cryptorchidism

Cryptorchidism is the absence of one or both testes from the scrotum. It is the most common birth defect of the male genitalia. In unique cases, cryptorchidism can develop later in life, often as late as young adulthood. About 3% of full-term and 30% of premature infant boys are born with at least one undescended testis. However, about 80% of cryptorchid testes descend by the first year of life (the majority within 3 months), making the true incidence of cryptorchidism only around 1%.

Undescended testes are associated with hypogonadism, reduced fertility, increased risk of testicular germ cell tumors, and psychological problems in adulthood. Undescended testes are also more susceptible to testicular torsion, infarction, and inguinal hernias. To reduce these risks, undescended testes are usually brought into the scrotum in infancy by an **orchiopexy**. If not corrected in early childhood, testicular malfunction and reduced testosterone production may result.

Many men born with undescended testes have reduced fertility, even after orchiopexy in infancy. The reduction with unilateral cryptorchidism is subtle, with a reported infertility rate of about 10%, compared with about 6% reported by the same study for the general population of adult men. The fertility reduction after orchiopexy for bilateral cryptorchidism is more common, about 38%, or six times that of the general population. The universal recommendation for early surgery is based on research showing degeneration of spermatogenic tissue and reduced spermatogonia counts after the second year of life in boys with undescended testes.

One contributing mechanism for reduced spermatogenesis and testosterone secretion in cryptorchid testes is the scrotal temperature. The temperature of testes in the scrotum is at least a couple of degrees cooler than in the abdomen. However, infertility is a more complex matter than can be explained simply by temperature. Subtle or transient hormone deficiencies that result in lack of descent also impair the development of spermatogenic tissue. An additional factor contributing to infertility is the high rate of anomalies of the epididymis in boys with cryptorchidism (over 90% in some studies). Even after orchiopexy, these factors may also affect sperm maturation and motility as the boy ages.

One of the strongest arguments for early orchiopexy is prevention of testicular cancer. About 1 in 500 men born with one or both testes undescended develop testicular cancer, roughly a 4- to 40-fold increased risk. The peak incidence occurs in the third and fourth decades of life. The risk is higher for intra-abdominal testes and somewhat lower for inguinal testes, but even the man with one normally descended testis has a 20% higher cancer risk than do other men. The most common type of testicular cancer occurring in men with undescended testes is a seminoma. Cancer developing in an intra-abdominal testis is unlikely to be recognized before it has grown considerably and metastasized. One of the advantages of orchiopexy is that a mass developing in a scrotal testis is far easier to recognize than an intra-abdominal mass.

Leydig Cell Aplasia

Leydig cell aplasia is a rare, autosomal recessive syndrome affecting an estimated 1 in 1,000,000 males. It is characterized by an inability of the testes to respond to LH due to absence of the Leydig cells, and therefore, testosterone and other androgen sex hormones are not produced. The condition is recognized by underdeveloped male genitalia, low serum testosterone levels, and elevated FSH and LH levels.

Leydig cell aplasia is caused by genetic mutations in the *LHCGR* gene, which encodes the LH/hCG receptor. LH normally acts through the LH/hCG receptor to stimulate the growth of Leydig cells in the testicles and the production of androgens, such as testosterone and DHT, by these cells. In Leydig cell aplasia, however, the capacity for the LH/hCG receptor to respond to LH is reduced, resulting in hypoplasia or absence of Leydig cells, testicular atrophy, and low androgen levels. In the most severe form of the condition, androgen production by the testicles is negligible, and secondary sexual characteristics fail to develop at puberty.

The symptoms of Leydig cell hypoplasia include feminized, ambiguous, or relatively mildly underdeveloped male genitalia. These individuals may have a micropenis, severe hypospadias, cryptorchidism, complete sterility, tall stature (due to delayed epiphyseal closure), eunuchoid skeletal proportions, delayed or absent bone maturation, and osteoporosis.

Individuals with Leydig cell hypoplasia should be treated with androgen replacement therapy, which will result in normal sexual development and the resolution of most symptoms. In the case of 46,XY individuals who are completely phenotypically female and/or identify with the female gender, estrogens may be given instead. Surgical correction of the genitals in 46,XY males may be required, and, if necessary, an orchidopexy performed.

Gonadotropin-Receptor Mutation

Mutations in the LH or FSH receptor lead to high levels of gonadotropins. Because FSH acts on Sertoli cells, patients with an FSH-receptor mutation will have low sperm counts and low levels of inhibin. Patients with an LH-receptor mutation will have Leydig cell hypoplasia and low levels of testosterone. Because the testosterone deficit occurs in the first trimester, these patients may present with ambiguous genitalia. Other signs and symptoms are those that are seen in individuals with low levels of testosterone.

Defects in Testicular Biosynthesis

Primary hypogonadism can also result from a mutation in one of the enzymes involved in testosterone synthesis. The mutations can occur at various enzymatic stages, most commonly at 3β-hydroxysteroid dehydrogenase (3β-HSD) and 17α-hydroxylase (17α-OHase) in the adrenal gland, and 17β-HSD in the testes. Each of these mutations results in a first-trimester deficit of testosterone, incomplete virilization, and different presentations of ambiguous genitalia. These defects are discussed in more detail in Chapter 15.

An autosomal recessive mutation in the 5α-R enzyme results in impaired conversion of testosterone to DHT, resulting in external female genitalia because DHT normally stimulates the development of male external genitalia. Due to appropriate testosterone and MIH production, these individuals have normal internal male genitalia. Because these newborns appear female at birth, they are usually reared as females. At puberty, however, these individuals develop primary amenorrhea and virilization, which may include testicular descent, hirsutism (facial/body hair considered normal in males—not to be confused with **hypertrichosis**), voice deepening, and clitoral enlargement. As adults, these individuals do not experience male-pattern baldness. Because DHT is more potent than testosterone, virilization in those lacking DHT may be absent or reduced compared to males with functional 5α-R deficiency. It is hypothesized that rising testosterone levels at the start of puberty (around age of 12 years) are able to generate sufficient levels of DHT, either by the action of 5α-R type I (active in the adult liver, nongenital skin, and some brain areas) or through the expression of low levels of 5α-R type II in the testes. Not unexpectedly, however, individuals with 5α-R deficiency may have gender-identity problems.

5α-R deficiency is characterized biochemically by a normal serum testosterone level, low DHT level, elevated testosterone/DHT ratio, and normal gonadotropin levels.

There is an increased risk of cryptorchidism in 5α-R deficiency, causing infertility and a higher risk of testicular cancer. Fertility is further compromised by the underdevelopment of seminal vesicles and the prostate gland. On the other hand, fertility depending on female characteristics is impossible. Although the external genitalia may be female, the vagina consists of only the lower two thirds of a normal vagina, creating a blind-ending vaginal pouch. Due to the normal action of MIH produced by the testes in utero, individuals with 5α-R deficiency lack a uterus and fallopian tubes and are, therefore, unable to carry a pregnancy. Because they have testes and not ovaries, they are likewise unable to produce ova, which precludes infertility treatments using a surrogate mother.

Partial 5α-R deficiency may also occur. The phenotype depends on the degree of the mutation of the enzyme.

Androgen-Receptor Defects

Androgen insensitivity, or *testicular feminization syndrome*, results from a defect in the androgen receptor. Functional testosterone is present, but the faulty receptor is unable to mediate its effects. The varying degrees of androgen insensitivity and receptor defects are reflected in different clinical presentations. Individuals with complete androgen insensitivity appear externally female. Testes may be present in the abdomen or elsewhere, the vagina may be short, and the clitoris and labia undeveloped. A uterus is absent, but due to the presence of elevated androgens and the aromatase enzyme, estrogen is effectively produced (due to peripheral conversion of androgen to estrogen), and breast development is normal. These individuals are typically raised as females and develop psychologically feminine characteristics. They usually present to medical attention because of amenorrhea and absence of adrenarche, despite having appropriate breast development. These individuals have elevated gonadotropin levels because the abnormal androgen receptors in the pituitary cannot recognize testosterone feedback.

Partial androgen insensitivity may also occur. In these cases, the phenotype depends on the degree of mutation in the androgen receptor. The variation ranges from virilized women to undervirilized men and varying degrees of ambiguous genitalia.

Because the phenotypes are highly variable in cases of complete or incomplete androgen insensitivity, laboratory tests are helpful in establishing the correct diagnosis. Once the individual is at the appropriate age for puberty, testosterone levels are elevated as is the serum LH level because the brain senses low effective testosterone.

PRIMARY HYPOGONADISM (ACQUIRED)

Acquired primary hypogonadism may clinically resemble the congenital forms if it occurs prior to the onset of puberty. When it occurs prior to the onset of puberty, these individuals will not progress through puberty. If the hypogonadism occurs after puberty, male individuals will already have signs of puberty but may be infertile and have a decrease in energy, body hair, and muscle mass. Some of these men may have permanent clinical manifestations, whereas others have only temporary findings until the underlying cause is treated. The most common causes of acquired primary hypogonadism are secondary to infection, trauma, and autoimmune destruction.

Infection

Orchitis is inflammation of the testes that most likely results from an infection that started in the epididymis and spread to the testis or began initially in the testis. The infection and subsequent inflammation may damage the Leydig cells, reduce testosterone secretion and sperm production, and increase gonadotropin levels. If the inflammation is severe, testicular atrophy and permanent hypogonadism may occur. The most common organism associated with orchitis is the mumps virus, although strict vaccination has made this occurrence less common during the past 20 years. Other organisms causing orchitis include the sexually transmitted *Neisseria gonorrheae* and *Chlamydia trachomatis*. The symptoms of orchitis are similar to that of testicular torsion and include testicular pain and swelling and hematuria. Once the infection has been treated or subsides, testicular function usually returns to normal. If the orchitis is due to a bacterial infection, nonsteroidal anti-inflammatory therapy for pain should be administered in addition to the antibiotic therapy. If the orchitis is due to a viral infection, only anti-inflammatory therapy is needed.

Trauma

Any testicular trauma that is significant enough to damage the seminiferous tubules or Leydig cells can result in hypogonadism with a reduced sperm count or low testosterone production and an increase in gonadotropins. Although not necessarily due to trauma, testicular torsion can lead to ischemic orchitis and testicular atrophy. Trauma or spontaneous torsion can lead to twisting of the spermatic cord, thereby reducing blood flow to the testis (Figure 13-5). Prolonged blood flow restriction can damage the testes, leading to a reduced sperm count or even infarction of the affected testicle.

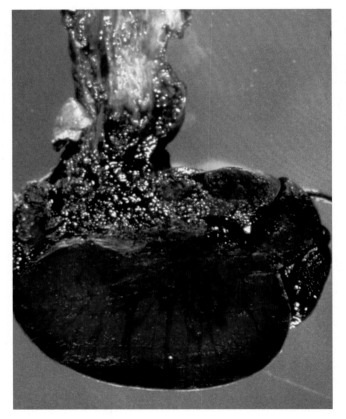

FIGURE 13-5. Testicular torsion. A cut section of the testicle from a man who experienced sudden excruciating scrotal pain shows diffuse hemorrhage and necrosis of the testis and adnexal structures. (Image from Rubin E, Farber JL. Pathology. 3rd ed. Philadelphia, PA: Lippincott Williams & Wilkins; 1999.)

Autoimmune Destruction

Primary hypogonadism may develop due to autoimmune destruction of the Leydig cells. These individuals have similar clinical and biochemical findings to those with hypogonadism due to trauma or orchitis but do not have swelling or pain of the testes. Individuals who develop this usually have an autoimmune polyglandular syndrome (see Chapter 16) and should be evaluated for other hormonal abnormalities.

CENTRAL HYPOGONADISM (CONGENITAL)

Inherited defects that occur in the hypothalamus or pituitary gland can lead to central hypogonadism. Individuals may have an inability to secrete GnRH or gonadotropins, which will ultimately result in low testosterone production. The congenital causes include gene mutations and genetic syndromes that hamper GnRH, FSH, and/or LH secretion.

Gene Mutations

Mutations have been identified in the GnRH prohormone and the GnRH receptor in the hypothalamus. These mutations inactivate GnRH or its receptor and cause variable phenotypes, ranging from partial to complete gonadotropic deficiencies. Some of these mutations are sporadic; others are heritable, with variable patterns of inheritance and penetrance.

In addition to the GnRH-related mutations, there are a number of transcription factors that are important for proper pituitary development, and mutations in some of these transcription factors can lead to hypopituitarism, including GnRH, LH, and FSH deficiency. An example of such a transcription factor, PROP-1, is necessary for differentiation of the gonadotroph cells from their precursor cells. This mutation will result in hypopituitarism and subsequent hypogonadism.

Inactivating mutations of the gene coding for the β-subunit of LH is extremely rare but has been described in five men. All presented with normal male genitalia at birth, but all of them failed to enter puberty and were infertile. Individuals with this mutation have a eunuchoid habitus, soft voice, gynecomastia, scant pubic hair, a micropenis, and underdeveloped testes.

Kallmann Syndrome

Kallmann syndrome is a heritable form of isolated hypogonadotropic hypogonadism. The initial step in the testosterone production pathway is the pulsatile release of GnRH from the hypothalamus. GnRH travels down the portal system of the hypothalamic stalk and depolarizes gonadotropes of the anterior pituitary that release FSH and LH. Boys with Kallmann syndrome have a deficiency of gonadotropin release due to a defect in GnRH, which is, in turn, due to the failure of the GnRH neurons to migrate from their initial location in the olfactory bulb to the hypothalamus. Although there have been a number of reported gene mutations, the most common is the *KAL-1* gene, located on the X chromosome. Kallmann syndrome has a prevalence of 1 in 7,500 males and 1 in 50,000 females. The mutated gene encodes a protein that mediates migration of neural cells of GnRH-producing neurons from the olfactory bulb during development. This leads to the two major abnormalities in these individuals: anosmia and GnRH deficiency. GnRH is present in those with Kallmann syndrome, but the impairment is in the pulsatility of GnRH release. The pulsatile release of GnRH is necessary to produce the increase in testosterone required to enter puberty. Thus, the GnRH "deficiency" is manifested as delayed puberty. If the GnRH deficiency is severe, testosterone deficiency can impair masculinization of the male fetus, resulting in an infant born with a micropenis.

The diagnosis is suggested by the clinical features described above and confirmed by biochemical analysis and imaging studies. Serum levels of FSH, LH, and testosterone are low. The gonadotropins are inappropriately low because, in the presence of a low testosterone level, they should be markedly elevated. The inability to respond to low testosterone is due to the dysfunction of GnRH. Imaging studies should be performed to exclude lesions in the hypothalamus and pituitary; however, with the exception of an abnormal olfactory region in 50% of the individuals with Kallmann syndrome, most individuals have a normal hypothalamus and pituitary gland. Treatment consists of administration of hormone replacement therapy. Males are treated with either hCG or testosterone.

These different mutations highlight the importance of a normally functioning hypothalamic–pituitary axis, which is abnormal in many cases of hypogonadism. Many of the discoveries of the mutations in this axis were uncovered in studies of Kallmann syndrome. Kallmann syndrome is isolated because the pituitary can respond to exogenous GnRH. Other clinical signs include micropenis, cryptorchidism, cleft palate, short metacarpals, renal agenesis, low testosterone, and low gonadotropin levels.

Prader-Willi Syndrome

Prader-Willi Syndrome (PWS) is another cause of central hypogonadism, but the constellation of genetic defects and symptoms is more global than in other more specific causes of central hypogonadism. PWS is characterized by hypotonia, mental retardation, central hypogonadism, marked obesity, and characteristic facial features. Boys who do not receive androgen replacement therapy have a small penis; undescended, small testes; and incomplete virilization (Figure 13-6). The genetic abnormality is most commonly associated with a deletion of the paternal 15q11-13 chromosome region.

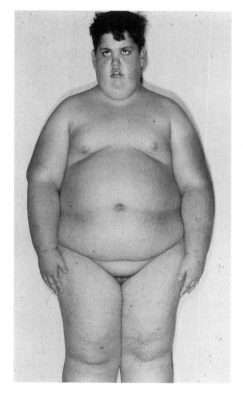

FIGURE 13-6. Prader-Willi syndrome. Patient with Prader-Willi syndrome resulting from a microdeletion on paternal chromosome 15. (Courtesy of Dr. R. J. Gorlin, Department of Oral Pathology and Genetics, University of Minnesota.)

CENTRAL HYPOGONADISM (ACQUIRED)

Like the congenital causes of central hypogonadism, the acquired causes can originate at any level of the hypothalamic–pituitary axis. They are also associated with low levels of gonadotropins and low testosterone levels. The causes are classified as those that damage the cells responsible for gonadotropin secretion and those that suppress gonadotropin section.

Gonadotropin Cell Destruction or Disruption

Sellar masses are a common cause of secondary hypogonadism. These masses can cause hypogonadism by mass effect or by hormone secretion and subsequent gonadotropin suppression. These masses may result in headaches, visual changes, hormonal changes, and other neurological findings. The most characteristic and classic visual change is bitemporal hemianopsia, due to compression of the optic chiasm.

A pituitary adenoma is the most common type of a sellar mass and a common cause of hypogonadism. The adenoma is usually benign and nonfunctioning but may lead to hypopituitarism and hypogonadism by placing pressure on the pituitary gland and decreasing FSH and/or LH secretion. Genetic influences are important in the evaluation of any tumor but are especially critical with pituitary adenomas, which may be part of the multiple endocrine neoplasia type 1 (MEN-1) syndrome (see Chapter 17). Individuals with MEN-1 syndrome classically have tumors in the parathyroid glands, pancreatic islets, and the pituitary gland, and may present with hypopituitarism.

Pituitary adenomas are not the only benign tumor that may cause central hypogonadism. Craniopharyngiomas, a benign tumor arising from the Rathke pouch, may also result in pituitary gland hormone abnormalities. These individuals will have other clinical signs associated with their sellar masses.

Malignancies arising in the sellar area are rare and include germ cell tumors, sarcomas, chordomas, lymphomas, and carcinomas. Metastases to the sellar area affecting pituitary or hypothalamic function are also rare. The hypothalamus is more likely than the pituitary gland to harbor a metastatic lesion. The most common source of metastases in men is lung cancer. Other structural sources of hypopituitarism that may result in central hypogonadism are cysts, abscesses, lymphocytic hypophysitis, and arteriovenous malformations.

Other causes of acquired central hypogonadism not due to a mass compression effect of the pituitary gland include infiltrative diseases such as sarcoidosis and hemochromatosis, trauma, and severe pituitary hemorrhage. The most common traumatic cause is damage to the pituitary stalk from a car accident or damage to the hypothalamus from a fracture of the skull that leads to hypothalamic hormone deficiency and subsequent hypopituitarism. Hypopituitarism has also been associated with subarachnoid hemorrhage.

Gonadotropin Suppression

An elevation of prolactin can lead to hypogonadism by suppressing the hypothalamic–pituitary axis and, subsequently, the levels of gonadotropins. This suppression may be due to any cause of hyperprolacinemia. The mechanism is not well understand but most likely involves prolactin feedback at the hypothalamus, thus altering secretion of GnRH. This causes LH and FSH secretion to become inappropriately low relative to testosterone levels. Reduction in the normal LH pulsatility also occurs.

Exogenous hormone therapy may affect the hypothalamic–pituitary axis, leading to central hypogonadism. Prolonged or continuous administration of GnRH analogs that are administered for the treatment of precocious puberty will suppress gonadotropin and testosterone levels. The administration of exogenous gonadal steroids has occurred with athletes who attempt to enhance their performance. These men experience suppression of gonadotropin secretion as well as endogenous testicular function. Withdrawal of these gondadal steroids can lead to prolonged hypogonadism. The chronic use of glucocorticoids may also cause hypogonadism and decreased testosterone and LH levels.

MIXED PRIMARY AND CENTRAL HYPOGONADISM

Some factors such as medical therapy, chronic illness, and aging cause hypogonadism by both primary and central mechanisms.

Iatrogenic

Chemotherapy or radiation therapy for the treatment of cancer can interfere with both testosterone and sperm production. The effects of either treatment are usually temporary, but permanent infertility may occur. Although many men regain their fertility within a few months after treatment ends, preserving sperm before starting cancer therapy is an option that many men should consider. In addition to chemotherapeutic agents and radiation therapy, a number of other pharmacologic agents can cause hypogonadism. These agents with their proposed mechanism for causing hypogonadism are listed in Table 13-2.

TABLE 13-2.	Pharmacologic Agents and their Proposed Mechanism that Cause Male Hypogonadism
Agent	**Proposed Mechanism**
Glucocorticoids	Suppression of LH secretion
Alkylating agents	Damage to Leydig and germ cells
Ketoconazole, spironolactone, metrinidazole, etomidate	Inhibits steroidogenic enzymes (17α-OHase/17,20-desmolase)
Spironolactone	Blocks receptor binding of testosterone Displaces estradiol from SHBG
Digitalis, clomiphene, delousing powder, marijuana	Binds to estrogen receptor
Flutamide, bicalutamide, finasteride, cyproterone, zanoterone	Blocks androgen action in peripheral tissues
Cimetidine, ranitidine	Blocks androgen receptors
Opiates	Suppression of LH secretion
GnRH analogs	Interrupts normal pulsatile stimulation of GnRH Desensitizes GnRH receptors Directly downregulates secretion of FSH/LH
Psychotropic agents	Inhibits GnRH release

Notes: LH, luteinizing hormone; SHBG, sex hormone–binding globulin; GnRH, gonadtropin-releasing hormone; FSH, follicle-stimulating hormone.

BOX 13-1.	Most Common Chronic Conditions that Cause Male Hypogonadism

Hemochromatosis	Obesity	Cushing syndrome
Renal failure	Type 2 diabetes	Cirrhosis
Hyperprolactinemia	Cardiovascular disease	Alcoholism

Chronic Illness

Men suffering from a chronic, systemic disease are prone to develop hypogonadism that may either be primary, with a direct adverse effect on the testes, or secondary, by suppression of the hypothalamic–pituitary axis. The most common chronic diseases that cause male hypogonadism are listed in Box 13-1.

Cirrhosis is a relatively common condition that can cause hypogonadism. Many of the cirrhotic findings such as gynecomastia or palmar erythema are due to increased circulating levels of estrogen, but cirrhosis can also cause direct damage to the testes or a reduction in gonadotropin secretion, both of which reduce testosterone levels. Hypogonadism that occurs in men with cirrhosis is reversed following liver transplantation.

Many alcoholics also have features of hypogonadism because ethanol affects testicular biosynthesis. Ethanol and its metabolite acetaldehyde have both a direct toxic effect on Leydig cells and disrupt the HPG axis. Chronic alcohol exposure decreases circulating LH levels and reduces the response of LH to GnRH. The disturbance of the HPG axis persists for months after cessation of alcohol intake.

Chronic renal failure also causes major adverse effects on the male reproductive system, notably impairment of spermatogenesis, steroidogenesis, and sexual function. These effects occur at all levels of the HPG axis.

Hemochromatosis results in central hypogonadism with testicular atrophy in 50% of patients. Hypogonadism results from iron deposits in the gonads and selective impairment of gonadotropin secretion. Patients may present with impotence or infertility, low testosterone levels, azoospermia or low semen volume, and low sperm motility.

Circulating testosterone levels are reduced in massively obese men. Several studies have confirmed that total testosterone levels decrease as body mass increases. The major reason for the low levels is the reduced level of SHBG, but free and non-SHBG-bound testosterone levels are also reduced in massive obesity. Leydig cell function is normal in obese individuals, but there is a lower mean LH level and lower pulse amplitude. The leading hypothesis for these findings is that reduced LH pulse amplitude in obesity results from increased estrogen production, because estradiol suppresses the pituitary LH response to GnRH stimulation in males. Testosterone is then converted to estradiol by the aromatase enzyme. Aromatase activity may be increased in obesity because of increased subcutaneous adipose tissue mass, or adipose-derived factors upregulating aromatase in selected tissues. Because the majority of men with cardiovascular disease, type 2 diabetes, and Cushing syndrome are obese, they, too, are at higher risk for developing hypogonadism.

Aging

Older men generally have lower testosterone levels than younger men. As men age, testosterone production slowly and continuously decreases, although the rate of decline varies greatly among men. Up to 30% of men who are aged 75 years and older have a testosterone level below the normal range. Treatment with testosterone replacement therapy has not proven to be uniformly effective.

CASE FOLLOW-UP

Initial laboratory evaluation reveals that the young man has a serum testosterone level of 45 ng/dL, FSH level of 0.5 IU/L, and LH level of 0.3 IU/L. Further questioning reveals that he is not sure if he has a sense of smell. He does not recall noticing the difference between good and bad smells.

A smell test is performed in which he is unable to identify the smell of coffee beans, cinnamon, or nail polish remover.

A head MRI with and without contrast is performed. Special views for visualization of the hypothalamus, pituitary gland, and olfactory bulbs are obtained and all are normal.

The biochemical findings suggesting hypogonadotropic hypogonadism, together with anosmia, provide indisputable evidence that he has Kallman syndrome. For this young man, the GnRH neurons, embryologically located in the olfactory bulb, likely failed to migrate to their final location in the hypothalamus.

He is started on IM testosterone cypionate at a dose of 50 mg every 28 days. After 6 months of therapy, he develops more pubic hair, a deeper voice, and a larger penis. The dose is then increased to 100 mg every 28 days for 6 months; to 100 mg every 14 days for the next 6 months; and, finally, to 200 mg every 14 days. He reports no adverse effects but is concerned about the lack of increase in the size of his testes.

Because he is unable to adequately stimulate LH secretion, his testes will not develop. With concerns over the size of his testes, he is referred to a urologist for consideration of scrotal implantation of prosthetic testes.

REFERENCES and SUGGESTED READINGS

Adams PC, Deugnier Y, Moirand R, Brissot P. The relationship between iron overload, clinical symptoms, and age in 410 patients with genetic hemochromatosis. Hepatology 1997;25:162–166.

Bianco SD, Kaiser UB. The genetic and molecular basis of idiopathic hypogonadotropic hypogonadism. Nat Rev Endocrinol. 2009;5:569–576.

Chevrier L, Guimiot F, deRoux N. GnRH receptor mutations in isolated gonadotropic deficiency. Mol Cell Endocrinol. 2011;346(1–2):21–28.

Darby E, Anawalt BD. Male hypogonadism: an update on diagnosis and treatment. Treat Endocrinol. 2005;4(5):293–309.

Karagiannis A, Hargoulis F. Gonadal dysfunction in systemic diseases. Eur J Endocrinol. 2010;152:501–513.

Layman LC. Hypogonadotropic hypogonadism. Endocrinol Metab Clin North Am. 2007;36:283–296.

Lofrano-Port A, Buro GB, Giacomiri LA, Nascimento PP, Latronico AC, Casulgri LA. Luteinizing hormone beta mutation and hypogonadism in men and women. N Engl J Med. 2007;357(9):897–904.

Mitchell AL, Dwyer A, Pitteloud N, Quinton R. Genetic basis and variable phenotypic expression of Kallmann syndrome: towards a unifying theory. Trends Endocrinol Metab. 2011;22:249–258.

Nachtigall LB, Boepple PA, Pralong FP, Crowley WF. Adult-onset idiopathic hypogonadotropic hypogonadism – a treatable form of male infertility. N Engl J Med. 1997;336:410–415.

Phillip M, Arbelle JE, Segar Y, Pavari R. Male hypogonadism due to a mutation in the gene for the B subunit of follicle stimulating hormone. N Engl J Med. 1998;338(24):1729–1732.

Segal TY, Mehta A, Anazodo A, Hindmarsh PC, Dattani MT. Role of gonadotropin-releasing hormone and human chorionic gonadotropin stimulation tests in differentiating patients with hypogonadotropic hypogonadism from those with constitutional delay of growth and puberty. J Clin Endocrinol Metab. 2009;94(3):780–785.

Smyth CM, Bremner W.J. Klinefelter syndrome. Arch Intern Med. 1998;158(12):1309–1314.

Wu FCW, Tajar A, Beynon JM, Pye SR, Silman AJ, Finn JD, et al. Identification of late-onset hypogonadism in middle-aged and elderly men. N Engl J Med. 2010;363:123–135.

Young J. Approach to the male patient with congenital hypogonadotropic hypogonadism. J Clin Endocrinol Metab. 2012;97:707–718.

CHAPTER REVIEW QUESTIONS

1. A tall and thin 14-year-old boy with lack of pubertal development presents with gynecomastia and small, hard testes. What is the best test to confirm the diagnosis?

   A. MRI of the brain
   B. Serum gonadotropin levels
   C. IQ test
   D. Karyotype
   E. Serum ACTH and cortisol levels

2. A 52-year-old man complains of decreased sexual function. Initial laboratory tests reveal a low testosterone and elevated gonadotropin levels. All of the following could be causes of his condition except:

   A. Mumps infection
   B. Anorchia
   C. Radiation therapy
   D. Kallman syndrome
   E. Testicular trauma

3. A 40-year-old man complains that over the past month he has developed softening of his voice, weakness, testicular atrophy, and the need to shave less. His past medical history is significant for receiving 6 months of chemotherapy for cancer. Which biochemical finding would not be consistent with his presentation?

   A. Low serum testosterone level
   B. Elevated serum inhibin level
   C. Decreased sperm production
   D. Elevated serum LH level
   E. Low serum dihydrotestosterone (DHT) level

4. Which of the following conditions is not associated with hypogonadotropic hypogonadism?

   A. Kallman syndrome
   B. Cleft-lip-palate
   C. Closed-head injury after an automobile accident
   D. LH-receptor defect
   E. Craniopharyngioma

5. All of the following statements are probable factors as to why a 43-year-old obese man develops gynecomastia except:

   A. Obese men have normal Leydig cell function.
   B. Obese men have lower serum LH levels.

C. Obese men have a high ratio of testosterone to estrogen.

D. Estrogen suppresses the LH response to GnRH stimulation.

E. Obese men have excess conversion of testosterone to estrogen by the aromatase enzyme.

CHAPTER REVIEW ANSWERS

1. The correct answer is D. This boy has Klinefelter syndrome (KS) as evidenced by the clinical constellation of tall stature, delayed or absent puberty, and small, firm testes. The diagnosis is confirmed with a karyotype showing at least one extra X chromosome.

An MRI of the brain (**Choice A**) would not be very helpful in this condition, as the hypothalamus and pituitary gland are typically normal in boys with KS. Serum gonadotropin levels, if measured (**Choice B**) would be elevated, but would not distinguish KS from other causes of hypergonadotropic hypogonadism. An individual with KS may experience challenges in cognition and behavior and may have a low IQ, however, many "normal" individuals have a low IQ. An IQ test (**Choice C**) would not help in making the diagnosis of KS. Serum ACTH and cortisol levels (**Choice E**) would not be helpful in establishing the diagnosis of KS, but would be most helpful in a patient suspected of having adrenal insufficiency.

2. The correct answer is D. Individuals with Kallman syndrome have central hypogonadism due to failure of the GnRH neurons to migrate from their embryologic location in the olfactory bulb to the hypothalamus during embryogenesis. In addition to anosmia, individuals with Kallman syndrome have low serum gonadotropin and low serum testosterone levels.

All of the other choices, mumps infection (**Choice A**), anorchia (**Choice B**), radiation therapy (**Choice C**), and bilateral testicular torsion (**Choice E**) cause primary hypogonadism with elevated serum gonadotropin levels and low serum testosterone levels.

3. The correct answer is B. A man with a history of chemotherapy treatment who develops clinical manifestations of hypogonadism has primary testicular failure. Inhibin is secreted from the Sertoli cells in the testes, and therefore, primary testicular failure due to chemotherapy would result in a lower production and secretion of inhibin.

All of the other choices are biochemical findings consistent with primary gonadal failure. Low serum testosterone (**Choice A**) and dihydrotestosterone (DHT) (**Choice E**) levels are consistent with hypogonadism. With primary testicular failure, sperm production would be decreased (**Choice C**) and serum FSH and LH levels (**Choice D**) would be elevated.

4. The correct answer is D. Individuals with an LH-receptor defect will have elevated LH levels due to the lack of negative feedback from low testosterone. Testosterone levels are low in these individuals because despite the increase in LH secretion, without a functional receptor, the Leydig cells are unable to be stimulated to release testosterone. Therefore, these individuals have a hypergonadotropic form of hypogonadism.

All of the other choices are consistent with hypogonadotropic hypogonadism. In Kallman syndrome (**Choice A**), individuals have central hypogonadism due to failure of the GnRH neurons to migrate from their embryologic location in the olfactory bulb to the hypothalamus during development. In addition to anosmia, individuals with Kallman syndrome have low serum gonadotropin and low serum testosterone levels.

Individuals who are born with or develop a central midline defect such as a cleft-lip-palate (**Choice B**), a closed-head injury (**Choice C**), or a brain tumor, such as a craniopharyingioma (**Choice E**) are at risk for developing central hypogonadism.

---

5. The correct answer is C. Obese men usually have normal serum testosterone levels. The excess adipose tissue, however, results in increased estrogen production through the effect of the aromatase enzyme on testosterone in adipose tissue. Therefore, these men usually have a lower than normal testosterone/estrogen ratio.

The other choices are all correct statements in regard to gynecomastia in an obese male. Leydig cell function is normal (**Choice A**) confirming that the production of testosterone is not deficient in obesity. The serum LH level is lower (**Choice B**), and the LH response to GnRH is also lower than normal (**Choice D**) due to the increased production of estrogen from the conversion of testosterone by the aromatase enzyme in adipose tissue (**Choice E**).

Pediatric Growth and Development 14

Geoffrey S. Kelly
Eric I. Felner

CASE

An 8.5-year-old boy was brought by his parents to his pediatrician with concerns regarding his short stature. The child has no obvious constitutional symptoms, but he and his parents are concerned about his small size in relation to his peers. Although he had always been one of the shorter children in the class dating back to nursery school, it now seems to affect him because he is being ridiculed by other kids in his school. The basketball coach recently told him that he was too small to even try out for the team. His younger brother (6.5 years) is only an inch shorter than he is. He is an otherwise healthy child and performs exceptionally well in school. Dietary history is elicited and is unremarkable. Family history reveals normal height in first-degree relatives, although the father recalls that he was short until high school. His vital signs are normal, and, other than appearing shorter than the average boy his age, his physical examination is normal.

This chapter reviews normal pediatric growth and development as well as the normal changes associated with puberty, followed by a discussion of the normal and abnormal causes of short stature. The abnormal causes will be classified as endocrine and nonendocrine, allowing the reader to develop hypotheses that focus on the etiology of this child's short stature. At the end of this chapter, a summary of the work-up and management of this child's condition is provided.

OBJECTIVES

1. Recognize normal and abnormal patterns of childhood growth and development.

2. List the timing and the changes that occur during puberty.

3. Develop a differential diagnosis for causes of short stature.

(continued)

PHYSIOLOGY

Growth is a tightly regulated dynamic process that involves the interplay of hormones, nutrition, bone development, family history, and a number of other physiologic factors. One of the central goals of routine pediatric care is to optimize the growth potential of a child and to promptly identify and manage potential growth-related abnormalities. Therefore, knowledge of the normal patterns of growth is essential to the comprehensive care of children.

Normal Growth and Development

Normal growth and development refers to the progressive changes in height, weight, head circumference, and physical maturity that fall within the established standards of a particular population. Normal growth is a reflection of the overall health and nutritional status of an individual. Regular surveillance of growth is a central aspect in the care of the pediatric patient, and deviations from the normal growth pattern can alert the clinician to the presence of an underlying problem.

Assessment of growth begins with proper measurement of the major growth parameters—height, weight, and head circumference—to provide a snapshot of an individual's growth at any point in time. Whenever the information is available, growth parameters should always be compared to the previously measured values. The rate of change of growth is referred to as **growth velocity**, a much more sensitive index for the detection of abnormal growth than a single measurement. Growth velocity varies greatly between infancy, childhood, and adolescence for each of the growth parameters (Table 14-1).

Growth Charts

Growth charts are the most powerful tools in the assessment of growth. Growth charts present a set of normal standards for a population. Males and females are presented on

TABLE 14-1.	Height and Growth Velocity of Boys and Girls			
Age (y)	Boys		Girls	
	50th Percentile (cm)	Growth Velocity (cm/y)	50th Percentile (cm)	Growth Velocity (cm/y)
Birth	50	N/A	49	N/A
1	76	26	74	25
2	87	8.3	86	8.6
3	98.3	7.4	94.6	7.6
4	102.7	6.8	102.2	6.8
5	109.5	6.4	109	6.4
6	115.9	6	115.4	6.1
7	121.9	5.8	121.5	5.9
8	127.7	5.4	127.4	5.7
9	133.1	5.2	133.1	5.8
10	138.3	5.1	138.9	6.7
11	143.4	5.3	145.6	8.3
12	148.7	6.8	153.9	5.9
13	155.5	9.5	159.8	3
14	165	6.5	162.8	0.9
15	171.5	3.3	163.7	0.1
16	174.8	1.5	163.8	0

separate charts, reflecting the different patterns of growth between the sexes. The World Health Organization (WHO) growth charts are widely used standards and describe optimal growth patterns for children aged 0 to 59 months based on a pooled, international sample. The Centers for Disease Control and Prevention (CDC) publishes growth charts for children aged 0 to 19 years based on national health surveys done within the United States. Additionally, separate growth charts exist for low-birth-weight infants, premature infants, and a variety of disorders known to alter growth (e.g., Down syndrome [DS], Turner syndrome [TS], Klinefelter syndrome, and achondroplasia). In the United States, children are plotted on WHO growth charts until age 2 years (Figure 14-1), at which point they are typically transferred to CDC growth charts (Figures 14-2 and 14-3).

A growth chart presents several percentile curves, which show cross-sectional distributions of values for weight, length, head circumference, weight for length (or height), and body mass index (BMI) for a range of ages. The utility of the growth chart gives the clinician an opportunity to track changes in these parameters over time. In general, healthy individuals tend to track along a percentile line as they grow. A normal exception may occur between the ages of 6 and 24 months, when infants may shift upward or downward and follow a new percentile for weight and/or height. This shift represents the waning influence of the intrauterine environment on the child's growth and the increasing influence of genetics in determining growth potential.

The major percentile lines of a growth chart define boundaries for normal and abnormal growth. Abnormal growth on CDC growth charts is defined as below the 5th percentile or greater than the 95th percentile. WHO charts use 2 standard deviations (SDs) as a cutoff: 2.3% and 97.7%. The percentile lines are also used in the definition of some pathologic states, such as failure to thrive (FTT), which can be defined as a fall in weight that crosses two major percentile lines, weight below the 5th percentile, or weight-for-height below the 5th percentile. For short stature, a definition of less than 2 SDs is generally used (corresponding to 2.3%). Care must be taken in interpretation, because percentiles represent statistical cutoffs rather than biological thresholds. Nevertheless, growth charts provide a simple and easily reproducible method for describing patterns of growth and identifying abnormalities.

Linear Growth and Patterns of Growth

Linear growth is expressed in terms of length or height. Proper measurement requires a firm, flat surface with perpendicular measurement surfaces at either end. *Length* refers to the measurement of children younger than age 2 years, whom are measured in the recumbent position. *Height* (stature) is measured in children older than age 2 years who can stand and cooperate with the operator taking the measurement. Ideally, this is done using a stadiometer and a trained operator. Surrogate measurements for height may be used in the case of children who cannot be measured in this way such as those with cerebral palsy. In such cases, arm span, tibial length, or knee length may be used, and height is then estimated according to the established formulas.

Linear growth can be divided into three phases: infantile, childhood, and pubertal. The timing of the first two phases is essentially the same for both sexes, but the timing and tempo of the pubertal phase differ significantly between the sexes.

Height velocity is greatest during the **infantile period** of growth, reaching approximately 25 cm/year in the first year (see Table 14-1). Within this year, the first few months of life show the most rapid growth at rates of up to 3 cm/month. Following this rapid growth phase, there is a deceleration in growth velocity to around 10 cm/year by the second year of life.

The **childhood phase** occurs following infancy and lasts until the onset of puberty. This phase of growth was previously referred to as the "latent" period, due to the fact that

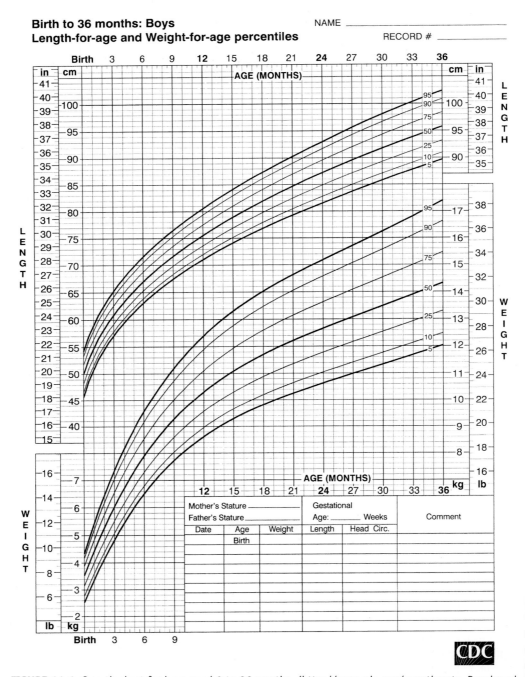

Birth to 36 months: Boys
Length-for-age and Weight-for-age percentiles

NAME _____

RECORD # _____

FIGURE 14-1. Growth chart for boys aged 0 to 36 months. (http://www.cdc.gov/growthcarts. Developed by the National Center for Health Statistics in collaboration with the National Center for Chronic Disease Prevention and Health Promotion (2000). Revised April 20, 2001.)

there is a gradual deceleration of growth velocity beginning around the age of 2 years. Growth during this period occurs discontinuously in a series of three to six growth spurts per year. Normal growth velocity during this period is 5 to 8 cm/year. A growth velocity of less than 5 cm/year between childhood and the onset of puberty is abnormal and merits attention.

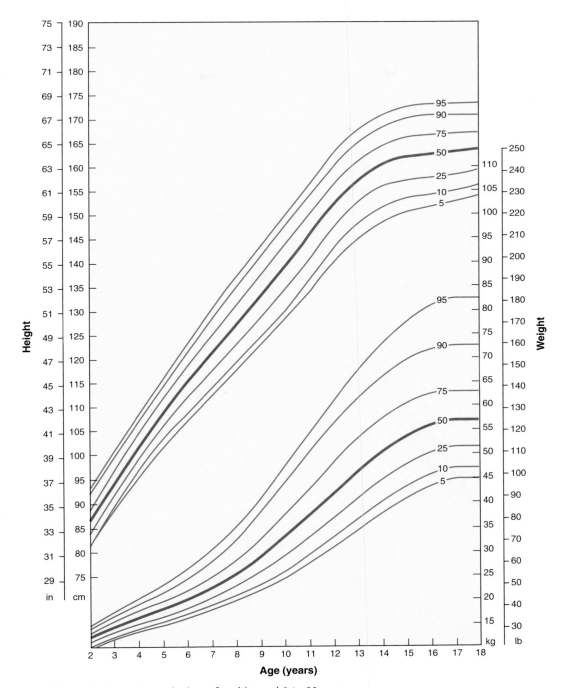

FIGURE 14-2. Physical growth charts for girls aged 2 to 20 years.

The **pubertal growth phase** occurs alongside the changes in body composition, sexual characteristics, and cognitive maturation that occur during puberty. This phase is characterized by a series of growth spurts that last approximately 8 weeks, followed by intercessions of relatively slower growth. Growth during this period accounts for approximately 20% of adult height. There are considerable differences between the sexes during this phase. Growth velocity increases up to a peak of approximately 8 cm/year at

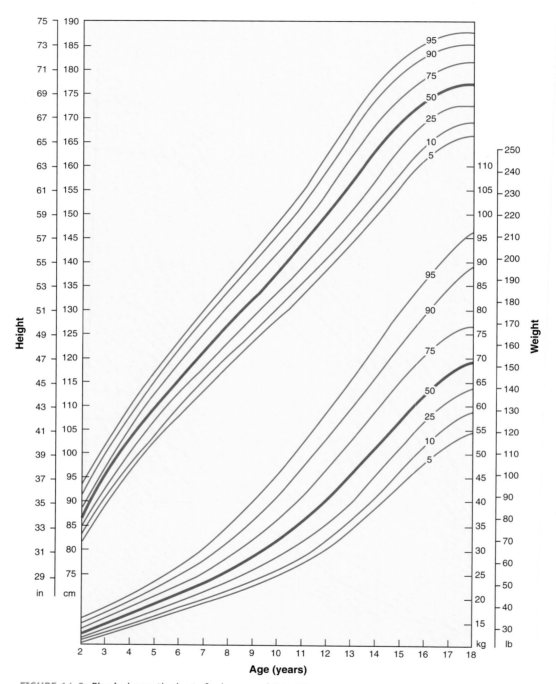

FIGURE 14-3. Physical growth charts for boys aged 2 to 20 years.

age 11.5 years in girls. Boys reach their peak velocity of 9.5 to 10 cm/year at age 13.5 years. This disparity during puberty between the peak velocities is largely responsible for the difference in the adult height of males and females. Following the pubertal phase, growth again decelerates until adult height is reached. The cessation of linear growth corresponds to the closure of the epiphyseal plates of long bones.

The pubertal phase is heavily influenced by sex hormones and is mediated by the functional hypothalamic–pituitary–gonadal (HPG) axis. In addition to linear bone growth, the calcium content of bones increases during puberty, which is reflected in a rapid increase in bone mineral density (BMD). Peak bone mineral content is achieved 9 to 12 months following peak height velocity. The rate of bone mineral deposition and the number and size of ossification centers form the basis for the concept of skeletal maturity or "bone age," which normally coincides closely with chronologic age, except in conditions of abnormal growth.

It is important to remember that the values of height velocity reflect averages based on cross-sectional data. Their interpretation must be carefully analyzed, insofar as they represent population averages not individual, longitudinal trajectories. As a consequence, there may be significant interindividual variability based on a number of factors, the most important of which is the timing and tempo of puberty. Individuals that vary from the normal timing of puberty can be categorized as "early" and "late" bloomers based on the timing of their peak growth velocity.

Predictors of Height

Height estimation is a useful parameter both in the preventive care setting and in the assessment of response to therapy in abnormal growth states. Adult height potential represents a constellation of factors, including genetic, nutritional, socioeconomic, and psychosocial, as well as the presence or absence of disease.

Several methods have been developed for estimating a child's ultimate adult height. A widely used metric is the midparental height. This midparental height is an average of the height of the child's parents with an added corrective factor for sex of the child, represented mathematically as: (father's height + mother's height + male or female factor)/2, where the corrective factor is +5 in/+13 cm for males or −5 in/−13 cm for females. Midparental height may better reflect a child's growth potential than population-derived averages and, therefore, can be used to generate more realistic target heights. Correcting for midparental height refers to plotting this value on the right-hand side of a growth chart and drawing SDs about the calculated height.

Another method of height prediction involves comparing the skeletal maturity (bone age) as determined by radiographic comparison of the hands and wrists to a standard bone age atlas. Compare the open epiphyses and potential room for bone growth in the bone age of a child (Figure 14-4A) to those of an adult (Figure 14-4B). In the adult, the epiphyses are fused, leaving no room for bone growth, whereas in the child, the epiphyses are open with plenty of room for growth. Throughout life and particularly during puberty, ossification centers and BMD progress at a predictable rate, which allows for derivation of an observed bone age to be measured and compared against a set of standards. The two most widely used standards are the Greulich and Pyle atlas and the Tanner and Whitehouse maturity scoring system. Assessment of bone age may help uncover pathologic states or determine estimates of growth potential, most notably in conditions such as growth hormone (GH) deficiency and constitutional delay of growth (CDG). All methods of height prediction have shortcomings, but accuracy increases with advancing patient age.

Hormones as Mediators of Growth

The most important hormones that play a role in linear growth of the growing and developing child are GH, insulin-like growth factor 1 (IGF-1), thyroid hormones, glucocorticoids, and sex hormones.

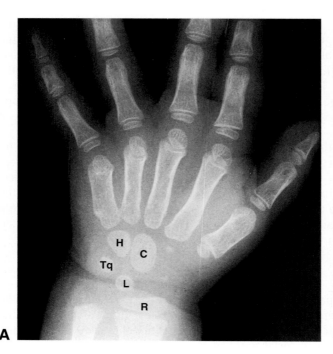

A

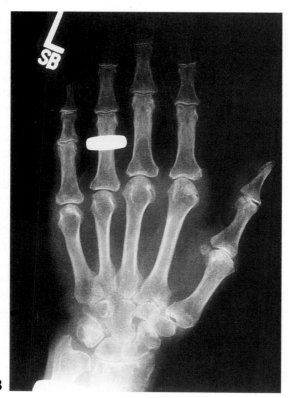

B

FIGURE 14-4. Skeletal age of a child. **(A)** Posteroanterior view of the distal end of the forearm and the hand of a 2.5-year-old child. Ossification centers of only four carpal bones appear. Radiographs of the hand and wrist are often used to assess skeletal age. C, capitate; H, hamate; Tq, triquetrum; L, lunate; R, distal radial epiphysis. **(B)** Skeletal age of an adult. The hand radiograph of an adult female with complete fusion of all epiphyses. (**A:** From Moore KL, Dalley AF. Clinically Oriented Anatomy. 4th ed. Baltimore, MD: Lippincott Williams & Wilkins; 1999; **B:** From Koopman WJ, Moreland LW. Arthritis and Allied Conditions: A Textbook of Rheumatology. 15th ed. Philadelphia, PA: Lippincott Williams & Wilkins; 2005.)

Human Growth Hormone

GH and its main downstream mediator, IGF-1, are critical to the process of linear growth and skeletal maturation. GH is a polypeptide hormone produced by somatotrophs in the anterior pituitary; its secretion is controlled by the hypothalamus via hypothalamic GH–releasing hormone (GHRH). Its release is under the inhibitory control of a number of factors, including negative feedback from IGF-1, somatostatin, and GH itself via autoinhibition. Its secretion is promoted primarily by hypoglycemia and sleep. GH is released in a pulsatile fashion, with peak concentrations being achieved during sleep stages 3 and 4. The majority of GH circulates bound to GH–binding protein (GHBP).

GH mediates its effects on target cells via the GH receptor, which is linked to the JAK/STAT pathway. GH receptors are present in the liver, bone, kidney, skeletal muscle, brain, and heart. The major targets of GH with respect to growth are bone and liver. In the liver, the effect of GH is to promote the production and secretion of IGF-1, a small 70–amino acid protein, that circulates bound to insulin-derived growth factor binding protein (IGFBP)-3. In long bones, GH acts directly (and indirectly via IGF-1) to stimulate osteoblasts and chondrocytes in the epiphyseal plates. It accelerates chondrogenesis, causing widening of the epiphyseal plates, subsequent bony matrix deposition, and linear growth of long bones. In addition to growth, BMD increases due to the promotion of mineral deposition. GH has several other physiologic functions, such as promotion of gluconeogensis, mobilization of free fatty acids, and protein synthesis.

Deficiencies in the production, receptors, or mediators of GH may result in various abnormal growth states, including GH deficiency (GHD) and GH insensitivity (GHI) syndromes that are discussed in detail later in this chapter.

Other Hormones

GH and IGF-1 are the major endocrine mediators of linear growth, but there are several other hormones that influence growth. Thyroid hormone, glucocorticoids, and sex hormones also affect growth primarily during pathologic situations. These hormones are not the common causes of abnormal bone growth but are amenable to treatment and merit prompt investigation if suspected.

Thyroid hormone contributes to linear growth in its role as a global regulator of metabolism. Hypothyroid states from any cause may lead to growth failure. A particularly dramatic example occurs with congenital hypothyroidism, which leads to markedly poor growth and developmental delay. Hyperthyroid states may cause a paradoxical accelerated early growth phase but lead to earlier closure of epiphyseal plates.

Glucocorticoids have pleiotropic effects and may exert a linear growth-retarding effect in a number of glucocorticoid excess states. Growth retardation occurs in children being treated for prolonged time periods with supraphysiologic glucocorticoid therapy and in those with Cushing syndrome.

Sex hormones normally exert their primary influence during puberty, when they lead to increase in skeletal maturity via timing of peak height velocity, increase in BMD, and gradual closure of epiphyseal plates. Estrogens, in particular, promote epiphyseal closure. In pathologic states such as precocious puberty (PP), congenital adrenal hyperplasia (CAH), and obesity, accelerated linear growth at an early age with rapid epiphyseal closure may result in ultimate short stature.

Evaluation of Growth

Abnormal growth may require investigation. Although there are pathologic causes of excessive linear growth, most referrals and clinic visits are due to real or perceived growth retardation. Prior to undertaking an extensive work-up, it is essential to establish whether or not an abnormal pattern truly exists. The initial step in an evaluation should confirm measurements of growth parameters and should be compared to previous values if available. They then should be plotted onto appropriate growth charts. In order to ensure accuracy, multiple measurements should be taken by a skilled operator on properly calibrated equipment. This is particularly important in fidgety infants and young children, because inaccurate measurements are a common cause of apparent growth failure.

A careful history and physical examination may help narrow the differential diagnosis. A dietary history may identify nutritional deficiencies, such as micronutrient deficiency or global undernutrition. Past medical history may reveal chronic disease or the use of medications known to interfere with growth, such as glucocorticoids and certain chemotherapeutic agents. A family history should include heights of first-degree relatives, history of shortness compared to peers, and timing and tempo of puberty. A thorough review of systems may identify subtle signs and symptoms indicative of organic etiologies. Physical examination may reveal chromosomal abnormalities such as DS and TS that exhibit specific physical exam findings that suggest their diagnosis and guide subsequent work-up.

After a careful history and physical examination, further evaluation and diagnostic testing may be warranted if stature and growth velocity are decreased. Short stature is defined as more than 2 SDs below the population average. This should be explained to patients and families in cases in which reassurance is appropriate such as when a child may be perceived as short (e.g., 10th percentile) but does not meet the standard for short stature. The work-up of short stature is detailed in sections on pathophysiology that follow. Finally, it should be emphasized that short stature should not be reflexively thought of as a disease, because there is considerable variation in the distribution of normal human height among the population.

Puberty

Puberty is the transition period from the sexually immature state to the potentially fertile stage during which secondary sexual characteristics appear. **Adolescence** is commonly used as a synonym for puberty but is often also used to convey a psychosocial coming of age, whereas puberty is a physical state in which a change occurs in the growing and maturing child. Just as some children grow at a more rapid velocity earlier or later than their peers, likewise some children enter puberty earlier or later than age-matched peers. The average age range for pubertal development in girls (Table 14-2) and boys (Table 14-3) centers amid **thelarche** (breast development), **adrenarche** (pubic hair development), and **gonadarche** (testicular enlargement). Pubertal stages are rated from I to V using the **Tanner staging system** in girls (Figure 14-5A,B) and boys (Figure 14-6A,B).

TABLE 14-2.	Ages of Pubertal Development in Girls	
Pubertal Parameter	**Average Age of Onset (y)**	**Age Range (y)**
Breast budding	10	8–13
Pubic hair appears	11	8–14
Growth spurt	11	9.5–14.5
Menarche	12.5	10–16.5

TABLE 14-3.	Ages of Pubertal Development in Boys	
Pubertal Parameter	**Average Age of Onset (y)**	**Age Range (y)**
Testes enlarge	11	9–14
Pubic hair appears	12	10–15
Penile enlargement	13	11–14.5
Growth spurt	13.5	10.5–16

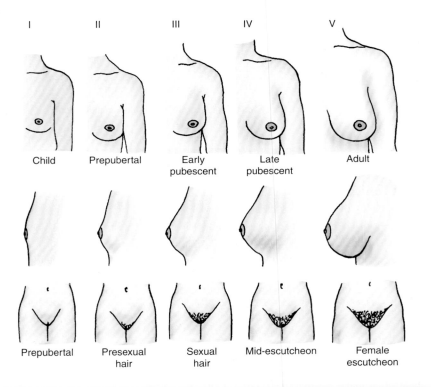

A

Tanner stages in the female		
Stage	**Breast**	**Pubic hair**
I	Prepubertal, evaluation of papilla only	Prepubertal
II	Enlargement of areola, evaluation of breast and papilla (breast bud)	Sparse, long, straight, slightly, pigmented hair along labia
III	Further enlargement of breast and areola with no separation of contour	Hair is darker, curlier, and coarser with increased distribution of pubes
IV	Areola and papilla form a second mount above the breast	Adult-type hair limited to pubes with no extension to medial thigh
V	Mature breast	Mature distribution of inverse triange with spread to medial thighs

B

FIGURE 14-5. Tanner staging in females. **(A)** Illustrative. (From MediClip Clinical OB/GYN, CD-ROM. Baltimore, MD: Lippincott Williams & Wilkins; COG01013.) **(B)** Descriptive. (From Stedman TL. Stedman's Pediatric Words. Baltimore, MD: Lippincott Williams & Wilkins; 2001.)

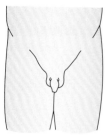 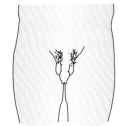 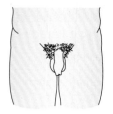

I. Preputertal   II. Down hair later to penis   III. Hair across pubis

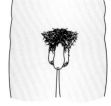 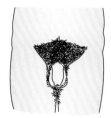

IV. Curled, adult distribution   V. Adult configuration
but less abundant

A

Tanner stages in the male		
Stage	**Gential development**	**Pubic hair**
I	Prepubertal	Prepubertal
II	Enlargement of testes (>4 mL volume) and scrotum with reddening of scrotal skin	Sparse, long, straight, slightly pigmented hair at base of penis
III	Growth of penis, primarily in length, with further increase in size of testes and scrotum	Hair is darker, curlier, and coarser with increased distribution of pubes
IV	Further increase in length and breadth of penis with development of glands, increase in size of testes and scrotum	Adult-type hair limited to pubes with no extension to medial thigh
V	Adult size and shape	Mature distribution with spread to medial thighs and lower abdomen

B

FIGURE 14-6. Tanner staging in males. **(A)** Illustrative. (From LifeART Nursing 1, CD-ROM. Baltimore, MD: Lippincott Williams & Wilkins; NU118014.) **(B)** Descriptive. (From Stedman TL. Stedman's Pediatric Words. Baltimore, MD: Lippincott Williams & Wilkins; 2001.)

In girls, the physical initiation of puberty occurs when the ovary enlarges and secretes estrogen, with resulting breast development from estrogen stimulation. In most girls, thelarche is the first sign of puberty, occurring between ages of 9 and 10 years. This is usually followed by adrenarche at age 11 years and menarche at ages 12 to 13 years. The average girl completes linear growth by age 15 years. In boys, the physical initiation of puberty occurs when the testes enlarge and secrete testosterone. In most boys, gonadarche is the first sign of puberty, occurring between ages of 9.5 to and 10.5 years. Adrenarche usually occurs between ages 11 to 12 years. The average boy completes puberty and linear growth at age 18 years. The Tanner staging system plots breast and pubic hair development in girls (see Figure 14-5A,B) and testicular volume and pubic hair in boys (see Figure 14-6A,B). Tanner stage II is the earliest pubertal stage.

The biochemical manifestations of puberty are the result of hormone secretion from the hypothalamus, pituitary gland, and gonads. Gonadotropin-releasing hormone (GnRH) is secreted from the hypothalamus and reaches the pituitary gland through the portal system. It is released episodically in varying amplitudes and frequencies during the various stages of development. The pulsatile activity originates in the arcuate nucleus. If the pulsatile nature of GnRH secretion is altered so that flow is constant, the pituitary gonadotrope decreases its affinity for GnRH, and the number of GnRH receptors decrease and gonadotropin secretion is reduced.

SHORT STATURE: PHYSIOLOGIC CAUSES

A child may be of shorter stature than his or her peers because of physiologic reasons or a number of pathologic conditions. The two physiologic causes, familial short stature (FSS) and constitutional delay of growth (CDG), are the most common causes of short stature.

Familial (Genetic) Short Stature

Children with FSS demonstrate a lifelong pattern of reduced height for age with respect to population means. Implicit in this diagnosis is that metabolic, endocrine, inflammatory, syndromic, and psychosocial causes of short stature have been excluded via history, physical examination, or diagnostic studies. Affected children have a height of 2 standard deviations (SDs) below the mean for age with respect to population norms but exhibit normal or low–normal growth velocities.

Several key features define FSS: the hallmark is that bone age and chronologic age are concordant, distinguishing FSS from a constitutional delay (discussed later). These children typically have a normal birth length and begin to exhibit a pattern of short stature beginning by 12 to 24 months of life. Growth velocity is normal, which is a helpful distinguishing feature from pathologic causes of growth retardation. A pubertal child brought in for evaluation will typically reveal normal timing of puberty and pubertal growth spurts. Parental height is useful to consider when interpreting the growth of these children. The midparental height should be used to generate a target height, which will be lower than the population height if the parents are also short. A child more than 2 SDs below the mean for height may be within 2 SDs of height corrected for midparental height, which suggests that the child is growing consistently with the genetic pattern of his or her family. The natural history of these children shows that they ultimately achieve an adult height that is below the population norms.

GH therapy is available as a treatment option in the United States, although its use is controversial. It may increase the adult height by 4 to 6 cm compared with the predicted height, although this gain requires long-term therapy. There is also an increase in short-term growth velocity when GH is administered to children with FSS, but this is not predictive of a final height increase. In addition, there is little evidence to suggest any significant change in psychosocial, academic, or quality-of-life outcomes in treated versus untreated children. Furthermore, due to the high cost and burdensome treatment schedule, there are issues of access, social justice, and the large financial burden placed on families seeking GH therapy.

FSS is best viewed as a variation of the normal height distribution rather than a pathologic cause of short stature. Objective parameters are consistently normal (growth velocity, bone age, pubertal timing, and metabolic parameters). These children simply achieve a lower adult height because of the genetic factors that are usually appreciable after meeting the parents.

Constitutional Delay of Growth

CDG refers to a slower pace of growth and development compared to normal individuals. Similar to FSS, this is not a disease process, but rather a pattern of growth that can be viewed as a variation of normal. Along with FSS, CDG forms the second major form of physiologic short stature and implies no identifiable underlying or pathologic cause.

Children with CDG usually seek medical attention because of a pattern of reduced height, generally 2 SDs below the population norm. The hallmark of CDG is that bone age is reduced with respect to chronologic age, suggesting that physical maturity is delayed. Similar to FSS, these children generally have a normal birth length. The short stature is manifested by ages 12 to 24 months by a drop in the height percentile. During the childhood growth phase, these children maintain normal or low–normal growth velocities and follow a trajectory parallel to, but below, the major percentile lines. A salient feature of CDG is that the onset of puberty is delayed with respect to chronologic age but generally occurs at a normal time when corrected for bone age. Commonly, family history reveals one or more "late bloomers" in the family. Parents and other family members are of normal height, which also helps to distinguish this condition from FSS. The natural history of these children shows that they usually achieve normal adult heights (corrected for midparental height). However, some of these individuals may attain only low–normal adult height because the pubertal growth velocities are less than expected.

Treatment for CDG is conservative and is usually limited to reassurance and appropriate follow-up. Assuming the correct diagnosis was made, there is no role for GH therapy in these children. These children and their parents should be reassured that growth will occur at a later date than their peers.

SHORT STATURE: PATHOLOGIC CAUSES (ENDOCRINE)

Normal linear growth is a reflection of overall health status; therefore, many endocrine conditions associated with growth hormone deficiency (GHD) or growth hormone insensitivity (GHI), hypothyroidism, and Cushing syndrome may cause poor linear growth.

Growth Hormone Deficiency

GHD is either a congenital or an acquired deficit of GH. With a congenital deficit, there is a primary dysfunction along the hypothalamic–pituitary–GH/IGF-1 axis. Acquired GHD is the result of an insult to the hypothalamic–pituitary–GH/IGF-1 axis and includes pituitary tumors (e.g., craniopharyngioma), irradiation to the hypothalamic–pituitary region, and trauma to the central nervous system (CNS).

Etiology

Mutations in several genes have been identified that lead to GHD and varying degrees of hypopituitarism. These genes include *POU1F1/Pit-1*, which encodes a pituitary-specific factor responsible for transcription of GH and other pituitary hormones. A number of transcription factors necessary for POU1F1 expression also lead to GHD, the most commonly affected being Prop-1. Other mutations that cause GHD include GHRH receptor gene defects, *GH-1* deletions (the gene encoding GH), and mutations producing inactive GH. The incidence of congenital GHD in the United States is found in approximately 1 in 10,000. Most cases are sporadic, but in 5% to 30% of cases, the child with congenital GHD has an affected relative.

Pathophysiology

The physiologic effects of GH are diminished or absent in GHD. Serum concentrations of GH, IGF-1, and IGFBP-3 are reduced. The most prominent pathophysiologic effect of GHD is postnatal growth failure, due to the central role of GH/IGF-1 in promotion of linear growth. Affected children have a normal birth length but exhibit a striking postnatal growth failure that is usually evident by the first year of life. Skeletal maturation is also affected, manifested as a delayed bone age. Hypoglycemia, sometimes severe and life threatening, is present due to the diminished counterregulatory effect of GH. Similarly, the lipolytic effect of GH is lost, and affected children have increased adiposity with a pudgy appearance despite a normal weight for height (Figure 14-7). Hypothyroidism, adrenal insufficiency, diabetes insipidus, and hypogonadism may be present due to the type and degree of associated hypopituitarism.

Clinical Findings

There is a spectrum of clinical findings in children with GHD. Children with the mild form may only have short stature, whereas those with the complete form may present with life-threatening hypoglycemia or frank growth failure during early infancy. Fasting hypoglycemia may present as poor feeding, lethargy, or vomiting. In more severe forms, hypoglycemia may present as apnea, seizures, or coma. Hypoglycemia in GHD is markedly worse if adrenocorticotropic hormone (ACTH) deficiency is also present.

In congenital GHD, children have a normal birth weight and length; growth deceleration occurs after the first few months of postnatal life. GHD may also present later in childhood as short stature or decreased growth velocity in the absence of an apparent cause. In older children, serial height measurements are required to confirm a decrease in height for age or growth velocity. In male children, a microphallus and/or cryptorchidism may be present, especially if there is concurrent GnRH deficiency. Children with GHD generally demonstrate normal intelligence and only moderately delayed motor

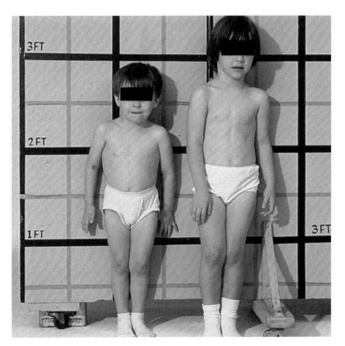

FIGURE 14-7. Childhood growth hormone deficiency. A 5.5-year-old boy (*left*) with growth hormone deficiency (GHD) was significantly shorter than his fraternal twin sister (*right*), with discrepancy beginning early in childhood. Notice his chubby immature appearance compared with his sister. (Shulman D, Bercu B. Atlas of Clinical Endocrinology, Neuroendocrinology, and Pituitary Diseases, Korenman, S, ed. Philadelphia, PA: Current Medicine; 2000.)

milestones, unless there is an anatomic defect, chronic hypoglycemia, or an unrecognized hypothyroid state that precludes normal intellectual development.

In acquired forms of GHD, growth failure is often severe and temporally associated with the inciting insult. Clinical findings vary according to the etiology. A child with an intracranial mass lesion, such as a craniopharyngioma, may present with headache, visual disturbances, vomiting, and cranial nerve palsy in addition to symptoms of absent GH. Arrest or regression of sexual development may occur and present as amenorrhea, hypogonadism, or regression of axillary and pubic hair. Cranial irradiation may cause symptomatic GHD usually 12 to 18 months following the radiation in a dose-dependent fashion, usually occurring with >20 Gy.

Diagnostic Studies

The diagnosis of GHD is established using a combination of the clinical features described above: characteristic growth patterns of short stature (>2 SDs below the median for growth velocity) and abnormal serum levels of GH, IGF-1, and IGFBP-3. The laboratory diagnosis of GH status is complicated by the fact that basal GH is low in both affected children and healthy controls, due to the relatively short half-life and pattern of pulsatile secretion. For this reason, a random GH level has little utility, and provocative testing is required, for which multiple secretagogues are used. This may also complicate the interpretation of results insofar as no single method is considered the gold standard. Pharmacologic stimuli used include arginine, clonidine, glucagon, and insulin. After administration of one of these agents, a response is normal if there is a rise in GH ≥ 10 ng/mL. The sensitivity and specificity of each individual test is variable; therefore, an abnormal GH response in two tests is required for diagnosis. Prepubertal and obese children exhibit lower rises in GH, which may be a false positive.

Measurements of serum IGF-1 and IGFBP-3 are additional diagnostic tools. In GHD, IGF-1 and IGFBP-3 levels are reduced due to their dependence on the action of GH. The serum concentration of these two proteins correlates well with overall GH status. Compared to GH, both IGF-1 and IFGBP-3 have longer half-lives, which precludes the need for provocative testing. However, there are shortcomings in using these measurements as surrogates for provocative GH testing. IGF-1 is occasionally normal in GHD patients and may represent a false-negative result, whereas IGF-1 varies with nutritional status and may incorrectly suggest a diagnosis of GHD in the setting of undernutrition. Finally, IGF-1 and IFGBP-3 should be compared to normative values based on bone age, rather than chronologic age. Despite these limitations, these are useful studies to obtain as they can corroborate the diagnosis of GHD and assist in distinguishing GHD from GHI.

Radiologic studies provide valuable diagnostic information. Bone age should be established with plain radiographs of the hand and wrist. When comparing a patient's radiograph to a standard bone age atlas, patients with GHD demonstrate delayed skeletal maturity with respect to chronologic age. Magnetic resonance imaging with and without contrast should be performed if an intracranial mass lesion is suspected.

Due to the strong association of GHD with other pituitary abnormalities, it is useful to search for other endocrinopathies by measuring thyroid-stimulating hormone, ACTH, thyroxine, cortisol, and gonadotropins because therapy for GHD is less effective if comorbid pituitary abnormalities are not concurrently treated.

Treatment

GH replacement therapy consists of recombinant human GH (hGH) administered subcutaneously 6 or 7 days a week. In order to maximize the potential for growth, treatment should begin as soon as the diagnosis of GHD is established. The greatest increase in height is usually seen within the first year of initiation, and an appropriate response to therapy is established when growth velocity is above the 75th percentile for age. Response to therapy is tracked by serial measurement of growth and IGF-1 levels. In children who have entered puberty, adjunct therapy with a GnRH agonist may also be used to delay epiphyseal closure and allow a greater period of time for linear growth. Therapy is continued until near-final height is achieved or linear growth slows to <1 in/year.

Prognosis

In the United States, the National Child Growth Study examined patients with GHD receiving recombinant hGH in order to quantify and track the results of treatment. A good response to therapy was predicted by young age, early diagnosis and initiation of therapy, [GH dose (0.3 mg/kg/week)], and above-average midparental height. Treatment is generally safe and allows patients to achieve a height within the patient's target height range (which must be adjusted for midparental height). The risk for long-term sequelae of GH therapy appears to be low. Possible complications of therapy include development of type 2 diabetes mellitus, pseudotumor cerebri, pancreatitis, slipped capital femoral epiphysis, and swelling of the distal extremities as well as an increased risk for leukemia and colorectal cancer. Historically, there was a risk for antibody development and Creutzfeldt-Jakob disease when GH was obtained from cadaveric pituitaries, but the risk for these complications has disappeared with the advent of recombinant hGH.

Growth Hormone Insensitivity

GHI is characterized by an absence of the effects of GH despite normal serum levels, which is the difference between GHI and GHD, in which GH levels are low.

Etiology

GHI is rare with an autosomal recessive inheritance pattern. The most common cause of GHI is a loss-of-function mutation or deletion in the GH receptor, which is known as *Laron syndrome*. Other causes include mutations in the IGF-1 gene, postreceptor signaling cascade proteins such as STAT5b, the IGF-1 receptor, or in the acid-labile subunit (ALS) responsible for stability of the circulating IGF-1:IGFBP-3 complex.

Pathophysiology

The pathophysiology of GHI is similar to that of GHD; in both conditions, there is no biologic response to the GH–GH receptor interaction. The major difference is that GH levels are normal to elevated in GHI. Loss of the response to GH leads to decreased circulating levels of IGF-1 in all of the GHI syndromes, with the exception of IGF-1-receptor mutations in which IGF-1 levels are normal or increased. Decreased or ineffective IGF-1 may produce the findings and complications described below.

Clinical Findings

Mild to severe postnatal growth failure is the principal clinical manifestation of GHI. Analysis of growth patterns shows a height more than 2 SDs below the mean for age and low–normal growth velocity. Bone age is also delayed. The more severe forms of growth failure exist in the homozygous loss-of-function mutations of the GH receptor and dysregulation of the postreceptor cascade seen in mutations of STAT5b. These infants have normal birth lengths, with the exception of IGF-1 loss-of-function mutations, which produce prenatal growth failure and neurocognitive deficits. Metabolic abnormalities due to the impaired effects of GH include hypoglycemia and hyperlipidemia. Children with classic Laron syndrome exhibit a characteristic pattern of dysmorphic features, including "saddle nose," prominent forehead, small head circumference, short limb length, and microphallus.

Diagnostic Studies

Nonendocrine pathologic causes of growth failure must be explored and excluded before considering GHI. The diagnosis of GHI is made by evidence of short stature, poor growth, normal to elevated serum levels of GH, and low serum levels of IGF-1 and IGFBP-3. Bioinactive IGF-1 due to a mutation of the IGF-1 gene is the exception, with normal or elevated serum levels of IGF-1/IGFBP-3. This rare form of GHI is suspected when an infant presents with prenatal growth failure and a normal growth hormone binding protein (GHBP). Provocative GH testing is not necessary for diagnosis of GHI but may be useful to distinguish GHI from GHD. A normal GH response is typically seen (i.e., GH >10 ng/mL rise in response to secretagogue administration). IGF-1 testing may also be used in cases in which the diagnosis remains unclear. In this test, an exogenous dose of GH is given; a positive result shows that the IGF-1 level will remain low in GHI, whereas a rise would be expected in healthy children.

Treatment

The mainstay of treatment for GHI is recombinant IGF-1 administration, which is useful in the treatment of most forms of GHI, including Laron syndrome, GH postreceptor defects, and IGF-1 gene mutations. It is less efficacious in treatment of the rare form of GHI that is due to IGF-1 receptor defects.

Prognosis

When treated, children with GHI exhibit a period of rapid catch-up growth, with corresponding improvements in BMD, body composition, head circumference, and hypoglycemia. In a large, open-label study of children with GHI, investigators noted an increase in growth velocity of 2.8 cm/year at baseline to 8.0 cm/year posttreatment. Although there is a vigorous growth response to IGF-1 therapy, the response is less in children with GHD who receive hGH replacement therapy because the actions of GH and IGF-1 are both required for normal growth, and only the latter is modifiable in children with GHI.

Hypothyroidism

Hypothyroidism exhibits deleterious effects on growth whether congenital or acquired. *Congenital hypothyroidism* causes severe postnatal growth failure, intellectual impairment, and delayed bone age. It affects 1 in 3,000 to 4,000 live births. The most common cause worldwide is dietary iodine deficiency. In the United States and many other developed countries, intellectual impairment has been virtually eliminated by newborn screening and early initiation of replacement therapy. Although the growth failure is partially reversible, recognition of congenital hypothyroidism is critically important because of the effects of thyroid hormone on normal brain development. Delay in treatment may lead to sustained intellectual deficits. Most sporadic cases of congenital hypothyroidism are due to thyroid dysgensis (i.e., agenesis, hypoplasia, or ectopy). Other causes include dysregulation of the hypothalamic–pituitary–thyroid axis, insensitivity syndromes, and defects in thyroid hormone synthesis or secretion. *Acquired* forms of hypothyroidism can be classified into autoimmune, systemic, and iatrogenic. Hypothyroidism is discussed in greater detail in Chapter 3.

Glucocorticoid Excess

Glucocorticoid excess exerts growth-retarding effects in children. **Cushing syndrome**, the state of excess glucocorticoids, is classified according to source as endogenous or exogenous. The most common etiology of Cushing syndrome that results in growth retardation is iatrogenic administration of glucocorticoids. Growth failure may be seen following the commencement of glucocorticoid therapy and depends on the dose and frequency of administration. Sustained deficits in growth may persist despite the cessation of therapy. Diagnosis is suggested by the presence of clinical features of Cushing syndrome and can be confirmed by laboratory testing, discussed in Chapter 19. Cushing syndrome is discussed in greater detail in Chapter 10.

SHORT STATURE: PATHOLOGIC CAUSES (NONENDOCRINE)

Normal linear growth is a reflection of overall health status; therefore, many nonendocrine conditions associated with malnourishment, chronic disease states, osteochondrodysplasias, and genetic syndromes may cause poor linear growth.

Malnutrition and Undernutrition

Undernutrition refers specifically to inadequate intake or absorption of food. **Malnutrition**, the broader term, refers to the spectrum of nutritional derangements that include undernutrition, micronutrient deficiencies, and obesity. Weight is usually affected before height in individuals with suboptimal nutritional status, but prolonged deficits of macro- or micronutrients may lead to stunting (permanent loss of linear growth potential). Malnutrition is a relatively uncommon cause of short stature in the United States; however, in the developing world, where access to nutritious food sources may be tenuous and the disease burden of parasites much greater, malnutrition may cause short stature. In the ensuing discussion, malnutrition refers to inadequate caloric intake, although, in the United States, obesity is rapidly becoming the leading cause of malnutrition in children.

The diagnosis of malnutrition as the etiology of short stature requires abnormal weight gain that precedes retardation of linear growth. This is readily apparent when growth parameters are plotted on growth charts. A clear downward trend across percentile lines can be seen in weight, height, and weight-for-height (assuming previous values are available for comparison). Malnutrition can also be diagnosed by history and physical examination; no specific laboratory testing is required. The WHO defines degree of malnutrition on the basis of **z-scores** (SDs) of height for age, with moderate occurring between 2 and 3 SDs below the mean and severe, occurring more than 3 SDs below the mean.

The most apparent cause of malnutrition is food insecurity, in which children have insufficient access to food to sustain normal growth. However, even in the presence of adequate food security, factors such as sanitation, access to potable water, and knowledge of proper feeding behaviors can lead to growth failure and stunting. In the developing world, infectious diseases are a significant cause of malnutrition, particularly parasitic infections (i.e., *Giardia lamblia*, *Ascaris lumbricoides*, and *Trichuris trichuria*). Dietary habits (e.g., veganism), dietary fads, and anorexia nervosa can also result in poor growth. In each of these examples, growth retardation is reversible, following a period of catch-up growth, if the cause is identified and appropriately corrected. However, growth potential may be permanently lost depending on the etiology, duration, and degree of malnutrition.

There are also several micronutrient deficiencies that result in growth failure and stunting. Iodine, iron, zinc, folate, vitamin B12, and vitamin A are the most common micronutrients. The mechanism of growth failure varies among these nutrient deficiencies. For example, iodine deficiency leads to growth failure by causing hypothyroidism, whereas zinc deficiency can lead to anorexia, diarrhea, and susceptibility to infection. Work-up and treatment depend upon which macronutrient is suspected.

Chronic Disease States

Chronic disease states involving any organ system in the body can cause linear growth retardation by a variety of overlapping mechanisms. Growth failure may be the presenting sign of many underlying abnormalities; therefore, careful attention to growth parameters may not only aid in uncovering an occult lesion but also assess its response to therapy. Several clinically important and representative conditions follow.

Cystic Fibrosis

Cystic fibrosis (CF) is the prototypical chronic disease that results in growth failure. CF is an autosomal recessive disorder caused by mutation of the CF transmembrane conductance–regulator protein, a chloride-ion channel located on the surface of epithelial cells. Growth failure in CF is multifactorial. In the gastrointestinal (GI) tract, maldigestion due to pancreatic insufficiency and subsequent malabsorption occur, resulting in malnutrition and increases in fecal caloric losses. Impaired mucociliary clearance in the respiratory tract leads to chronic pulmonary infections and also causes energy loss from the increased work of breathing. Management of the pulmonary complications and a high-calorie diet with vitamin supplementation (especially A, D, E, and K) can allow for an improvement in height outcome. GH therapy has not shown clear long-term benefit.

Celiac Disease

Celiac disease (*gluten-sensitive enteropathy*) is another chronic disease that may cause growth failure that results from a vigorous immune response to wheat gluten and related proteins, causing inflammation of the intestinal mucosa, leading in turn to remodeling and flattening of the mucosa. This results in macro- and micronutrient deficiencies, failure to thrive, anemia, fatigue, and various problems related to nutritional deficiencies or the abnormal immune response. Strict adherence to a gluten-free diet and the subsequent appropriate micronutrient supplementation may normalize growth and prevent stunting.

Cancer

Cancer may lead to growth failure either due to poor intake or due to increased caloric utilization. Treatment with chemotherapeutic agents and radiation may cause nausea, vomiting, anorexia, and/or impaired absorption, which may further exacerbate growth retardation. For example, the treatment of primary or metastatic brain tumors with excision or radiation may damage the hypothalamus or pituitary gland, resulting in growth impairment by disruption of the hypothalamic–pituitary–GH/IGF-1 axis or other hypothalamic homeostatic functions. Optimizing growth is an important consideration of pediatric oncologic care; cancer survivorship has been steadily improving over the past decades, and many children now survive into adulthood.

Other Diseases

Many other chronic disease states including renal, cardiac, inflammatory, autoimmune, and metabolic diseases can adversely affect growth. In some cases, the treatment for the underlying problem (e.g., chemotherapy) may actually accelerate growth retardation. This is particularly true for conditions requiring chronic steroid use, including inflammatory conditions such as Crohn's disease or severe asthma. Any child with a chronic disease (or receiving treatment) known to affect growth should have its growth parameters carefully monitored.

Osteochondrodysplasias

Osteochondrodysplasias are a group of rare disorders of bone and cartilage that cause the skeleton to develop abnormally. The most common and severe is achondroplasia, followed by hypochondroplasia.

Achondroplasia

Achondroplasia is a member of a larger family of disorders known as the *skeletal dysplasias*. It is a relatively rare disorder, with a birth prevalence of approximately 1 in 10,000 to 30,000. The diagnosis is suggested by the characteristic pattern of macrocephaly, elongated trunk, and short limbs (Figure 14-8A–C) and is readily confirmed with radiographs. The causative mutation occurs in the gene for fibroblast growth factor receptor 3 (FGFR3). Affected children display markedly abnormal linear bone growth, and rapidly fall behind unaffected children in height and weight by age 3 years. These children eventually reach adult heights of 120 to 140 cm and 110 to 130 cm for men and women, respectively. Achondroplasia-specific growth charts are available. Treatment options include surgical limb-lengthening and GH treatment. However, both options are imperfect, insofar as surgical limb-lengthening carries the burden of numerous complications from the surgery itself, and GH therapy has not shown clear long-term benefit.

Hypochondroplasia

Hypochondroplasia is similar to achondroplasia, but the features are milder. The final adult heights range from 140 to 165 cm and 130 to 150 cm for men and women, respectively. Individuals have disproportionately short arms and legs and broad, short hands and feet. Other clinical features include macrocephaly, limited range of motion at the elbows, and lordosis. The signs are less pronounced than in those with achondroplasia and may not be noticeable until early or mid-childhood.

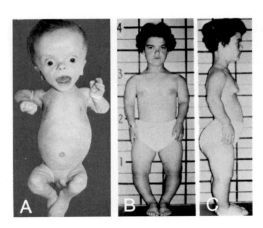

FIGURE 14-8. (A) Achondroplasia. Three-month-old infant with achondroplasia. Note the large head, short extremities, and protruding abdomen. **(B, C)** Achondroplasia in a 15-year-old girl. Note dwarfism of the short limb type, the limbs being disproportionately shorter than the trunk. The limbs are bowed; there is an increase in lumbar lordosis; and the face is small relative to the head. (From Sadler T. Langman's Medical Embryology, 9th ed. Image Bank. Baltimore, MD: Lippincott Williams & Wilkins; 2003.)

Genetic Syndromes

There are numerous genetic syndromes in which short stature is a significant component. A comprehensive list is beyond the scope of this chapter, but several common and representative syndromes are described in this section.

Turner Syndrome

TS is a chromosomal abnormality (classically, 45, XO) in which short stature is a major feature. The incidence is found in approximately 1 in 2,000 live births. The short stature is attributable to the loss or mutation of the short stature homeobox (*SHOX*) gene, located on the X chromosome. Short stature is rarely the presenting feature because the syndrome is recognized early, and there are opportunities for early and/or prenatal diagnosis. However, a karyotype analysis should be ordered in a girl with short stature of unknown etiology and clinical features suggestive of TS, such as delayed puberty, amenorrhea, and characteristic body features. Bone age is typically slightly delayed with respect to chronologic age due to the deficiencies in estrogen production. Children with TS should be plotted onto syndrome-specific growth charts. TS is the prototypical model for GH therapy insofar as early initiation of therapy will lead to improvement of adult height; therefore, GH therapy is routinely recommended.

Down Syndrome

DS, or *trisomy 21*, is the most common chromosomal abnormality of live-born infants, affecting approximately 1 in 730 live births in the United States. In addition to the dysmorphic features, intellectual impairment, heart disease, growth retardation, and short stature are prominent features of DS. Compared to unaffected children, children with DS demonstrate lower length, weight, and head circumference at any age and achieve a reduced final adult height. The pathophysiologic mechanism of causing the blunted height in DS is unclear. Deficiency of GH is uncommon, and the reduced growth is usually attributable to comorbidities, such as cardiac or GI problems that preclude optimal growth; therefore, growth optimization depends on proper management of the comorbidities. In the United States, DS-specific growth charts are available.

Prader-Willi Syndrome

Prader-Willi syndrome (PWS) is a rare genetic disorder in which seven genes on chromosome 15q are deleted or unexpressed on the paternal chromosome. The incidence is found in approximately 1 in 18,000 live births. The characteristic features include low muscle tone, short stature, hypogonadotropic hypogonadism, cognitive disabilities, and hypothalamic obesity. Growth failure may be evident at birth but is generally more impressive postnatally. The cause of growth failure is unclear. Low serum GH levels may reflect the impact of obesity or that these children have true defective pituitary dysfunction. GH is approved for children with PWS but the benefits are not solely related to increasing linear growth. In addition to reducing visceral fat, GH therapy has also been shown to improve muscle tone and strength.

PRECOCIOUS PUBERTY

Precocious puberty (PP) is premature sexual development, which occurs at an age more than 2.5 SDs below the mean age of puberty. Premature increases in androgens and estrogens cause acceleration of growth in the short term but ultimately compromise adult final height due to premature closure of the epiphyseal growth plates. For girls, PP is defined by the presence of breast development and/or pubic hair before age 8 years. For boys, it is defined by the presence of testicular enlargement and pubic hair before age 9.5 years. The appropriate cutoff age is controversial because many boys and girls do not have true pathology but, rather, a benign variant.

Etiology

PP may be due to a benign variant (premature adrenarche or thelarche), a central cause (gonadotropin-dependent PP), or a peripheral cause (gonadotropin-independent PP). Central PP results in early activation of the HPG axis, whereas peripheral PP is due to excessive administration of exogenous sex steroids or endogenous production of adrenal- or ovarian-derived sex steroids.

Benign Variants

Children with early signs of puberty who do not meet the criteria for PP may have a benign variant of PP. Girls may develop premature thelarche, whereas both girls and boys may develop premature adrenarche. Despite the presence of early signs of puberty, children with these variants usually do not require therapy and are not at risk for reaching a less-than-expected final height at an earlier-than-expected age.

Premature Thelarche

Premature thelarche is a condition of isolated breast development in a girl with no other signs of puberty or growth acceleration. Growth velocity and bone age are within normal limits, and the onset of puberty occurs within a normal age range. The breast tissue may resolve, persist, or enlarge but does not usually surpass Tanner stage III development until the girl reaches age 12 years.

Premature Adrenarche

Premature adrenarche refers to isolated pubic hair development in boys and girls. Body odor, acne, and axillary hair may also be present. Bone age may be slightly advanced but is usually within 2 SDs of the mean. These children may have elevated androgen levels, but those do not interfere with the onset of normal puberty.

Central Precocious Puberty

Central PP refers to puberty occurring via activation of the HPG axis at a younger than normal age. In childhood, the pituitary gland is physiologically unresponsive to GnRH. Once central puberty has been activated, the pituitary gland responds to GnRH by secreting gonadotropins, and the gonads enlarge in response to luteinizing hormone (LH) and follicle-stimulating hormone (FSH) stimulation. Although random levels of LH and FSH are not always helpful in confirming the diagnosis of central PP, a GnRH-stimulation test can be performed to determine whether there is a brisk rise in LH secretion or not. Central PP can be caused by congenital CNS anomalies, such as septo-optic dysplasia, hypothalamic hamartoma, or neurofibromatosis, or, by acquired CNS insults, such as infection, ischemia, trauma, or neoplasm. In 90% of girls and 50% of boys, the etiology of premature activation of the HPG axis is idiopathic. For girls and boys with idiopathic central PP, treatment with a GnRH analog is considered if predicted final height is compromised, or if the child is not psychosocially ready or able to handle the pubertal changes. The GnRH analog downregulates the GnRH receptors on the pituitary gland such that they no longer respond to GnRH pulses. After a brief surge of GnRH, the agonist desensitizes the pituitary to GnRH by GnRH-receptor downregulation. With monitoring of LH after repeated GnRH agonist injections, LH levels should drop to prepubertal levels. Serial radiographic studies of bone age every 3 to 6 months with monitoring of breast and pubic hair development should also help determine treatment efficacy.

Noncentral (Peripheral) Precocious Puberty

Peripheral PP is initiated by a process outside the HPG axis that results in either endogenous or exogenous androgen/estrogen exposure. Because the central axis is still immature, gonadotropin levels are low and do not respond to GnRH stimulation. In addition to exogenous administration of androgen or estrogen therapy, congenital adrenal hyperplasia (CAH), tumors, the McCune-Albright syndrome, and ovarian cysts are the most common causes.

Although females with CAH commonly present with ambiguous genitalia at birth, boys and girls may not present until infancy or childhood with signs of PP because presentation depends on the severity of the enzyme block. Because adrenal glands directly secrete androgens but not estrogen, premature breast development does not occur in girls with PP due to CAH. These children should be treated with glucocorticoids. CAH is described in detail in Chapter 15.

Adrenal, ovarian, or testicular tumors can produce androgen, estrogen, or human chorionic gonadotropin (hCG) and cause PP in boys or girls. hCG, which is very similar in structure to LH, can stimulate testes to produce testosterone. Functional ovarian or adrenal tumors usually require surgical excision, whereas hCG-secreting tumors may require chemotherapy or adjunctive radiation.

The McCune-Albright syndrome is due to a G-protein abnormality in which a gain-of-function mutation of the G_α subunit causes gonadal cells to behave as though they are constantly stimulated with FSH and LH, despite low gonadotropin levels. The gonadal cells continue to produce testosterone (testis) and estrogen (ovary) even though the FSH and LH receptors are not occupied. The clinical findings in patients with MAS include the triad of peripheral PP, polyostotic fibrous dysplasia of bone, and irregular café au lait spots. These children are usually treated with drugs that inhibit steroidogenesis or hormonal action such as aromatase inhibitors and/or anti-estrogens. Familial testotoxicosis is an autosomal dominant condition in which there is a mutation in the LH receptor. Boys with testotoxicosis can be treated with ketoconazole as it inhibits steroidogenic enzymes required for androgen synthesis.

Functional ovarian cysts can produce estrogen, causing acute onset of breast development in girls. The cysts resolve spontaneously but often result in withdrawal bleeding from the estrogen-stimulated endometrium, after which the breast tissue regresses. The diagnosis is made by ultrasound, and if the cysts persists and do not involute, surgery may be necessary to remove them.

CASE FOLLOW-UP

The boy's medical records show that his height at previous well-child visits was recorded as follows:

- Age 6 years: 43 in (109.2 cm)
- Age 7 years: 45 in (114.3 cm)
- Age 8 years: 47 in (119.4 cm)

(*continues*)

CASE FOLLOW-UP *(continued)*

The patient's height measurements are plotted onto the CDC height-for-age chart for boys. Short stature is confirmed by demonstration of a consistent pattern of stature along the 5th percentile for age, but the growth velocity is consistent. History and physical examination are not suggestive of any treatable pathologic etiology for growth failure. Therefore, he should undergo conservative laboratory testing (complete blood count, serum chemistries, and thyroid-function tests) and a plain radiograph of his hand and wrist.

Laboratory testing is unremarkable. He does not have electrolyte disturbances, thyroid dysfunction, hypoglycemia, anemia, or renal dysfunction. His bone age is consistent with a bone age of a boy aged 6.5 years. On the basis of the history and physical examination, growth velocity, normal laboratory studies, and a delayed bone age, a diagnosis of CDG is made. The patient and parents acknowledge the diagnosis and decide to forgo further testing at the moment, but they will return for periodic follow-up.

The child remains of short stature for several subsequent well-child visits, but his growth begins to accelerate around age 13 years, and he progressively crosses percentile lines on the height-for-age chart. He continues to consistently grow and achieves a final height at age 21 years of 70 in (177.8 cm), consistent with the 50th percentile.

REFERENCES and SUGGESTED READINGS

Albertsson-Wikland K, et al. Dose-dependent effect of growth hormone on final height in children with short stature without growth hormone deficiency. J Clin Endocrinol Metab. 2008;93:4342–4350.

Blethen SL, et al. Factors predicting the response to growth hormone therapy (GH) in prepubertal children with GH deficiency. J Clin Endocrinol Metab. 1993;76:574–579.

Carel JC, Ecosse E, Landier F, Meguellati-Hakkas D, Kaguelidou F, Rey G, et al. Long-term mortality after recombinant growth hormone treatment for isolated growth hormone deficiency or childhood short stature: preliminary report of the French SAGhE study. J Clin Endocrinol Metab. 2012;97:416–425.

Centers for Disease Control and Prevention, National Center for Health Statistics. CDC growth charts: United States. http://www.cdc.gov/growthcharts/. May 30, 2000.

Cohen P, Rogol AD, Deal CL, Saenger P, Reiter EO, Ross JL, et al. Consensus statement on the diagnosis and treatment of children with idiopathic short stature: a summary of the Growth Hormone Research Society, the Lawson Wilkins Pediatric Endocrine Society, and the European Society for Paediatric Endocrinology Workshop. J Clin Endocrinol Metab. 2008;93:4210–4217.

Lai H-C, Fitzsimmons SC, Allen DB, Kosorok MR, Rosenstein BJ, Campbell PW, et al. Growth impairment after alternate-day prednisone treatment in children with cystic fibrosis. N Engl J Med. 2000;342:851–859.

Laron Z. Laron syndrome (primary growth hormone resistance or insensitivity): the personal experience 1958-2003. J Clin Endocrinol Metab. 2004;89:1031–1044.

Lee MM. Idiopathic short stature. N Engl J Med. 2006;354:2576–2582.

Mahoney CP. Evaluating the child with short stature. Pediatr Clin North Am. 1987;34:825–849.

Lee JM, et al. Estimated cost-effectiveness of growth hormone therapy for idiopathic short stature. Arch Pediatr Adolesc Med. 2006;160:263–269.

Shah BC, Moran ES, Zinn AR, Pappas JG. Effect of growth hormone therapy on severe short stature and skeletal deformities in a patient with combined Turner syndrome and Langer mesomelic dysplasia. J Clin Endocrinol Metab. 2009;94:5028–5033.

Stephenson LS, Latham MC, Ottesen EA. Malnutrition and parasitic helminth infections. Parasitology 2000;121:S23–S38.

Styne D. Chapter 6. Growth. In: Gardner DG, Shoback D, eds. Greenspan's Basic & Clinical Endocrinology. 9th ed. New York, NY: McGraw-Hill; 2011.

Sybert VP, McCauley E. Turner's syndrome. N Engl J Med. 2004;351:1227–1238.

CHAPTER REVIEW QUESTIONS

1. Which of the following statements regarding growth velocity is *true*?

   A. Growth velocity is greatest during the first year of postnatal life.
   B. Growth velocity is relatively constant throughout childhood.
   C. Male and female children have roughly equal growth velocities.
   D. Deceleration of growth velocity between 18 and 24 months should trigger a work-up.
   E. Growth velocity always increases with administration of exogenous GH.

2. A 6-year-old girl presents to your office for the evaluation of short stature. She has no other complaints and has otherwise been developing normally. She is below the 3rd percentile for height when plotted on the growth chart. The child was adopted and the height of her parents is unknown. All of the following should be considered as potential causes of her short stature *except*:

   A. Constitutional delay of growth
   B. Down syndrome
   C. Familial short stature
   D. Growth hormone deficiency
   E. Turner syndrome

3. A 10-year-old boy was found to have constitutional delay of growth on the basis of clinical features and diagnostic testing. Which of the following statements most accurately reflects the natural history of this condition?

   A. He will begin puberty at the same age as his peers.
   B. He will require growth hormone therapy in order to reach his target height.
   C. He will exhibit a degree of intellectual impairment.
   D. He will have concordant chronologic and bone ages.
   E. He will reach a normal adult height.

4. A 9-year-old boy and his parents present to your office for a second opinion regarding abnormal laboratory studies. When administered arginine and insulin, rises in serum GH of 1.9 ng/mL and 2.8 ng/mL (normal serum GH level poststimulation $\geq$10 ng/mL) were observed, respectively. Serum IGF-1 and IGFBP-3 are also low. Which of the following statements regarding his condition is most likely *true*?

   A. Clonidine administration would produce a rise in GH of 10.6 ng/mL.
   B. He will require therapy with recombinant IGF-1 to achieve normal height.
   C. Radiographs of the hands and wrist would reveal delayed bone age.
   D. He will eventually achieve a normal adult height, corrected for midparental height.
   E. He had decreased birth weight and length.

5. An 8-year-old girl is undergoing testing for growth hormone deficiency. As part of her work-up, she is scheduled to undergo provocative testing using two different secretagogues. All of the following are limitations of provocative testing *except*:

   A. Lack of gold standard for the diagnosis of GH deficiency
   B. Suppression of GH release after carbohydrate of fat ingestion
   C. Long half-life of GH in serum
   D. Nonphysiologic nature of provocative test
   E. Blunted GH response in overweight and obese children

CHAPTER REVIEW ANSWERS

1. The correct answer is A. Growth velocity varies throughout childhood. The two peaks of growth velocity occur during infancy and puberty. Of the two, infancy (25 cm/year) is a more rapid period of growth than puberty (8 to 9 cm/year for girls, 9 to 10 cm/year for boys). All other choices are incorrect.

Growth is a dynamic process, which varies throughout childhood rather than being constant (**Choice B**). Growth can be divided into infant, childhood, and pubertal phases, which exhibit distinct patterns of growth. Male and female children have similar growth velocities during infancy and early childhood (**Choice C**), but the sexes diverge during puberty. Girls generally enter puberty earlier than boys, and reach a lower peak growth velocity during this period. Although growth deceleration can be worrisome, a modest acceleration or deceleration between the ages of 18 and 24 months is considered a variant of normal (**Choice D**). This represents the declining influence of maternal/gestational factors on growth and the rising influence of genetic makeup. In the absence of clinical features, this finding alone should not trigger a work-up for growth retardation. Human growth hormone (hGH) treatment is an accepted treatment for many of the causes of short stature, but it is most commonly used for growth hormone deficiency (GHD), with a resultant rapid rise in growth velocity following administration (**Choice E**). There are some disorders that do not respond to exogenous growth hormone, most notably the variants of growth hormone insensitivity.

2. The correct answer is B. In this scenario, a child has only a single measurement of height. Growth velocity cannot be adequately established, however, short stature is confirmed by a height below the 3rd percentile. This scenario generates a broad endocrine and nonendocrine differential diagnosis. Short stature can occur in all of the conditions listed, but short stature due to Down syndrome (DS) is least likely given that the child has otherwise normal development and has not shown other stigmata of DS, such as intellectual impairment, hypotonia, delayed milestones, or congenital anomalies.

Constitutional delay of growth (CDG) (**Choice A**) should always be considered in an otherwise normal, healthy child presenting for the evaluation of short stature. Previous height measurements, family history of "late bloomers," normal parental height, and radiographs demonstrating delayed bone age are valuable in making this diagnosis. Familial short stature (**Choice C**) is also a potential diagnosis in this child. Previous height measurements, reduced parental height, and radiographs demonstrating normal bone ages are required to make this diagnosis. Isolated growth retardation can be seen in mild-moderate forms of growth hormone deficiency (GHD) (**Choice D**). This child has no complaints that suggest pituitary abnormalities or midline defects, but GHD remains a diagnostic possibility. Radiographs, provocative GH testing, and determination of insulin-like growth factor 1 (IGF-1) and IGFBP-3 levels would assist in making this diagnosis. Occasionally, short stature can be the presenting sign of Turner syndrome (**Choice E**). This diagnosis should remain a consideration in a healthy prepubertal girl with growth deceleration or failure. Karyotype would assist in diagnosis.

3. The correct answer is E. In constitutional delay of growth (CDG), children eventually reach normal adult heights (corrected for sex and mid-parental height). They lag behind their peers through most of childhood, but eventually catch up. This sequence contrasts with that of familial short stature where only a less-than-average adult height is achieved. All other choices are incorrect.

Children with CDG have delayed puberty (**Choice A**). This is depicted as a delayed peak growth velocity seen on growth charts, which typically occurs at 11.5 years of age in girls and 13.5 years of age in boys. Administration of human growth hormone (hGH) is controversial in CDG. In general, it has no role because of the natural history of this condition, which results in normal adult height without any intervention (**Choice B**). Children with CDG display normal intelligence and lead healthy, productive lives (**Choice C**). The associated finding of intellectual impairment suggests an anatomic defect or chromosomal abnormality. Children with familial short stature (FSS) have concordant chronologic and bone ages (**Choice D**) but children with CGD have a delayed bone age compared to chronologic age.

---

4. The correct answer is C. The patient has classic laboratory findings for growth hormone deficiency (GHD) together with provocative testing, using two secretagogues, that failed to result in a normal rise in GH as expected. One of the characteristics of GH deficiency is a delayed bone age, due to the absent or diminished effects of GH on skeletal maturity. All of the other choices are incorrect.

Clonidine is a secretagogue used in provocative GH testing, but is unlikely to produce a normal rise in GH in the above scenario (**Choice A**). The lack of a gold standard for provocative testing and laboratory assays, however, makes a definitive diagnosis less concrete. Recombinant insulin-like growth factor 1 (IGF-1) is the treatment of choice for most forms of growth hormone insensitivity (**Choice B**). This patient likely has GHD as suggested by the laboratory values and the response to human growth hormone (hGH) therapy. In the absence of treatment, this child would not be expected to achieve a normal adult height (**Choice D**). Due to the central role of GH/IGF-1 in promoting linear growth, children with deficiencies in the production, secretion, or action of these hormones do not achieve normal adult height without intervention. Children with GHD generally have normal birth length and weight (**Choice E**) and gradually exhibit growth deceleration during the first few months of postnatal life. This contrasts to growth hormone insensitivity, where children generally present with reduced birth weight and length as in Laron syndrome.

---

5. The correct answer is C. A major limitation of provocative testing for growth hormone deficiency (GHD) is the short (not long) half-life of GH in serum. Due to this short half-life and pulsatile secretion of GH, a random level does not provide diagnostic information since it is low in both children with GHD and healthy children. Therefore, it requires alternative, nonphysiologic methods for assessing GH status. All of them have various limitations. All of the other choices are incorrect.

Lack of a gold standard is a problem with the diagnosis of GHD (**Choice A**). In order to counteract this problem, this test, with two secretagogues, is required to make an accurate diagnosis. GH release is suppressed by the ingestion of carbohydrates and fats. This may result in a false-positive test if the patient recently ate (**Choice B**). Therefore, the patient should fast 8 to 10 hours prior to the test. Provocative testing, however, is not physiologic (**Choice D**). The physiologic stimuli for GH release include growth hormone–releasing hormone (GHRH), sleep (stages 3 and 4), fasting, and various other inhibitory and stimulatory neuropeptides, such as somatostatin and ghrelin. Normally, GH is released in short pulses. The GH response in obese and overweight children is blunted (**Choice E**). The GH response is blunted under several physiologic situations. In obese and overweight children, and in those who are entering puberty, results may be falsely positive. When interpreting test results, the child's weight must be accounted for.

Pediatrics II: Disorders of Sexual Differentiation and Ambiguous Genitalia

15

Robert S. Gerhard

Eric I. Felner

CASE

A healthy, full-term baby is born by spontaneous vaginal delivery to a healthy mother. The baby is active, well perfused, and crying appropriately. The baby has no dysmorphic features. Upon close inspection, the baby has ambiguous genitalia. It is difficult to determine whether the baby has an enlarged clitoris or a small penis. Further examination reveals labioscrotal fusion. Gonads are not palpable.

The mother was followed carefully throughout pregnancy and had no discernible problems. She denied alcohol, tobacco, or drug use during pregnancy. She gained weight appropriately and did not develop signs of virilization during her pregnancy.

This chapter begins with a review of the embryology of the reproductive system for both males and females and is followed by a review of the causes of ambiguous genitalia to help the reader develop hypotheses regarding this baby's condition. The chapter has been organized to review disorders that result in virilization of females and undervirilization of males. Some conditions are only mentioned but are described in more detail in other chapters.

OBJECTIVES

1. Recognize the steps involved in sexual differentiation.

2. Discuss the most common enzyme deficiencies in the steroidogenesis pathway.

CHAPTER OUTLINE

(continues)

EMBRYOLOGY AND PHYSIOLOGY

In the developing fetus, the urogenital system arises from the intermediate mesoderm that ultimately gives rise to the internal and external genitalia. The presence or absence of a Y chromosome represents the genetic determination of gender, which is established at the moment of fertilization. For the first 8 weeks of gestation, the gonads are identical, regardless of the sex. This is referred to as the "indifferent stage" of gonadal development. After 8 weeks, the testes and ovaries begin to develop and to produce hormones, which drive the determination of male or female genitalia. The development of the sexual organs is referred to as *sexual differentiation*. In the normal fetus, sex determination is determined by the presence or absence of the sex-determining region on the Y chromosome (SRY).

The gonads (ovaries and testes) originate from the genital ridge of the fetus. The single step that determines the development of the gonadal sex is the presence or absence of the *SRY* gene. At 8 weeks' gestation, during the indifferent stage of gonadal development and in the presence of the *SRY* gene, the indifferent gonad differentiates into a testis. If the *SRY* gene is not present or expressed, the indifferent gonad develops into an ovary. Therefore, the female sex represents the default pathway, and, in the absence of the *SRY* gene, an ovary will develop (Figure 15-1).

Under the influence of the *SRY* gene, the primitive sex cord develops into a testis. Two different cells within the testis produce hormones essential for sexual development: the Sertoli cells and the Leydig cells. The Sertoli cells are the first to appear and produce Müllerian-inhibiting hormone (MIH), which causes involution of the Müllerian ducts and regression of the female internal genital structures. The Leydig cells produce testosterone, which stimulates the differentiation of the Wolffian duct, thereby triggering the development of the male internal genitalia system. In addition, testosterone produced from the Leydig cells must be converted to dihydrotestosterone (DHT) by the 5α-reductase (5α-R) enzyme in order to complete virilization of the male external genitalia. The embryologic genital structures give rise to homologous male and female genital structures (Table 15-1).

In the absence of the *SRY* gene, the testes, Leydig cells, and Sertoli cells do not form; therefore, testosterone and MIH are not secreted. Without testosterone, DHT does not form, the male external genitalia do not develop, and the Wolffian ducts involute. Without

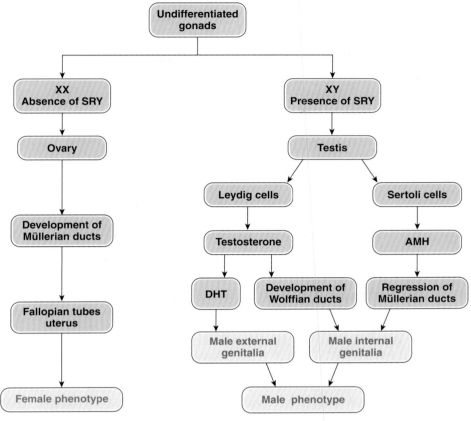

FIGURE 15-1. Sex determination and differentiation of the gonads. DHT, dihydrotestosterone; AMH, anti-Müllerian hormone.

MIH, the internal female genitalia system remains. The indifferent gonad of the genetic female, who lacks the *SRY* gene, will therefore develop into an ovary.

The gonads, the primary reproductive organs, serve two functions: gametogenesis (ova and sperm development) and sex-hormone production. In males, the testes produce testosterone, whereas, in females, the ovaries produce estrogen.

Sex hormone production by the gonads is controlled by the hypothalamic–pituitary–gonadal (HPG) axis. Androgen production from the adrenal cortex is under the influence of the hypothalamic–pituitary–adrenal (HPA) axis. The details of the hypothalamic and pituitary influences on the gonads and adrenal cortex have been reviewed in Chapters 2, 12, and 13.

TABLE 15-1.	Homologous Structures	
Female Structure	**Embryologic Structure**	**Male Structure**
Clitoris	Genital tubercle	Head of penis
Labia minora	Genital folds	Ventral aspect of penis
Labia majora	Genital swellings	Scrotum

Steroidogenesis

As previously discussed in Chapter 10, glucocorticoids and mineralocorticoids are produced and secreted by the adrenal cortex. The sex steroids, androgens and estrogens, are either directly or indirectly secreted by the adrenal cortex, testis, and ovary. All of these steroid hormones are derived from cholesterol and share various enzymes and intermediary hormones. The primary glucocorticoid is cortisol (hydrocortisone), and the primary mineralocorticoid is aldosterone. The conversion of cholesterol to cortisol, aldosterone, and androstenedione requires many enzymes and intermediary hormones (Figure 15-2). A defect in any of these enzymes may result in a hormone deficiency or excess. The functions of cortisol and aldosterone have been discussed in Chapter 10, and androgen functions have been discussed in Chapter 13.

Although describing each step of the steroid biosynthetic pathway is beyond the scope of this chapter, it is essential to understand which enzyme defects result in hormone deficiencies. Because this chapter focuses primarily on sexual differentiation and ambiguous genitalia, it is necessary to review the enzyme defects that cause virilization of the female newborn and undervirilization of the male newborn.

In order for the adrenal cortex to adequately produce and secrete cortisol, cholesterol must be converted to four intermediary hormones via five enzymes and a regulatory protein in the following sequence (also outlined in Figure 15-2): 1) steroidogenic acute regulatory protein (StAR) facilitates cholesterol transport across the mitochondria to the enzyme cholesterol desmolase; 2) cholesterol is then converted to pregnenolone by cholesterol desmolase; 3) pregnenolone is then converted to 17-hydroxypregnenolone by 17-hydroxylase (17-OHase); 4) 17-hydroxypregnenolone is then converted to 17-hydroxyprogesterone (17-OHP) by 3β-hydroxysteroid dehydrogenase (3β-HSD); 5) 17-OHP is then converted to 11-deoxycortisol by 21-hydroxylase (21-OHase); and 6) 11-deoxycortisol is converted to cortisol by 11-hydroxylase (11-OHase). A defect in any of these steps will result in congenital adrenal hyperplasia (CAH). Because a deficiency in cortisol secretion will result in a loss of negative feedback at the hypothalamus and pituitary gland, corticotropin-releasing hormone (CRH) and andrenocorticotropic hormone (ACTH) will be increased and will result in both overproduction and secretion of adrenal androgens. A defect in any of these enzymes will result in excess androgen production in newborn females but will not have an effect on male newborns. This is because newborn male infants produce more testosterone from their testes (via the HPG axis) than from an overstimulated adrenal cortex (due to CAH).

For adequate adrenal androgen production, cholesterol must be converted to at least three intermediary hormones via four enzymes in the following sequence: 1) cholesterol is converted to pregnenolone by cholesterol desmolase; 2) pregnenolone is converted to 17-hydroxypregnenolone by 17-OHase; 3) 17-hydroxypregnenolone is converted to the first and weakest androgen, dehydroepiandrosterone (DHEA), by 17,20 lyase; and 4) DHEA is converted to androstenedione by 3β-HSD. Androstenedione is, thus, the final step in androgen production by the adrenal cortex, but it, in turn, is converted to testosterone by 17β-HSD in the periphery, testis, and ovary. Female newborns produce a very small amount of androgen from their adrenal gland; therefore, a female with a defect in androgen production is not apparent in the newborn period. In the male newborn, however, without appropriate production and secretion of testosterone and, ultimately, DHT, the external genitalia will appear either ambiguous or like that of a normal female.

AMBIGUOUS GENITALIA (VIRILIZED FEMALES)

Virilization of the newborn female is most commonly due to a defect in steroid biosynthesis or to the presence of a virilizing disorder in the mother. Although there are a few

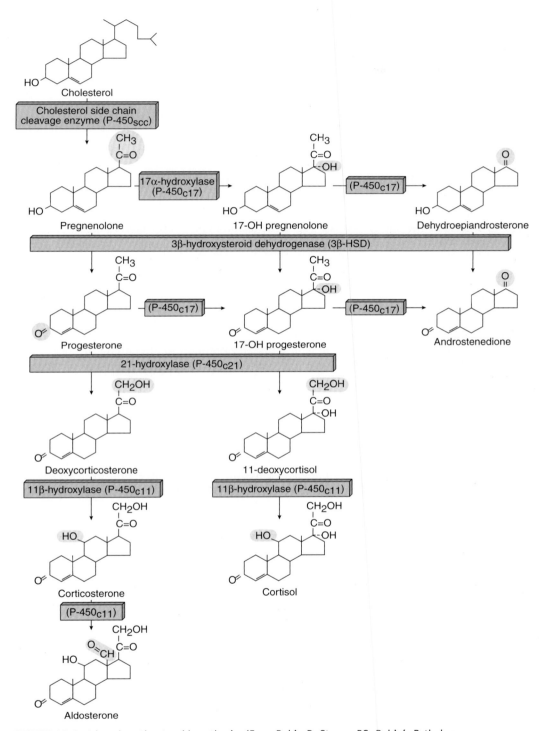

FIGURE 15-2. Adrenal corticosteroid synthesis. (From Rubin R, Strayer DS. Rubin's Pathology: Clinicopathologic Foundations of Medicine. 5th ed. Philadelphia, PA: Lippincott Williams & Wilkins; 2008.)

other disorders that affect the development of female genitalia, only those that result in ambiguous genitalia or virilizing disorders will be discussed in this chapter. The defects of female sexual differentiation that do not result in virilization or ambiguous genitalia are discussed in Chapter 12.

Defects in Steroid Biosynthesis

Autosomal recessive genetic disorders may disrupt any of the steps in the steroidogenesis pathway (see Figure 15-2). Most of these disorders result in diminished cortisol synthesis. In response to adrenal insufficiency, the pituitary gland synthesizes increased amounts of propiomelanocortin (POMC) and ACTH, which promote increased steroidogenesis. ACTH also stimulates adrenal hypertrophy and hyperplasia. Thus, CAH refers to a group of diseases resulting from the deficiency of one of the enzymes required for cortisol synthesis by the adrenal cortex. A genetic lesion in one of the steroidogenic enzymes may interfere with normal steroidogenesis. The signs and symptoms of the disease derive from the deficiency of the steroidal end-product and the effects of accumulated steroidal precursors proximal to the blocked step. By understanding the steroidogenesis pathway and the biologic effects of each steroid, the clinician should be able to deduce the manifestations of the disease.

The most common cause of CAH and virilization of female newborns is 21-OHase deficiency, which accounts for more than 90% of cases. Deficiency of 3β-HSD and 11β-OHase can also cause virilization of the female fetus and premature adrenarche in both sexes. The clinical and biochemical findings for each enzyme defect that results in virilization of females are shown in Table 15-2.

21-Hydroxylase Deficiency

Steroid 21-OHase (*CYP21*, also termed *CYP21A2* and *P450c21*) is a cytochrome P450 enzyme, located in the endoplasmic reticulum. It catalyzes both the conversion of 17-OHP to 11-deoxycortisol, a precursor of cortisol, and the conversion of progesterone to deoxycorticosterone (DOC), a precursor of aldosterone (see Figure 15-2). Individuals with 21-OHase deficiency cannot synthesize cortisol efficiently, resulting in overstimulation of the adrenal cortex by ACTH, which overproduces cortisol precursors. Some of these precursors are diverted to the biosynthesis of sex hormones, which may cause signs of androgen excess (e.g., ambiguous genitalia) in newborn girls and rapid postnatal growth in both sexes. The associated aldosterone deficiency may cause salt wasting and result in failure to thrive, hypovolemia, and shock. Three phenotypes have been observed. A severe form, with a concurrent defect in aldosterone biosynthesis (**salt-wasting type**) and a form with normal aldosterone biosynthesis (**simple virilizing type**) are termed *classic 21-OHase deficiency*. There is also a mild, *nonclassic 21-OHase deficiency* form in which individuals may be asymptomatic or display signs of postnatal androgen excess. Because the majority of individuals with CAH have 21-OHase deficiency, most are referred to as having the classic, salt-wasting form of CAH; the classic, simple-virilizing form of CAH; and the nonclassic form of CAH.

Classic 21-OHase deficiency is detected in approximately 1 in 16,000 births. The nonclassic form occurs in approximately 0.2% of the general white population but is more frequent (1% to 2%) in certain populations such as Eastern European Jews. Approximately 75% of individuals with classic 21-OHase deficiency have severely impaired 21-hydroxylation of progesterone and, therefore, cannot adequately synthesize aldosterone. The severity of the 21-OHase gene mutation determines whether an individual develops the salt-wasting, simple-virilizing, or nonclassic type. Classic salt wasters have a complete loss of enzyme function with a deficiency of both glucocorticoids and mineralocorticoids.

TABLE 15-2.	Defects in Steroid Biosynthesis				
Defect	**Genitalia**	**Presentation**	**Elevated Hormone Levels**	**Decreased Hormone Levels**	**Treatment**
Lipoid hyperplasia stAR	Undervirilized male / Normal female	Salt-wasting crisis	ACTH, PRA	Aldosterone, cortisol, DHEA, androstenedione, testosterone, DHT	GC / MC / Androgens[a]
Cholesterol desmolase[b]	Undervirilized male / Normal female	Salt-wasting crisis	ACTH, PRA	Aldosterone, cortisol, DHEA, androstenedione, testosterone, DHT	GC / MC / Androgens[a]
3β-HSD	Undervirilized male / Virilized female	Salt-wasting crisis	ACTH, 17-OH-pregnenolone, DHEA, androstenedione, testosterone, DHT	Cortisol, 17-OHP, aldosterone	GC / MC
21-OHase	Normal male / Virilized female	**Classic** Salt water / Simple virilizer	**SW** ACTH, 17-OHP, PRA, DHEA, androstenedione, Testosterone, DHT **SV** ACTH, 17-OHP, DHEA, androstenedione, testosterone, DHT	**SW** Cortisol, aldosterone **SV** Cortisol	**SW** GC / MC **SV** GC
11β-OHase	Normal male / Virilized Female	Hypertension	ACTH, DOC, 11-deoxycortisol	Cortisol, PRA	GC
17α-OHase 17,20-Lyase	Undervirilized male / Normal female	Hypertension Hypokalemia	Progesterone, DOC, corticosterone	DHEA, androstenedione, testosterone, DHT, cortisol	Androgens[a]
17β-HSD	Undervirilized male / Normal female		Androstenedione	Testosterone, DHT	Androgens[a]
5α-R	Undervirilized male / Normal female		Testosterone	DHT	Variable
Placental aromatase	Normal male / Virilized female		DHEA Androstenedione Testosterone		

[a]Androgen replacement for males but may or may not be used in females.
[b]No mutations have been identified.

Notes: GC, glucocorticoid (hydrocortisone); MC, mineralocorticoid (fludrocortisone); SW, salt water; SV, simple virilizer; 5α-R, 5α-reductase; DHT, dihydrotestosterone; ACTH, adrenocorticotropic hormone; 17-OHP, 17-hydroxyprogesterone; PRA, plasma renin activity; DHEA, dehydroepiandrosterone; DOC, deoxycorticosterone; StAR, steroidogenic acute regulatory protein; 3β-HSD, 3β-hydroxysteroid dehydrogenase; 17β-HSD, 17β-hydroxysteroid dehydrogenase; 17α-OHase, 17α-hydroxylase.

Individuals with the simple virilizing form do not have aldosterone deficiency, insofar as they maintain at least 5% activity of the 21-OHase enzyme. Individuals with nonclassic 21-OHase deficiency retain 20% to 50% of enzyme function, which is enough to produce sufficient cortisol but not enough to completely inhibit ACTH. Therefore, these individuals commonly show early signs of adrenarche.

In the female, the diagnosis of 21-OHase deficiency is manifested clinically by virilization of the genitalia and biochemically by an elevated 17-OHP level, low cortisol level, and hypoglycemia. The individual with the salt-wasting type will also have a low aldosterone level, elevated plasma renin activity (PRA), hyponatremia, and hyperkalemia. The diagnosis is confirmed by an elevated 17-OHP level ($>$500 µg/dL). In the United States, 17-OHP measurement is included in all neonatal screening tests.

Girls with classic 21-OHase deficiency are exposed to high systemic levels of adrenal androgens from approximately the seventh week of gestation. These girls have ambiguous genitalia: a large clitoris, rugated and partially fused labia majora, and a common urogenital sinus in place of a separate urethra and vagina (Figure 15-3A). The uterus, fallopian tubes, and ovaries are normally formed, and there is no development of the Wolffian duct. A general pediatric surgeon or pediatric urologist experienced in reconstructive genital surgery can perform a clitoroplasty and vaginoplasty (Figure 15-3B). In contrast, affected boys have no overt signs of the disease except variable and subtle hyperpigmentation and penile enlargement.

11β-Hydroxylase Deficiency

11β-Hydroxylase (11β-OHase) deficiency is the next most common cause of CAH, with an incidence of 1 in 100,000 births. The mutation results in complete loss of enzyme function and causes accumulation of DOC and 11-deoxycortisol. Like females with

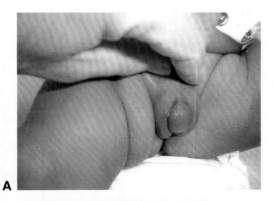
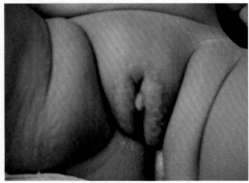

FIGURE 15-3. Virilized female with 21-OHase deficiency. **(A)** First day of life. **(B)** Postoperation at age 6 months. (Courtesy of Eric Felner, MD, Department of Pediatrics, Division of Endocrinology, MSCR Tulane University School of Medicine.)

21-OHase deficiency, these female newborns may have ambiguous genitalia. Unlike those with 21-OHase deficiency, these newborns are hypertensive due to the accumulation of the mineralocorticoid DOC. Affected boys have no overt signs of the disease except for variable and subtle hyperpigmentation and penile enlargement, but they are hypertensive. The diagnosis is confirmed by a cortrosyn-stimulated 11-deoxycortisol level three times higher than the upper limit of normal.

3β-Hydroxysteroid Dehydrogenase Deficiency

3β-HSD shares activity in the mineralocorticoid, glucocorticoid, and androgen pathways. A deficiency of this enzyme is extremely rare. DHEA, the earliest and weakest androgen, accumulates and cannot be converted to androstenedione, resulting in virilization of females and undervirilization of males. The diagnosis of 3β-HSD deficiency is suggested by an infant with adrenal insufficiency and features of ambiguous genitalia. Due to the wide and variable fluctuation of 17-hydroxypregnenolone, the diagnosis of 3β-HSD deficiency is established by calculating the ratio of 17-hydroxypregnenolone to 17-OHP. The condition should be suspected in any individual with a ratio greater than 10 standard deviations above the upper limit of normal.

Aromatase Deficiency

The aromatase enzyme converts androgens (DHEA, androstenedione, and testosterone) to estrogens (estriol, estrone, and estradiol). This enzyme is located in the gonads, muscles, liver, brain, adipose tissue, and placenta. A mutation of the placental aromatase gene, another rare autosomal recessive disorder, prevents androgen conversion to estrogen. Therefore, both the female newborn with this mutation and her mother during pregnancy will be virilized. Once the baby is born, however, the mother's virilizing features will resolve. The baby, on the other hand, may require surgical reconstruction of the external genitalia but will not require hormone therapy. Males with this condition are unaffected.

Management

The goal of treatment for individuals with CAH is to supplement glucocorticoid therapy with cortisol (hydrocortisone) in order to normalize androgen production and administer the mineralocorticoid fludrocortisone to prevent salt wasting and hypotension. With appropriate hydrocortisone therapy, ACTH production is reduced that decreases the driving force for adrenal production and secretion of androgens. Treatment is monitored by titrating replacement to normal blood 17-OHP levels. Surgical reconstruction of the vagina and clitoral reduction is also commonly necessary. If the mother undergoes prenatal testing, likely because of a family history or a previously affected newborn, virilization may be prevented if dexamethasone is administered early in pregnancy to suppress excess ACTH production.

Maternal Hyperandrogenism

Maternal hyperandrogenism may affect the genitalia of female newborns as the result of endogenous androgen production or exogenous use of androgenic hormones. Genital development of male fetuses is not affected. The endogenous causes include maternal CAH, adrenal tumors, ovarian tumors, and human chorionic gonadotropin (hCG)-dependent luteomas of pregnancy. Maternal hyperandrogenism may usually be differentiated from placental aromatase deficiency by the persistence of maternal virilization after pregnancy.

AMBIGUOUS GENITALIA (UNDERVIRILIZED MALES)

Ambiguous genitalia that occurs in the newborn genetic male is due to undervirilization. The external male genitalia develop in the presence of DHT. Because DHT is converted from testosterone by the 5α-R enzyme, normal male external genitalia occurs only if there is adequate testosterone and DHT available, and, the androgen receptor functions normally. The causes of ambiguous genitalia in the newborn male include abnormalities in any of the following: steroid biosynthesis, the androgen receptor, gonadal differentiation, the hypothalamus, and the pituitary gland. In addition to affecting the genitalia of female newborns, the use of pharmacologic agents by the mother during pregnancy may also cause undervirilization in male newborns.

Defects in Steroid Biosynthesis

Inborn errors of testosterone and/or DHT synthesis occur due to decreased activities of any of the following: StAR, cholesterol desmolase, 17α-hydroxylase (17α-OHase), 17,20-lyase, 3β-HSD, 17β-HSD, and 5α-R. The clinical and biochemical findings for each enzyme defect that results in undervirilization of males are shown in Table 15-2.

Lipoid CAH (StAR Deficiency) and Cholesterol Desmolase

Lipoid CAH is the most severe genetic disorder of steroid hormone synthesis. It is characterized by markedly reduced concentrations of all corticosteroids, high basal ACTH and PRA, and grossly enlarged adrenal glands with cholesterol and cholesterol esters. Unlike all of the other causes of CAH, lipoid CAH is not caused by a disrupted steroidogenic enzyme but, rather, by the reduced activity of StAR. StAR promotes steroidogenesis by facilitating cholesterol transport from the outer to the inner mitochondrial membrane. In the absence of StAR, steroidogenesis proceeds at less than 20% of the StAR-induced level. The loss of StAR leads to a deficiency in all corticosteroids that, in turn, leads to a compensatory rise in ACTH and luteinizing hormone (LH). These hormones increase cyclic adenosine monophosphate, increasing biosynthesis of low-density lipoprotein (LDL) receptors, their uptake of LDL cholesterol, and de novo synthesis of cholesterol. In the absence of StAR, this increased intracellular cholesterol accumulates and leads to mitochondrial and cellular damage caused by the accumulated cholesterol, cholesterol esters, and their auto-oxidation products. Without the ability to produce androgens, male newborns with lipoid CAH are undervirilzed and appear to have normal external female genitalia.

It was originally believed that lipoid CAH was due to impaired activity of cholesterol desmolase (side-chain cleavage P450scc), which catalyzes the 20α-hydroxylation, 22-hydroxylation, and scission of the cholesterol side chain. However, no mutations have been identified in the gene coding for cholesterol desmolase, but mutations in the StAR gene have been identified in individuals with lipoid CAH.

Because all three hormone pathways (mineralocorticoid, glucocorticoid, and androgen) are blocked, treatment requires both glucocorticoid and mineralocorticoid replacement therapy. Males should undergo an orchiectomy in order to prevent the likely development of a gonadoblastoma. They are usually raised as females. Genetic females have normal external genitalia.

17α-Hydroxylase and 17,20-Lyase Deficiencies

CYP17 encodes a single enzyme with both 17α-OHase and 17,20-lyase activities. This single gene mediates two separate steps in the steroidogenic pathway. In rare instances, gene mutations can result in either isolated 17α-OHase or isolated 17,20-lyase deficiency.

Most cases, however, are the result of a combined loss of enzyme function and referred to as *CYP17* deficiency, a very rare disorder, affecting 1 in 50,000 newborns. Isolated deficiency of 17α-OHase, although extremely rare, results in decreased cortisol synthesis, overproduction of ACTH, and stimulation of the mineralocorticoid pathway. These individuals may have mild symptoms of glucocorticoid deficiency, but the disorder is not life threatening, because there is overproduction of corticosterone, a mineralocorticoid that also has glucocorticoid activity.

The absence of 17α-OHase and 17,20-lyase activities prevents the synthesis of adrenal and gonadal sex steroids. In genetic males, this will result in absent or incomplete development of the external genitalia and hypertension. The diagnosis is made by low or absent biochemical levels of DHEA, androstenedione, testosterone, DHT, 17-hydroxypregnenolone, 17-OHP, 11-deoxycortisol, and cortisol with elevated levels of DOC and corticosterone. Due to the elevated level of DOC, infants have hypokalemia, hypertension, and low levels of aldosterone and PRA. In isolated *CYP17* deficiency, the mineralocorticoid excess is minimal and does not cause the individual to seek medical attention. Treatment involves glucocorticoid replacement therapy to suppress ACTH and DOC levels, so that aldosterone, PRA, potassium concentration, and blood pressure return to normal. Similar to lipoid CAH, genetic males are usually raised as females with appropriate surgical removal of the testes and estrogen supplementation.

17β-Hydroxysteroid Dehydrogenase Deficiency

17β-Hydroxysteroid dehydrogenase (17β-HSD) converts androstenedione to testosterone in the testes. Loss-of-function mutations result in testosterone deficiency and undervirilization of genetic males. The genitalia of genetic females is unaffected. The step mediated by 17β-HSD is exclusive to androgen synthesis, and, therefore, glucocorticoid and mineralocorticoid production are unaffected. Both testosterone and DHT are distal to 17β-HSD; therefore, deficiency results in low or absent levels. In the genetic male, testes develop, and Sertoli cells produce MIH, leading to the involution of Müllerian remnants. Without testosterone, the testes fail to descend and are commonly found in the inguinal canal. The diagnosis is confirmed by elevated androstenedione levels coupled with hCG stimulation that causes an increased ratio of plasma androstenedione to testosterone.

Treatment depends on the sex assignment the family desires. These individuals have historically been raised as either female or male. Recent evidence, however, suggests that male assignment produces the best results. This is achieved by early testosterone supplementation and surgical genitoplasty to achieve an acceptable male phallus. At the desired age of puberty, testosterone supplementation is reinitiated and maintained throughout life.

5α-Reductase Deficiency

5α-R is expressed in the genital skin and male accessory glands. This enzyme converts testosterone, produced in the testes, to DHT in the peripheral tissues. Two forms of the enzyme exist: type 1 and type 2. Type 2 is expressed in the developing fetus during critical phases of male sexual differentiation, and type 1 becomes more prominent during puberty. DHT is a potent androgen and important in sexual differentiation of male external genitalia and accessory glands. Under the influence of DHT, the primordial male phallus undergoes elongation and fusion of the urethra and scrotal walls at the midline. In the absence of DHT, as a result of a mutation in 5α-R type 2, and, despite the presence of adequate testosterone, external male genitalia will not develop. The internal male genitalia, however, do develop due to the presence of testosterone and MIH. This condition is also discussed in Chapter 13.

Disorders of the Androgen Receptor: Androgen Insensitivity (Testicular Feminization) Syndrome

Proper endocrine function depends on both normal hormone levels and intact receptor and intracellular messaging pathways. Complete androgen insensitivity syndrome (CAIS) occurs in a genetic male who has a nonfunctioning androgen receptor. The androgen receptor is encoded on the X chromosome and is a ubiquitous intracellular receptor responsible for binding testosterone. Individuals with CAIS have sufficient circulating testosterone levels, but the tissues that lack a functioning androgen receptor fail to respond. This results in an apparent testosterone deficiency. Seventy percent of cases are inherited as an X-linked recessive disorder with the other 30% arising from a de novo mutation. The prevalence ranges from 1:20,000 to 1:100,000 live born genetic males.

During male sexual development, testosterone action is required for proper differentiation of the Wolffian ducts and virilization of the external genitalia. In CAIS, the *SRY* is intact, and the testes develop, but the androgen receptor is dysfunctional, causing the Wolffian duct structures (epididymis, vas deferens, and seminal vesicles) to be underdeveloped. In addition to binding testosterone, the androgen receptor also binds DHT. Without proper DHT action, male external genitalia does not develop, but, because the Sertoli cells of the testes are present and produce MIH, the Müllerian structures involute. At birth, newborns have bilateral undescended testes that are located in the inguinal canal or within the labial folds, female-appearing external genitalia, and a blind vaginal pouch.

Genetic males with CAIS are reared as females. In the incomplete form, undervirilization occurs, and there is the potential to rear these individuals as males. Before age 12 years, there is an approximate 2% risk of gonadal malignancy. Therefore, an orchiectomy should be performed prior to age of 12 years to avoid the risk of developing a gonadoblastoma. For individuals being reared as females, leaving the gonads in place so that testosterone production induces endogenous estrogen production (via the aromatase enzyme), at least until puberty is initiated, is an option. Regardless of the age in which the orchiectomy is performed, supplemental estrogen replacement therapy will be required for individuals reared as females. A vaginoplasty of the blind vaginal pouch may be considered to achieve normal vaginal depth. This condition is also discussed in Chapters 12 and 13.

Disorders of Gonadal Differentiation: Testicular Dysgenesis

The testes develop in the eighth week of gestation under the control of the *SRY*. There are various genetic mutations that can result in disruption of testicular development despite the presence of the *SRY* gene. The most common of these are due to single gene mutations that drive fetal development and may also be part of a more encompassing syndrome that affects many organ systems. Many of the conditions involving abnormal testicular differentiation, such as the vanishing testes syndrome, Leydig cell dysfunction, and Klinefelter syndrome, are discussed in Chapter 13. In this section, the disorders of gonadal differentiation will focus on the undervirilized males who have testicular dysgenesis and ovotestes.

Gonadal dysgenesis refers to the abnormal formation of the gonads. Testicular dysgenesis can be complete or partial and result in a variety of presentations. Although many genes are involved in the development of the testes, the *SRY*, *SOX9* (SRY-related HMG box-9), and *WT1* (Wilms tumor 1) are the most important ones. Mutations that affect these genes result in gonadal dysgenesis.

The most common mutation affects the *SRY* gene and accounts for almost 20% of the cases of female external genitalia in a genetic male. The *SRY* gene provides the initial instruction for the undifferentiated gonad to develop into a testis. Absence of this gene causes the undifferentiated gonad to develop into an ovary. Despite the male genotype, absence of the testes prevents production of testosterone and MIH; therefore, these individuals appear female and have internal and external female genitalia.

Shortly after the onset of *SRY* activation, *SOX9*, a fundamental testis-differentiation gene common to all vertebrates, is activated. *SOX9* is an SRY-box-containing gene that encodes a transcriptional activator. *SOX9* expression is restricted to the Sertoli cell lineage and persists into adulthood. Humans with heterozygous mutations in *SOX9* develop a skeletal syndrome known as *campomelic dysplasia,* and most genetic male *SOX9* heterozygotes show variable male-to-female sex reversal, implicating *SOX9* in testis development.

The *WT1* gene encodes a zinc finger transcription factor expressed in gonadal and kidney tissues. The Denys-Drash and Frasier syndromes are both due to *WT1* gene mutations. Individuals with the Denys-Drash syndrome have a point mutation in the *WT1* gene. The syndrome consists of gonadal dysgenesis, nephropathy, and Wilms tumor development. It typically presents in the first three years of life with a rapid decline in kidney function that ultimately results in renal failure. The Frasier syndrome is caused by a mutation in the donor splice site of exon 9 of the *WT1* gene. It is more deleterious to testicular development, resulting in complete testicular dysgenesis. Individuals with this syndrome have a 46,XY karyotype but have internal and external female genitalia. Like individuals with the Denys-Drash syndrome, they too develop nephropathy, but not until the second decade of life. These individuals are at a high risk for gonadal malignancy.

Disorders of the Hypothalamus and Pituitary Gland

Undervirilized males with central hypogonadism have hypogonadotropic hypogonadism. They may have ambiguous genitalia at birth that is due to a gene mutation resulting in a deficiency of gonadotropin-releasing hormone (GnRH), follicle-stimulating hormone (FSH), or luteinizing hormone (LH). Due to the absence of these central gonadal hormones, testis differentiation and hormone (testosterone, DHT, and MIH) production are affected. The most common causes are due to Kallman syndrome, a GnRH mutation, a *PROP-1* mutation, and an LH mutation. These conditions are discussed in more detail in Chapter 13.

OVOTESTICULAR DISEASE

Ovotesticular disease (OTD), previously referred to as *true hermaphroditism,* is defined by the presence of both ovarian and testicular tissue within the same gonad. This gonad is referred to as the "ovotestis." This condition is extremely rare with only about 500 reported cases worldwide. The ovotestis can be present in the labioscrotal folds, inguinal canal, or abdomen. The external and internal genitalia are usually abnormal. The ovarian portion of the ovotestis is usually more functional than the testicular portion. Almost 60% of individuals with OTD are genetic females and 30% genetic males; the remaining 10% are mosaics.

The diagnosis of OTD should be considered in all newborns with ambiguous genitalia. Hormonal stimulation tests are needed to confirm the presence of testis-producing testosterone. Testicular function is tested by hCG stimulation. The gold standard for making the diagnosis of OTD is a tissue biopsy revealing the presence of both testicular and ovarian tissue. Stimulation testing is discussed in Chapter 19.

Management is often complicated by age of diagnosis, gender identity, and external/internal genitalia. Genetic females with a uterus are usually reared as females with surgical removal of functional testicular tissue. Individuals with phallic development and absence of female internal structures can be reared as males. Regardless of the sex of rearing, the gonad should be removed before puberty. If raising the child as a male, the gonad should be removed to prevent both estrogen secretion and the risk for developing a gonadoblastoma. If raising the child as a female, the gonad should be removed to prevent both testosterone secretion and the risk for developing a gonadoblastoma. Despite undergoing an orchiectomy, close monitoring of these individuals is required because occasionally not all of the testicular tissue (which has the propensity to become malignant) is located and removed.

Gender of Rearing

While awaiting results of the initial laboratory studies, attention is focused on the main decision: **gender of rearing**. A pediatric endocrinologist, psychologist, pediatric urologist with expertise in reconstructive surgery, and the parents need to participate in discussions and decision-making regarding the options for gender assignment and possible surgical interventions. Although the child is a silent partner in the decision-making process, as the child matures, honest explanations regarding the medical condition are essential. Decisions on the appropriate sex of rearing should be based on the specific pathophysiology, prognosis for spontaneous pubertal development, risk for gonadal tumors, capacity for sexual intercourse and orgasm, and potential for fertility.

Evaluation and Management

The evaluation, determination, and management of newborns with ambiguous genitalia can be very difficult. The diagnosis should be made as quickly as possible so that the family understands what the birth defect is and how the child should be reared. Depending on the presence of palpable gonads, an algorithm can be followed to determine what tests should be performed and what the corresponding diagnosis is (Figure 15-4).

CASE FOLLOW-UP

It is obvious that our patient has ambiguous genitalia. A broad differential diagnosis is required, however, that can be narrowed considerably after collecting special studies. The cause of the ambiguous genitalia can be categorized as either a virilized female or an undervirilized male. Because the baby appears healthy, time should be taken to inform the family of the plan for care. A pediatrician, pediatric endocrinologist, and pediatric urologist should be consulted, and appropriate laboratory and radiologic studies should be ordered.

In addition to the standard newborn screen, blood should be collected to determine karyotype, and an ultrasound of the baby's abdomen and pelvis should be performed to determine the internal genital structures.

In less than 1 hour, the radiologist reports that the baby has a normal-appearing uterus with a gonad on either side of the uterus. A few hours later, the genetics laboratory reports that the baby has a 46,XX karyotype.

At this point, based on the presence of female internal genitalia and a female genotype (XX), the differential can be narrowed to only include causes of a virilized female. The causes include a defect in steroidogenesis (3β-HSD, 21-OHase,

(continues)

CASE FOLLOW-UP *(continued)*

or 11-OHase), an aromatase deficiency, or a maternal virilizing disorder. It is unlikely that the baby has an aromatase deficiency or that the mother has a virilizing disorder insofar as she denied using any medications during pregnancy, and she did not develop signs of virilization during her pregnancy. Therefore, the etiology is most likely a defect in steroidogenesis. Because 21-OHase is by far the most common cause of CAH, it is presumed to be the most likely cause.

An ACTH stimulation test is performed. Immediately after blood is sampled for baseline 17-hydroxyprogesterone and ACTH levels, cortrosyn is administered to the baby. Sixty minutes later, blood is sampled for an ACTH-stimulated 17-hydroxyprogesterone level. The results of the stimulation test are shown below:

Hormone	Baseline	Normal Baseline	60 Minutes	Normal 60 Minutes
ACTH (pg/mL)	320	10–60		
17-OH-Progesterone (µg/dL)	22,355	10–200	25,780	500–1,000

The levels confirm classic 21-OHase deficiency. With the impressive virilization and ambiguity, in addition to the elevated ACTH and 17-OH levels, the baby likely has the salt-wasting form. Most newborns do not experience significant electrolyte abnormalities until 10 to 21 days of life.

The family is informed of the diagnosis and introduced to clinicians from the endocrine, genetics, and surgical teams. Serum sodium, potassium, and glucose levels are collected and are all within normal limits. Hydrocortisone (three times a day) and fludrocortisone (twice a day) are started.

The baby is discharged from the hospital 2 days later, and the family is given appointments to see the geneticist to discuss the risk for recurrence in subsequent pregnancies; a pediatric endocrinologist to monitor electrolytes, hormone levels, and therapy; and a pediatric urologist to discuss the plan for performing a vaginoplasty and clitoroplasty.

REFERENCES and SUGGESTED READINGS

Auchus RJ, Chang AY. 46,XX DSD: the masculinised female. Best Prac Res Clin Endocrinol Metab. 2010;24(2):219–242.

Barrett, EJ. Chapter 50: Adrenal gland. In: Medical Physiology: A Cellular and Molecular Approach. Edited by Boron WF, Boulpaep EL. Philadelphia, PA: Saunders/Elsevier; 2009.

Carlson BM. Chapter 16: Urogenital system. In: Human Embryology and Developmental Biology. St. Louis, MO: Mosby; 2004.

Gardner DG, Shoback DM, Greenspan FS. Chapter 14: Disorders of sex determination and differentiation.

In: Greenspan's Basic & Clinical Endocrinology. New York, NY: McGraw-Hill Medical; 2007.

Houk CP, Lee PA. Approach to assigning gender in 46,XX congenital adrenal hyperplasia with male external genitalia: replacing dogmatism with pragmatism. J Clin Endocrinol Metab. 2010;95:4501–4508.

Hughes I. Disorders of sex development: a new definition and classification. Best Prac Res Clin Endocrinol Metab. 2008;22(1):119–134.

Maclaughlin DT, Donahoe PK. Sex determination and differentiation. N Engl J Med. 2004;350:367–378.

Mendonca, BB, Domenice S, Arnhold IP, Costa EF. 46,XY disorders of sex development (DSD). Clin Endocrinol. 2009;70(2):173–187.

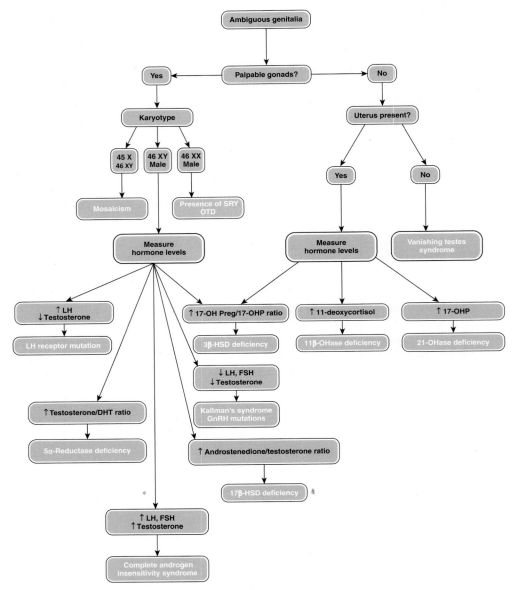

FIGURE 15-4. Algorithm for the approach to evaluating the newborn with symmetric ambiguous genitalia. OTD, ovotesticular disease; SRY, sex-determining region on the Y chromosome; FSH, follicle-stimulating hormone; LH, luteinizing hormone; 17-OHP, 17-hydroxyprogesterone; 17-OH Preg, 17-hydroxypregnenolone; 3β-HSD, 3β-hydroxysteroid dehydrogenase; 11β-OHase, 11β-hydroxylase; 21-OHase, 21-hydroxylase; FSH, follicle-stimulating hormone; DHT, dihydrotestosterone; 17β-HSD, 17β-hydroxysteroid dehydrogenase.

Rosler, A. Male Pseudohermaphroditism due to 17-beta-hydroxysteroid dehydrogenase deficiency: Studies on the natural history of the defect and effect of androgens on gender role. J Steroid Biochem. 1983; 19.1:663–674.

Saenger P. Turner's syndrome. N Engl J Med. 1996; 335(23):1749–1754.

Smyth CM, Bremner WJ. Klinefelter syndrome. Arch Intern Med. 1998;158(12):1309–1314.

Speiser PW, White PC. Congenital adrenal hyperplasia. N Engl J Med. 2003;349:776–788.

Stoler JM, Leach NT, Donahoe PK. Sex determination and differentiation. N Engl J Med. 2004;351: 2319–2326.

Williams RH, Wilson JD. Disorders of sex development. Williams Textbook of Endocrinology. 12th ed. Edited by Melmed S, Polonsky KS, Larsen PR, Kronenberg HM. Philadelphia, PA: Saunders; 2011:868–934.

CHAPTER REVIEW QUESTIONS

1. A 48-hour-old fetus is born with ambiguous genitalia. The newborn screening exam in your state reveals elevated 17-hydroxyprogesterone (17-OHP). What is the diagnosis?

   A. 3β-HSD deficiency
   B. 21-OHase deficiency
   C. 17α-OHase deficiency
   D. Turner syndrome
   E. 5α-Reductase deficiency

2. An infant is born with a small penis, hypospadias, a bifid scrotum, and a blind vaginal pouch. Hormonal analysis reveals elevated testosterone levels. Stimulation testing with hCG results in an increase in the ratio of testosterone to dihydrotestosterone (DHT). What is the diagnosis?

   A. 17,20 lyase deficiency
   B. 17β-HSD deficiency
   C. 5α-Reductase deficiency
   D. Leydig cell dysfunction
   E. Klinefelter syndrome

3. You are called to see a newborn with ambiguous genitalia. The baby's phallus is very small, the gonads are not palpable, and the scrotum is very small. The child also has a cleft lip and palate. What hormone profile would you expect?

	FSH	LH	Testosterone
A.	↑	↑	↑
B.	↑	↑	↓
C.	↓	↓	↑
D.	↓	↓	↓
E.	Normal	Normal	Normal

4. A 16-year-old female presents to your office because she has failed to have her first period despite full breast development and normal external female genitalia. She does not have pubic hair. On physical exam she has a blind vaginal pouch. There are palpable masses within the inguinal canals. Hormone analysis reveals extremely high levels of plasma testosterone. Chromosomal analysis reveals a 46,XY karyotype. What is the diagnosis?

   A. Turner syndrome
   B. Complete androgen insensitivity syndrome
   C. 5α-Reductase deficiency
   D. 17β-HSD deficiency
   E. 11β-OHase deficiency

5. What hormone profile would be expected in an individual with a 46,XX karyotype and ambiguous genitalia due to an 11β-hydroxylase deficiency?

	ACTH	Cortisol	Deoxycorticosterone	Testosterone
A.	↑	↓	↑	↑
B.	↓	↓	↑	↓
C.	↓	↑	↓	↓
D.	↓	↓	↓	↑
E.	↑	↓	↓	↑

CHAPTER REVIEW ANSWERS

1. The correct answer is B. 21-OHase deficiency is the most common cause of congenital adrenal hyperplasia (CAH) and ambiguous genitalia in the genetic female. This deficiency blocks synthesis of both cortisol and aldosterone while shunting substrate down the androgen pathway. Androgen excess masculinizes the female genitalia and a mineralocorticoid deficiency presents as a salt-wasting crisis early in life. Currently, all states include the measurement of the hormone, 17-OHP, which accumulates in 21-OHase deficiency, to their standard newborn screening protocol. This hormone level is chosen in particular because it is by far the most common cause of CAH and because in males, in whom the genitalia appears normal, the diagnosis would otherwise be missed until life-threatening salt wasting occurs in the first 2 weeks of life. Knowledge of the enzymes and hormones of the steroidogenesis pathway is required to correctly answer this question.

3β-HSD deficiency (**Choice A**) leads to accumulation of dehydroepiandrosterone (DHEA) and 17-OH pregnenolone and low production of 17-OHP. The low levels of androgen would not cause virilization of the external genitalia. 17α-OHase deficiency (**Choice C**) blocks production of 17-OHP; therefore, it would be low and not elevated. Turner syndrome (**Choice D**) is not due to a defect in steroidogenesis but to absence of an X chromosome and results in gonadal dysgenesis. These females have normal external female genitalia. 5α-Reductase (**Choice E**) converts testosterone to dihydrotestosterone (DHT). Individuals with this defect have a normal 17-OHP level.

2. The correct answer is C. 5α-Reductase (5α-R) is found in peripheral tissues and converts testosterone to dihydrotestosterone (DHT). DHT is critical for the development of external genitalia in the developing fetus. A deficiency in 5α-R results in the characteristic genitalia described in the question. Blocking the conversion of testosterone to DHT would elevate the testosterone level. Stimulation with hCG would further increase testosterone production and the ratio of testosterone to DHT.

17,20 lyase deficiency (**Choice A**) rarely occurs in isolation and usually exists with 17α-OHase deficiency since both enzymes are found on the same protein. Its deficiency blocks the entry of 17-OH steroids into the androgen pathway resulting in low levels of testosterone and DHT that do not respond to hCG stimulation. 17β-HSD deficiency (**Choice B**) blocks the conversion of androstenedione to testosterone. Leydig cells of the testis produce testosterone; therefore, Leydig cell dysfunction (**Choice D**) results in low levels of testosterone and a minimal response to hCG. Individuals with Klinefelter syndrome (**Choice E**) have a normal to hypoplastic male phallus and small testicles, which does not mimic the genital description in the question.

3. The correct answer is D. This baby has ambiguous genitalia that may be the result of being virilized (genetic female) or undervirilized (genetic male). The cleft lip and palate provides a clue that this child has a central midline defect and potentially has a problem with hormone production from the hypothalamus and/or anterior pituitary gland. Given that information, the baby is likely a genetic male with a deficiency in a central hormone. This deficiency results in an inability to stimulate testicular descent and testosterone production. Therefore, low gonadotropin levels (FSH and LH) lead to low testosterone production.

Elevated gonadotropins and testosterone (**Choice A**) would be expected in a child with precocious puberty but unlikely to be seen in a newborn. A baby with an abnormality of the testes but intact hypothalamic and pituitary gland hormones would have elevated gonadotropin levels and low testosterone (**Choice B**). A newborn with low gonadotropin levels and an elevated testosterone level (**Choice C**) likely has an adrenal, rather than testicular cause for an elevated testosterone level. The baby could be an overvirilized female due to congenital adrenal hyperplasia (CAH), but with the central findings of a midline defect, it is more likely that this baby is an undervirilized male. Normal gonadotropin levels with a normal testosterone level (**Choice E**) would not be likely in this child given the genital ambiguity.

4. The correct answer is B. Complete androgen insensitivity syndrome (CAIS) is caused by a dysfunctional androgen receptor. Without a functioning receptor, tissues are incapable of responding to circulating testosterone, which phenotypically results in an apparent lack of testosterone. The tissues cannot respond to testosterone. Therefore, without testosterone action, the male internal genitalia do not develop. Without testosterone (or its action), the hypothalamus, due to the absence of negative feedback, produces high levels of GnRH, FSH, and LH that act on the testes to further drive testosterone production. The extreme levels of testosterone are aromatized to estrogen in the periphery, which drive female secondary sexual characteristics (female breasts).

Girls with Turner syndrome (**Choice A**) may present with primary amenorrhea; however, these girls, due to ovarian dysgenesis from lack of an X chromosome, usually do not have significant breast development. In addition, these girls do not have elevated testosterone levels. The karyotype for these girls is not 46,XY but usually 45,XO. Individuals with 5α-reductase deficiency (**Choice C**) may have normal female genitalia at birth, but when they enter puberty, the increase in testosterone causes virilization of the external genitalia. The girl in this question has normal external female genitalia. 17β-HSD converts androstenedione to testosterone and a deficiency in 17β-HSD (**Choice D**) results in low levels of testosterone but would not have an effect on ovarian production of estrogen. A 46,XY individual with 11β-OHase deficiency (**Choice E**) would have normal male genitalia and no breast development. These individuals are hypertensive due to the accumulation of deoxycorticosterone.

5. The correct answer is A. 11β-OHase mediates conversion of deoxycorticosterone (DOC) to corticosterone and 11-deoxycortisol to cortisol. A deficiency of this enzyme leads to an accumulation of DOC, shunting of substrate down the androgen pathway (elevated testosterone), and a low serum cortisol. With low levels of cortisol, the HPA axis responds by increasing ACTH secretion. The expected hormonal profile consists of a low cortisol with compensatory elevation of ACTH, elevated testosterone from shunting, and elevated DOC insofar as it is just proximal to the enzymatic block.

Autoimmune Polyglandular Syndromes

16

Elicia D. Skelton
Kristina M. Cossen
Eric I. Felner

CASE

A 39-year-old woman presents to the emergency department complaining of fever, nausea, vomiting, abdominal pain, and near-syncope 4 hours earlier. Prior to the episode, she admits to 2 days of a nonproductive cough and nasal congestion. She took over-the-counter cold remedy treatment but did not improve. Over the past 3 months she has been tired and anorexic and has lost 10 lb. Her past medical history is significant for hypothyroidism for which she has taken levothyroxine since she was diagnosed at age 15 years. Until 2 months ago, when her thyroid function studies revealed a need for a higher dose of levothyroxine, she had been taking the same dose for the previous 5 years. Her family history is significant. Her sister has type 1 diabetes and her mother also has hypothyroidism. Her vital signs are: temperature, 98.1°F; respiratory rate, 12 breaths per minute; blood pressure (supine), 110/78 mmHg; pulse (supine), 80 beats per minute; blood pressure (standing), 84/55 mmHg; and pulse (standing), 105 beats per minute. On examination, she is thin and cachectic and appears older than her stated age. The only abnormal finding is hyperpigmentation of her gums and fingernails. Her chemistry profile is remarkable for a low serum sodium level (127 mEq/L), low serum chloride level (95 mEq/L), and elevated serum potassium level (5.9 mEq/L).

This chapter reviews the autoimmune polyglandular syndromes (APSs), which comprise endocrine and nonendocrine disorders. We give a brief overview of autoimmune physiology followed by a review of the pathophysiology of the two major types of APSs to help the learner develop hypotheses that explore the etiology and pathophysiology of this woman's condition. We advise reviewing autoimmune endocrine disorders discussed in earlier chapters. The chapter is organized by: 1) immune dysfunction; 2) characteristics; and 3) screening recommendations of these syndromes.

CHAPTER OUTLINE

Autoimmune Polyglandular Syndromes

Physiology: Immune System
  Central Tolerance
  Peripheral Tolerance

Physiology: Autoimmunity
  Human Leukocyte Antigen Genes
  Nonhuman Leukocyte Antigen Genes
  Environmental Triggers
  Faulty Apoptosis

(continues)

OBJECTIVES

1. Describe the factors that contribute to immunologically mediated endocrine conditions.

2. Describe the role of the autoimmune regulator protein in autoimmune disorders.

3. Compare and contrast the four types of autoimmune polyglandular syndromes.

4. Describe the evaluation and management of patients with a suspected autoimmune polyglandular syndrome.

AUTOIMMUNE POLYGLANDULAR SYNDROMES

Polyendocrine failure has been recognized for more than 150 years. In 1886, Oegle discovered a patient with both adrenocortical insufficiency and diabetes mellitus. The patient's adrenal insufficiency, however, was secondary to tuberculosis, not autoimmune destruction. In 1910, Parkinson had a patient with diabetes mellitus and pernicious anemia. A few years later, Schmidt had two patients with both adrenocortical insufficiency and lymphocytic thyroiditis (now known as *Schmidt syndrome*). Rowntree and Snell, in 1931, described several patients with adrenal insufficiency, Graves disease, and type 1 diabetes mellitus (T1D). Shortly thereafter, Gowen reported a patient with adrenal insufficiency, T1D, and Hashimoto thyroiditis. It was not until 1974 when Bottzaao and Doniach found islet cell autoantibodies in a patient with T1D, that an autoimmune process was considered. The term autoimmune polyglandular syndrome (APS) eventually evolved to describe a group of syndromes that involve both endocrine and nonendocrine autoimmune diseases. In 1980, Neufeld and Blizzard published an official classification scheme for these syndromes, identifying four types: APS 1 to 4. Despite their similar nomenclature, the pathogenesis, clinical presentation, and inheritance patterns of each type is very different.

PHYSIOLOGY: IMMUNE SYSTEM

Autoimmune disease is fairly common, affecting approximately 3% of the general population. Understanding the basics of the immune system is necessary for understanding autoimmune disorders. **Immune tolerance** is the ability to distinguish between self and nonself. If tolerance is present, the immune system does not mount a reaction against self-antigens. With a loss of tolerance, however, the immune system will attack self-antigens. The mechanisms that underlie normal immunologic tolerance occur at both central and peripheral levels and involve the T and B lymphocytes (T cells and B cells). **Central tolerance** is the mechanism by which newly developing T cells and B cells are rendered nonreactive to self-antigens. It is different than **peripheral tolerance** insofar as it occurs while the cells are still present in the primary lymphoid organs (thymus, T cells; bone marrow, B cells) and prior to their export into the periphery. Peripheral tolerance is generated after cells reach the periphery (Figure 16-1).

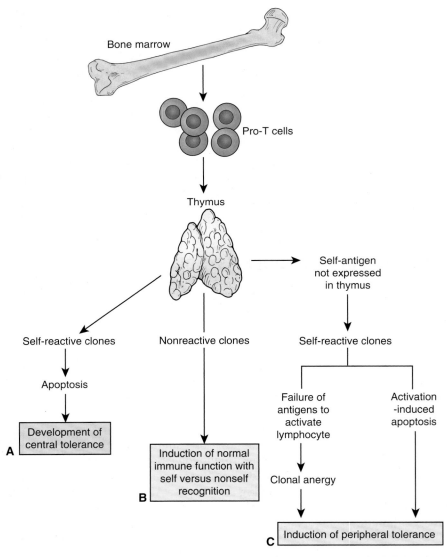

FIGURE 16-1. Development of immunologic tolerance. **(A)** Development of central tolerance with deletion of self-reactive T lymphocytes in the thymus. **(B)** Nonreactive lymphocytes with development of normal immune function. **(C)** Induction of peripheral tolerance in self-reactive cells that are not eliminated in the thymus. (From Pathology. 3rd ed. Philadelphia, PA: Lippincott-Rave; 102.)

Central Tolerance

In the thymus, immature T cells, whose role is to recognize nonself-antigens, randomly construct **T cell receptors (TCRs)** via gene rearrangements. These TCRs encounter self-antigens (within the thymus) and autologous antigens (from peripheral tissue) that are either brought to the thymus by **antigen-presenting cells (APCs)** or created in the thymus by the **autoimmune regulator (AIRE) protein**. Through negative selection, any T cells with self-reactive TCRs will be eliminated. The AIRE protein is crucial to the process of negative selection by eliminating autoreactive T cells that bind to antigens not traditionally found in the thymus, thereby reducing the threat of autoimmunity.

In the bone marrow, immature B cells undergo a similar process to that in the thymus, known as **receptor editing**. During this process, any B cell receptor that demonstrates a strong reaction against a self-antigen will be rearranged to create new receptors not specific for self-antigens. If receptor editing does not occur, the self-recognizing B cells are eliminated by the process of apoptosis.

Peripheral Tolerance

In the peripheral tissue, there are several mechanisms in place to silence any self-reactive T and/or B cells that have evaded central tolerance, including anergy, clonal deletion, and immunoregulation. **Anergy** involves the inactivation or immune unresponsiveness of lymphocytes following an antigen encounter under very specific conditions. For example, if the antigen is presented by a cell that does not have the necessary co-stimulatory molecule, then the T cell will be inactivated. **Clonal deletion** is a process by which B cells and T cells are deactivated after they have expressed receptors for self-antigens and before they develop into fully immunocompetent lymphocytes. **Immunoregulation** is the suppression of reaction against self-antigens by regulatory T cells. Regulatory T cells develop in response to recognition of self-antigens.

B cells also have an important role in deterring autoimmunity. Once the self-antigens have been recognized by T cells and APCs, the immune attack depends on B cells. These B cells create antibodies against the autoantigens that begin the self-perpetuating war of autoimmunity.

PHYSIOLOGY: AUTOIMMUNITY

Immune reactions against self-antigens may disrupt immune tolerance at any point in its pathway. Autoimmunity may be due to genetic, environmental, or apoptotic factors.

Human Leukocyte Antigen Genes

The *human leukocyte antigen (HLA)* gene complex, located on chromosome 6, encodes cell surface antigen-presenting proteins and plays a critical role in the regulation of immune tolerance and the ability of T cells to differentiate between self- and nonself-antigens. The *HLA* genes are the human versions of the *major histocompatibility complex (MHC)* genes that are found in most vertebrates. The major *HLA* genes are essential elements for immune function. These genes are divided into three classes (I, II, or III) with each class encoding a different function. HLAs corresponding to MHC class I present antigens from inside the cell. These antigens are peptides produced from digested proteins that are broken down in the proteasomes. They attract cytotoxic T cells that destroy cells. HLAs corresponding to MHC class II present antigens from outside the cell to T cells. These antigens stimulate the multiplication of T-helper cells that in turn stimulate B cells to produce antibodies to that specific antigen. HLAs corresponding to MHC class III encode components of the complement system.

Nonhuman Leukocyte Antigen Genes

A number of non-HLA genes are also vital to the maintenance of a normal immune response. Autoimmune diseases have been associated with defects in the *AIRE*, *cytotoxic T-lymphocyte antigen-4* (*CTLA4*), *forkhead box P3 of the fox protein family* (*FOXP3*), and *protein tyrosine phosphatase, nonreceptor type 22* (*PTPN22*) genes.

The *AIRE* gene is the primary non-HLA gene implicated in autoimmune diseases. It is mapped to chromosome 21q22.3 and consists of several domains that are important for transcription regulation. *AIRE* is predominantly expressed in the medullary thymic epithelial cells (mTECs) as well as bone marrow–derived dendritic cells. The protein from AIRE is a punctuate structure that is located in the nucleus of these mTECs. AIRE may regulate gene expression by coordinating and recruiting components of the transcription complex. The *AIRE* gene binds to several classes of molecules, including proteins involved in nuclear transport, chromatin binding, transcription, and pre-mRNA processing. The ability of *AIRE* to influence the expression of tissue-restricted antigens identifies mTECs as the primary mediators of central tolerance. *AIRE* expression can, therefore, be viewed as an epigenetic modifier of transcription. The loss of function of the *AIRE* gene is focused primarily at central tolerance mediators, specifically the negative selection process (Figure 16-2).

The CTLA4 is a molecule expressed on the surfaces of activated T cells. It allows for the modification of T cell activation and functions as a negative regulator of T cell activation. The FOXP3 is a transcription factor necessary for the maturation of regulatory

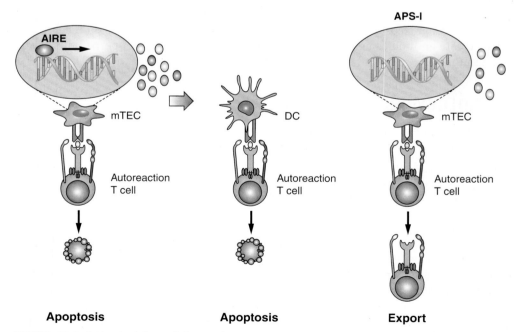

Apoptosis   **Apoptosis**   **Export**

FIGURE 16-2. Pathophysiology of the autoimmune regulator protein and its relationship to autoimmune polyglandular syndrome type 1. APS-1, autoimmune polyglandular syndrome type 1; AIRE, autoimmune regulator; mTEC, medullary thymic epithelial cell; DC, dendritic cell.

T cells. The PTPN22 is a lymphoid tyrosine phosphatase protein that is involved in regulatory inhibition of the TCR-signaling pathway.

Environmental Triggers

In addition to genetic predisposition, environmental factors play an equally important role in the pathogenesis of autoimmune diseases. Environmental factors produce their effect on the autoimmune response through molecular mimicry and bystander activation. With molecular mimicry, infectious agents with structural similarity to host antigens may trigger an immune response, not only to foreign antigens, but also to self-antigens. With bystander activation, the cytokines that are released during an inflammatory response (i.e., infectious agents and psychosocial factors) drive the recruitment of T cells that result in the activation of anergic T cells.

Faulty Apoptosis

Apoptosis, in which cells undergo self-destruction, is another crucial factor in regulation of the immune system. A defect in apoptosis permits autoreactive antibodies and faulty T cells to evade the regulatory mechanisms of destruction and increase the susceptibility to autoimmunity. The process of apoptosis involves the interaction between multiple enzymes and molecules, including DNAse-1 and caspase. DNase-1 is the nuclease responsible for DNA fragmentation, whereas caspase is a protease that is required for the maturation of lymphocytes.

AUTOANTIBODIES IN ORGAN-SPECIFIC AUTOIMMUNE DISEASES

The APSs comprise a variety of diseases involving immune attacks on organ-specific autoantigens. A variety of characteristic autoantibodies and autoantigens have been identified and subsequently linked to specific autoimmune diseases and APS types (Table 16-1). Although these autoantigens may aid in establishing the diagnosis, they do not explain the underlying pathophysiology of these syndromes.

Autoimmune Polyglandular Syndrome Type 1

The most common components of APS type 1 (APS-1) are mucocutaneous candidiasis, hypoparathyroidism, and primary adrenocortical insufficiency. In order to make the diagnosis, two of these three components must be present. APS-1 is also known as *Whitaker syndrome*, polyglandular autoimmune syndrome type 1, and autoimmune polyendocrine-candidiasis-ectodermal dystrophy.

Epidemiology

In the general US population, APS-1 is an extremely rare syndrome with an annual incidence of <1:100,000. It is inherited in an autosomal recessive fashion with a higher prevalence among Finish, Iranian, Jewish, and Sardinian populations. Males and females are equally affected.

Pathophysiology

APS-1 is a monogenic syndrome due to mutations in the *AIRE* gene. There are more than 60 mutations in the *AIRE* gene that can result in APS-1. These mutations tend to cluster

TABLE 16-1.	Autoimmune Polyglandular Syndrome Diseases and Autoantibodies	
Autoantibody	**Associated Disease**	**APS Type(s)**
21-Hydroxylase	Adrenocortical insufficiency	APS-1, APS-2
Tyrosine hydroxylase	Alopecia	APS-1–APS-3
P450 IID6; P450 IA2	Autoimmune hepatitis	APS-1
Tissue transglutaminase	Celiac disease	APS-1
Thyroid-stimulating hormone receptor	Graves disease	APS-2, APS-3
Thyroid peroxidase Thyroglobulin	Hashimoto thyroiditis Idiopathic myxedema	APS-2 APS-3
17-Hydroxylase P450 side-chain cleaving enzyme	Hypogonadism	APS-1
Calcium-sensing receptor	Hypoparathyroidism	APS-1
Intrinsic factor H^+-K^+ ATPase	Pernicious anemia Atrophic gastritis	APS-1 APS-3
Glutamic acid decarboxylase Tyrosine-phosphatase Islet cell Insulin	T1D	APS-1 APS-2 APS-3
Tyrosinase SOX9, SOX10	Vitiligo	APS-2 APS-3

around three regions of the gene that display a high degree of evolutionary conservation. Each mutation can lead to different phenotypes, even within families with similar mutations. The AIRE protein plays a critical role in preservation of central immune tolerance. This loss of central tolerance may result in the development of autoantibodies against the adrenal cortex, parathyroid glands, islet cells, parietal cells, intrinsic factor, liver, hair follicle keratinocytes, and melanocytes (see Table 16-1).

Despite the clear genetic link in this disease, genetics cannot explain the entire picture as evidenced by the approximately 6% of those affected without a genetic mutation. In addition, despite the discovery of many mutations in the *AIRE* gene, no clear genotype–phenotype link has been found. Among members of the same family with identical mutations, the clinical presentation is not always identical. This suggests that other factors, such as environmental triggers, may influence this syndrome.

Clinical Manifestations

APS-1 typically manifests during the first decade of life and only rarely after the second. Sixty percent of patients with APS-1 develop the classic triad of chronic mucocutaneous candidiasis, hypoparathyroidism, and adrenocortical insufficiency. Patients generally present with mucocutaneous candidiasis in infancy or early childhood. On average, hypoparathyroidism develops at age of 7 years and adrenocortical failure at

TABLE 16-2.	Classification of Autoimmune Polyglandular Syndrome Types 1 and 2	
	APS-1	**APS-2**
Diagnostic criteria	At least 2: • Mucocutaneous candidiasis (73–100%) • Hypoparathyroidism (77–89%) • Adrenocortical insufficiency (60–86%)	Adrenocortical insufficiency and at least 1: • AITD (70%) • T1D (41–52%)
Endocrine	• T1D (4–18%) • AITD (8–40%) • Ovarian failure (30–60%) • Testicular failure (7–17%)	• Ovarian failure (3–10%) • Testicular failure (5%)
Nonendocrine	• Ectodermal dysplasia (77%) • Pernicious anemia (12–15%) • Vitiligo (4–13%) • Alopecia (27%) • Hepatitis (10–15%)	• Pernicious anemia (2–25%) • Vitiligo (4–5%) • Alopecia (2%)

Notes: AITD, autoimmune thyroid disease; T1D, type 1 diabetes mellitus.

age 13 years. In a recent review on APS-1, by the fourth decade of life, 97% had chronic mucocutaneous candidiasis, 85% had hypoparathyroidism, and 78% had adrenocortical failure. In addition to these characteristic clinical features, there are minor endocrine and nonendocrine conditions associated with APS-1 (Table 16-2).

Major Endocrine Conditions

Hypoparathyroidism is usually the first endocrinopathy to manifest. Between 75% and 95% of patients with APS-1 have a component of hypoparathyroidism. Males develop hypoparathyroidism less frequently than do females and tend to present with symptoms at an older age. When this syndrome presents early in life, it is necessary to differentiate the autoimmune dysregulation from DiGeorge syndrome, in which affected children are born without functional parathyroid glands. The genetic mutation in DiGeorge syndrome can be detected by using fluorescence in situ hybridization. In those with autoimmune hypoparathyroidism, autoantibodies are detected in only 11% to 38%. Presenting symptoms can range from asymptomatic hypocalcemia to tetany and seizures. Sometimes symptoms can be precipitated by decreased calcium or increased phosphorous intake. To distinguish APS-1 from other causes of hypocalcemia, a low serum parathyroid hormone level with an elevated serum phosphate level is diagnostic for hypoparathyroidism. Hypocalcemia due to hypoparathyroidism is discussed in detail in Chapter 4.

Clinical adrenocortical insufficiency usually manifests during early adolescence. Autopsies from patients diagnosed with APS-1 reveal significant adrenal cortical abnormalities including severe fibrosis and atrophy. Deficiencies in cortisol and aldosterone can occur simultaneously or several years apart depending on the degree of autoimmune activity and organ damage. Autoantibodies to the cortex and steroid-producing cells can be detected in almost 100% of patients with adrenocortical insufficiency. These autoantibodies can be detected before overt disease occurs and are usually highest at diagnosis but decrease in subsequent years. Because adrenocortical insufficiency is rare in childhood, a child presenting with primary adrenocortical failure should raise the suspicion for APS. The diagnosis can be confirmed with a suboptimal cortisol response to cortrosyn (synthetic ACTH). The Cortrosyn test is performed in the early morning after an overnight fast with collection of baseline serum ACTH and cortisol levels immediately prior to the administration of Cortrosyn. Serum cortisol levels are measured 30 and 60 minutes after administration. A stimulated cortisol level ≥ 18 μg/dL indicates an appropriate glucocorticoid response. Stimulation tests used for the evaluation of adrenal insufficiency are described in detail in Chapter 21. Symptoms associated with primary adrenal failure include nausea, vomiting, fatigue, and postural dizziness. Signs include hyperpigmented lesions and hypotension. Laboratory tests reveal hypoglycemia, hyponatremia, hyperkalemia, and metabolic acidosis. Adrenocortical insufficiency is discussed in detail in Chapter 10.

Minor Endocrine Conditions

Hypergonadotrophic hypogonadism is a minor endocrine manifestation of APS-1 and is commonly present with adrenocortical failure. Approximately 20% to 60% of patients with APS-1 have primary hypogonadism and virtually all have autoantibodies to steroid-producing cells. The onset of gonadal failure usually occurs prior to the fifth decade of life. Women (30% to 60%) are affected more frequently than men (7% to 17%). Half of the APS-1 female patients who have primary hypogonadism present with primary amenorrhea. Laboratory tests reveal elevated serum follicle-stimulating hormone (FSH) and luteinizing hormone (LH) levels and low estrogen (female)/testosterone (male) levels.

T1D occurs in <12% of patients with APS-1. Autoantibodies to islet cells and glutamic acid decarboxylase are typically present in up to 30% of individuals without diabetes. These autoantibodies do not affect pancreatic function, but are markers of the inflammatory process within the pancreas. T1D is more common in APS-2.

Hashimoto thyroiditis is the most common form of thyroid disease in APS-1. Only 2% to 13% of patients with APS-1 have hypothyroidism, however, insofar as it is a more common component of APS-2.

In a very small percentage of patients with APS-1, pituitary failure may occur and present as deficiencies in growth hormone, gonadotropins, vasopressin, and adrenocorticotropic hormone (ACTH).

Nonendocrine Conditions

In addition to chronic mucocutaneous candidiasis, the other nonendocrine components of APS-1 are pernicious anemia, autoimmune hepatitis, ectodermal dysplasia, alopecia, and vitiligo.

Mucocutaneous candidiasis, a superficial infection due to **Candida albicans**, presents as the earliest manifestation of APS-1 and is the most frequent of the three major components. It affects 73% to 100% of patients and peaks in early childhood, where it is usually found on oral (most common), vaginal, and esophageal mucous membranes. It can occasionally occur on the nails. Less than 5% of the body surface is usually affected, and rarely do patients develop fungemia. Candidiasis may range from mild to severe. In the mild form, ulceration and soreness is present on the mucous membranes, whereas a severe infection involves the entire mouth. In the hyperplastic form, white plaques form on the mucous membranes. Squamous cell carcinoma is a severe complication and is usually of the atrophic form that results in the mucous membranes developing erythematous and leukoplakic areas.

Pernicious anemia is present in 12% of patients with APS-1, with a higher percentage in those with T1D. Macrocytic anemia results from autoantibodies directed at the H^+-K^+ ATPase pump or intrinsic factor. If untreated, these patients develop decreased absorption of vitamin B12. Patients with pernicious anemia may exhibit pallor, ataxia, glossitis, and an impaired vibratory sense.

Autoimmune hepatitis was originally believed to be a rare component of APS-1, but recent prevalence studies indicate that up to 15% of patients with APS-1 develop chronic autoimmune hepatitis after the second decade of life. Autoantibodies directed at liver smooth muscle and mitochondria have been detected. If this complication is not detected early, rapid deterioration from fulminant hepatic failure may develop.

Ectodermal dysplasia causes dental enamel hypoplasia that is not a result of hypocalcemia. The defect never involves the deciduous teeth. Evidence of some degree of ectodermal dystrophy is found in 40% to 75% of patients with APS-1.

Alopecia occurs in approximately 30% of these patients and is typically a late finding. Autoantibodies are directed at the keratinocytes of hair follicles. They may cause a loss of hair from anywhere on the body.

Vitiligo, the depigmentation of skin, occurs in approximately 10% of patients with APS-1. It usually occurs in either the first or second decade of life and is due to autoantibodies to both melanocytes and tyrosinase-related protein-2.

Diagnostic Studies

The clinical diagnosis of APS-1 is made when two of the three major clinical components of the syndrome are present. More than 10% of infants may develop a minor component prior to developing a major component. Therefore, infants and children who have vitiligo and/or alopecia should be closely monitored for the development of the other autoimmune processes associated with APS-1.

The diagnosis of candidiasis may be made by microscopic examination of skin or nails. Potential hormone deficiencies such as hypoparathyroidism, adrenocortical deficiency, T1D, hypothyroidism, or hypopituitarism should be evaluated according to the recommendations in the previous chapters.

In patients who have at least two of the major components of APS-1, or in children with some of the minor components, reactive autoantibodies interferon-ω and interferon-α_2 should be collected. If a thymoma and myasthenia gravis can be clinically ruled out, the presence of these autoantibodies confirms the diagnosis of APS-1. The presence of autoantibodies against specific glands or tissues that are known components of APS-1 is also diagnostic of APS-1.

Treatment

For chronic candidiasis, antifungal therapy should be administered. Oral candidiasis must be treated early because it can lead to esophageal strictures and oral and esophageal squamous cell carcinoma.

For the endocrine components of APS-1, the management involves appropriate hormone replacement therapy as well as monitoring. For more information on the treatment of these diseases, please refer to previous chapters.

The role of immunosuppressive therapy in APS-1 is a topic of current research, insofar as the benefits of immunosuppression are unclear. Treatment consists of managing the phenotypic manifestations and providing supportive therapy.

Follow-up and Screening

The presence of autoantibodies often precedes the clinical manifestations. Therefore, patients with clinical components of APS-1 should be routinely screened for the development of additional autoimmune diseases. In addition to genetic testing, it is recommended that these patients undergo screening for autoimmune diseases every 1 to 2 years until age 40 years. Patients with APS-1 need to follow up with an endocrinologist annually and be knowledgeable of the types of symptoms they may develop. Current and potential hormone deficiencies should be evaluated by monitoring the specific hormone levels.

Detection of *AIRE* gene mutations has also proved very useful in identifying those at risk for developing APS-1. In addition to caring for the affected patient, screening of relatives of individuals with APS-1 should be carried out.

Prognosis

Overall mortality has improved over recent years due to early treatment and appropriate screening for other autoimmune disorders. The course of the disease varies greatly from individual to individual given the number of organ systems involved and how the glandular abnormalities can be controlled. In a study of Finnish patients with APS-1, the major factor contributing to early demise was the lack of a social support system. Oral squamous cell carcinoma secondary to uncontrollable candidiasis and acute adrenal failure prior to diagnosis are also important factors related to mortality in patients with APS-1.

Autoimmune Polyglandular Syndrome Type 2

The most common components of the APS type 2 (APS-2) are adrenocortical insufficiency, autoimmune thyroid disease (AITD), and T1D. In order to make the diagnosis of APS-2, an individual must have adrenocortical insufficiency and either AITD (Schmidt syndrome) or T1D (Carpenter syndrome).

Epidemiology

APS-2 is a rare, polygenic, inherited disorder with a prevalence of 1:20,000 in the general US population. The annual incidence of APS-2 is up to 10- to 20-fold greater than that of APS-1. APS-2 has a 3:1 predilection for women over men and tends to manifest in the fourth or fifth decade of life. Its inheritance is autosomal dominant with incomplete penetration.

Pathophysiology

The tendency for APS-2 to occur within families suggests that genetic factors are fundamental to this syndrome, but environmental triggers play a role. Approximately one in seven relatives of individuals with APS-2 develops an autoimmune disease.

APS-2 is a polygenic disease, involving both HLA and non-HLA genes. The HLA haplotypes *HLA-AI*, *HLAB8*, *HLA-DR3*, and *HLA-DR4* are among those commonly involved. Mutations in a variety of these HLA genotypes are strongly associated with the development of adrenocortical insufficiency, T1D, and celiac disease and may explain the basis for the grouping of these conditions in APS-2 (see Table 16-2).

In addition to the HLA haplotypes, errors in the immune tolerance pathway, encoded by non-HLA genes, provide another pathogenetic mechanism. Non-HLA genes such as *MICA*, *PTPN22*, and *CTLA4* have been associated with various components of APS-2.

Clinical Manifestations

Clinically, APS-2 can be diagnosed if there is primary adrenocortical insufficiency and AITD (Hashimoto thyroiditis or Graves disease) or T1D. These three diseases are the major components of APS-2 with AITD more common (69% to 88%) than T1D (23% to 52%). The most classic combinations are adrenocortical insufficiency with Hashimoto thyroiditis (56%), adrenocortical insufficiency with Graves disease (21%), and adreno-cortical insufficiency with T1D (11%). Less common is a combination of all three. The prevalence of adrenocortical insufficiency with Hashimoto thyroiditis and T1D (10%) occurs more commonly than adrenocortical insufficiency with Graves disease and T1D (2%). Similar to APS-1, APS-2 has minor endocrine and nonendocrine components.

The onset of each autoimmune disease correlates with age. Vitiligo, T1D, and hyper-gonadotropic hypogonadism tend to appear before the fourth decade of life, whereas Graves disease, adrenocortical insufficiency, pernicious anemia, and alopecia tend to occur during the fourth decade. Hashimoto thyroiditis and chronic atrophic gastritis occur in the first half of the fifth decade, and autoimmune chronic hepatitis occurs between the fifth and sixth decade.

Major Endocrine Conditions

Primary adrenocortical insufficiency must be present in order to consider the diagnosis of APS-2. Fifty percent of patients with APS-2 have adrenocortical insufficiency as the presenting sign of the disease. The signs, symptoms, and biochemical findings are the same as in APS-1 and are discussed in detail in Chapter 10.

AITD manifests as hyper- or hypothyroid autoimmune disease, with Hashimoto thyroiditis more common than Graves disease. Thyroid autoimmune disease is fairly common in the general population, but only 1% of patients with Hashimoto thyroiditis develop adrenocortical insufficiency. Thyroid disease is discussed in detail in Chapter 3.

In T1D, individuals develop autoantibodies prior to the clinical onset of diabetes. Insu-lin autoantibodies are generally presented first, followed by glutamic acid decarboxylase (GAD65), and islet cell antibodies. T1D is discussed in detail in Chapter 7.

Minor Endocrine Conditions

Lymphocytic hypophysitis can lead to the empty sella syndrome, panhypopituitarism, or isolated failure of the anterior pituitary. Infiltration of lymphocytes in the pituitary gland leads to loss of pituitary function involving growth hormone, ACTH, thyroid-stimulating hormone (TSH), FSH, and LH. Pituitary disease is discussed in detail in Chapter 2.

As in APS-1, hypergonadotrophic hypogonadism is more common in women. It causes premature ovarian failure and secondary amenorrhea in women younger than 40 years of age. Testicular failure occurs in only 4% to 9% of men. Female and male reproductive disorders are discussed in detail in Chapters 12 and 13, respectively.

Nonendocrine Conditions

APS-2 is also associated with several minor clinical components: vitiligo (12%), alopecia (4%), chronic autoimmune hepatitis (3%), pernicious anemia (2%), arthritis (2%), and myasthenia gravis (1%).

Individuals with T1D and APS-2 are six times more likely to develop celiac disease; only 1% of the general population has celiac disease. Immunoglobulin A (IgA) auto-antibodies to endomysium and transglutaminase are sensitive and specific markers for celiac disease. IgA endomysium autoantibodies are almost 100% sensitive and specific for celiac disease. A small intestine biopsy showing crypt hyperplasia and increased intraepithelial lymphocytes confirms celiac disease. Common symptoms include diar-rhea, bloating, and skin rashes as well as failure to thrive.

Diagnosis

The diagnosis of APS-2 should be made clinically based on the endocrine and nonen-docrine criteria. Confirmation of the autoimmune nature of each component revolves around the presence of 21-hydroxylase antibodies. Because the presence of adrenocortical insufficiency is necessary for the diagnosis, these antibodies are typically present in patients with APS-2. Thyroid antibodies, such as antithyroid peroxidase (anti-TPO) and antithyroglobulin (anti-TG) are present in those with AITD. Insulin, GAD65, and islet cell antibodies are present in those with T1D.

Treatment

As with APS-1, treatment depends on which organs are involved. Replacement of any hormone deficiency requires hormone replacement therapy. Treatment of hypothyroidism may induce an adrenal crisis, insofar as hypothyroidism may mask adrenal insufficiency by extending the half-life of cortisol. Therefore, in all patients with hypothyroidism who have been diagnosed with or who are suspected of having APS-2, screening for adrenal insufficiency should be performed before initiating thyroid hormone replacement therapy. Also, a reduced insulin requirement in a patient with T1D may be an early sign of adrenal insufficiency. Specific treatment modalities for each of the endocrinopathies in patients with APS-2 are discussed in detail in the appropriate chapters.

Similar to APS-1, immunotherapies that suppress the body's autoimmune response are presently a fruitful area of research. Antigen-specific and nonspecific therapies are being used to treat patients with APS-2.

Follow-up and Screening

Patient education is essential in the management of APS-2. Emergency cards or bracelets should be given to all patients with APS-2. A patient with antibodies to 21-hydroxylase needs annual screening with a cortrosyn stimulation test to monitor for the development of adrenocortical insufficiency. In patients with T1D, even in the absence of APS-2, annual screening for the development of thyroid and celiac disease should be performed, insofar as their prevalence in patients with T1D is approximately 20% and 3%, respectively. These percentages are much higher than in the general population. Once the diagnosis of APS-2 is established, all first-degree relatives should be screened every 1 to 2 years for AITD and T1D until they reach their sixth decade of life. A screening scheme for a patient newly diagnosed with adrenal insufficiency is illustrated in Figure 16-3.

Prognosis

Patients with primary adrenal insufficiency have a mortality rate double that of the general population because of the chance of acute adrenal crises. The mortality rate is present regardless of the cause or association with other syndromes.

Other Autoimmune Polyglandular Syndromes

APS-1 and APS-2 are the major forms of APS, but two other forms, APS-3 and APS-4, have also been described. APS-3 is present when an individual with an autoimmune thyroid disorder develops a second autoimmune condition other than adrenocortical insufficiency or hypoparathyroidism. The second condition in APS-3 is usually T1D, atrophic gastritis, pernicious anemia, vitiligo, alopecia, or myasthenia gravis. Patients with APS-3 may later progress to APS-2 if they develop autoimmune adrenocortical insufficiency.

APS-4 is present when an individual develops two or more autoimmune conditions that cannot be classified as APS-1, APS-2, or APS-3. Examples include the combination of T1D and autoimmune growth hormone deficiency or adrenocortical insufficiency and celiac disease.

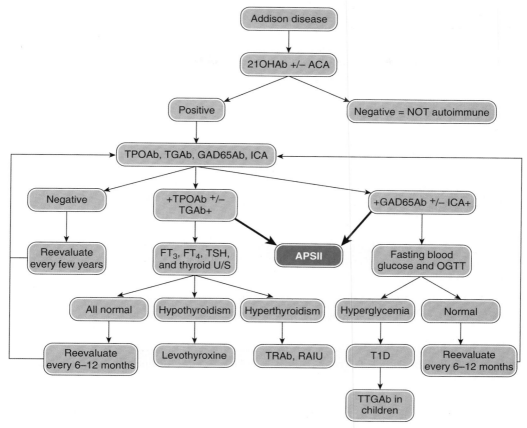

FIGURE 16-3. Screening scheme for autoimmune polyglandular syndrome type 2 after diagnosis of Addison disease. 21 OHAb, 21-hydroxylase antibody; ACA, adrenocortical antibody; TPOAb, thyroid peroxidase antibody; TGAb, thyroglobulin antibody; GAD65Ab, glutamate decarboxylase 65 antibody; ICA, islet cell antibody; FT_3, free triiodothyronine; FT_4, free thyroxine; TSH, thyroid-stimulating hormone; U/S, ultrasound; OGTT, oral glucose tolerance test; RAIU, radioactive iodine uptake; TRAb, thyrotropin receptor antibody; T1D, type 1 diabetes mellitus; TTGAb, transglutaminase antibody.

CASE FOLLOW-UP

A patient who presents with nausea, vomiting, and orthostatic hypotension coupled with the biochemical findings of hyponatremia, hypochloremia, and hyperkalemia most likely has adrenocortical insufficiency.

The treatment of our patient should include fluid replacement therapy with a bolus infusion of normal saline, maintenance fluid to improve hydration status, and corticosteroids to correct adrenocortical insufficiency. Her history of one autoimmune disease (Hashimoto thyroiditis) and family history of autoimmune endocrine diseases (T1D and Hashimoto thyroiditis) makes it extremely likely that she also has autoimmune adrenocortical insufficiency.

Her presentation with acute adrenal crisis was likely triggered by her recent infection manifested by cough and nasal congestion, and the recent increase in thyroid replacement therapy.

(continues)

CASE FOLLOW-UP *(continued)*

In addition to the emergent therapy, additional biochemical studies were collected in an attempt to confirm the diagnosis of adrenocortical insufficiency and to evaluate her thyroid function:

Serum cortisol	1.7 µg/dL (normal = 8 to 22)
Plasma ACTH	213 pg/mL (normal = 10 to 60)
Free thyroxine (FT$_4$)	1.3 ng/dL (normal = 0.9 to 1.4)
TSH	2.2 mIU/L (normal = 0.5 to 4.3)
21-Hydroxylase antibody	Positive

Although she did not present in the early morning when ACTH and cortisol levels peak, the fact that her plasma ACTH was much higher than normal and her serum cortisol was very low confirms the presence of primary adrenocortical failure. Her thyroid studies were within normal limits indicating that her levothyroxine dose was appropriate.

A few hours after receiving fluid replacement in the emergency department, her hydration status, heart rate, and blood pressure improved and she was admitted to the hospital. She was also given a stress dose of intravenous hydrocortisone (100 mg/m^2), and she was continued on oral hydrocortisone, every 6 hours, for the next 48 hours. She was discharged home 3 days after admission on oral hydrocortisone (three times a day) and oral fludrocortisone (once a day). She was also advised to continue the current dose of levothyroxine once a day.

She saw her endocrinologist every 3 months in order to monitor her adrenocortical insufficiency and hypothyroidism as well as to watch for the development of other autoimmune conditions. Adrenocortical insufficiency is best monitored by history, physical examination, and biochemical studies including electrolyte, glucose, ACTH, and plasma renin activity levels. Thyroid function is monitored using serum FT$_4$ and TSH levels. Surveillance for the development of other autoimmune conditions is best accomplished by a thorough history and physical examination.

Our patient developed adrenocortical insufficiency after being treated for hypothyroidism due to Hashimoto thyroiditis. The presence of these two autoimmune endocrinopathies is evidence for a diagnosis of APS-2. In addition to managing both adrenocortical insufficiency and hypothyroidism, her physicians must look for other autoimmune disorders, such as T1D, pernicious anemia, and ovarian failure that may develop in this syndrome.

Finally, although it appears that her mother and sister already have one endocrinopathy, their physicians must also realize that other autoimmune conditions, particularly adrenocortical insufficiency, may develop, insofar as failure to recognize it may prove lethal. Each family member should undergo adrenal function screening with collection of pre- and post-Cortrosyn cortisol levels and 21-hydroxylase autoantibody testing. Other family members, even those without an obvious autoimmune disorder should be evaluated and possibly screened for adrenocortical insufficiency, AITD, and T1D.

REFERENCES and SUGGESTED READINGS

Anderson MS. Update in endocrine autoimmunity. J Clin Endocrinol Metab. 2008;93:3663–3670.

Ballotti S, Chiarelli F, de Martino M. Autoimmunity: basic mechanisms and implications in endocrine diseases. Part 1. Horm Res. 2006;66(3):132–141.

Betterle C, Lazzarotto F, Presotto F. Autoimmune polyglandular syndrome Type 2: the tip of an iceberg? Clin Exp Immunol. 2004;137(2):225–233.

Chen QY, Kukreja A, Maclaren NK. Classification of the autoimmune polyglandular syndromes. In: Gill RG, Harmon JT, Maclaren NK, eds. Immunologically Mediated Endocrine Diseases. Philadelphia, PA: Lippincott Williams & Wilkins; 2002:167–187.

Dittmar M, Kahaly GJ. Genetics of the autoimmune polyglandular syndrome type 3 variant. Thyroid. 2010;20(7):737–743.

Eisenbarth GS, Gottlieb PA. Autoimmune polyendocrine syndromes. N Engl J Med. 2004;350(20):2068–2079.

Husebye ES Perheentupa J, Rautemaa R, Kampe O. Clinical manifestations and management of patients with autoimmune polyendocrine syndrome type I. J Intern Med. 2009;265(5):514–529.

Jaume JC. Endocrine autoimmunity. In: Gardner DG, Shoback D, eds. Greenspan's Basic & Clinical Endocrinology. 9th ed. New York, NY: McGraw-Hill; 2011:Chapter 2 (Online). http://www.accessmedicine.com/content.aspx?aID = 8400184. Accessed November 21, 2011.

Kahaly GJ. Polyglandular autoimmune syndromes. Euro J Endocrinol. 2009;161(1):11–20.

Kahaly GJ, Dittmar M. Autoimmune polyglandular syndrome type 2. In: Weetman AP, ed. Contemporary Endocrinology: Autoimmune Diseases in Endocrinology. Totowa, NJ: Humana Press; 2008:411–425.

Lankisch TO, Jaeckel E, Strassburg, CP. The autoimmune polyendocrinopathy-candidiasis-ectodermal dystrophy or autoimmune polyglandular syndrome type 1. Semin Liver Dis. 2009;29(3):307–314.

LeBoeuf N, Garg A, Worobec S. The autoimmune polyendocrinopathy-candidiasis-ectodermal dystrophy syndrome. Pediatr Dermatol. 2007;24:529–533.

Loyd RV. Polyglandular autoimmune diseases. In: Loyd RV, ed. Endocrine Pathology: Differential Diagnosis and Molecular Advances. 2nd ed. New York, NY: Springer Science+Business Media; 2010:Chapter 25.

Michels AW, Eisenbarth GS. Autoimmune polyendocrine syndrome type 1 (APS-1) as a model for understanding autoimmune polyendocrine syndrome type 2 (APS-2). J Intern Med. 2009;265:530–540.

Michels AW, Gottlieb PA. Autoimmune polyglandular syndromes. Nat Rev Endocrinol. 2010;6(5):270–277.

Perterson, P. Autoimmune polyglandular syndrome type 1. In: Weetman AP, ed. Contemporary Endocrinology: Autoimmune Diseases in Endocrinology. Totowa, NJ: Humana Press; 2008:393–410.

CHAPTER REVIEW QUESTIONS

1. A 16-year-old female patient has had T1D since age 7 years and has been stable on her current insulin regimen. She presents to the clinic with increasing fatigue, weight gain, constipation, and changes in her menses. Based on an elevated TSH level, low free T_4 level, and the presence of anti-TPO and anti-TG antibodies, you make the diagnosis of autoimmune hypothyroidism and start her on levothyroxine. A week later, she presents to the emergency center with hypotension and altered mental status. With the exception of low serum levels of glucose and sodium, and an elevated potassium level, all other biochemical parameters are within normal limits. Which is the most likely cause?

   A. She has not taken her insulin for the past 24 hours.
   B. She has not taken her levothyroxine in the past 3 days.
   C. She has acute liver failure.
   D. She has primary adrenal insufficiency.
   E. She has acute renal failure.

2. Which of the following statements regarding APS-1 and APS-2 is true?

   A. Individuals with APS-1 tend to present at a later age than patients with APS-2.
   B. Both APS-1 and APS-2 affect women at a significantly higher rate than men.

C. APS-1 is associated with hypoparathyroidism.

D. APS-2 is a monogenic syndrome.

E. Hypothyroidism occurs more commonly in APS-1 than in APS-2.

3. Which of the following screening tests should not be performed on patients recently diagnosed with primary adrenocortical insufficiency to assess for other autoimmune disorders?

A. Autoantibodies to the parathyroid glands

B. Serum calcium level

C. Thyroid function tests

D. Autoantibodies to insulin

E. Autoantibodies to TPO

4. For individuals affected by *AIRE* gene mutations, which of the following statements is true?

A. Individuals usually present with thyroid disease as the first endocrinopathy.

B. The inheritance pattern is autosomal dominant.

C. Mutations result in dysregulation of the negative selection of T cells in the thymus.

D. There is a higher prevalence in the Hispanic population.

E. The leading cause of mortality is systemic infection.

5. A 10-year-old boy is diagnosed with T1D. His mother is curious about the possibility that he will develop other autoimmune conditions. Of the following, which screening study should be collected within the following year?

A. *HLA-DR2*

B. Transglutaminase antibodies

C. Antibody to interferon-ω

D. 21-Hydoxylase autoantibody

E. Serum calcium level

CHAPTER REVIEW ANSWERS

1. The correct answer is D. The woman arrived at the emergency department in an adrenal crisis as evidenced by hypotension, altered mental status, and biochemical abnormalities. The administration of levothyroxine (thyroid hormone replacement therapy) in an individual with adrenal insufficiency may precipitate an adrenal crisis by stimulating increased metabolism of corticosteroids.

If she had not taken her insulin in the past 24 hours (**Choice A**), she would be hyperglycemic rather than hypoglycemic. Likewise, although not taking her levothyroxine for the past 3 days (**Choice B**) is not recommended, due to the long half-life of the medication, it is unlikely that she would develop significant symptomatology or biochemical abnormalities. Although autoimmune hepatitis is a nonendocrine autoimmune component of both APS-1 and APS-2, it is unlikely that she has liver failure (**Choice C**) given that her only abnormal biochemical findings include hypoglycemia, hyponatremia, and hyperkalemia. In addition, she would likely have abnormal liver function studies and physical findings such as jaundice and hepatomegaly. Acute renal failure (**Choice E**) is not a component of any type of APS and, given the abnormal biochemical findings, would be an unlikely cause of her presentation.

2. The correct answer is C. The major components of APS-1 are mucocutaneous candidiasis, hypoparathyroidism, and primary adrenocortical insufficiency. The major components of APS-2 are primary adrenocortical insufficiency and either autoimmune thyroid disease (AITD) or type 1 diabetes mellitus (T1D).

Individuals with APS-1 do not present at a later age than do those with APS-2 (**Choice A**). Individuals with APS-1 usually present in childhood or adolescence (before the third decade of life), whereas those with APS-2 are usually diagnosed between ages of 20 and 40 years (between the third and fifth decades of life). Both APS-1 and APS-2 do not affect females at a significantly higher rate than males (**Choice B**). APS-2 is three times more likely to occur in females, but in APS-1, males and females are equally affected. APS-2 is not a monogenic disease (**Choice D**) but, rather, a polygenic syndrome involving human leukocyte antigen (HLA) and non-HLA genes. APS-1, on the other hand, is a monogenic syndrome due to mutations in the *AIRE* gene. Hypothyroidism does not occur more commonly in APS-1 than in APS-2 (**Choice E**). In APS-1, hypothyroidism occurs in less than 15%, whereas in APS-2, it occurs in approximately 75%.

3. The correct answer is A. When an individual presents with isolated adrenocortical insufficiency, there should be a low threshold for screening for other autoimmune processes such as hypoparathyroidism, autoimmune thyroid disease (AITD), and type 1 diabetes mellitus (T1D). In some of the autoimmune endocrine diseases, collection of autoantibodies is useful, but in others, hormone levels are more reliable. Collection of autoantibodies to the parathyroid glands has very low sensitivity and specificity and therefore would not be useful for diagnosis or as a screening test for hypoparathyroidism, a major component of APS-1.

Collection of a serum calcium level (**Choice B**) would be useful in the evaluation for hypoparathyroidism. Collection of thyroid function tests (**Choice C**) is an appropriate screening modality for assessing thyroid function. Autoantibodies to thyroid peroxidase (TPO) (**Choice E**) and thyroglobulin (TG) are also acceptable screening markers for AITD. Collection of autoantibodies to insulin (**Choice D**) in addition to glutamate decarboxylase 65 (GAD65) and the islet cell are also acceptable screening tests for T1D.

4. The correct answer is C. The autoimmune regulator (AIRE) protein plays a critical role in preservation of central immune tolerance. This loss of central tolerance may result in the development of autoantibodies against the adrenal cortex, parathyroid glands, islet cells, parietal cells, intrinsic factor, liver, hair follicle keratinocytes, and melanocytes. A mutation in the gene results in APS-1 but does not appear to have a role in APS-2. Mutations in the *AIRE* gene result in dysregulation of the negative selection of T cells in the thymus.

Autoimmune thyroid disease (AITD) occurs rarely in APS-1 and therefore is unlikely to be the first endocrinopathy to present in an individual with a mutation of the *AIRE* gene (**Choice A**). APS-1, which results from a mutation in the *AIRE* gene, follows an autosomal recessive pattern, not a dominant pattern (**Choice B**). APS-1 is more prevalent in Finnish, Iranian, Jewish, and Sardinian populations but not in Hispanic populations (**Choice D**). Patient mortality is not due to systemic infections (**Choice E**) but, rather, to oral squamous cell carcinoma and adrenal crises.

5. The correct answer is B. Individuals with type 1 diabetes mellitus (T1D) are at an increased risk of other autoimmune disorders, especially autoimmune thyroid disease (AITD) and celiac disease. Approximately 15% to 30% of individuals with T1D develop AITD and 6% develop celiac disease. As the risk for developing celiac disease in those with T1D is six times greater than in the general population, collection of transglutamin-ase antibodies is an appropriate screening method in an individual with T1D.

Although T1D is associated with several human leukocyte antigen (HLA) genes such as *HLA-DR3* and *DR4*, *HLA-DR2* (**Choice A**) is a protective genotype from T1D and would not be an appropriate screening test. Antibodies to interferon-ω (**Choice C**) would only be appropriate if the patient had either hypoparathyroidism or primary adrenocortical insufficiency, insofar as interferon-ω is associated with APS-1. T1D is more likely to be associated with APS-2 rather than APS-1. Adrenocortical insufficiency occurs at only a slightly higher rate in those with T1D compared to the general population, and, therefore, collection of 21-hydroxylase antibodies (**Choice D**) would not be an appropriate screening test. Collection of serum calcium level (**Choice E**) is appropriate if the patient is at risk for hypoparathyroidism as in APS-1, but T1D is more likely to be associated with APS-2 rather than APS-1. Therefore, the measurement of a serum calcium level or other test to evaluate parathyroid function is not an appropriate screening test for APS-2 in an individual with T1D.

Multiple Endocrine Neoplasia Syndromes

17

Kristina M. Cossen
Eric I. Felner

CASE

A 28-year-old woman presents to the outpatient clinic with general malaise and diffuse aches and pains that began 2 months ago. For the past week, she has had abdominal pain with diarrhea that has not responded to over-the-counter medicines. She also complains of fatigue that has prevented her from doing her usual activities but attributes it to the stress of having three kids at home. She states that her clothes are fitting more loosely lately. Her past medical history is significant only for a tonsillectomy and adenoidectomy at age 8 years. She takes oral contraceptive pills for birth control. She has no drug allergies and has no history of illicit drug use. Her family history is significant. Her mother was diagnosed with hyperparathyroidism at age 29 years and recently was diagnosed with lung cancer. Both of her brothers have stomach ulcers and cutaneous lipomas. Her vital signs are normal. Physical examination reveals a diffusely tender abdomen with hyperactive bowel sounds.

Her chemistry profile reveals the presence of hypercalcemia (13.8 mg/dL), normal albumin (3.9 g/dL), and hypophosphatemia (1.7 mg/dL). An intact serum parathyroid hormone level is elevated (246 pg/mL). Thyroid studies are within normal limits.

This chapter reviews the main types of multiple endocrine neoplasias (MENs) to help the learner develop hypotheses that explore the etiology and pathophysiology of this patient's condition. We recommend reviewing the details of endocrine disorders discussed in earlier chapters. The organization of this chapter facilitates a review of the: 1) genetics, 2) clinical characteristics, 3) screening recommendations, and 4) treatment of MEN syndromes.

OBJECTIVES

1. Review the role of proto-oncogenes and tumor suppressor genes in the development of cancer.

2. Compare and contrast the three main types of MEN syndromes.

3. Describe the evaluation and management of patients with possible MEN syndromes.

CHAPTER OUTLINE

(continues)

MULTIPLE ENDOCRINE NEOPLASIA

Multiple endocrine neoplasia (MEN) syndromes are rare, inherited conditions in which several endocrine glands develop benign or malignant tumors or hyperplasia without forming tumors. They are classified into two broad categories: MEN type 1 (MEN 1) and MEN type 2 (MEN 2). The MEN 2 syndrome is further subcategorized into MEN 2A and MEN 2B. Understanding of the MEN syndromes has evolved through the following three phases: 1) descriptive phase to describe the clinical syndromes along with their genetic patterns, 2) screening phase to identify the syndromes to reduce morbidity and mortality, and 3) elucidation phase to determine the genetic and molecular basis of these syndromes.

Characteristics

The MEN syndromes share certain characteristics but have different mechanisms for tumor development. The similar characteristics between the syndromes include their cell type, histologic progression, development of hyperplasia, and mode of inheritance.

The tumor of all MEN syndromes is composed of one or more specific polypeptide- and biogenic amine-producing cell types known as the **amine precursor uptake and decarboxylation (APUD) cell**. The APUD cells are derived embryologically from the neural crest and are able to take up and metabolize tryptophan. The MEN syndromes also share a similar histologic progression from hyperplasia to adenoma, and occasionally, to carcinoma. The third similar characteristic between the MEN syndromes is that the development of hyperplasia is a multicentric process, with each tumor derived from a single clone. The last feature is that they all have an autosomal dominant inheritance pattern.

The syndromes have different mechanisms in tumorigenesis. Genetic alterations that cause neoplastic transformation fall into one of two categories: activating mutations of a proto-oncogene or loss of function of a tumor suppressor gene.

Proto-oncogenes

An **oncogene** is a gene that has the potential to cause cancer. In tumor cells they are often mutated or expressed at high levels. A **proto-oncogene** is a normal gene that can become an oncogene due to mutations or increased expression. Proto-oncogenes code for proteins that help regulate cell growth and differentiation. Through their protein products, proto-oncogenes are often involved in signal transduction and execution of mitogenic signals. Upon activation, a proto-oncogene (or its product) becomes a tumor-inducing agent, or an oncogene. This is the result of a relatively small modification of its original function. There are three basic scenarios in which proto-oncogenes become activated: 1) a mutation within a proto-oncogene causes a change in protein structure that increases protein activity and loss of regulation, 2) an increase in protein concentration, and 3) a chromosomal translocation.

Tumor Suppressor Genes

A **tumor suppressor gene**, or **anti-oncogene**, prevents tumor development, regulates cell division, and may cause cellular apoptosis if there is a gene mutation. The proteins for which tumor suppressor genes code have a dampening effect on the regulation of the cell cycle and/or promote apoptosis. Tumor suppressor genes generally follow the "two-hit" hypothesis in which both alleles that code for a particular protein must be affected before an effect is manifested. If only one allele for the gene is damaged, the second can still produce the correct protein. Inactivating mutations of tumor suppressor genes impair normal regulation of growth or cellular function. The regulatory functions lost are varied.

Multiple Endocrine Neoplasia Syndrome Type 1

The major clinical manifestations of MEN 1 are referred to as the "3 Ps": primary hyperparathyroidism, pancreatic and duodenal neuroendocrine tumors, and pituitary tumors. To confirm the diagnosis, two of these three major manifestations must be present. In individuals with known MEN 1 relatives, the presence of one major manifestation is diagnostic. Genetic testing confirms the clinical diagnosis.

Epidemiology

MEN 1, also known as **Wermer syndrome**, is inherited as an autosomal dominant disorder that has the potential to affect tumorigenesis in at least eight endocrine and nonendocrine tissues. The prevalence of MEN 1 is probably underestimated but is approximately 1 in 50,000. Expression of MEN 1 rarely occurs before the second decade of life; most often, the syndrome presents between the third and fifth decades of life. There is no gender predilection. Penetrance for MEN 1 is nearly 100% by the sixth decade of life, but there is no association between the affected individual's genotype and phenotype.

Pathophysiology

Genetic factors play a major role in the development of MEN 1, but up to 15% of cases occur sporadically in individuals without a family history. MEN 1 is caused by a mutation in the tumor suppressor gene found on chromosome 11q13. The MEN 1 gene encodes a nuclear protein referred to as **menin**. Overexpression of menin in animal models leads to increased apoptosis and inhibits proliferation. A lack of menin leads to reduced apoptosis.

Menin functions as a DNA-binding nuclear protein and regulates transcription, division, and proliferation. Menin also interacts with histone proteins involved in DNA structure and transcription, causing deacetylation by a specific histone methyltransferase that represses transcription. When this function cannot be performed by menin, the histones remain acetylated and DNA is left unwound for unregulated transcription.

There are approximately 500 mutations of the menin protein. In the presence of a mutated *menin* gene, there is neoplastic clonal expansion of cells with increased chromosomal breakage. Without menin, apoptosis is dysfunctional within these mutated cells.

Clinical Manifestations

The clinical manifestations of MEN 1 include major endocrine, minor endocrine, and nonendocrine associations.

Major Endocrine Associations

The most common endocrine conditions include pituitary adenomas, pancreatic endocrine tumors, and parathyroid adenomas. Individuals with MEN 1 share the clinical presentation and biochemical findings of individuals who develop these neoplasms sporadically. The most common tumor of MEN 1 is a parathyroid adenoma, with approximately 90% of patients developing hyperparathyroidism by the third decade of life. This is a few years earlier than the average onset for sporadic hyperparathyroidism. Of all the cases of hyperparathyroidism, less than 5% are due to a mutation of the *menin* gene.

The islet cell neoplasm is the second most common endocrine tumor, and approximately 50% of individuals develop at least one of the pancreatic/duodenal neuroendocrine tumors. Individuals with MEN 1 usually develop symptoms of the islet cell/duodenal neuroendocrine tumors by the fifth decade of life. The tumors are multicentric, consisting of both micro- and macroadenomas. They can be invasive and even metastatic at the time of diagnosis. Similar to the parathyroid adenoma of MEN 1, the neoplastic islet cells are secretory and may secrete chromogranin A or B, pancreatic polypeptide, glucagon, insulin, proinsulin, somatostatin, gastrin, vasoactive intestinal peptide (VIP), serotonin, calcitonin, growth hormone–releasing factor, or neurotensin. Gastrinomas are the most common islet cell neoplasms. They occur in up to 40% of individuals with MEN 1 and approximately 75% are malignant at diagnosis. In contrast to the parathyroid adenoma, up to 25% of individuals with a gastrinoma have a mutation of the *menin* gene. Most gastrinomas are located in the so-called gastrinoma triangle with its three borders: 1) the confluence of the cystic and common bile duct, 2) the junction of the second and third portions of the duodenum, and 3) the junction of the neck and body of the pancreas. Individuals with gastrinomas may present with severe diarrhea and may develop gastric ulcers. Gastrinomas usually develop after the parathyroid adenoma but may actually be the result of the parathyroid adenoma. Although the exact mechanism is not known, prolonged periods of hypercalcemia may elevate gastrin levels and may contribute to the development of a gastrinoma or peptic ulcer disease. If the hypercalcemia is treated with a parathyroidectomy, the development of a gastrinoma or symptoms related to elevated gastrin levels can potentially be diminished.

Pituitary adenomas occur less frequently (~35%) than primary hyperparathyroidism or pancreatic/duodenal neuroendocrine tumors. Individuals with MEN 1 usually develop symptoms of pituitary adenomas by the end of the fourth decade of life. Most of these pituitary tumors are macroadenomas with prolactinomas accounting for approximately 60% of them.

Minor Endocrine Associations

Five to ten percent of individuals with MEN 1 develop carcinoid tumors during their lifetime. They originate from the foregut and secrete serotonin. The most common symptoms of carcinoid syndrome include flushing, diarrhea, cramping, edema, and wheezing. Excess serotonin may also cause heart valvular lesions and arthritis. Most of the symptoms are not specific and may result in delayed diagnosis. The three most common types of carcinoid tumors are thymic, bronchial, and type II gastric entoerchromaffin-like tumor. Females are more likely to develop bronchial carcinoids and males, thymic carcinoids. The thymic carcinoid is frequently aggressive and carries a poor prognosis. Approximately 30% of individuals with MEN 1 develop adrenal lesions and tumors, but most of these lesions are nonfunctional.

Nonendocrine Associations

Cutaneous and visceral lipomas are present in approximately 30% of individuals with MEN 1, as compared to only 6% in the general population. Cutaneous manifestations may be helpful in identifying those individuals, or their asymptomatic family members, who should also be screened for MEN 1. Collagenomas are due to overgrowth of collagenous tissue and appear as cutaneous nodules usually on the upper torso with a symmetrical arrangement.

Diagnostic Studies

The essential diagnostic studies for MEN 1 are both genetic and biochemical testing. Genetic testing for a *menin* gene mutation is the most accurate method for diagnosis of MEN 1. The genetic test, however, is only 90% sensitive for most of the known mutations; therefore, if a *menin* gene mutation is not discovered, biochemical testing for the major conditions associated with MEN 1 should be performed.

The diagnostic studies ordered should relate to the symptoms the individual is experiencing. Biochemical and imaging studies can be performed on the three most common endocrine conditions associated with MEN 1.

In patients with hyperparathyroidism due to parathyroid adenomas, serum calcium and parathyroid hormone (PTH) levels should be measured. In those with elevated serum calcium and PTH levels, a technetium sestamibi scan can determine the presence of parathyroid tumor(s). Hyperparathyroidism is discussed in detail in Chapter 5.

Pancreatic and pituitary tumors should be considered based on clinical presentation. Biochemical studies should be performed prior to the imaging studies. For pancreatic/duodenal neoplasms, biochemical studies should reveal the following:

- Gastrinoma—Elevated serum gastrin,
- Insulinoma—Low serum glucose with inappropriately normal or elevated serum insulin and C-peptide levels,
- Glucagonoma—Elevated serum glucagon level,
- VIPoma—Elevated serum VIP level,
- Somatostatinoma—Elevated serum somatostatin level, and
- Carcinoid tumor—Elevated serum serotonin level.

If these biochemical studies indicate an elevated hormone level, imaging studies, such as an abdominal or endoscopic ultrasound, computed tomography (CT), magnetic resonance image (MRI), or an octreotide scan, can be performed to localize the neoplasm. For gastrinomas, elevated serum gastrin levels may require other biochemical studies such as basal acid output and secretin-stimulated gastrin levels prior to performing imaging studies.

For the two most common pituitary adenomas, the biochemical studies include

- Prolactinoma—Elevated serum prolactin level and
- Acromegaly—Elevated insulin-like growth factor (IGF)-1 and growth hormone levels.

Once the biochemical studies have confirmed an elevated pituitary or target organ hormone level, an MRI of the pituitary gland should be performed to localize the tumor. Hypo- and hyperfunctioning pituitary tumors are discussed in detail in Chapter 2.

Treatment

Despite the fact that individuals with a *menin* gene mutation will develop MEN 1, and those individuals with MEN 1 will develop neoplasms, it is not possible to predict what types of neoplasms an individual will develop. Prophylactic resections, therefore, are not performed. Individuals with an identifiable macroscopic tumor should be treated as if highly malignant with surgical removal. Individuals with hyperparathyroidism should undergo a subtotal parathyroidectomy.

Individuals with prolactinomas and most patients with small gastrinomas (<2.5 cm) may be managed medically. Dopamine receptor agonists (e.g., bromocriptine or cabergoline) can be used to treat prolactinomas. Small gastrinomas should be treated with proton-pump inhibitors (e.g., omeprazole). Only 16% of individuals undergoing surgical resection for a gastrinoma are disease free a year later, and only 6% are disease free 5 years after surgery. Due to the increased risk of malignancy, large gastrinomas (>2.5 cm) should be removed surgically. Surgical treatment of endocrine conditions is discussed in detail in Chapter 21.

Individuals with MEN 1 should be evaluated at least semi-annually to monitor their current problems as well as screened for potential ones.

Follow-up and Screening

A cost-effective screening schedule for MEN 1 is shown in Table 17-1. Those individuals with MEN 1 or at increased risk for MEN 1 include:

- Age <30 years with at least one MEN 1–associated tumor,
- Presence of ≥2 MEN 1–associated tumors, and
- Any first-degree relative of an individual with MEN 1.

For those individuals meeting the screening criteria above, screening studies should begin at the following ages and continue throughout their lifetime:

- Age 5 years—Annual pituitary neoplasm testing (serum prolactin and IGF-1 levels) and insulinoma testing (serum glucose, insulin, and C-peptide levels),
- Age 8 years—Annual parathyroid testing (serum calcium and PTH levels),
- Age 20 years—Annual pancreatic neoplasm testing (serum gastrin, chromogranin A, insulin, C-peptide, and glucagon levels) and imaging for foregut carcinoids.

Prognosis

The prognosis for individuals with MEN 1 has improved over the past decade due to more accurate testing methods and frequent screening for affected individuals and their relatives. The most common cause of death is from a malignant endocrine neoplasm or a carcinoid tumor. For the various phenotypes of MEN 1, a lack of effective screening previously contributed to mortality. Mortality due to hyperparathyroidism

TABLE 17-1.	MEN Screening and Follow-up After Establishment of a Positive Gene Carrier Status	
Syndrome	**Test**	**Frequency**
MEN 1	Serum calcium[a]	Every 3–5 y
	Serum prolactin	Every 3–5 y
	Serum gastrin	Every 3–5 y
	Imaging of pituitary[b]	Every 5–10 y
MEN 2A	Serum calcitonin	Every 1–2 y, then every 5 y
	Urine epinephrine and norepinephrine[c]	Yearly
	Serum calcium[a]	Every 2 y
MEN 2B	Serum calcitonin	Every 1–2 y, then every 5 y
	Urine epinephrine and norepinephrine[c]	Yearly

[a]This could be either a serum ionized calcium or an albumin-adjusted serum calcium.
[b]Pituitary imaging studies are controversial, especially if anterior pituitary hormone levels are normal.
[c]Urine epinephrine and norepinephrine levels should be collected as a 12-hour or 24-hour specimen.

and gastrinomas has decreased due to the use of aggressive metabolic and surgical management.

Identification of individuals who are at risk for developing MEN 1 is extremely important. The time of onset of tumor symptoms to diagnosis for each specific neoplasm associated with MEN 1, is the most important determinant for prognosis.

Multiple Endocrine Neoplasia Syndrome Type 2

The MEN 2 syndrome is divided into two subgroups: MEN 2A (75%) and MEN 2B (25%). The differences lie in the type of *RET* (REarranged during Transfection) proto-oncogene mutation and the clinical manifestations. The prevalence of MEN 2 is 1 per 30,000 people. The endocrine disorders that are similar in MEN 2A and MEN 2B are medullary carcinoma of the thyroid gland (MTC) and pheochromocytoma. The differences between the two syndromes include parathyroid tumors (MEN 2A only) and the nonendocrine manifestations. The epidemiology, pathophysiology, and clinical manifestations of MEN 2A and MEN 2B will be discussed separately, and the diagnostic studies, treatment, follow-up, and prognosis of MEN 2 will follow.

MEN Type 2A

MEN 2A is also known as **Sipple syndrome**.

Epidemiology

MEN 2A is inherited as an autosomal dominant condition that usually presents at the end of the second decade of life. There is no predilection for gender.

Pathophysiology

The *RET* proto-oncogene encodes a receptor tyrosine kinase for members of the glial cell line–derived neurotrophic factor family of extracellular signaling molecules. It is a 1,100 amino acid protein found near the centromere at chromosome 10q11.2 and is expressed in cells derived from neurocrest cells; thyroid C cells; adrenal medulla, and sympathetic, parasympathetic, and enteric ganglia. Loss-of-function mutations of the *RET* proto-oncogene are associated with the development of Hirschprung disease, whereas gain-of-function mutations are associated with various tumors including MTC, pheochromocytoma, and parathyroid hyperplasia. Activating point mutations in *RET* can give rise to MEN 2 that has three subtypes based on the clinical presentation: MEN 2A, MEN 2B, and **familial MTC (FMTC)**. There is a high degree of correlation between the position of the point mutation and the phenotype of the disease (Figure 17-1). Over 50 different mutations have been identified in the *RET* proto-oncogene.

The *RET* mutation that gives rise to MEN 2A is within the extracellular cysteine-rich domain of the protein. The most common mutation is a cysteine residue at codon 634 (exon 11), which is present in 85% of MEN 2A patients. Ninety-five percent of MEN 2A patients have an identifiable mutation in the *RET*. Only 5% of patients have a *de novo* mutation.

Clinical Manifestations

The primary endocrine clinical manifestations of MEN 2A include MTC, pheochromocytomas, and parathyroid tumors.

Endocrine Associations

Over 90% of all individuals with MEN 2A will develop MTC, which is usually the first endocrine manifestation, occurring in the third decade of life. Individuals with sporadic FMTC usually present in the fifth decade of life. Of all cases of MTC, 25% are due to a *RET* mutation and a manifestation of MEN 2. MTC is caused by the calcitonin-producing parafollicular cells (C cells). The C cells originate from neural crest cells that migrate to

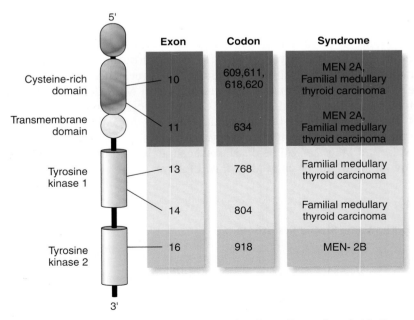

	Exon	Codon	Syndrome
Cysteine-rich domain	10	609,611, 618,620	MEN 2A, Familial medullary thyroid carcinoma
Transmembrane domain	11	634	MEN 2A, Familial medullary thyroid carcinoma
Tyrosine kinase 1	13	768	Familial medullary thyroid carcinoma
	14	804	Familial medullary thyroid carcinoma
Tyrosine kinase 2	16	918	MEN- 2B

FIGURE 17-1. *RET* proto-oncogene mutations in MEN 2. (Image from Rubin E, Farber JL. Pathology. 3rd ed. Philadelphia, PA: Lippincott Williams & Wilkins; 1999.)

branchial pouches and are separated from the thyroid interstitium by the follicular basal lamina. The growth begins with C-cell hyperplasia that eventually leads to a neoplasm. FMTC is typically multicentric and its histology in individuals with MEN 2 is indistinguishable from those with sporadic disease. Individuals with MTC usually present with neck pain and a palpable neck mass. They may also experience diarrhea, likely due to excessive calcitonin secretion. Serum calcitonin levels are elevated, but thyroid function studies are usually normal.

Pheochromocytomas are neuroendocrine tumors of the adrenal medulla or extra-adrenal chromaffin tissue that failed to involute after birth. They develop in approximately 50% of individuals with MEN 2A and secrete excessive amounts of catecholamines (i.e., norepinephrine and epinephrine). Most are bilateral and rarely are malignant. Pheochromocytomas in MEN 2 present similarly to those in individuals with the sporadic form. Individuals with pheochromocytomas present with symptoms of sympathetic nervous system hyperactivity and include palpitations, anxiety, diaphoresis, headaches, pallor, and weight loss. The characteristic signs of a pheochromocytoma are headache, tachycardia, and hypertension. For individuals with MEN 2, 65% of pheochromocytomas occur bilaterally, but each adrenal gland can develop a pheochromocytoma independently of the other. Only 3% of pheochromocytomas are malignant, and only 3% are extra-adrenal. In contrast to pheochromocytomas due to MEN 2, sporadic pheochromocytomas are less likely to occur bilaterally (10%), are more commonly malignant (10%), and are more likely to be extra-adrenal (15%). There are no histologic markers to distinguish it from the sporadic type.

Multiglandular parathyroid tumors occur in only approximately 25% of individuals with MEN 2A. The mutation in codon 634 has a higher incidence of parathyroid tumors than other mutations associated with MEN 2A. The hyperparathyroidism that occurs in individuals with MEN 2A is usually due to bilateral tumors, whereas sporadic hyperparathyroidism is more commonly unilateral. Hyperparathyroidism and hypercalcemia is discussed in detail in Chapter 5.

Nonendocrine Associations

Individuals with MEN 2A can develop nonendocrine conditions, such as pruritic cutaneous lichen amyloidosis and Hirschsprung disease. Pruritic cutaneous lichen amyloidosis is an erythematous, pruritic rash that develops on the upper portion of the back. It develops prior to MTC and is virtually pathognomonic for MEN 2A. Only individuals with MEN 2A who have a *RET* mutation at codon 634 develop pruritic cutaneous lichen amyloidosis.

Individuals with a loss-of-function *RET* mutation of exon 10 (codons 609, 611, 618, and 620) have a 10% to 15% risk of developing Hirschsprung disease. Hirschsprung disease is due to the congenital absence of the autonomic ganglia of the colon. The absence of the ganglia occurs because neurocrest cells fail to migrate into the intestine during embryogenesis. Symptoms are typically present in the newborn period and include constipation and obstipation. Imaging studies confirm colonic dilation and megacolon. Usually the ganglia are absent from only a small portion of the sigmoid colon, but, occasionally, the entire colon is affected. In the general population, Hirschsprung disease affects 1 in 5,000 live births.

Multiple Endocrine Neoplasia Type 2B

Individuals with MEN 2B differ from those with MEN 2A in their lack of development of parathyroid tumors and their Marfan syndrome–like appearance and mucosal neuromas.

Epidemiology

MEN 2B is also inherited in an autosomal dominant fashion and presents during the first decade of life. As in MEN 2A, there is no predilection for gender.

Pathophysiology

The *RET* mutation for MEN 2B is found in the intracellular tyrosine kinase domain. The most common mutation is found at codon 918, comprising 95% of mutations. Individuals with a codon 918 mutation develop pheochromocytomas. In cases of MEN 2B, 98% have an identifiable *RET* mutation, whereas 50% of individuals have de novo mutations.

Clinical Manifestations

The primary endocrine clinical manifestations of MEN 2B include MTC and pheochromocytomas.

Endocrine Associations

Most individuals with MEN 2B are similar in age at presentation (third decade of life) to those with MEN 2A. Most individuals (90%) with MEN 2B develop MTC that is similar to MEN 2A. Unlike MEN 2A, individuals with MEN 2B are usually younger and have a much more aggressive form of MTC.

The pheochromocytomas that develop in individuals with MEN 2B are similar in location (65% bilateral adrenal gland and 3% extra-adrenal) and risk for malignancy (low, 3%) to the pheochromocytomas that occur in individuals with MEN 2A.

Nonendocrine Associations

The most obvious clinical characteristic that differentiates individuals with MEN 2B from those with MEN 2A is the presence of a Marfan syndrome–like appearance associated with mucosal neuromas and ganglioneuromatosis. Individuals with MEN 2B are lanky, have decreased subcutaneous fat, and have increased joint laxity. Mucosal neuromas are present on the tongue, lips, and eyelids (Figure 17-2). The tongue is bumpy,

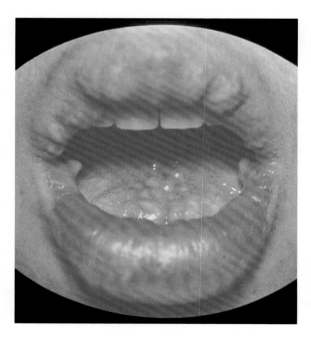

FIGURE 17-2. Mucosal Neuromas in a patient with MEN 2B. Multiple neuromas thicken the lips. (From Gold DH, Weingeist TA. Color Atlas of the Eye in Systemic Disease. Baltimore, MD: Lippincott Williams & Wilkins; 2001.)

lips are enlarged, and eyelids are everted. Ganglioneuromas are found throughout the gastrointestinal tract and can cause obstipation, constipation, diarrhea, and abdominal distension.

Diagnostic Studies

The laboratory tests used for the diagnosis of MEN 2 include genetic, biochemical, imaging, and histologic studies. Individuals with dermatologic features, such as cutaneous lichen amyloidosis or mucosal neuromas, should have skin biopsies of the affected areas. The most accurate method for establishing the diagnosis of MEN 2 is with genetic testing for a *RET* proto-oncogene mutation.

Nongenetic studies include biochemical, imaging, and histologic studies that relate to MTC, pheochromocytoma, and parathyroid tumors.

The diagnostic test for MTC is measurement of serum calcium and calcitonin levels. Depending on the stage of the thyroid cancer, calcitonin levels may be normal (less aggressive stage) or elevated (more aggressive stage). Ultrasonography, CT, and MRI of the neck are performed to localize a suspected tumor. A biopsy of the thyroid gland and/ or adjacent lymph nodes should be performed and the specimen stained with a calcitonin and carcinoembryogenic antigen (CEA). The presence of a positive stain with either of these antigens is diagnostic for MTC (Figure 17-3).

The diagnosis of a pheochromocytoma can be established by measuring serum and 24-hour urine catecholamines (epinephrine, norepinephrine) and metanephrines (epinephrine metabolites). Once the presence of elevated catecholamines and metanephrines is established, the lesion(s) can be localized with a CT or MRI of the head, neck, chest, and abdomen. A scintigraphic method to provide additional information in localizing the lesion is an I-123-marked metaiodobenzylguanidine (MIBG) scan (Figure 17-4). In this scan, a guanethidine analog that resembles norepinephrine is taken up by sympathomimetic tissues by a noradrenergic transport system, and then actively transferred into catecholamine storage vesicles. When these vesicles are present in sufficient amounts, scintigraphic images from the distribution of MIBG can be detected. The MIBG scan has a sensitivity of

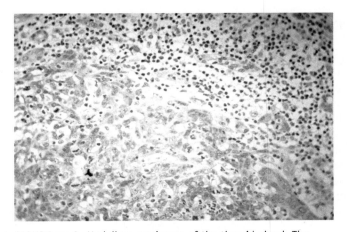

FIGURE 17-3. Medullary carcinoma of the thyroid gland. The malignant cells are pleomorphic and grow in solid sheets, forming a blunt margin. There is no gland formation. Numerous mitoses are present. The tumor is surrounded by a dense lymphocytic infiltrate. (Image from Rubin E, Farber JL. Pathology. 3rd ed. Philadelphia, PA: Lippincott Williams & Wilkins; 1999.)

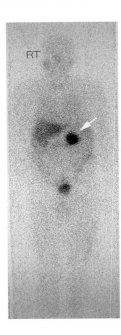

FIGURE 17-4. Metaiodobenzylguanidine scan of a patient with a pheochromocytoma. The metaiodobenzylguanidine (MIBG) scan shows the location of the pheochromocytoma and its relationship to surrounding structures. (From Mulholland MW, Lillemore KD, Doherty GM, et al. Greenfield's Surgery Scientific Principles and Practice. 4th ed. Philadelphia, PA: Lippincott Williams & Wilkins; 2006.)

77% to 90% and specificity of 88% to 99% for localizing a pheochromocytoma. Thus, it is superior in specificity to other radiologic studies; however, it is not a sensitive enough test to exclude a pheochromocytoma. Any individual with a pheochromocytoma and an elevated serum calcitonin level warrants testing for a mutation of the *RET* proto-oncogene.

Treatment

At the time an individual is diagnosed with a *RET* proto-oncogene mutation, or once the diagnosis of MTC is made, she/he should undergo an extracapsular total thyroidectomy with lymph node dissection. Unlike papillary and follicular thyroid cancer, radioablative therapy is not a therapeutic option because C cells are unable to take up iodine. An individual with a *RET* mutation should undergo surgery as soon as possible, regardless of the calcitonin level, to prevent development or progression of the thyroid cancer. There are four reasons for this approach: 1) early treatment drastically reduces mortality; 2) surgery is well tolerated in infants and young adults; 3) calcitonin is a good marker for disease and recurrence of disease but, has up to a 10% false-positive rate for MTC; and 4) the *RET* genetic test is highly sensitive with a low rate of false-negative and false-positive tests.

The current therapy for treatment of a pheochromocytoma in a patient with MEN is a unilateral cortex-sparing adrenalectomy and total contralateral adrenalectomy in an attempt to preserve some adrenal function. Surgeons previously performed bilateral adrenalectomies, but, with improved surgical techniques, the sparing procedure provides a low risk for developing a recurrence and eliminates the need for lifelong glucocorticoid and mineralocorticoid replacement therapy. Prior to performing a thyroidectomy for MTC, evaluation for a pheochromocytoma must be done because a pheochromocytoma must be operated on first to prevent the unopposed catecholamine surge that occurs after the thyroid gland is removed.

The treatment for hyperparathyroidism due to parathyroid tumors is the same as for individuals with MEN 1 described earlier in this chapter.

Tyrosine kinase inhibitor therapies (sunitinibmalate, sorafenib tosylate, ZD 6474, and imatinib) are currently in development. They are direct *RET* mutation agonists and should be excellent medical treatment for MEN 2.

Follow-up and Screening

MEN 2 is one of the few genetic disorders in which genetic testing of infants can significantly reduce morbidity and mortality. Individuals who require screening include those with: 1) an MTC or two or more MEN 2 endocrine tumors, 2) one MEN 2–associated tumor and age <30 years, 3) mucosal neuromas or somatic features that are unique to MEN 2B, and 4) a first-degree relative with MEN 2. All first-degree relatives should be tested before age of 5 years. An algorithm for screening and follow-up for individuals and relatives of individuals with MEN 2 is shown in Figure 17-5.

Once diagnosed, the individual will need collection of laboratory studies several times a year. Biochemical tests should be obtained every 3 to 6 months. These tests include thyroid function tests (TSH and free T_4), MTC monitoring (calcitonin), parathyroid monitoring (serum calcium and PTH), and pheochromocytoma monitoring (urine and plasma catecholamines and metanephrines). Imaging tests should be performed one to two times a year and should include an ultrasound of the neck and abdomen; CT or MRI of neck and abdomen; or, when a pheochromocytoma is suspected, a MIBG scan.

After a total thyroidectomy for MTC, the individual should continue to be tested for serum calcitonin level and the presence of CEA. Calcitonin is extremely useful because it is almost entirely produced by C cells of the thyroid, and the calcitonin levels rise significantly when MTC is present. After successful removal of the gland, the calcitonin level drops significantly to almost undetectable levels. Calcitonin levels are typically only elevated during states of sepsis and inflammatory states. Calcitonin secretion by C cells can be stimulated by calcium and pentagastrin. Previously these agents were used for the diagnosis of MTC, but the side effects of diarrhea, vomiting, flushing, and abdominal cramps and the presence of false-positive and false-negative tests decreased their efficacy. The stimulation tests are now only used if persistent or recurrent MTC is suspected.

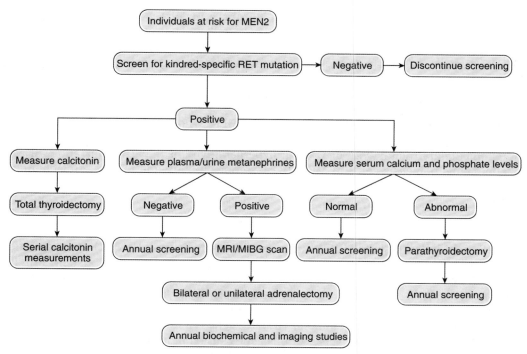

FIGURE 17-5. MEN 2 screening and follow-up. MEN 2 - multiple endocrine neoplasia type 2; MRI, magnetic-resonance image; MIBG, I-123-marked metaiodobenzylguanidine.

If an individual has undergone the cortex-sparing adrenalectomy, he/she will still require follow-up for the potential recurrence of a pheochromocytoma. All of these individuals should have an adrenocorticotropic hormone–stimulation test postoperatively to assess for adrenal insufficiency.

Relatives of affected individuals should be screened for the *RET* mutation. If they do not have a *RET* mutation, they will not require lifelong screening tests. A cost-effective screening schedule for MEN 2 is shown in Table 17-1.

Prognosis

The leading cause of mortality for individuals with MEN 2 syndromes is related to MTC. Around 15% to 25% of these individuals will succumb to MTC because of the high chance of metastasis: 80% to central cervical lymph nodes, 75% to the ipsilateral jugular lymph nodes, and 47% to the contralateral lymph nodes. Metastatic MTC 10-year survival rate, however, is 40% to 50% because the tumor can be slow growing. Lymph node dissection has improved survival rates. The mean survival from diagnosis of MTC is 28 years with the age of onset being a strong predictor of outcomes. The risk of mortality from MTC increases 5.2% every year.

Patients following cortical-sparing adrenalectomy for pheochromocytomas have a 66% chance of becoming steroid dependent, and 10% will have recurrence of their disease. Fortunately, death from pheochromocytomas has decreased in recent years because of medical treatment, but these individuals are still at risk for life-threatening adrenal insufficiency after successful surgery.

After a subtotal parathyroidectomy, 5% to 10% of MEN 2A patients will have persistently elevated PTH levels, and 10% to 20% will become hypoparathyroid.

Multiple Endocrine Neoplasia of Mixed Type

Hereditary MEN syndromes that do not fit the MEN 1 or MEN 2 categorization fall into four major categories: 1) overlap syndromes, 2) familial occurrence of an unusual combination of endocrine organ neoplasias that does not fit MEN 1 or MEN 2, 3) MEN 1 or MEN 2 variants, and 4) syndromes that do not fit into any clear pattern.

Overlap Syndromes

As the name implies, individuals with overlap MEN syndromes have features of both MEN 1 and MEN 2. In single patients, carcinoid and either MEN 1 or MEN 2, pituitary and adrenomedullary tumors with or without hyperparathyroidism, gastrinoma and MEN 2, adenomatous polyposis coli and MEN 2B, posterior pituitary and MEN 1, prolactinoma and MEN 2A, and a pheochromocytoma and MEN 1, have been reported.

Familial Occurrence of Two or More Endocrine Neoplastic Disorders

Von Hippel-Lindau disease (VHL) and **neurofibromatosis type 1 (NF 1)** are neoplastic syndromes that not only affect the nervous system but also the endocrine system. VHL is characterized by the presence of hemangioblastomas of the central nervous system, retinal angiomas, renal cell carcinomas, visceral cysts, pheochromocytomas, and islet cell tumors. About 25% to 35% of these individuals have unilateral or bilateral pheochromocytomas and 15% to 20% have islet cell tumors. The *VHL* gene is a tumor suppressor gene so that inactivating mutations of both alleles of this gene cause tumor formation.

NF 1 is associated with pheochromocytoma, hyperparathyroidism, somatostatin-producing carcinoid tumors, MTC, and hypothalamic or optic nerve tumors that cause precocious puberty.

Multiple Endocrine Neoplasia 1 or 2 Variants

MEN 1 kindred have been recognized in which prolactinoma, insulinoma, or acromegaly is the predominate manifestation. It is unclear whether these disorders are MEN 1 variants or the result of another molecular abnormality.

Well-defined variants of MEN 2A include FMTC and familial pheochromocytoma. The majority of families with FMTC have mutations in the *RET* proto-oncogene, although there is considerable overlap with MEN 2A (see Figure 17-1).

Multiple Endocrine Neoplasia Syndromes without a Clear Pattern

Carney complex is characterized by myxomas, spotty pigmentation, and generalized endocrine overactivity transmitted as an autosomal dominant trait. Patients with this disorder have myxomas of the heart, skin, and breast; spotty pigmentation; testicular, adrenal, and pituitary tumors; and peripheral nerve schwannomas.

CASE FOLLOW-UP

The laboratory test results together with her history make primary hyperparathyroidism the most likely cause of her symptoms. Given her family history (hyperparathyroidism, likely bronchial carcinoid, and symptoms consistent with a gastrinoma) and the complaints of diarrhea, a fasting gastrin level (400 pg/mL; normal = 0 to 200) is collected and noted to be elevated. An endoscopic ultrasound is performed and reveals four microadenomas (<2.5 cm) in her duodenum.

The elevated serum calcium level is a result of her elevated serum PTH level due to adenomas or hyperplastic parathyroid glands. The elevated gastrin level is consistent with peptic ulcer disease, diarrhea, and multiple gastrinomas.

MEN 1 is the most likely diagnosis. She is started on a proton-pump inhibitor and admitted for subtotal parathyroidectomy. Surgery is carried out without complications, and 3.5 parathyroid glands are removed. During surgery, her PTH levels were monitored 5, 10, and 15 minutes after parathyroid gland removal. The levels were 101, 12, and 11 pg/mL, respectively, indicating a successful operation. These intraoperative PTH levels are consistent with hyperparathyroidism that responds appropriately to a parathyroidectomy, as her PTH levels dropped to the normal range within 10 minutes after parathyroid gland removal.

She remained in the hospital for 4 days to monitor and control her serum calcium and phosphate levels.

A month after the operation, her repeat gastrin level (25 pg/mL) is in the normal range. A repeat endoscopic ultrasound shows a decrease in size of each of the gastrinomas.

Due to the above findings and family history, our patient was screened and found to have a mutation in the *menin* gene, confirming MEN 1. Her first-degree relatives now must be tested for the mutation as well. She is followed annually by an endocrinologist. The following tests are performed each year to look for recurrence of hyperparathyroidism, gastrinomas, and/or development of new areas of neoplasia: 1) serum calcium and PTH levels; 2) serum gastrin level; 3) serum chromogranin A, glucose, insulin, and glucagon levels; 4) serum prolactin and IGF-1 levels; and 5) CT imaging for foregut carcinoids.

REFERENCES and SUGGESTED READINGS

Akerstrom G, Stalberg P. Surgical management of MEN-1 and -2: state of the art. Surg Clin North Am. 2009;89(5):1047–1068.

Almeida MQ, Stratakis CA. Solid tumors associated with multiple endocrine neoplasias. Cancer Genet Cytogenet. 2010;203:30–36.

Brandi ML, Gagel RF, Angeli A, et al. Guidelines for diagnosis and therapy of MEN type 1 and type 2. J Clin Endocrinol Metab. 2001;86(12):5658–5671.

Burgess J. How should the patient with multiple endocrine neoplasia type 1 (MEN 1) be followed? Clin Endocrinol. 2010;72:13–16.

Callender GG, Rich TA, Ferrier ND. Multiple endocrine neoplasia syndromes. Surg Clin North Am. 2008;88:863–895.

Dreijerink KMA, Lips CJM, Timmers HTM. Multiple endocrine neoplasia type 1: a chromatin writer's block. J Intern Med. 2009;266:53–59.

Falchetti A, Marini F, Luzi E, Tonelli F, Brandt ML. Multiple endocrine neoplasms. Best Pract Res Clini Rheumatol. 2008;22(1):149–163.

Fendrich V, Langer P, Waldmann J, Bartsch DK, Rothmund M. Management of sporadic and multiple endocrine neoplasia type 1 gastrinomas. Brit J Surg. 2007;94:1331–1341.

Frank-Raue K, Raue F. Multiple endocrine neoplasia type 2 (MEN 2). Euro J Cancer. 2009;45(supp 1):267–273.

Lakhani VT, You YN, Wells SA. The multiple endocrine neoplasia syndromes. Ann Rev Med. 2007;58:253–265.

Mensah-Osman EJ, Veniaminova NA, Merchant JL. Menin and JunD regulated gastrin gene expression through proximal DNA elements. Am J Physiol Gastrointest Liver Physiol. 2011;301(5):G783–G790.

Moore SW, Zaahl SW. Multiple endocrine neoplasia syndromes, children, Hirschsprung's disease and RET. Pediatr Surg Inter. 2008;24:521–530.

Piecha G, Chudek J, Wiecek A. Multiple endocrine neoplasia type 1. Euro J Intern Med. 2008;19:99–103.

Raue F, Frank-Rue K. Update multiple endocrine neoplasia type 2. Fam Cancer. 2010;9:449–457.

Rubinstein WS. Endocrine cancer predisposition syndromes: hereditary paraganglioma, multiple endocrine neoplasia type 1, multiple endocrine neoplasia type 2, and hereditary thyroid cancer. Hematol Oncol Clin North Am. 2010;24(5):907–937.

Spiegel AM. Focus on hereditary endocrine neoplasia. Cancer Cell. 2004;6:327–332.

Thakker RV. Multiple endocrine neoplasia. Medicine. 2009;37(9):450–453.

Thakker RV. Multiple endocrine neoplasia type 1 (MEN1). Best Pract Res Clin Endocrinol Metab. 2010;24:355–370.

Waguespack SG, Rich TA, Perrier ND, Jimenez C, Cote GJ. Management of medullary thyroid carcinoma and MEN2 syndromes in childhood. Nat Rev. 2011;7:596–607.

Westphal SA. Diagnosis of a pheochromocytoma. Am J Med Sci. 2005;329(1):18–21.

White ML, Doherty GM. Multiple endocrine neoplasia. Surg Oncol Clin North Am. 2008;17:439–459.

Wohllk N, Schweizer H, Erlic Z, Schmid KW, Walz MK, Raue F, et al. Multiple endocrine neoplasia type 2. Best Pract Res Clin Endocrinol Metab. 2010;24:371–387.

Wu T, Hua X. Menin represses tumorigenesis via repressing cell proliferation. Am J Cancer Res. 2011;1(6):726–739.

CHAPTER REVIEW QUESTIONS

1. A 9-year-old boy presents to his pediatrician for his yearly checkup. He is in good health. Family history includes a diagnosis of MEN 1 with a *menin* gene mutation found by screening his 35-year-old mother, after she was diagnosed with MEN 1. His vital signs and physical examination are normal. Which of the following tests are recommended at this time?

    A. Abdominal CT to evaluate for a carcinoid tumor

    B. Urine collection for metanephrines

    C. Serum basal prolactin for pituitary testing

    D. Endoscopic ultrasound to evaluate his pancreas

    E. DNA analysis for a *RET* proto-oncogene mutation

2. Which of the following statements about islet cell neoplasms in MEN 1 is true?

    A. Twenty-five percent of all gastrinomas can be linked to MEN 1.

    B. Hypercalcemia does not stimulate the production of gastrin.

    C. Insulinomas are most commonly malignant.

D. Islet cell neoplasms are found in <20% of MEN 1 cases.

E. Islet cell neoplasms are generally small and localized when diagnosed.

---

3. All of the following statements about MEN syndromes are true *except*:

A. MEN 2 is due to a mutation in a proto-oncogene.

B. MEN 1 is due to a mutation in a tumor suppressor gene.

C. Prophylactic parathyroidectomy is recommended for all patients with MEN 1.

D. Pheochromocytomas can present in patients with MEN 2, but not in MEN 1.

E. Hyperparathyroidism is not a component of MEN 2B.

---

4. Regarding screening for MEN 2, which of the following statements is true?

A. Serum calcitonin levels do not need to be monitored after thyroidectomy for MTC.

B. Medullary carcinoma of the thyroid can be treated effectively with radiation.

C. The specific *RET* mutation is indicative of the phenotype of the patient.

D. Cortex-sparing adrenalectomies do not require annual pheochromocytoma screening.

E. Fasting glucose and insulin levels should be monitored yearly.

---

5. In regards to treatment of patients with MEN 1, which of the following statements is true?

A. Surgery is not indicated for macroscopic pancreatic tumors.

B. Pancreatic surgery is indicated in patients diagnosed with MEN 1 to prevent malignancies.

C. All pituitary adenomas require transsphenoidectomies to prevent mass effect.

D. Gastrinomas are generally treated medically, unless >2.5 cm.

E. Gastrinomas are successfully removed by surgery 70% of the time.

CHAPTER REVIEW ANSWERS

---

1. The correct answer is C. This young patient has a known *menin* mutation. Screening is of critical importance in these young patients. In an individual older than age 8 years, screening for MEN 1 should include: 1) annual pituitary testing with basal prolactin and IGF-1 levels, 2) annual testing for insulinoma with fasting glucose and insulin levels, and 3) annual parathyroid testing with ionized calcium and parathyroid hormone tests. Periodic MRI for pituitary adenomas can also be considered. All first-degree relatives of both the mother and her son should be screened for a mutation of the *menin* gene.

An abdominal CT to evaluate for a carcinoid tumor (**Choice A**) is not an appropriate screening test for this patient because of his young age. Since carcinoid tumors usually do not occur in children, screening is not necessary until the patient reaches his/her third decade of life. Urine collection for metanephrines (**Choice B**) screens for a pheochromocytoma that is a component of MEN 2. Endoscopic ultrasound to evaluate his pancreas (**Choice D**) screens for and localizes pancreatic neoplasms that usually do not develop until after the third decade of life. In addition, an abdominal ultrasound would not be obtained until after biochemical tests confirm an insulinoma or gastrinoma. DNA analysis for a mutation of the *RET* proto-oncogene (**Choice E**) is used to screen for MEN 2.

---

2. The correct answer is A. It has been estimated that 25% of all gastrinomas are found in patients with MEN 1, and 40% of patients with MEN 1 will develop a gastrinoma.

There is a definite link between gastrinomas and hyperparathyroidism; 90% of patients with MEN 1 have hyperparathyroidism and all will have elevated levels of calcium. The elevated calcium induces gastrin secretion from gastrinomas (**Choice B**). If hypercalcemia is treated, the symptoms and rapid progression of gastrinomas is reduced. Insulinomas are most likely to be benign (**Choice C**). Patients with MEN 1 have a 30% to 75% chance of developing an islet cell tumor (**Choice D**) and an additional 5% will have an islet cell neoplasm at autopsy. Islet cell neoplasms associated with MEN 1 are multicentric, consist of macroadenomas and microadenomas, and are not small and localized (**Choice E**). The most common place to find the neoplasms is in the duodenum.

---

3. The correct answer is C. Because there is no established relationship between the genotype of MEN 1 and the phenotype, prophylactic parathyroidectomy is not performed. However, in MEN 2, since medullary carcinoma of the thyroid is a very aggressive cancer, prophylactic thyroidectomy is part of the standard of care.

RET, the protein mutated in MEN 2, is a proto-oncogene (**Choice A**). Menin, the protein mutated in MEN 1, is a tumor suppressor gene (**Choice B**). Pheochromocytomas are the major endocrine tumors in MEN 2A and MEN 2B, but are not found in patients with MEN 1 (**Choice D**). Parathyroid adenomas are the major endocrine tumors in MEN 1 and MEN 2A, but are absent from the MEN 2B syndrome (**Choice E**).

---

4. The correct answer is C. Unlike *menin* mutations, *RET* mutations provide insight into a patient's phenotype. Such examples are *RET* exon 10, which is associated with Hirschsprung disease and codon 634 and its association with hyperparathyroidism.

Calcitonin is an excellent marker for MTC recurrence. It is almost solely produced by C cells of the thyroid; therefore, calcitonin levels should be undetectable after a thyroidectomy. A patient with MTC will have significantly elevated calcitonin levels. If calcitonin levels are measureable after thyroidectomy, then MTC cells are still present. Calcitonin levels should be monitored every 6 to 12 months after thyroidectomy for the presence of MTC. Therefore, not monitoring calcitonin levels after surgery for MTC (**Choice A**) is an incorrect choice. Surgery is the only effective therapy for MTC; radiation therapy is not a method of treatment (**Choice B**). The C cells do not absorb iodine; therefore, MTC is not effectively treated with radiation therapy as are papillary or follicular thyroid cancer. Patients with a cortex-sparing adrenalectomy must be screened for pheochromocytomas and monitored for adrenal function to assess the need for steroid replacement therapy (**Choice D**). Fasting glucose and insulin levels (**Choice E**) are not used to screen for MEN 2 but, rather, for MEN 1.

---

5. The correct answer is D. The success rate for gastrinoma surgery is <20%. Therefore, most small gastrinomas (<2.5 cm) are treated medically. Surgery is reserved for larger gastrinomas (>2.5 cm) because, the larger the gastrinoma, the more likely it is malignant.

Macroscopic tumors are more likely to be malignant and, therefore, should be treated surgically (**Choice A**). The phenotype of a patient with MEN 1 cannot be predetermined by genotype or by family history. Having a mutation of the *menin* gene does not determine which neoplastic endocrine condition an individual will develop. Therefore, prophylactic surgery, at any age (**Choice B**), should not be undertaken. Microscopic adenomas can be managed medically and not by transsphenoidectomy (**Choice C**). Surgical intervention is required when there is a mass effect or a macroadenoma. Gastrinoma surgery only has a 16% success rate, not a 70% success rate (**Choice E**). Therefore, medical management is the treatment of choice for gastrinomas <2.5 cm.

Endocrine Assays

18

Steven C. Kim
Milton R. Brown

CASE

A healthy 10-year-old female presents to the clinic with her mother, who is concerned that her child is short for her age. The child states she gets made fun of at school because of her height, but otherwise does well in school and has had a "normal" childhood. In the physician's office her vital signs are as follows: heart rate 85 beats per minute, blood pressure in both arms 135/86 mmHg, respiratory rate 16, and temperature 37.0°C. The patient's height is 4 ft 1 in (<5th percentile), and weight is 45 lb (<5th percentile). Her physical examination demonstrates a short female with a low posterior hairline, prepubertal breast and pubic hair, and a high-arched palate. There is no significant past medical, surgical, family, or social history.

Initial laboratory studies included a normal blood count and metabolic panel. In addition, an endocrine work-up for short stature included collection of thyroid studies and growth factors. Her thyroid studies included an elevated thyroid-stimulating hormone ([TSH] 21.0 µIU/mL; normal range 0.4 to 4.0 µIU/mL) and low free thyroxine ([T_4] 0.5 ng/dL; normal range 0.9 to 1.6 ng/dL). Her insulin-like growth factor (IGF)-1 and IGFBP-3 levels were within normal limits. A karyotype was also collected, but the results were not yet available.

This chapter addresses the common endocrine assays and their clinical uses to help the reader make appropriate decisions when ordering these studies. The chapter will also allow the reader to explore the various etiologies of a child with short stature and aid in developing a differential diagnosis, work-up, and therapy.

OBJECTIVES

1. Describe the basic concepts of common immunoassays used to evaluate endocrine disorders.

2. Describe the advantages and limitations of immunoassays.

3. List the immunoassays used in the evaluation of a patient with an endocrine disorder.

ASSAY BASICS

Clinical endocrinology is predicated on the measurement of hormones, metabolites, ions, and pH. Hormone concentrations are determined as the basis for diagnosis and for monitoring treatment. Some of the assays such as blood glucose and hemoglobin A_{1c} levels are routine and robust and can be performed by the patient at home using approved devices. This chapter is not intended to provide an overview of all assay modalities available to the clinician but rather to describe the basic principles of assays typically used for measuring circulating hormones. Table 18-1 lists the assays that are currently used to measure hormones and proteins that are routinely ordered to evaluate endocrine disorders.

Bioassays

Bioassays are rarely used today but have historical significance because they were the earliest methods to measure hormone concentrations and test potency of biological compounds. During the development of insulin for treatment of type 1 diabetes mellitus

TABLE 18-1.	Most Common Assays Used to Measure Hormone	
Test	**Assay**
Sex hormones	
Follicle-stimulating hormone	Direct ELISA
Luteinizing hormone	Direct ELISA
Estradiol	LC-MS
Testosterone	LC-MS
β-Human chorionic gonadotropin	Direct ELISA
Thyroid hormones	
Free T_4	RIA
Thyroid-stimulating hormone	Direct ELISA
Thyroperoxidase antibody	Indirect ELISA
Thyroglobulin antibody	Indirect ELISA

(continues)

TABLE 18-1. Most Common Assays Used to Measure Hormone (*Continued*)

Test	Assay
Thyroid-binding globulin	ICMA
T_3 uptake	Resin uptake[a]
Glucose metabolism	
HbA_{1c}	HPLC
Glucose	Chemical assay (photometric)
Insulin	Direct ELISA
Calcium metabolism	
Parathyroid hormone	Direct ELISA
Calcium	Chemical assay (photometric)
Phosphorus	Chemical assay (photometric)
25-OH-vitamin D_3	LC-MS
1,25-$(OH)_2$-vitamin D_3	LC-MS
Growth-related hormones	
GH-binding protein	Indirect ELISA
Growth hormone	Direct ELISA
Insulin-like growth factor-1	Direct ELISA
IGFBP-3	Direct ELISA
Adrenal hormones	
Cortisol	LC-MS
Aldosterone	LC-MS
Adrenocorticotropic hormone	ICMA
Plasma renin activity	RIA

[a]Most T_3 uptake assays are currently performed using an indirect ELISA rather than the resin.

Notes: LC-MS, liquid chromatography–mass spectroscopy; HPLC, high-performance liquid chromatography; RIA, radioimmunoassay; ICMA, immunochemiluminescent assay; ELISA, enzyme-linked immunosorbent assay; T_3, triiodothyronine; T_4, thyroxine; HbA_{1c}, hemoglobin A_{1c}; GH, growth hormone; IGF, insulin-like growth factor.

(T1D) in the 1920s, preparations of extracted porcine insulin were standardized by determining the amount of extract required to cause hypoglycemic shock in a 1-kg fasted rabbit. In 1927, a pregnancy test was developed that required injection of a woman's urine into a female rabbit. Later, the ovaries of the rabbit were examined for maturation in response to the amount of human chorionic gonadotropin (hCG) present in the pregnant woman's urine. The assay remained in use until the 1970s. Beginning in 1943, in attempts to isolate growth hormone (GH) from pituitary glands, extracts were tested for human growth hormone (hGH) activity by measuring the growth of femur cartilage of hypophysecotmized rats following injection with the extracts. In each case, the bioassay was eventually replaced with an antibody-based assay.

Currently, bioassays are limited to three uses: 1) standardizing hormone preparations, such as World Health Organization international reference concentrations of GH and leptin; 2) testing biological effectiveness of new agents in preclinical models; and 3) testing biological activity of circulating hormones such as bioactive GH or TSH. However, with advances in laboratory techniques, bioassays have played a less prominent role in clinical medicine and diagnostics.

Polyclonal and Monoclonal Antibody Production

In order to understand the clinical relevance of assay measurements, it is important to distinguish between polyclonal and monoclonal antibodies and their production. The body produces millions of different types of B lymphocytes (or B cells), and each type of B cell expresses a different surface receptor that can interact with an antigen. When the immune system is challenged with an antigen, the antigen interacts with the B cell surface receptors. If the antigen is recognized by the receptor, the cell engulfs the antigen and cleaves it into small fragments. The fragments are bound to the major histocompatability complex (MHC) molecules and transferred to the surface of the cell. This MHC–antigen complex attracts T cells that recognize the antigen and produce cytokines that activate the B cell. The B cells proliferate and secrete a free form of the receptors as antibodies that recognize the antigen fragment. Antigenic fragments are termed **epitopes**. Many different fragments of the antigen are presented. This results in many different B cells that may expand into clones; each clone produces a specific antibody against different epitopes. Therefore, the blood contains a heterogeneous or polyclonal mixture of antibodies each with different affinity for different parts or epitopes of the antigen.

Small polypeptides (<10 kd) and nonprotein antigens usually do not produce a strong immune response. To generate antibodies against very small proteins and nonproteins, the antigen must be attached to an immunogenic carrier protein that can be processed into T-cell epitopes. For example, T_4 is a small molecule that cannot be used as an antigen but can be conjugated to albumin to produce antibodies.

Polyclonal antibodies are obtained by purifying the target substance, the "antigen," and subcutaneously injecting it into an animal (e.g., rabbit), which then mounts an immunologic response to the antigen. Purified antigens are often poor immunogens and must be complexed with an adjuvant to improve immune response. Adjuvants may contain a detergent or oil that solubilizes the antigen and provides slow release. These immunostimulatory agents provoke an enhanced and prolonged immune response. Over a period of weeks, additional booster shots of antigen are administered to increase the immunological response. An aliquot of blood from the animal is then collected, and the serum is tested for antibodies to the antigen (Figure 18-1).

When an animal exhibits the desired antibody, serum is collected, and the antibodies that recognize the antigen are then purified. The antibodies collected from the animal are a heterogenous or polyclonal mixture of antibodies against the multiple epitopes that

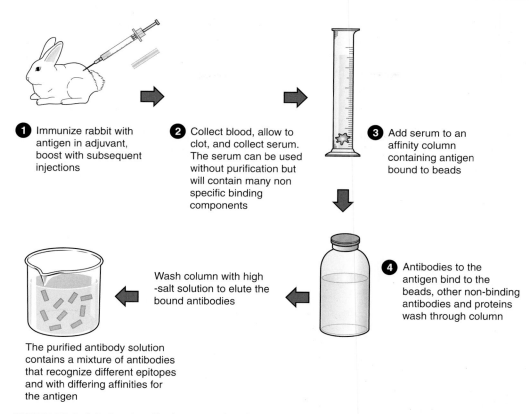

1 Immunize rabbit with antigen in adjuvant, boost with subsequent injections

2 Collect blood, allow to clot, and collect serum. The serum can be used without purification but will contain many non specific binding components

3 Add serum to an affinity column containing antigen bound to beads

4 Antibodies to the antigen bind to the beads, other non-binding antibodies and proteins wash through column

Wash column with high -salt solution to elute the bound antibodies

The purified antibody solution contains a mixture of antibodies that recognize different epitopes and with differing affinities for the antigen

FIGURE 18-1. Polyclonal antibody preparation. (Based on art by Milton Brown, PhD, Department of Pediatrics, Division of Pediatric Endocrinology, Emory University School of Medicine.)

were derived from the antigen molecule. Antibody production can also be explained as follows: 1) an antigen may have 100 different epitopes (regions within the antigen for which an antibody can be specific for) that can create 100 different specific antibodies to match each epitope; 2) each epitope has 100 different subtypes; and, as a result 3) polyclonal antibodies will have greater assay-to-assay variation and greater cross-reactivity with other antigens. This will decrease their binding specificity.

Monoclonal antibodies are specific to a single epitope within an antigen. Unlike a polyclonal antibody, monoclonal antibodies are produced by a single clone of a B lymphocyte cell that is specific to just one epitope of an antibody. In the 1970s, Kohler and Milstein developed a method to produce monoclonal antibodies using hybrid cells of mouse B lymphocytes and "immortal" myeloma cells. Mice are injected with the target antigen to induce B lymphocyte proliferation. When a sufficient antibody titer is reached in the serum, the mice are euthanized. The spleen is harvested and dissociated into single cells, and the B lymphocytes are collected. Each B lymphocyte produces a unique antibody that is specific for an epitope. By isolating a single B lymphocyte from the spleen, a homogeneous population of antibodies can be produced. The isolated B lymphocytes are then fused with immortalized myeloma cells. The B lymphocytes that successfully fuse into hybrid cells are selected and individually cultured. Each clone of the hybrid lymphocyte–myeloma complex is screened for production of antibodies against the antigen. Each clone containing a specific antibody is propagated in culture and can produce an unlimited supply of the monoclonal antibody. These monoclonal antibodies from each clone are specific for a single epitope. They have consistent binding-site affinity, do not require a purified antigen, and provide a limitless supply of cells to produce the specific monoclonal antibody (Figure 18-2).

Radioimmunoassay

The assays used in hormone measurement in clinical practice today are very sophisticated. Even the smallest alterations in hormone structure can evoke antibody production. Techniques have now been developed that take advantage of this highly sensitive reactive potential of antibodies produced in response to hormones.

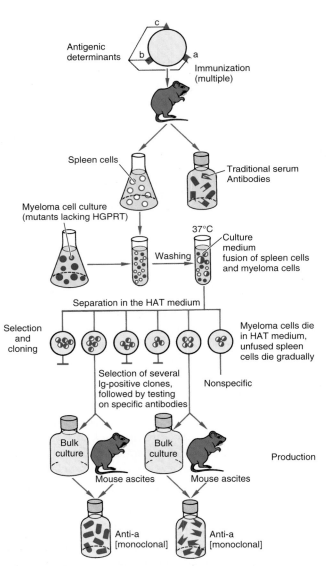

FIGURE 18-2. Monoclonal antibody preparation.

HGPRT, hypoxanthine-guanosine-phosphoribosyl transferase
HAT, hypoxanthine, aminopterin, and thymidine

When an antibody binds to a hormonal antigen, it forms an antibody–antigen complex that has a unique set of physical properties different from either the antibody or antigen alone. These properties include various precipitation qualities, electrophoresis behavior, and binding capacity. A **radioimmunoassay (RIA)** works on the principle that radio-labeled iodine is readily incorporated into the tyrosine residues of hormones, thereby permitting detection and quantification of very small amounts of hormone. By mixing a known amount of radiolabeled and unlabeled hormone, two forms of hormone compete for a finite number of binding sites. This is the basis of the RIA.

A plasma sample containing an unknown amount of unlabeled hormone is taken from a patient and mixed with a known amount of radioactive hormone (radiolabeled hormone) and a known amount of antibody. The two forms of hormone compete for the limited number of antibody binding sites in vitro. These competing reactions dictate whether or not the antibodies bind more unlabeled hormone or more radiolabeled hormone. The more unlabeled hormone in the biological patient sample, the more unlabeled hormone–antibody complexes will form, because the radiolabeled hormone is displaced from the antibody complexes.

Following the mixture step, radiolabeled hormone–antibody complexes are separated from the unbound radiolabeled hormone by a physicochemical technique (Figure 18-3). The last step is to determine the ratio of bound to unbound radioactive hormone and esti-mate the amount of unlabeled hormone that was initially available in the plasma sample. This amount is determined by the use of a standard curve, based on known amounts of unlabeled hormone (Figure 18-4).

RIAs are robust and relatively simple to perform, but the radioisotope I-125 typically used has a short half-life (60 days). Therefore, assays must be performed in a matter of weeks from the time of radiolabeling. Other requirements for using these agents include the administrative ability to use radioactivity, obtain a radiation permit, maintain ade-quate facilities for use and storage, and proper dispose of waste.

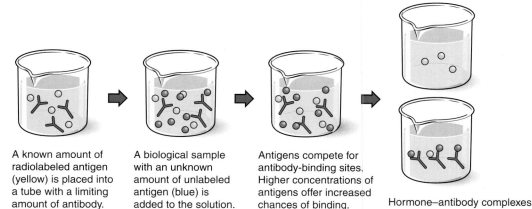

A known amount of radiolabeled antigen (yellow) is placed into a tube with a limiting amount of antibody.

A biological sample with an unknown amount of unlabeled antigen (blue) is added to the solution.

Antigens compete for antibody-binding sites. Higher concentrations of antigens offer increased chances of binding.

Hormone–antibody complexes are then separated from the unbound antigens and the radioactivity in each fraction is measured. The bound to unbound radioactive antigen ratio is used to estimate the amount of unlabeled antigen in biological sample.

FIGURE 18-3. Radioimmunoassay (RIA) experiment flow.

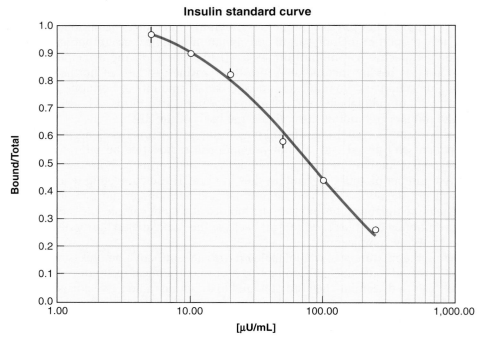

FIGURE 18-4. Competitive radioimmunoassay standard curve. The fraction of bound radiolabeled antibody is inversely related to the concentration of the antigen. Signal intensity is inversely proportional to the concentration of the antigen. This assay is optimized for physiological concentrations of injected Lispro™ insulin in serum and does not show the typical 4- to 5-log concentration range of RIA.

Immunoradiometric and Immunochemiluminescent Assays

Although RIAs rely on the competitive properties of antibody binding to hormone peptides, a range of noncompetitive assays of diagnostic value also are available and are 10 times more sensitive than RIAs. **Immunoradiometric assays (IRMAs)** and **immunochemiluminescent assays (ICMAs)** utilize radioactive or fluorescent reporter molecules coupled to the antibodies. They provide specific and sensitive detection and quantification.

These assays use two separate antibodies that have different binding-site properties. When used in tandem, they allow for two binding steps for hormone level detection. These assays use one population of antibodies (the capture antibody) that are attached to a solid support such as polymer beads, walls of a test tube, plastic culture dishes, or multi-well assay plates. The biological sample containing the hormone under investigation is then added to the assay. The level of antibody is kept very high relative to the amount of unknown hormone to ensure that almost all of the hormone in the sample will ultimately be bound by the antibody.

After ensuring that the hormone in the biological sample has had adequate opportunity to bind completely by the first antibody, a second antibody (the detection antibody) is added. This second antibody group is different from the first in two ways: 1) the antibody's binding site is specific for a region of the hormone that is not bound by the first antibody population that was mounted to a solid structure and 2) the detection antibody is labeled with a reporter that allows for detection and quantification of bound second antibody after excess antibody has been removed. The radioactivity of the IRMA can be measured when the detection antibody binds to the hormone. In the ICMA, fluorescence is measured after binding of the detection antibody.

Then, after measuring either the radioactivity (IRMA) or fluorescence (ICMA) released upon the binding of the detection antibody to hormone, one is able to determine the concentration of hormone in the biological sample that was tested. The amount of antibody-linked detection that is measured from the solid support system is directly proportional to the amount of hormone that was present in the biological sample (Figure 18-5). These assays are often referred to as "sandwich assays," because the hormone of interest is bound by both a first and a second antibody. Both antibodies serve different functions in the assay.

Enzyme-linked Immunosorbent Assay

A specific example of a sandwich assay is the **enzyme-linked immunosorbent assay (ELISA)**. In this assay, the same principles of IRMA and ICMA apply. A capture antibody provides a method in which a hormone or antigen is immobilized to a solid support system. Then, with application of a detection antibody, the hormone level can be quantified. The detection antibody has an enzyme attached to it that causes a quantifiable color change when a substrate is added. By measuring the color change after adding substrate to the mixture that contains the hormone-bound detection antibody, the amount of hormone can be calculated. Polyclonal or monoclonal antibodies can be used for ELISA, but monoclonal antibodies yield more consistent results. An ELISA can typically detect less than 1 ng (10^{-9} g) of target antigen because each enzyme–antibody molecule can convert many molecules of the substrate to product and thus amplifies the signal of the capture antibody.

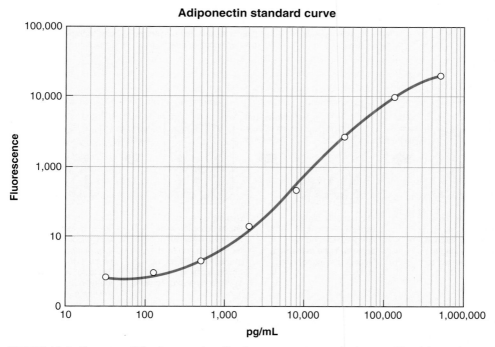

FIGURE 18-5. Noncompetitive immunochemiluminescent assay standard curve. Signal intensity is proportional to the concentration of the antigen. Note log–log scales. The assay has a four-log usable range.

Direct Enzyme-linked Immunosorbent Assay

In the **direct ELISA**, the capture antibody is mounted to a solid surface support similar to the IRMA and ICMA methods. After mixing with the biological sample, the antigen or hormone is immobilized by forming a complex with the solid-bound capture antibodies. The secondary detection antibody has a binding site that is specific for the hormone of interest; therefore, the enzyme-linked detection antibody directly binds to the immobilized antigen that is bound to the capture antibody on the solid support system. Substrate for the enzyme is added to the mixture and is converted to a colored or fluorescent product. The rate of color formation is proportional to the amount of enzyme–antibody complex bound to the antigen and to the amount of antigen present (Figure 18-6A).

Indirect Enzyme-linked Immunosorbent Assay

Several diseases of the endocrine system, such as T1D, Hashimoto thyroiditis, Addison disease, and Graves disease, are caused by the production of autoantibodies against normal tissue or cellular proteins. The autoantibodies can be detected using an

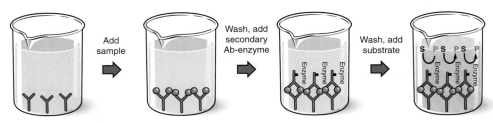

Primary capture antibodies are immobilized on a solid support surface such as a reaction well.

The patient's plasma sample is added to the reaction and capture antibodies bind to the antigen of interest (blue circles).

Secondary enzyme-linked detection antibodies are then added to the reaction well and bind to the immobilized antigen bound to capture antibodies.

Substrate (S) for the enzyme-linked detection antibody is added to the mixture and the color change of the product (P) is measured. The color is proportional to the amount of antigen in the sample.

A

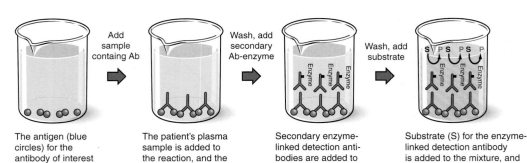

The antigen (blue circles) for the antibody of interest is coated along the inside of a reaction well.

The patient's plasma sample is added to the reaction, and the antibody to be measured binds to the immobilized antigen.

Secondary enzyme-linked detection antibodies are added to the mixture and bind to the immobilized antibody that is bound to the antigen-coated well.

Substrate (S) for the enzyme-linked detection antibody is added to the mixture, and the color change of the product (P) is measured. The color is proportional to the amount of antibody in the sample.

B

FIGURE 18-6. (A) Direct enzyme-linked immunosorbent assay experiment flow. Direct enzyme-linked immunosorbent assay (ELISA) experiment flow. (Based on art by Milton Brown, PhD, Department of Pediatrics, Division of Endocrinology, Emory University.) **(B)** Indirect enzyme-linked immunosorbent assay experiment flow. (Based on art by Milton Brown, PhD, Department of Pediatrics, Division of Endocrinology, Emory University.)

indirect ELISA. In an indirect ELISA, it is not the capture antibody that is bound to the solid surface, but rather the antigen of interest. This utilizes the same principles of sandwich assays for measuring hormone or antigen levels in patients' plasma in order to measure a specific amount of antibody present in a sample. In an indirect ELISA, a patient's serum is added to the antigen-coated wells of the assay plate. The binding complex forms between specific antibodies in the sample, and the target antigens attached to the solid support. After washing to remove unbound components, enzyme-linked detection antibodies against immunoglobulin (Ig)G molecules are added and bind to the primary antibodies bound to the target antigen. The color formation is proportional to the amount of autoantibodies bound to the target antigen (Figure 18-6B).

Nonantibody-binding Assays

Abnormalities in the measurement of hormones bound to proteins may occur because of a decreased or increased level of binding protein. In patients with thyroid-binding globulin (TBG) abnormalities, the measurement of an elevated or decreased level of total T_4 may actually have elevated serum TBG rather than a decreased production of T_4. A standard antibody assay for T_4 will not distinguish between altered TBG and T_4 levels. TBG can be measured with an antibody assay or resin-binding assay. The resin-binding assay is an indirect measure of TBG-binding capacity in the blood and can indicate altered levels of TBG. The competitive binding assay uses radiolabeled triiodothyronine (T_3) and a synthetic resin in place of an antibody to measure T_4 binding. In this assay, a small amount of tracer I-125-T_3 is added to a serum sample. A binding resin with low affinity for T_3 is then added. The I-125-T_3 tracer partitions between TBG-binding sites in the serum and on the resin. The supernatant containing TBG and the resin are separated using centrifugation, and the I-125-T_3 present in resin fraction and total I-125-T_3 added are measured. The binding is calculated as the percentage of the total I-125-T_3 added that is bound to the resin. In the presence of an elevated serum T_4 level and normal serum TBG levels, T_4 saturates TBG-binding sites and shifts binding of the tracer I-125-T_3 to the resin so the percent bound is elevated. Conversely, a low T_4 allows more of the I-125-T_3 to bind to the TBG and decreases the percent of I-125-T_3 bound to the resin.

Beyond Antibody-based Assays

Antibody assays are the predominate modality for measuring hormone concentrations; however, the immunoassays do have several limitations. They are subject to interference and require availability of specific antibodies against the target molecule. Most clinical immunoassays detect only single targets, and current multiplex assays require specialized instruments and specialized antibody reagents. Antibodies made against a purified, denatured protein may not react with the native or posttranslationally modified state of the protein. Additionally, antibody binding may be sensitive to normal variations in amino acid sequence caused by DNA polymorphisms and are not present in the antigen used to produce the antibody. The difficulties of producing antibodies against nonprotein or low-molecular-weight compounds limit the development of immunoassays for these compounds. In many instances, high-resolution liquid or gas chromatography coupled with mass spectrometry can provide another assay approach that is independent of antibodies.

Although once considered too expensive and complex for routine clinical use, **mass spectrometry** has rapidly moved into the clinical lab as instruments became smaller and less expensive, and the analyses became more robust and user-friendly. Mass spectrometric assays offer high sensitivity and specificity and can rapidly identify and measure the abundance of multiple targets in a single sample. Reagent costs for mass spectrometry are very low relative to immunoassay costs. For some endocrine assays, mass spectrometric analysis is already an alternative or a replacement for antibody and chemical assays. Commercial labs offer mass spectrometric assays for numerous nonprotein hormones, such as the adrenal and gonadal steroid hormones, sex steroids, thyroid hormones, vitamin D metabolites, and gonadotropin-releasing hormone.

Mass spectrometers move ionized molecules through a magnetic or electric field so the ions are separated according to their mass-to-charge (m/z) ratios. The collection of ions produced from the parent molecule produce a characteristic pattern of m/z peaks that uniquely identify the parent molecule. Mass spectrometers for clinical use are composed of a gas or liquid chromatograph to separate the individual components in a sample and inject them into the mass spectrometer. Under a high vacuum, the injected material is ionized and moved through a magnetic mass filter to separate the ions by m/z ratios. The selected ions are then focused onto a detector. The detector signal identifies the m/z ratio for the ions, and the signal intensity provides the abundance of the ions. The pattern of m/z peaks are then compared to known m/z spectra to identify the individual components in the sample.

FACTORS THAT INTERFERE WITH IMMUNOASSAYS

There are a number of factors that interfere with immunoassays. In addition to the limitations of the assay itself, physiologic factors, antibodies, and binding proteins may interfere with immunoassays.

Assay Limitations

There are limitations to all immunoassays. Endocrine immunoassays measure a hormone's immunologic activity and not its biologic activity. The portion of the hormone recognized by the antibody in the assay may be different from the portion of the hormone recognized by its endogenous receptor. Both competitive and noncompetitive immunoassays can be sensitive to cross-reactions with closely related antigens, nonspecific binding, and monoclonal antibodies.

Very high antigen levels in a sandwich assay can create a "hook" effect and overwhelm the binding kinetics of the assay. The excess antigen can inhibit interaction of the antibodies. Below the hook point, the signal increases as the concentration increases but then declines as the higher antigen levels exceed the hook point. If assay values are very low and inconsistent with other clinical data, the laboratory should determine whether serial dilutions of the specimen need to be assayed again to confirm a questionable low value.

Physiologic Factors

There are multiple factors that affect the reliability of an immunoassay. These factors may be due to patient features and others to the fluctuating nature of hormone levels in biologic systems. For example, some hormone levels (e.g., GH) fluctuate with pulsatile episodic secretions throughout a 24-hour cycle. Therefore, any single assay reading may reflect a nadir or peak of the fluctuated levels instead of an accurate steady state reading. In addition, some hormones are elevated in settings of physiological stress (e.g., cortisol), which may be a confounding factor in accurate measurements of these immunoassays.

Circadian rhythm and diurnal variation play roles in fluctuating hormone levels. These occurrences may cause difficulty in accurately measuring hormones. Hormones such as luteinizing hormone (LH), follicle-stimulating hormone (FSH), prolactin, TSH, dehydroepiandrosterone (DHEA), estradiol, testosterone, and leptin are examples of hormones that can be highly variable based on what time of day or month the samples are drawn. Seasonal variation can also have an effect on the measured levels of vitamin D due to its dependence on sunlight exposure for synthesis.

Behavioral changes play roles in certain hormone level measurements by immunoassays. Postural changes can affect plasma levels of aldosterone, renin, norepinephrine, and epinephrine because of the need to maintain blood pressure. Nutritional status and food intake affect the levels of many hormones including, leptin, IGF-1, IGFBP-1, IGFBP-3, insulin, C-peptide, proinsulin, glucagon, thyroxine-binding globulin, and adiponectin. Activity level and acute stresses can also lead to drastic changes in levels of norepinephrine, epinephrine, adrenocorticotropic hormone, cortisol, vasopressin, and glucagon in the blood.

Antibodies

The two types of antibodies that affect immunoassays are heterophile antibodies and autoantibodies.

Heterophile Antibodies

Because immunoassays rely on known amounts of antibodies mixed with a biologic sample, any level of interference with antibody binding can affect the accuracy of these diagnostic tools. Even in healthy patients, natural antibodies and autoantibodies are produced that have the capacity to weakly bind heterogenous, poorly defined antigens with low affinity called **heterophile antibodies**. Heterophile antibodies can affect the accuracy of immunoassays by either a competitive or noncompetitive mechanism. For instance, heterophile antibodies may affect the competitive binding of antigen to antibody by binding to the antigen of interest itself; conversely, heterophile antibodies may also have a low affinity–binding capacity for the assay antibodies themselves. Therefore, in the sandwich assays that rely on capture antibodies immobilized on a solid support, these heterophile antibodies may bind to the capture antibodies instead of the antigen of interest. Then, upon addition of the detection antibody and substrate, color production from bound detection antibodies may be due to their binding to the heterophile antibodies rather than the antigens of interest, which provides a falsely elevated reading.

Autoantibodies

A unique condition that can cause elevated TSH levels by immunoassay is **macro-TSH**, in which anti-TSH IgG autoantibodies form complexes with endogenous TSH to falsely elevate the level of TSH on immunoassay. These IgG autoantibodies are especially prevalent in autoimmune thyroid diseases. Although the TSH level by immunoassay will be markedly elevated, the free T_3 and T_4 levels will be within normal range.

The presence of macro-TSH complexes can be identified by using the **polyethylene glycol (PEG) precipitation test**. This test determines a recovery rate of TSH from the biologic sample after the serum sample is mixed with a 25% solution of PEG. A decreased recovery rate of TSH after mixing suggests that the levels measured by the assay have been altered by high-molecular-weight proteins, usually Igs. Further testing with electrophoretic methods, such as gel filtration chromatography, allows the exact molecular weight of the complexes to be determined whether or not the complexes being formed are from macro-TSH or other elevated TSH levels.

The **protein G addition test** can also be helpful by using protein G agarose's absorptive properties to bind the serum IgG in the sample, which may form macro-TSH complexes and elevate the measured TSH level. After the addition of protein G agarose, the patient's serum is processed and the TSH level re-measured.

Hormone-binding Proteins

Hormone-binding globulins are circulating proteins that can change the concentration of the analyte of interest by binding to them and effectively removing or blocking them. For example, sex hormone–binding globulin can decrease the amount of measured steroid in a plasma sample by binding to it. Additionally, cortisol-binding globulin can bind cortisol in a patient's plasma and prevent an accurate measurement of cortisol. Furthermore, endogenous hormone-binding proteins, such as TBG, can be bound by substances in the patient's blood other than the hormone of interest. For example, elevated levels of free fatty acids can displace free T_4 from TBG and lead to a false reading.

CASE FOLLOW-UP

A week after the initial presentation, the laboratory result shows a 45,XO karyotype. A diagnosis of Turner syndrome (TS) is confirmed. Any female pediatric patient with short stature and phenotypic features such as a webbed neck, wide-spaced nipples, and low posterior hairline must have a karyotype analysis to first exclude TS. There are several different chromosomal combinations associated with TS including a single X, an X with an abnormal second X chromosome, or any form of mosaicism. The incidence of TS due to a loss of part or all of an X chromosome ranges from 1:2,000 to 1:5,000 live female births. Females with a structural abnormality of the second X chromosome have an X-isochrome (46,X,i(Xq)). The loss of the second X chromosome altogether is known as *monosomy X* (45,XO). A range of other abnormal karyotypes that constitute TS involving partial loss of the X chromosome exists, but most females with TS have the monosomy X karyotype.

Once the diagnosis of TS is established, a search for anomalies associated with the condition should be performed on physical examination and by appropriate laboratory studies. Most females with TS have a coexisting endocrine disorder. They are at a higher risk for developing autoimmune hypothyroidism and T1D. The relative risks for these endocrine conditions depend on the karyotype. Hashimoto thyroiditis, due to the production of thyroid autoantibodies occurs in up to 40% of females with TS who have an X-isochromosome karyotype, 14% who have the 45,XO karyotype, and only 6% who have other karyotypes. It is important to obtain TSH and free T_4 levels in these females to assess their thyroid function.

Females with TS also have many associated physical abnormalities including growth failure, gonadal dysgenesis, inverted and widely spaced nipples, webbed neck, nail dysplasia, defective dental development, and lymphatic obstruction. More serious complications such as left-sided cardiac anomalies and renal dysgenesis are present in over 50% of patients. More than 95% of these girls have ovarian failure due to gonadal dysgenesis and should be assessed with measurements of serum LH, FSH, and estradiol levels.

The endocrine tests that a female with TS should have collected include FSH, LH, estradiol, TSH, free T_4, thyroglobulin antibody, and thyroid peroxidase antibody; a karyotype should also be done. The assays used to measure these tests are shown in Table 18-1.

REFERENCES and SUGGESTED READINGS

Arkin MR, Glicksman MA, Fu H, Havel JJ, Du Y. Inhibition of protein-protein interactions: non-cellular assay formats. In: Sittampalam GS, Gal-Edd N, Arkin M, et al., eds. Assay Guidance Manual [Internet]. Bethesda, MD: Eli Lilly & Company and the National Center for Advancing Translational Sciences; 2004.

Carvalho VM. The coming of age of liquid chromatography coupled to tandem mass spectrometry in the endocrinology laboratory. J Chromatogr B Analyt Technol Biomed Life Sci. 2012;883-884:50-58.

Diamond FB, Bercu BB. Laboratory testing in pediatric endocrinology. In: Eugster C, Pescovitz O, eds. Pediatric Endocrinology: Mechanisms and Management. Philadelphia, PA: Lippincott Williams & Wilkins; 2004:775-779.

Dunlap DB. Thyroid function tests. In: Walker HK, Hall WD, Hurst JW, eds. Clinical Methods: The History, Physical, and Laboratory Examinations. 3rd ed. Boston, MA: Butterworths; 1990:666-676.

Elmlinger MW, Kühnel W, Wormstall H, Döller PC. Reference intervals for testosterone, androstenedione and SHBG levels in healthy females and males from birth until old age. Clin Lab. 2005;51(11-12):625-632.

Elmlinger MW. Laboratory techniques, quality management and clinical validation of hormone measurement in endocrinology. In Ranke MB, ed. Diagnostics of endocrine function in children and adolescents. 3rd ed. Basel:Karger; 2003:1-29.

Elsheikh M, Wass JA, Conway GS. Autoimmune thyroid syndrome in women with Turner's syndrome–the association with karyotype. Clin Endocrinol (Oxf). 2001;55(2):223-226.

Gravholt CH, Juul S, Naeraa RW, Hansen J. Morbidity in Turner syndrome. J Clin Epidemiol. 1998;51:147.

Grebe SK, Singh RJ. LC-MS/MS in the clinical laboratory—where to from here? Clin Biochem Rev. 2011;32(1):5-31.

Grebe SK, Singh RJ. Laboratory testing in hyperthyroidism. Am J Med. 2012;125(9):S2.

Kricka LJ. Human anti-animal antibody interferences in immunological assays. Clin Chem. 1999;45:942-956.

Norman JJ, Raviele NA, Brown MR, Prausnitz MR, Felner EI. Insulin Delivery using Hollow Microneedles in Children with Type 1 Diabetes Mellitus. Journal of Pediatric Diabetes, Scheduled for publication September 2013.

Sakai H, Fukuda G, Suzuki N, Watanabe C, Odawara M. Falsely elevated thyroid-stimulating hormone (TSH) level due to Macro-TSH. Endocr J. 2009;56: 435-440.

Tate J, Ward G. Interferences in immunoassay. Clin Biochem Rev. 2004;25:105-120.

Wild D. The Immunoassay Handbook. 3rd ed. Amsterdam, London: Elsevier; 2005.

CHAPTER REVIEW QUESTIONS

1. A company approaches you to help develop an assay for the detection of a newly discovered hormone peptide. They prefer a radioimmunoassay design but you explain that a sandwich assay would be better. All of the following statements are true regarding sandwich assays as compared to radioimmunoassays *except*:

    A. Higher sensitivity and specificity
    B. Less stable reagents
    C. Ease of implementing
    D. Use nonradioactive agents
    E. Requires very small amounts of target antigen

2. Which of the following choices depicts the correct order of steps in performing a radioimmunoassay?

    I. Determine bound/unbound radioactive antigen ratio.
    II. Add radioactive antigen with antibody to the reaction mixture.
    III. Remove radiolabeled antigen–antibody complexes from the reaction mixture.
    IV. Add unlabeled antigen to the reaction mixture.
    A. II, III, IV, I
    B. II, IV, III, I
    C. IV, II, III, I
    D. I, IV, II, III
    E. II, III, I, IV

3. An 8-year-old female comes to your office for work-up of short stature. You suspect
   Turner syndrome (TS) and order a karyotype. Her mother asks you what the likelihood
   is that her daughter has TS and what other tests you can order to rule out other causes
   of growth hormone deficiency. Which of the following statements is true?

   A. The incidence of TS is 1:2,000 to 1:5,000 live female births; order GH.
   B. The incidence of TS is 1:200 to 1:500 live births; order IGFBP-3 and IGF-I.
   C. The incidence of TS is 1:2,000 to 1:5,000 live female births; order IGFBP-3
      and IGF-I.
   D. The incidence of TS is 1:200 to 1:500 live female births; order GH.
   E. The incidence of TS is 1:200 to 1:500 live births; order GH.

4. A mother brings her 11-year-old child to see you for a second opinion. On a recent primary care visit, the child was diagnosed with hyperthyroidism. After taking a careful
   history and performing a physical examination, there are no signs or symptoms that
   suggest a clinical picture of hyperthyroidism. Previous laboratory values are available
   and show a TSH level of 0.1 μIU/mL (normal range = 0.5 to 4.5 μIU/mL). What is the
   most appropriate next step in work-up?

   A. Ask the patient what kinds of pets she has at home.
   B. Send for another TSH level using your preferred laboratory.
   C. Order a radioactive iodine uptake test (RAIU) and thyroid scan.
   D. Obtain the original sample to perform additional filtration techniques.
   E. Prescribe propylthiouracil.

5. All of the following physiological factors can affect the accurate readings of hormone
   levels determined by immunoassays *except*:

   A. Postural change
   B. Emotional stress
   C. Seasonal variation
   D. Time of day
   E. Weather

CHAPTER REVIEW ANSWERS

1. The correct answer is B. Sandwich assay designs (e.g., direct ELISA) have replaced
radioimmunoassays because of their increased sensitivity and specificity in detecting
very small amounts of a target antigen. Other advantages of sandwich assays include better precision at lower concentration of antigen, nonradioactive reagents, ease of handling
and disposing of reagents, less regulatory burden, and more stable reagents.

2. The correct answer is B. In performing a radioimmunoassay, a plasma sample from
a patient with an unknown amount of hormone (unlabeled hormone) is mixed with a
tube filled with both a known amount of radioactive iodinated hormone (radiolabeled
hormone) and a known amount of antibody. The two populations of hormones compete
for the known, limited number of antibody-binding sites in the test tube. Competing
reactions based on relative concentrations of unlabeled and radiolabeled hormones dictate whether or not the antibodies bind more unlabeled or radiolabeled hormone. The
more unlabeled hormone there is in the biological patient sample, the more unlabeled
hormone–antibody complexes will be formed. Following this mixture step, radiolabeled
hormone–antibody complexes are removed from the unbound radiolabeled hormone

by a physicochemical technique. Finally, the ratio of bound to unbound radioactive hormone must be determined. The amount of unlabeled hormone that was initially available in the plasma sample to compete for the antibody-binding spots can be estimated using a standard curve that is calculated based on known standard amounts of unlabeled hormone.

---

3. The correct answer is C. The incidence of Turner syndrome is 1:2,000 to 1:5,000 live female births. Baseline collection of IGF-1 and IGFBP-3 are the most appropriate screening tests for growth hormone (GH) deficiency. IGF-I and IGFBP-3 have higher sensitivities for predicting the diagnosis of GH deficiency in children younger than 10 years. To make the diagnosis of GH deficiency, a formal stimulation test must be performed.

---

4. The correct answer is A. Prolonged exposure to mice and rabbits can lead to the development of heterophile antibodies in humans—human anti-animal antibodies. These heterophile antibodies can affect accurate readings of immunoassays like TSH levels. Therefore, it is important to ask the patient what pets she has at home since a pet mouse or pet rabbits can cause an abnormal test value.

Always consider other possibilities in patients with no physical findings or clinical history to suggest hyperthyroidism. Therefore, it would not be appropriate to resend the TSH test (**Choice B**) or order additional tests that would expose the young patient to unnecessary radiation (**Choice C**). It is not necessary to obtain the original serum sample for further filtration since a thorough history and physical examination would obviate the need for further costly analysis (**Choice D**). Anti-thyroid medications such as propylthiouracil should not be given because this patient does not have hyperthyroidism (**Choice E**).

---

5. The correct answer is E. All of the listed factors (postural change, emotional stress, seasonal variation, and time of day) can affect the levels of hormones in blood because of the variable and pulsatile nature of hormone secretion. Although seasonal changes such as cold limits exposure to sunlight and may lower vitamin D levels, the weather itself has not been shown to affect hormone levels.

Stimulation and Suppression Testing

19

Bhavya S. Doshi
Eric I. Felner

CASE

A 9-year-old boy is brought to the clinic with a 2-week history of nocturnal enuresis. Both the child and his mother deny any other issues. A review of his birth history reveals that he was born full term without any complications. His past medical history is remarkable for otitis media as an infant and, just in the past month, has been diagnosed with otitis on three different occasions in both ears. He just recently completed a course of antibiotic therapy. He has not had surgery. On further questioning, the mother reports that he wakes up in the middle of the night after having wet his bed and drinks out of the sink for almost 5 minutes. His teachers have mentioned that he has asked to use the bathroom more frequently lately. On physical examination, his vital signs are normal and he appears thin but in no distress. Other than what appears to be scarring over his tympanic membranes, the rest of the examination is normal. A basic chemistry profile is normal, including serum sodium (145 mEq/L) and glucose (95 mg/dL). Urinalysis is remarkable for a low specific gravity (1.002), negative glucose, and negative ketones. After considering the possibilities, you inform the family that you would like to schedule the boy for formal endocrine testing.

This chapter reviews dynamic testing of endocrine function. Although the endocrine diseases and evaluation of endocrine disorders are discussed in preceding chapters, this chapter describes the dynamic testing of endocrine function in much greater detail. The detail of the testing also allows the learner to review and better understand endocrine physiology and pathophysiology. We provide a brief overview of dynamic testing followed by a review of endocrine physiology and diseases amenable to dynamic testing, helping the reader develop hypotheses that explore testing methods useful to determining the etiology of this boy's condition. Specific agents and protocols used for stimulation and suppression tests of different axes and their interpretations follow.

(*continued*)

OBJECTIVES

1. Describe the appropriate dynamic test for a given clinical scenario.

2. List the stimulation and suppression tests for hormonal abnormalities.

3. Recognize limitations of stimulation and suppression tests.

CHAPTER OUTLINE

Disorders of the Hypothalamic-Pituitary-Gonadal Axis
   Delayed Puberty
     Hypogonadotropic Hypogonadism
     Hypergonadotropic Hypogonadism
   Precocious Puberty
Disorders of Water Regulation
   Diabetes Insipidus
Combined Anterior Pituitary Testing

DYNAMIC ENDOCRINE TESTING OVERVIEW

Hormone secretion varies in response to a number of factors such as physiologic events, time of day, and posture. Dynamic tests that involve the stimulation or suppression of hormone production provide critical insight into hormone pathology. Stimulation tests are used when hypofunction is suspected and are designed to assess the reserve capacity to form and secrete hormones. These tests usually involve either the administration of an exogenous trophic hormone or stimulation of the endogenous production of a hormone (Table 19-1). Suppression tests are used when endocrine hyperfunction is suspected and are designed to determine whether or not the negative-feedback loop is intact (Table 19-2).

These dynamic tests are particularly useful for detecting subtle endocrine dysfunction and for localizing the site of the defect. The main problem in their interpretation, however, is that the range of normal responses has not been adequately defined either in suitable numbers of normal control subjects or in patients with concurrent diseases, particularly in the presence of coexisting endocrine disorders, other medical disorders, or psychiatric disease. Furthermore, a variety of drugs may interfere with dynamic testing. Even when a dynamic abnormality is documented, such information provides no insight into the natural history of the disorder.

DISORDERS OF THE HYPOTHALAMIC-PITUITARY-ADRENAL AXIS

The hormones in the adrenal gland including glucocorticoids, mineralocorticoids, and androgens have been described in detail in Chapters 10, 11, 13, and 15. All three hormone groups can be stimulated by adrenocorticotropic hormone (ACTH) and corticotropin-releasing hormone (CRH) from the anterior pituitary gland and hypothalamus, respectively. Aldosterone is primarily under the control of the renin–angiotensin system (RAS), and androgens are primarily secreted during puberty.

Cortisol (hydrocortisone), the primary glucocorticoid, is counterregulatory to insulin, so that during hypoglycemia, cortisol production and secretion are increased. In the absence of cortisol, hypoglycemia may occur due to the inability to stimulate gluconeogenesis. In addition, without cortisol, individuals may develop hypotension due to the inability of the vascular system to respond to the pressor effects of catecholamines.

Aldosterone is the main mineralocorticoid and governs retention and excretion of sodium and potassium and indirectly affects water balance. Aldosterone retains sodium; it acts on the collecting ducts in the kidney to cause increased exchange of sodium for

TABLE 19-1. Stimulation Testing

Condition	Deficient Hormone	Testing Agents
Glucocorticoid deficiency (primary)	Cortisol	Cortrosyn (high), insulin, metyrapone
Glucocorticoid deficiency (central)	CRH and/or ACTH	Cortrosyn (low), insulin, metyrapone
Mineralocorticoid deficiency	Aldosterone	Cortrosyn
GH deficiency	GHRH and/or GH	Insulin, arginine, clonidine, L-DOPA
Hypothyroidism (central)	TRH and/or TSH	TRH
Diabetes insipidus (central)	Vasopressin	Water deprivation and ADH Responds to DDAVP
Diabetes insipidus (nephrogenic)	None	Water deprivation and ADH Does not respond to DDAVP
Male hypogonadism (primary)	Testosterone	HCG
Hypogonadism (central)	GHRH and/or LH/FSH	LHRH

Notes: ACTH, adrenocorticotropic hormone; ADH, antidiuretic hormone; CRH, corticotropin-releasing hormone; DDAVP, desmopressin; GH, growth hormone; GHRH, growth hormone–releasing hormone; HCG, human chorionic gonadotropin; L-DOPA, L-3,4-dihydroxyphenylalanine; TRH, thyrotropin-releasing hormone; TSH, thyroid-stimulating hormone; LH, luteinizing hormone; FSH, follicle-stimulating hormone; LHRH, luteinizing hormone–releasing hormone.

TABLE 19-2. Suppression Testing

Condition	Excessive Hormone	Testing Agents
Cushing syndrome	Cortisol	Dexamethasone, CRH, DDAVP
Hyperaldosteronism	Aldosterone	Sodium
Acromegaly	GH	Glucose
Precocious puberty	Estradiol/testosterone	LHRH

Notes: CRH, corticotropin-releasing hormone; DDAVP, desmopressin; GH, growth hormone LHRH, luteinizing hormone-releasing hormone.

potassium and hydrogen ions, resulting in a loss of potassium and acidification of the urine. In retaining sodium, it maintains an individual's blood pressure.

Androstenedione and dehydroepiandrosterone (DHEA) are the two major androgens produced in the adrenal cortex. Androstenedione is a precursor of testosterone in men and estrogen in women. DHEA functions predominantly as a metabolic intermediate in the biosynthesis of the androgen and estrogen sex steroids. Both androstenedione and DHEA potentiate protein anabolism and virilization but are only about one fifth as potent

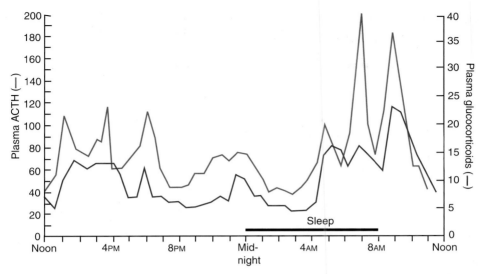

FIGURE 19-1. Diurnal oscillation of the hypothalamic–pituitary–adrenal axis. The amplitude of the pulses of ACTH and cortisol is lower in the evening hours and then increases during the early morning hours. (Modified from Krieger DT. Rhythms of CRF, ACTH and corticosteroids. In: Krieger DT, ed. Endocrine Rhythms. New York, NY: Raven; 1979:123–142.)

as testosterone. Unlike testosterone, secretion of androstenedione and DHEA is mediated by ACTH rather than the gonadotropin luteinizing hormone (LH).

CRH, potentiated by vasopressin (antidiuretic hormone [ADH]), stimulates release of ACTH from the anterior pituitary in a pulsatile and diurnal pattern. ACTH stimulates the adrenal cortex to produce cortisol, which in turn, inhibits release of CRH and ACTH via negative-feedback mechanisms. The lowest levels of CRH, ACTH, and cortisol occur in the late hours of the day, whereas peak levels occur in the early morning hours (Figure 19-1).

The adrenal cortex also releases aldosterone and adrenal androgens. Although aldosterone secretion is primarily regulated by the RAS, both CRH and ACTH can stimulate the release of aldosterone. Unlike cortisol, aldosterone is not secreted in diurnal fashion but, rather, in response to certain physiologic conditions (i.e., hypotension, standing) or biochemical abnormalities (i.e., hyponatremia, hyperkalemia, or hyperreninemia).

Adrenal Insufficiency

When clinical symptoms consistent with adrenal insufficiency do not correlate with biochemical findings, dynamic testing may be necessary to diagnose or rule out adrenal insufficiency. Stimulation of the adrenal cortex can be performed to assess for cortisol and aldosterone deficiency. The agents, dose, route of administration, and biochemical tests are shown in Table 19-3.

Glucocorticoid Deficiency

Glucocorticoid insufficiency can be classified as central (hypothalamus and/or pituitary) or primary (adrenal gland). An elevated serum concentration of ACTH in the presence of an inappropriately low serum cortisol concentration suggest primary adrenal insufficiency or adrenal insensitivity to ACTH. Low levels of ACTH in the presence of a low serum cortisol concentration suggests central adrenal insufficiency.

TABLE 19-3.	Adrenal-stimulation Testing		
Agent	Dose	Route	Baseline and Stimulated Tests
Cortrosyn (high dose)	10 µg/kg^a	IV	Serum ACTH, cortisol, aldosterone
Cortrosyn (low dose)	1–10 mg	IV	Serum ACTH, cortisol
Insulin (regular)	0.05–0.1 units/kg	IV	Serum ACTH, cortisol
Metyrapone	2–3 g^b	po	Serum ACTH, cortisol, 11-deoxycortisol
CRH	1 µg/kg	IV	Serum ACTH, cortisol

^{a}Maximum dose = 250 µg.
^{b}2 g (<70 kg), 2.5 g (70–90 kg), 3 g (>90 kg).
Notes: ACTH, adrenocorticotropic hormone; CRH, corticotropin-releasing hormone; IV, intravenous; po, oral (*per os*).

The standard high-dose ACTH (cortrosyn)–stimulation test and insulin–hypoglycemia test are the principal tests used in the evaluation of primary adrenal insufficiency. Cortrosyn is a synthetic polypeptide that is identical to the 24-amino acid segment at the N-terminal of ACTH. Cortrosyn is also known as *cosyntropin, tetracosactrin, tetracosactide,* and *tetracosapeptide.*

Primary Glucocorticoid Insufficiency

The high-dose (250 µg) cortrosyn test is performed in the early morning after an overnight fast with collection of baseline serum ACTH and cortisol levels immediately prior to the administration of cortrosyn. Serum cortisol levels are measured 30 and 60 minutes after administration. A stimulated cortisol level ≥18 µg/dL indicates an appropriate glucocorticoid response. The high-dose cortrosyn-stimulation test is highly sensitive (97%) and specific (95%) for primary glucocorticoid insufficiency but much less sensitive (59%) for central glucocorticoid insufficiency.

The insulin–hypoglycemia test is considered the gold standard (95% sensitivity, 97% specificity) for assessing the integrity of the hypothalamic–pituitary–adrenal (HPA) axis but, because it is potentially very dangerous and there is considerable intra-individual and inter-individual variation, the cortrosyn stimulation is more commonly utilized. Unlike the high-dose cortrosyn-stimulation test, the insulin–hypoglycemia test is used to assess primary and secondary glucocorticoid insufficiency. The insulin test should be performed in the early morning after an overnight fast. Baseline cortisol and glucose levels are collected immediately prior to the administration of regular insulin (0.05 to 0.1 U/kg). Cortisol and glucose levels are measured every 30 minutes, and a cortisol level <20 µg/dL, with either a 50% decrease in blood glucose or a simultaneous glucose level <40 mg/dL, suggests an inappropriate glucocorticoid response. Collection of ACTH levels in addition to cortisol and glucose levels allows the insulin–hypoglycemia test to be interpreted for central glucocorticoid insufficiency. If the ACTH level is <60 pg/mL, the cortisol level is <20 µg/dL, and the simultaneous glucose level is low, central glucocorticoid insufficiency should be suspected.

Central Glucocorticoid Insufficiency

Central (secondary) glucocorticoid insufficiency is the result of CRH and/or ACTH deficiency. Dynamic testing may be accomplished using the low-dose (1 to 10 µg) cortrosyn, CRH, or Metyrapone tests. The low-dose cortrosyn test is currently the most widely used. After collection of early morning basal ACTH and cortisol levels, 1 to 10 µg of cortrosyn is administered, and serum cortisol levels are measured 30 and 60 minutes later. Low baseline ACTH and cortisol levels with a peak serum cortisol level <15 µg/dL suggests central glucocorticoid insufficiency.

CRH-stimulation testing can distinguish between pituitary and hypothalamic glucocorticoid insufficiency. After a 4-hour fast, baseline samples are collected, synthetic ovine CRH is infused, and repeat measurements for cortisol and ACTH are carried out every 15 minutes for 1 hour. In individuals with normal glucocorticoid secretory capacity, the ACTH level should increase by 20% to 40%, and the cortisol level should stimulate to ≥18 µg/dL. Individuals with pituitary disease have subnormal responses. Individuals with hypothalamic disease have augmented and prolonged ACTH and reduced cortisol responses.

Due to limited access to metyrapone, it is rarely used but, may be useful in the identification of central or primary glucocorticoid insufficiency. Metyrapone inhibits the final step in cortisol biosynthesis by inhibiting the 11-β-hydroxylase enzyme. This enzyme catalyzes the conversion of 11-deoxycortisol to cortisol (see Figure 15-2). Because it is devoid of glucocorticoid activity, 11-deoxycortisol does not inhibit ACTH secretion. A fall in the serum cortisol, however, leads to sequential increases in ACTH secretion; adrenal steroidogenesis; and the secretion of cortisol precursors, in particular, 11-deoxycortisol. In blocking the final step of cortisol biosynthesis, and due to the HPA feedback mechanism, both CRH and ACTH should be stimulated to levels well above baseline levels. A failure of CRH and/or ACTH to increase in the absence of cortisol indicates CRH or ACTH deficiency. Metyrapone is taken orally with a small snack at midnight to reduce the nausea that commonly occurs with this drug. The following morning, serum ACTH, cortisol, and 11-deoxycortisol levels are measured. The results are reliable only if cortisol is effectively blocked, confirmed by an early morning cortisol level <5 µg/dL. Central glucocorticoid insufficiency is ruled out if the ACTH level is >60 pg/mL, and the 11-deoxycortisol level is >10.5 µg/dL. If, on the other hand, the ACTH level is <20 pg/mL, and the 11-deoxycortisol level is <10.5 µg/dL, central glucocorticoid insufficiency is likely. If the early morning cortisol level is <5 µg/dL, 11-deoxycortisol level is <7 µg/dL, and ACTH level is >60 pg/mL, primary glucocorticoid insufficiency should be considered in the differential diagnosis.

Mineralocorticoid Deficiency

In patients with primary glucocorticoid deficiency, the presence of hyponatremia and hyperkalemia suggests a lack of mineralocorticoid (aldosterone) secretion. Isolated mineralocorticoid deficiency accompanied by normal cortisol production is rare and is suspected in the presence of persistent hyperkalemia. It is important to exclude other causes of hyperkalemia, such as renal insufficiency or use of certain medications (angiotensin-converting enzyme inhibitors [ACE-I] or angiotensin-receptor blockers). The work-up includes evaluation of cortisol and aldosterone response to ACTH stimulation. The high-dose cortrosyn-stimulation test is used in a similar fashion to that for assessing glucocorticoid deficiency. Serum aldosterone levels are measured 30 and 60 minutes after administration of cortrosyn. An appropriate response for those older than age 2 years is a stimulated value that is >50 ng/dL, and a value that is >100 ng/dL for those age less than 2 years. Individuals with stimulated aldosterone levels below these are suspicious for mineralocorticoid deficiency.

Excess Secretion of Adrenal Hormones

When clinical symptoms are consistent with excess secretion of an adrenal hormone but do not correlate with biochemical findings, dynamic testing may be necessary to

TABLE 19-4.   Adrenal-suppression Testing

Agent	Dose	Route	Baseline and Suppression Tests
Dexamethasone (overnight)	30 μg/kg[a]	po	Cortisol[b]
Dexamethasone (low dose)	0.5 mg q6 h × 48 h	po	ACTH, cortisol
Dexamethasone (high dose)	2 mg q6 h × 48 h	po	ACTH, cortisol
CRH	1 μg/kg	IV	ACTH, cortisol
DDAVP	10 mg	IV	ACTH, cortisol
CRH (petrosal sinus sampling)	1 μg/kg	IV	ACTH[c]
Sodium load (IV)	500 mL/h × 4 h	IV	Aldosterone
Sodium load (po)	10–12 g × 5 d	po	24-h urine

[a]Maximum dose = 1 mg.

[b]Dexamethasone taken at 11 PM and cortisol collected between 7 and 8 AM the next day.

[c]ACTH is collected from both the petrosal sinus (central) and iliac vein (peripheral).

Notes: ACTH, adrenocorticotropic hormone; CRH, corticotropin-releasing hormone; DDAVP, desmopressin; IV, intravenous; po, oral (*per os*).

diagnose or rule out excess secretion of adrenal hormones. Suppression testing of the adrenal gland can be performed to assess for the presence of excess cortisol (Cushing syndrome) or aldosterone. The agents, dose, route of administration, lab values, and biochemical tests are shown in Table 19-4.

Glucocorticoid Excess (Cushing Syndrome)

The differential diagnosis between Cushing disease and ectopic ACTH syndrome relies on a composite of dynamic tests and imaging studies. The main objective of the dynamic tests is to address whether the presumed source of ACTH is the pituitary (Cushing disease), an adrenal adenoma, or an ectopic tumor; then direct the efforts to localize the tumors by appropriate imaging methods. Cushing syndrome results from exogenous glucocorticoid administration or endogenous glucocorticoid secretion. Due to the diurnal variation of ACTH and cortisol secretion and pathophysiologic causes of Cushing syndrome (i.e., ACTH dependent, ACTH independent, and pseudo-Cushing), a number of static and dynamic tests have been developed to assess for glucocorticoid excess. For the individual with signs of cortisol excess and an elevated 24-hour urine free cortisol level (>90 μg/m^2/day), one or more suppression tests should be performed. Suppression tests used in the evaluation of glucocorticoid excess include the overnight dexamethasone-suppression test, low-dose dexamethasone-suppression test, high-dose dexamethasone-suppression test, desmopressin (DDAVP), and CRH stimulation (with and without petrosal sinus sampling). In order to improve the accuracy, some tests are combined.

Dexamethasone-Suppression Testing

In the overnight dexamethasone-suppression test, oral dexamethasone is taken at 11 PM, and, between 7 and 8 AM the following morning, blood is collected and sampled for cortisol. If the cortisol level is <5 μg/dL, it is unlikely that the individual has glucocorticoid excess. Further testing is usually not necessary. If the cortisol level is >5 μg/dL, further testing is necessary, and suppressive testing is needed to confirm the diagnosis. In all other tests, baseline blood levels are collected, followed by blood collection at various time intervals. For the low- and high-dose dexamethasone-suppression tests, serum cortisol and urinary free cortisol levels are collected the morning prior to taking the initial dose of dexamethasone. This step is then repeated 12 to 14 hours after completing the last dose of dexamethasone. The low- and high-dose tests are used to differentiate between excess glucocorticoid due to a pituitary ACTH-secreting adenoma (Cushing disease) and, an adrenal adenoma or ectopic ACTH secretion. In those with Cushing disease, serum cortisol and urine free cortisol levels will not suppress after an overnight or a low-dose dexamethasone-suppression test but will suppress after a high-dose test. Excess glucocorticoid secretion that is due to either ectopic ACTH secretion or an adrenal adenoma will not suppress using any form of dexamethasone suppression. In differentiating Cushing disease from ectopic ACTH secretion, the high-dose dexamethasone-suppression test has a sensitivity and specificity of 80% and 85%, respectively.

Corticotropin-Releasing Hormone–Suppression Testing

The CRH-stimulation test is much more expensive than the dexamethasone-suppression tests and, therefore, is usually performed if the dexamethasone test is not confirmatory. The CRH test is based on the assumption that pituitary corticotrophic tumors are responsive to CRH as most of them express CRH receptors, whereas ectopic ACTH-producing tumors are not. The CRH test involves the collection of serum ACTH and cortisol levels before and 30 minutes after infusion of ovine CRH. In those with Cushing disease, more than 90% of patients will have an ACTH level two to three times above baseline, whereas those with ectopic or adrenal Cushing syndrome will have no ACTH or cortisol response. The CRH test is most useful for Cushing disease because a rise of 35% in ACTH levels (30 minutes after CRH injection) has a sensitivity and specificity of 93% and 100%, respectively. The cortisol response (a 20% rise) is less discriminatory with a sensitivity and specificity of 91% and 88%, respectively.

Desmopressin-Suppression Testing

DDAVP is a synthetic peptide, analogous to vasopressin, and stimulates the V_2 and V_3 vasopressin receptors. Pituitary ACTH-producing adenomas overexpress the pituitary-specific V_2 and V_3 receptors, whereas most of the ACTH-producing ectopic tumors do not. Due to its low cost, wide availability, and comparable accuracy, it was proposed as an alternative to CRH stimulation. The test involves injecting DDAVP intravenously (IV) and measuring serum ACTH and cortisol levels in basal and standardized times. Like the CRH test, DDAVP is most useful for Cushing disease but is less accurate. After DDAVP infusion, a rise of 35% in ACTH levels has a sensitivity and specificity of 77% and 73%, respectively. The cortisol response (a 20% rise) has a sensitivity and specificity of 84% and 83%, respectively. Because the DDAVP test may be less discriminative than CRH testing in differentiating Cushing disease from ectopic ACTH secretion, DDAVP should only be performed if the results from the dexamethasone and CRH tests are not definitive. The test is rarely used in clinical practice.

Combined Noninvasive Testing

The noninvasive dynamic tests have limitations in discriminating Cushing disease from ectopic ACTH secretion; therefore, combining different tests may be more discriminative than each test alone. Combining the high-dose dexamethasone test with the CRH test requires a negative cortisol response in the CRH-stimulation test plus a cortisol suppression of <50% in the dexamethasone test to exclude Cushing disease. The sensitivity and specificity of this combination is 99% and 94%, respectively.

Corticotropin-Releasing Hormone–Suppression Testing with Petrosal Venous Sampling

CRH-stimulation testing can also be performed with petrosal venous sinus sampling to determine if a patient has pituitary Cushing disease or ectopic ACTH production. The objective of this test is to assess whether or not the source of ACTH is the pituitary. Prior to administration of synthetic ovine CRH, sampling catheters are placed into both inferior petrosal veins (central) and in the iliac vein (peripheral). Simultaneous blood samples are drawn from all sites for plasma ACTH immediately before CRH infusion, and two sets are drawn at 2 to 3 minutes and 5 to 6 minutes after CRH infusion. A central-to-peripheral plasma ACTH gradient of 2.0 before CRH or 3.0 after CRH is diagnostic of pituitary ACTH production. A gradient of 1.4 to 1.5 between the two petrosal sinuses may predict the site of the adenoma but is only 70% accurate in lateralizing the adenoma. This test is very discriminative, with an overall sensitivity of 94% and a specificity of 100%. This procedure is not without complications and should only be performed if absolutely necessary.

Aldosterone Excess

In individuals suspected of having primary hyperaldosteronism, an aldosterone-suppression test is necessary. Suppressive agents include IV saline and oral sodium loading.

Salt Loading

In the saline-suppression test, the individual arrives in the early morning and should lie supine for at least 1 hour before receiving a 4-hour infusion of IV saline (500 cm³/hour). Prior to testing, all antihypertensive medications should be discontinued (2 weeks before) and serum potassium should be normalized to 3.5 mEq/L. Baseline samples for serum aldosterone, potassium, and sodium are collected immediately prior to, 2 hours after, and 4 hours after infusion. In normal individuals, post-saline suppression aldosterone levels drop 50% to 80% from baseline to <10 ng/dL and, usually, are suppressed to <5 ng/dL. Post-saline aldosterone levels >10 ng/dL are highly suggestive of hyperaldosteronism.

In the oral sodium–loading test, individuals add 10 to 12 g of salt (NaCl) to their diet for 5 days. On day 5, the individual collects a 24-hour urine that will be sampled for sodium and aldosterone excretion. If high sodium intake is verified (urine sodium ≥250 mEq/day), and the urine aldosterone excretion rate is ≥14 mg/day, a diagnosis of hyperaldosteronism is likely.

Corticotropin-Releasing Hormone Stimulation

A CRH-stimulation test with adrenal venous sampling can be performed to distinguish between an adrenal adenoma and adrenal hyperplasia in patients diagnosed with primary hyperaldosteronism. CRH is infused 30 minutes before and continued throughout testing. Measurements of cortisol and aldosterone levels are obtained on samples from the inferior vena cava (IVC) and both adrenal veins. Cortisol levels that are fivefold higher in the adrenal veins compared with that in the IVC constitute successful testing. A lateralizing response is defined as a serum aldosterone/cortisol ratio fourfold higher in the adrenal vein draining the secreting side. A ratio <3 is characteristic of bilateral aldosterone hypersecretion.

DISORDERS OF GROWTH HORMONE

Growth hormone (GH) secretion is regulated by the stimulatory effects of growth hormone–releasing hormone (GHRH) and the inhibitory effects of somatostatin; a peptide hormone produced in the brain and several cells in the digestive system. In the brain, somatostatin is produced by neuroendocrine neurons of the periventricular nucleus of the hypothalamus and inhibits GH secretion. GH is secreted in pulsatile bursts, especially during sleep; therefore, random single samples obtained during the day usually do not provide information regarding its secretory capacity. Dynamic testing is necessary to determine if a GH-related disorder is present. If the clinical history and physical findings are suggestive of a GH-related disorder, static screening studies such as insulin-derived growth factor (IGF)-1 and IGF-binding protein(BP)-3 may be collected. IGF-1, also known as *somatomedin C*, is a hormone similar in structure to insulin that plays an important role in childhood growth and continues to have anabolic effects in adults. It is produced by the liver, stimulated by GH, and the primary mediator of the effects of GH. Approximately 98% of IGF-1 is bound to one of six binding proteins, of which IGFBP-3 is the most abundant, accounting for 80% of all IGF-1 binding. The diagnosis of GH deficiency, however, cannot be confirmed or ruled out until dynamic testing is performed. The current GH-stimulation tests, with an upper limit of diagnostic sensitivity at 80% and a lower limit of specificity at 25%, may not be very accurate in predicting who has and who will respond to GH therapy. The sensitivity and specificity of GH-stimulation tests are attributable to broad inter-subject variation in GH clearance, rates of GH elimination, and GH volume of distribution.

Because GH is necessary for linear growth, evaluations for GH deficiency are most commonly performed in children who are short or who are growing poorly. Adults may also develop GH deficiency, but because they have generally completed linear growth, symptoms will determine the need for the evaluation of GH deficiency.

Growth Hormone Deficiency

The evaluation of GH deficiency is performed in the morning after an overnight fast. GH secretory status can be assessed by measurement of GH concentrations during physiologic conditions (e.g., sleep, fasting, and exercise) or in response to a pharmacologic agent (Table 19-5). Physiologic stimuli are not as reliable as pharmacologic stimuli. GH-stimulation testing is nonphysiologic, and cutoff levels of "normal" are arbitrary. These tests are age-dependent, have variable accuracy, questionable reproducibility, and are expensive. They should be limited to those individuals with a high index of clinical suspicion for GH deficiency, such as those with other pituitary hormone deficiencies, poor linear growth, or family history of growth problems. The tests should not be performed simply because a child is of short stature. Children require more GH than adults to promote linear growth. Therefore, in children, a stimulated GH level $\geq$10 ng/mL is normal, whereas in adults, a GH level $\geq$5 ng/mL is appropriate.

Dynamic testing of GH requires that the individual be referred to a specialized endocrine testing center in the morning, between 7 and 9 AM, after a minimum of a 10-hour fast. To allow for delivery of the pharmacologic agent and to obtain multiple, timed blood samples, an IV line is placed, and a baseline blood sample is collected. The insulin-induced hypoglycemia test is the most specific test for GH deficiency. After collection of the baseline sample, regular insulin is infused over 1 minute, and blood is collected every 15 minutes for the first hour and every 30 minutes for the second hour. GH levels that fail to stimulate to $\geq$10 ng/mL with a simultaneously low glucose level (either <50% of the previous level or $\leq$40 mg/dL) are diagnostic for GH deficiency.

TABLE 19-5.   Growth Hormone–stimulation Testing

Agent	Dose	Route	Baseline and Stimulated Serum Tests	Lab Frequency
Insulin (regular)	0.1 U/kg	IV	GH, glucose	q15 min × 4; q30 min × 2
Arginine	0.5 g/kg[a]	IV	GH	q30 min × 4
Clonidine	0.15 mg/m²	po	GH	q30 min × 4
L-DOPA	125–500 mg[b]	po	GH	q30 min × 4
Glucagon	1 mg	IM	GH, glucose	q30 min × 6
Premarin	5 mg BID[c]	po	N/A	N/A

[a]Maximum dose = 30 g.
[b]125 mg (<13.5 kg), 250 mg (13.5 to 35 kg), 500 mg (>35 kg).
[c]Used as a primer 2 to 3 days before GH testing with arginine.
Notes: GH, growth hormone; L-DOPA, L-3,4-dihydroxyphenylalanine; IM, intramuscular; po, oral (*per os*).

Arginine stimulates GH secretion by inhibiting somatostatin. After collection of a baseline sample, arginine hydrochloride is infused over 30 minutes, and blood is sampled every 30 minutes over 2 hours. False-positive results can be reduced by administering oral L-3,4-dihydroxyphenylalanine (L-DOPA) just prior to arginine. For men and postmenopausal women, the GH response to arginine may improve by pretreatment with premarin. Endogeneous GH secretion is increased during puberty, but estrogen priming has not proven to improve GH-stimulation tests in children.

Clonidine and L-DOPA stimulate GH secretion by binding to the central α2-adrenergic receptors, causing an increase in GH secretion. After collection of a baseline blood sample, clonidine or L-DOPA is taken orally, and GH levels are collected every 30 minutes for 2 hours. The clonidine test is not recommended because the side effects include hypotension and hypoglycemia.

Glucagon may also be used in the evaluation of GH deficiency. Glucagon causes transient hyperglycemia, stimulating endogenous insulin secretion and, ultimately, causing an in increase in GH secretion. This procedure is preferred over the insulin-induced hypoglycemia test in infants and younger children due to its enhanced safety profile. After glucagon administration, GH levels are drawn every 30 minutes for 3 hours. Side effects include nausea, vomiting, sweating, and headaches.

GH secretion may be subnormal due to hypothyroidism. Therefore, it is imperative that thyroid status be determined prior to GH-stimulation testing. If hypothyroidism is present, GH-stimulation testing should be postponed until the patient is biochemically euthyroid. The insulin-induced hypoglycemia test may provide the best accuracy in determining if an individual is GH deficient; it does require the patient to become significantly hypoglycemic. Because there is no gold standard, two tests are usually performed. The decision as to which tests to choose depends on the capabilities of the testing center and risks of the pharmacologic agents.

Acromegaly

In individuals with a compatible clinical history and physical appearance consistent with acromegaly, the diagnosis is relatively easy to confirm. In the absence of serious illness or malnutrition, serum levels of IGF-1 are uniformly elevated. The gold standard for making the diagnosis of acromegaly is the GH response to the oral glucose tolerance test (OGTT). GH secretion is a counterregulatory defense against hypoglycemia, and physiologic GH secretion is inhibited by hyperglycemia. In individuals with acromegaly, or children with gigantism, GH secretion is autonomous and does not suppress with hyperglycemia. Therefore, failure to suppress GH levels during the OGTT is diagnostic of acromegaly (adults) or gigantism (children). In the OGTT, after collecting baseline samples (GH and glucose), a glucose solution (1.75 g/kg, maximum 100 g) is given orally, and blood is collected every 30 minutes for 3 hours. Normally, GH levels suppress to <2 ng/mL within 2 hours. Today, using the newest available assays, including the immunoradiometric or immunochemiluminescent assays, GH levels in the nonacromegalic individual suppress to <0.4 μg/L. Values >1 μg/L are diagnostic of acromegaly. The majority of those with acromegaly have GH levels >2 μg/L.

DISORDERS OF THE HYPOTHALAMIC-PITUITARY-THYROID AXIS

The hypothalamus secretes thyrotropin-releasing hormone (TRH) to increase the secretion of thyroid-stimulating hormone (TSH) from the anterior pituitary gland. TSH is secreted into the circulation and stimulates secretion of the thyroid hormones, thyroxine (T_4) and triiodothyronine (T_3) from the thyroid gland. Thyroid hormones feedback at the level of the hypothalamus and pituitary and inhibit secretion of TRH and TSH, respectively.

Hypothyroidism

Central and primary hypothyroidism present in a very similar manner. Unlike GH and adrenal hormones, TSH and thyroid hormones have minimal fluctuation throughout the day. Therefore, static levels for TSH and T_4 are usually reliable and stable enough to make a diagnosis of hypo- or hyperthyroidism without dynamic testing. In rare instances, when an individual has a low T_4 and normal TSH, the TRH-stimulation test could be utilized to diagnose or rule out central hypothyroidism. In this test, after a baseline blood sample for TSH is collected, 400 to 500 μg of synthetic TRH is infused intravenously. Blood samples for TSH are collected 30 and 60 minutes after baseline. In the euthyroid patient, TSH normally rises by 2 to 20 mIU/L. In the patient with central hypothyroidism or isolated TSH deficiency, there is no rise in TSH. This test is not recommended for routine use because of its widely variable results and side effects including transient nausea, headache, dizziness, mild hypertension, gustatory sensations, flushing, and urinary urgency. TRH-stimulation testing should not be performed in individuals with epilepsy because it lowers the seizure threshold and in those with large pituitary tumors because it increases the risk for developing pituitary apoplexy.

DISORDERS OF THE HYPOTHALAMIC-PITUITARY-GONADAL AXIS

The hypothalamus secretes gonadotropin-releasing hormone (GnRH) in a pulsatile pattern to stimulate release of follicle-stimulating hormone (FSH) and LH from the anterior pituitary. GnRH secretion is regulated by dopamine, serotonin, endorphin, and norepinephrine. Hypogonadism that is the result of a hypothalamic or pituitary defect results in low gonadotropin levels (i.e., hypogonadotropic hypogonadism). Hypogonadism that is due to a primary gonadal insult results in elevated gonadotropin levels (i.e., hypergonadotropic hypogonadism). There are many causes of hypogonadism (see Chapters 12 and 13), and the biochemical evaluation involves both static and dynamic tests. In most cases of primary gonadal failure, dynamic testing is usually not necessary insofar as FSH and LH levels are usually well above the normal range. In central hypogonadism, however, stimulation testing with GnRH is generally required to determine if gonadotropin levels increase.

Delayed Puberty

Hypogonadism due to lack of gonadotropins (hypogonadotropic hypogonadism) or a primary gonadal failure (hypergonadotropic hypogonadism) results in delayed or absence of puberty. In hypergonadotropic hypogonadism, loss of negative feedback from gonadal sex steroids (estrogen in females, testosterone in males) and inhibin on the hypothalamus and pituitary gland results in increased gonadotropin levels. Therefore, stimulation testing is only necessary in those who have low gonadotropin levels.

Hypogonadotropic Hypogonadism

For an individual without signs of puberty or who has a bone age in which signs of puberty should be present (females by age 12 years, males by age 14 years), a serum FSH level <1.2 IU/L suggests hypogonadotropic hypogonadism. If the FSH level is ≥1.2 IU/L, a GnRH-stimulation test can be performed to evaluate the hypothalamic–pituitary–gonadal axis. GnRH is administered after basal levels of testosterone, FSH, and LH are determined. Serum FSH and LH are measured at 15, 30, 45, 60, and 120 minutes after luteinizing hormone–releasing hormone (LHRH) infusion to determine peak values and LH to FSH ratios. In the prepubertal state, levels increase two- to fourfold with a mean peak LH/FSH ratio of 0.7. In the pubertal state, LH levels increase six- to tenfold, and FSH increases four- to sixfold with a mean peak LH/FSH ratio of 3.5. If the peak FSH level is <4.6 IU/L, and peak LH level is <5.8 IU/L, the individual has hypogonadotropic hypogonadism. If FSH and LH levels are above those cutoff values, the individual likely has a constitutional delay of puberty (see Chapter 14).

Hypergonadotropic Hypogonadism

In adolescents with primary gonadal failure, a stimulation test is rarely necessary because as long as puberty should be occurring (based on bone age), static levels of gonadotropins should be elevated. In the neonate or infant male, however, because testosterone and gonadotropin levels rapidly decline to less than measurable levels by age 6 months, a stimulation test may be necessary. For those suspected of primary failure, a human chorionic gonadotropin (HCG)–stimulation test can be performed. The overall goal of HCG stimulation is to determine whether functioning testicular Leydig cells are present and capable of producing testosterone. The child presents in the morning but does not need to be fasting. Baseline blood samples are collected for FSH, LH, androstenedione, dehydroepiandrosterone-sulfate (DHEA-S), and dihydrotestosterone. Immediately after collection, HCG is delivered intramuscularly based on the age of the child (Table 19-6). The dose of HCG is repeated at the same time over the next 2 days, and, on the fourth day, 24 hours after the previous injection, baseline blood studies are repeated. A normal response is an HCG-stimulated testosterone level >250 ng/dL. An absent response with elevated LH/FSH levels confirms primary gonadal failure. If the androstenedione and DHEA-S levels are elevated with an absent testosterone response, there is likely a block in testosterone biosynthesis. A rise in testosterone without a rise in dihydrotestosterone suggests 5α-reductase deficiency.

TABLE 19-6.	Human Chorionic Gonadotropin Dosing in the Evaluation for Male Hypogonadism	
Age	**Dose of Human Chorionic Gonadotropin (Units)**
<6 mo	500
6 mo to <5 y	1,000
5 y to <10 y	1,500
≥10 y	2,000

Precocious Puberty

Children with precocious puberty can either have gonadotropin-dependent or gonadotropin-independent disease. In children with gonadotropin-dependent precocious puberty, gonadotropin levels will stimulate after receiving a dose of LHRH. In those with gonadotropin-independent precocious puberty, gonadotropin levels will not increase after LHRH stimulation. In the LHRH-stimulation test, baseline and stimulated serum LH levels are measured after administration of 100 µg of IV LHRH. Previous recommendations included the collection of FSH and LH levels prior to and every 15 minutes after (for 1 hour) receiving LHRH. Recent evidence indicates that a one-time measurement of an LH level, collected 40 minutes after receiving LHRH, is sufficient. If the LH level is ≥5 IU/L, central precocious puberty is confirmed. If the LH level is <5 IU/L, the child does not have gonadotropin-dependent precocious puberty but, rather, has gonadotropin-independent precocious puberty.

DISORDERS OF WATER REGULATION

The hypothalamus produces vasopressin, or anti-diuretic hormone (ADH), that is subsequently transported to the posterior pituitary gland, where it is stored for release. ADH is secreted into circulation in response to increased serum osmolality or decreased effective circulating volume by the posterior pituitary. It travels in circulation to the collecting ducts of the kidneys, where it binds to V_2 receptors and causes expression of aquaporin-2 water channel proteins on the apical membranes of these cells. Consequently, the sodium gradient drives water reabsorption.

Diabetes Insipidus

For those individuals with polyuria, polydypsia, a dilute urine, and normal serum glucose, the differential diagnosis is limited to diabetes insipidus (DI) or psychogenic polydypsia. In central DI there is inadequate release of ADH, whereas in nephrogenic DI, the kidneys fail to respond to ADH. A water-deprivation test is used to distinguish between psychogenic polydipsia and the two types of DI.

After an overnight fast, urine and plasma osmolality are measured, followed by water deprivation. Hourly weights, urine volumes, urine osmolality, serum osmolality, and serum electrolytes are measured. Once the urine or serum osmolality on three consecutive tests varies by <30 mOsm/kg, a serum ADH level is measured and then either IV or intranasal DDAVP is given. Urine osmolality is obtained at 30 and 60 minutes. In normal individuals, urine osmolality should be greater than plasma osmolality following water deprivation and should increase only minimally (<10%) after DDAVP. In those individuals with DI, urine osmolality is less than plasma osmolality following fluid restriction. DDAVP increases urine osmolality by >50% in central DI. In nephrogenic DI, urine osmolality does not change.

COMBINED ANTERIOR PITUITARY TESTING

This test is used to determine pituitary reserve function after pituitary surgery, radiation, and head trauma or, for patients previously on chronic hormone replacement after hormone withdrawal. CRH, GHRH, GnRH, and TRH are given IV sequentially over 30 seconds each. Blood measurements of ACTH, GH, LH, FSH, TSH, and prolactin are made at baseline, 15, 30, 60, 90, and 120 minutes after infusion. Results are interpreted according to individual tests as listed above.

CASE FOLLOW-UP

For individuals who present with polyuria and polydipsia, diabetes mellitus (DM) must be ruled out. This is usually simple because the individual with DM also has hyperglycemia and glycosuria. Our young boy has the classic symptoms except for the fact that he does not have any glucose abnormalities. Without hyperglycemia, the differential diagnosis for polyuria and polydipsia is limited to three conditions: central DI, nephrogenic DI, and psychogenic polydipsia. Individuals with DI who have an intact thirst mechanism, access to liquids, and the ability to urinate can maintain normal electrolytes assuming adequate liquid intake is maintained. Individuals with psychogenic polydipsia have polyuria because they drink excessively. If liquid intake is limited, urine output will decrease. A water-deprivation test was ordered to determine the etiology of our patient's problem. The test involves frequent blood and urine sampling during which time he is unable to eat or drink. He is brought to the hospital to perform the test, which begins at 8 AM. The following table reveals hourly urine osmolality, serum osmolality, serum sodium, urine output, weight, blood pressure, and hydration status:

Time	Serum Na (mEq/L)	Serum Osmolality (mOsm/kg)	Urine Output (cm³)	Urine Osmolality (mOsm/kg)	Weight (kg)	BP (mmHg)	Action
8 AM	145	295			35.0	95/60	
9 AM	147	315	100	305	34.5	92/58	
10 AM	148	330	130	110	34.0	90/55	
11 AM	151	335	110	90	33.5	85/50	
12 PM	154	340	115	65	33.0	82/47	
1 PM	157	345	135	50	32.0	78/45	DDAVP
2 PM	147	299	0	310	33.5	85/50	

Note: DDAVP, desmopressin.

(continues)

CASE FOLLOW-UP (*continued*)

From the table, it is obvious that despite depriving our patient of liquid, he continues to urinate, lose weight, lower his blood pressure, and maintain dilute urine. This case is now highly suspicious for DI. The next step is to determine if he has central DI or nephrogenic DI. A dose of subcutaneous DDAVP is given at 1 PM, and by 2 PM, he shows improvement, confirming that he has central DI, or a decrease in vasopressin secretion.

Further work-up in the evaluation for the etiology of his central DI revealed that he has histiocytosis X. Immune cells attacked the bone in his skull and around his ear canal, thus causing the frequent evaluations and treatment for otitis. His DI was easy to treat, because he maintained appropriate fluid intake, urination, and serum sodium levels on a twice-daily dose of intranasal DDAVP.

The histiocytosis X, however, was not as easy to treat, and our patient required both radiation therapy and chemotherapy. With proper follow-up in the oncology clinic, and because the histiocytosis was localized, the prognosis for this child is favorable.

REFERENCES and SUGGESTED READINGS

Berneis K, Staub JJ, Gessler A, Meier C, Girard J, Muller B. Combined stimulation of adrenocorticotropin and compound-S by single dose metyrapone test as an outpatient procedure to assess hypothalamic–pituitary–adrenal function. J Clin Endocrinol Metab. 2002;87(12):5470–5475.

Carmichael JD, Bonert VS, Mirocha JM, Melmed S. The utility of oral glucose tolerance testing for diagnosis and assessment of treatment outcomes in 166 patients with acromegaly. J Clin Endcorinol Metab. 2009;94(2):523–527.

Carroll TB, Findling JW. The diagnosis of Cushing's syndrome. Rev Endocr Metab Disord. 2010;11(2):147–153.

Cavallo A, Richards GE, Busey S, Michaela SE. A simplified gonadotropin-releasing hormone test for precocious puberty. Clin Endocrinol. 1995;42:641–646.

Fisher, DA. Endocrinology: Test Selection and Interpretation. 4th ed. San Juan Capistrano, CA: Quest Diagnostics; 2007.

Grinspon RP, Ropelato MG, Gottlieb S, Keselman A, Martinez A, Ballerini MG, et al. Basal follicle-stimulating hormone and peak gonadotropin levels after gonadotropin-releasing hormone infusion show high diagnostic accuracy in boys with suspicion of hypogonadotropic hypogonadism. J Clin Endocrinol Metab. 2010;95(6): 2811–2818.

Guistina A, Chanson P, Bronstein MD, Klibanski A, Lamberts S, Casanueva FF, et al. A consensus on criteria for cure of acromegaly. J Clin Endocrinol Metab. 2010;95(7):3141–3148.

Kandemir N, Demirbilek H, Ozon ZA, Gonc N, Alikasifoglu A. TGnRH stimulation test in precocious puberty: single sample is adequate for diagnosis and dose adjustment. J Clin Res Pediatr Endocrinol. 2011;3(1):12–17.

Kazlauskaite R, Evans AT, Villabona CV, Abdu TA, Ambrosi B, Atkinson AB, et al. Corticotropin tests for hypothalamic-pituitary- adrenal insufficiency: a metaanalysis. J Clin Endocrinol Metab. 2008;93(11):4245–4253.

Knoers NVAM. Hyperactive vasopressin receptors and disturbed water homeostasis. N Engl J Med. 2005;352(18):1847–1850.

Makaryus AN, McFarlane SI. Diabetes insipidus: diagnosis and treatment of a complex disease. Cleve Clin J Med. 2006;73(1):65–71.

Moncayo H, Dapunt O, Moncayo R. Diagnostic accuracy of basal TSH determinations based on the intravenous TRH stimulation test: an evaluation of 2570 tests and comparison with the literature. BMC Endocr Disord. 2007;7:5–10.

Pandian R, Nakamoto JM. Rational use of the laboratory for childhood and adult growth hormone deficiency. Clin Lab Med. 2004;24:141–174.

Petersenn S, Quabbe HJ, Schofl C, Stalla GK, von Werder K, Buchfelder M. The rational use of pituitary stimulation tests. Dtsch Arztebl Int. 2010;107(25):437–443.

CHAPTER REVIEW QUESTIONS

1. Which of the following conditions does not typically require dynamic testing to confirm its diagnosis?

   A. Addison disease
   B. Kallmann syndrome
   C. Septo-optic dysplasia
   D. Graves disease
   E. Diabetes insipidus

2. A 25-year-old woman presents with weight gain, difficulty climbing stairs, abnormal menses, and depression. On examination, she has a prominent dorsocervical hump, wide abdominal striae, and facial plethora. A 24-hour urine free cortisol level is 387 g/dL (normal = <90 g/dL). Inferior petrosal sinus sampling is performed during corticotropin-releasing hormone (CRH) infusion. Bilateral inferior petrosal sinus sampling with plasma adrenocorticotropic hormone (ACTH) levels before and after CRH administration are shown below. What is the most likely diagnosis?

	ACTH (before CRH) (pg/mL)	ACTH (3 min post-CRH) (pg/mL)
Right petrosal sinus	57	63
Left petrosal sinus	67	72
Peripheral vein	68	70
Normal range	10–60	50–100

   A. Lung carcinoma producing ACTH
   B. Adrenal carcinoma producing ACTH
   C. Hypothalamic hamartoma
   D. Exogenous glucocorticoid therapy
   E. Pituitary macroadenoma producing ACTH

3. A 50-year-old woman seeks evaluation for a complaint of increasing shoe size. Further history indicates severe arthritis in her knees and a 10-year history of type 2 diabetes. Examination shows prognathism and wide-spaced teeth. Which of the following is the best test to make the correct diagnosis?

   A. Oral glucose-suppression test
   B. Magnetic resonance imaging of the head
   C. Growth hormone level
   D. Fasting prolactin level
   E. Petrosal sinus and peripheral blood sampling after corticotropin-releasing hormone (CRH) infusion

4. An 8-year-old boy is brought to the clinic because of concerns regarding his small size. On examination, he is 116 cm (<1st percentile) and weighs 19.4 kg (<1st percentile). He has shown poor growth over the past 3 years. Which of the following is the best test to determine if he has growth hormone deficiency?

   A. Fasting growth hormone levels
   B. Oral glucose–suppression testing

C. Insulin-induced hypoglycemia

D. Clonidine-stimulation test

E. Intravenous desmopressin

5. A 36-year-old man has been treated for 3 years for hypertension. He is currently taking three different antihypertensive medications but is still hypertensive. An electrolyte panel collected prior to starting any of his medications is remarkable for an elevated sodium level (148 mEq/L) and low potassium level (3.0 mEq/L). You are concerned that he may have hyperaldosteronism. In regard to the saline-loading test, all of the following are true *except*:

A. He must be off his blood pressure medications for at least 2 weeks prior to the test.

B. He will receive a 4-hour infusion of 0.9% NaCl.

C. Blood should be collected for serum sodium, potassium, aldosterone, and plasma renin activity.

D. A serum aldosterone level <5 ng/dL after the 4-hour infusion confirms hyperaldosteronism.

E. Blood sampling should occur at baseline, 2 hours after infusion, and 4 hours after infusion.

CHAPTER REVIEW ANSWERS

1. The correct answer is D. Graves disease is caused by autoantibodies to the thyroid gland called *thyroid-stimulating immunoglobulins*. Diagnosis is via static testing of thyroid-stimulating hormone, free thyroxine, and antibodies. All of the other choices are incorrect.

Addison disease (**Choice A**) is most commonly caused by an autoimmune destruction of the adrenal cortex resulting in insufficient production of glucocorticoids and mineralocorticoids. Those with Addison disease may present with hyponatremia, hyperkalemia, hypoglycemia, and hypotension. It is the most common cause of primary adrenal insufficiency in the United States. Addison disease results in primary adrenal insufficiency and individuals suspected of having it should undergo stimulation tests with cortrosyn (high dose) or insulin. Kallmann syndrome (**Choice B**) results from a defect in migration of neurons from the olfactory placode to the hypothalamus. These individuals most commonly present with anosmia and hypogonadotropic hypogonadism. As these individuals are deficient in gonadotropin-releasing hormone, confirmation of hypogonadotropic hypogonadism can be made with luteinizing hormone–releasing hormone–stimulation testing. Septo-optic dysplasia (SOD) (**Choice C**) is a heterogenous condition that results in midline and forebrain anomalies, optic nerve hypoplasia, and pituitary hypoplasia. Patients with SOD may have multiple pituitary hormone deficits including growth hormone (GH) deficiency, central diabetes insipidus (DI), and adrenocorticotropic hormone (ACTH) deficiency. The evaluation for the suspicion of GH, ACTH, cortisol, or antidiuretic hormone (ADH) deficiency requires stimulation testing.

DI (**Choice E**) can either be central, due to deficient ADH secretion, or nephrogenic due to impaired renal response to ADH. Water-deprivation testing is used to distinguish between these etiologies.

2. The correct answer is A. This woman is presenting with signs of cortisol excess, or Cushing syndrome, which may result from exogenous glucocorticoids, an adrenocorticotropic hormone (ACTH)-producing adenoma or ectopic ACTH production. Small cell carcinoma of the lung can produce ectopic ACTH. With corticotropin-releasing hormone (CRH) testing, ectopic ACTH production causes no increase in ACTH levels, whereas patients with Cushing disease should have increased ACTH levels. All of the other choices are incorrect.

Adrenal carcinoma producing ACTH (**Choice B**) would result in elevated ACTH levels in the peripheral vein with normal levels in the petrosal sinuses. Hypothalamic hamarto-mas (**Choice C**) are malformations that can distort the lateral hypothalamus and pituitary gland. They may uncommonly cause ACTH deficiency but not ACTH excess. Exoge-nous glucocorticoid therapy (**Choice D**) causes secondary adrenal insufficiency with decreased serum ACTH levels. A pituitary macroadenoma producing ACTH (**Choice E**) results in a central to peripheral ACTH gradient of 3.0 after CRH administration. Here the ratio is nearly 1, ruling out a pituitary cause of ACTH excess.

3. The correct answer is A. The patient is presenting with signs of acromegaly. Dynamic testing for the evaluation for acromegaly involves the oral glucose–suppression test. In the normal individual, glucose loads should suppress the release of growth hormone (GH) from the pituitary gland. In individuals with acromegaly, the GH levels are not suppressed.

Magnetic resonance imaging of the head (**Choice B**) would be useful in locating a pitu-itary tumor only if the tumor were large (i.e., >9 mm). Most pituitary tumors, especially those secreting excess GH are microadenomas, and are difficult to pick up on imaging studies. Therefore, an oral glucose–suppression test is the most specific test for making the diagnosis of acromegaly. GH levels (**Choice C**) fluctuate with time of day and nutri-tional status and are rarely helpful as a static test.

Prolactinomas are the most common pituitary adenomas and result in visual field defects, loss of libido, abnormal menses, and galactorrhea. Prolactin levels do not fluctu-ate during the day, so a fasting prolactin level (**Choice D**) is unnecessary. Additionally, this patient is presenting with signs of GH, not prolactin, excess. Petrosal sinus and peripheral blood sampling after CRH infusion (**Choice E**) is used to detect pituitary or ectopic causes of cortisol excess not acromegaly.

4. The correct answer is C. Insulin-induced hypoglycemia is the most sensitive test for detection of growth hormone (GH) deficiency. Hypoglycemia triggers the release of counterregulatory hormones, such as glucagon, norepinephrine, cortisol, and GH. A GH level <10 µg/dL after insulin administration, in addition to the history of having poor growth confirms GH deficiency.

A fasting growth hormone level (**Choice A**) is incorrect because GH secretion is pulsa-tile with surges occurring at 3- to 5-hour intervals. Therefore, a static, one-time GH level is of little value in supporting the diagnosis of GH deficiency. An oral glucose–suppression test (**Choice B**) is used in evaluating an individual for acromegaly (GH excess) not GH deficiency. An increased glucose load should suppress GH release. Clonidine (**Choice D**) is a stimulating agent used in the evaluation of GH deficiency but is a less sensitive test than insulin for diagnosing GH deficiency. In the evaluation of GH deficiency, clonidine should be rarely used in children because it can cause hypotension. Intravenous or sub-cutaneous desmopressin (**Choice E**) is used to treat central diabetes (DI). It is also used during a water-deprivation test to differentiate between central and nephrogenic DI. It does not have a significant role in GH secretion.

5. The correct answer is D. This patient is being evaluated for hyperaldosteronism with a saline-suppression test. This statement is the only statement that is not true. In the normal individual, post-saline serum aldosterone levels are usually suppressed to

<5 ng/dL. In individuals with levels >10 ng/dL, hyperaldosteronism is highly likely. Therefore, an aldosterone level of <5 ng/dL after a saline infusion would be expected in an individual who does not have hyperaldosteronism. Although it is not always possible, in those individuals undergoing a saline-suppression test to rule out hyperaldosteronism, all antihypertensive medications should be discontinued for 2 weeks before testing (**Choice A**). For the saline-suppression test, a 0.9% NaCl solution is infused for 4 hours at a rate of 500 cm³/hour (**Choice B**). During the saline-suppression test, blood sampling should occur at baseline, 2 hours after infusion, and when the infusion is complete (after 4 hours) (**Choice E**). The blood is collected and sampled for serum sodium, serum aldosterone, serum potassium, and plasma renin activity (**Choice C**).

Nuclear Medicine Approaches to Endocrinology

20

Stanislav Polioshenko
Raghuveer Halkar

CASE

A 51-year-old female presents to her primary care physician with a history of extreme anterior neck pain radiating to her chest and ears for the past 2 weeks. She also admits to feeling weak, having jitteriness in her hands, and having difficulty in sleeping. Other than an upper respiratory tract infection that she developed 4 weeks ago, and resolved within a few days, she denies any significant past medical or surgical history. She is taking no medications. Her family history is unremarkable.

Her vital signs are as follows: temperature, 98.0°F; respiratory rate, 12 breaths per minute; blood pressure, 150/64 mmHg (both arms); and pulse, 114 beats per minute. On examination, she is sweating, appears nervous, and has an asymmetric thyroid gland with the right lobe larger than the left. There is a firm 2×2 cm nodule on the right. She also has a firm and enlarged right anterior cervical lymph node. She has poor proximal muscle strength.

A variety of tools are used to produce images including ultrasound waves, magnetic and radiofrequency fields, and photons of varying energies. The usefulness of each modality depends on the location in the body and/or type of disease being imaged. Many modalities are used to evaluate endocrine abnormalities; the most widely used involve nuclear medicine.

This chapter explains what therapeutic and imaging modalities are available to evaluate and treat this patient; at the end of the chapter, a table summarizing the radionuclides used in imaging and treating endocrine conditions is provided. This chapter has been organized to: 1) review the fundamentals of nuclear medicine and 2) review the imaging and therapeutic modalities available for evaluating and treating a patient with endocrine pathology.

(continues)

(continued)

OBJECTIVES

1. List the most common radionuclides used for imaging patients with suspected endocrine disorders.

2. List the indications for the use of nuclear imaging in specific endocrine disorders.

3. Recognize the role of nuclear medicine in the treatment of endocrine disorders.

CHAPTER OUTLINE

Iodine-123 and Iodine-131
  Metaiodobenzlguanidine
18-Fluorodeoxyglucose
Indium-111 OctreoScan
Clinical applications
Thyroid Gland
  Radioactive Iodine Uptake and
    Scintigraphy
  Patient Preparation
  Thyroid Nodule
  Ectopic Thyroid Tissue
  Thyroiditis
  Graves Disease
  Multinodular Goiter
Parathyroid Glands
  Parathyroid Scintigraphy
  Hyperparathyroidism
Adrenal Glands
  Adrenal Cortex
  Adrenal Medulla
Neuroendocrine Tumors

NUCLEAR MEDICINE

Nuclear medicine is a branch of medical imaging that uses small amounts of radioactive material to diagnose and determine the severity of heart disease, gastrointestinal, endocrine, and neurological disorders. It is also used for treatment of hyperthyroidism and differentiated thyroid cancer. Nuclear medicine procedures are able to pinpoint molecular activity within the body; therefore, they offer the potential of identifying disease in its earliest stages, guide therapeutic choices, and assess the response to therapeutic interventions.

Nuclear medicine imaging procedures are noninvasive and, with the exception of intravenous injections, are painless tests that help clinicians diagnose and evaluate medical conditions. These imaging scans use radioactive materials called **radiopharmaceuticals**, or *radiotracers*. Depending on the type of nuclear medicine examination, the radiotracer is either injected into the body, ingested, or inhaled as a gas and eventually accumulates in the organ or area of the body being examined. Radioactive emissions from the radiotracer are detected by a special camera or imaging device that produces pictures and detailed molecular information.

In many centers, nuclear medicine images can be superimposed with computed tomography (CT) or magnetic resonance imaging (MRI) to produce special views, a practice known as **image fusion**, or *co-registration*. These views allow the information from two different examinations to be correlated and interpreted on one image, leading to more accurate diagnoses. In addition, manufacturers are now making single photon–emission computed tomography (SPECT)/CT and positron-emission tomography (PET)/CT units that are able to perform both imaging examinations at the same time. An emerging imaging technology (but not yet readily available) is PET/MRI.

Nuclear medicine utilizes radioactive decay to produce an image. A radioactive label is attached to a biologically active molecule, such as glucose. When the radioactive substance spontaneously decays, a γ particle is released and recorded by an imaging device such as a γ camera.

Specific biologic agents are chosen depending on the area of the body to be studied. The biologically active molecule can localize to tissue by active transport, phagocytosis, or receptor binding. By choosing an agent utilized by a specific tissue, the radiotracer will congregate in that tissue and identify the area of activity when γ rays from the tracer are recorded. The image produced by a nuclear scan has a low spatial resolution and a high contrast. To overcome this problem of limited spatial resolution, nuclear medicine techniques are often combined with CT scans to create an image that overlays anatomy and function.

Scintigraphy is the name of a basic two-dimensional nuclear medicine image formed by detection of γ rays. SPECT and PET are two types of nuclear imaging techniques. Both capture multiple two-dimensional images in order to construct a three-dimensional image. They differ in that γ rays are measured directly in SPECT (i.e., the tracer itself emits γ rays that are detected by a γ camera). PET utilizes a tracer that emits positrons that disturb neighboring electrons, which then emit a pair of photons pointed in opposite directions. PET has the benefit of the using this pair of γ rays to record only rays detected at the same time (and at opposite sides of the camera), creating an image with less distortion and higher special resolution than SPECT. In the SPECT, the radionuclides pass safely through the body and are detected by a scanner. In the PET scan, the radionuclide remains in the blood stream rather than being absorbed by tissues, thereby limiting the image to locations where blood flows. Because SPECT and PET utilize different radioisotopes, SPECT is much less expensive than PET.

RADIATION

The radioactive isotopes or nuclides used in nuclear medicine are mainly emitters of γ rays and/or β particles. These are produced during radioactive decay as the nucleus moves toward its ground state. For a given isotope, there are characteristic energy emissions. The most frequent of these is referred to as its **peak energy**. Many of the isotopes used in nuclear medicine emit more than one β and/or γ particle. The emitted energy is measured in electron volts (eV), and most nuclides used in nuclear medicine emissions are in the kilo-electronvolts (keV) range.

Particles

A β particle is a high-velocity electron ejected from a disintegrating nucleus. This particle can have a negative charge (**negatron**, or β *emitter*) or a positive charge (**positron**). β Particles can be emitted with or without the simultaneous emission of a γ ray. Those emitted without γ rays are referred to as *pure β* emitters. These are used as therapeutic agents insofar as they deliver a localized dose of radiation. β Emitters with γ rays can be used for both therapy and imaging, whereas γ emissions are used for diagnostic imaging only. They provide electromagnetic energy and have no charge. They have a wavelength corresponding to very short X-rays. γ Rays differ from X-rays in their origin; γ rays come from the nucleus, whereas X-rays originate from the electron shell. When γ rays encounter certain detectors, a flash of light, or **scintillation**, is produced.

Positrons are positively charged β particles. After ejection from the nucleus, positrons almost immediately undergo an annihilation reaction by collision with an electron. Two photons of the same energy are emitted at 180° to one another.

Rate of Decay

The rate of decay of radioactive materials is measured in disintegrations/unit of time. The traditional unit is the Curie (3.7×10^{10} disintegrations/second). The international system unit is the becquerel (Bq) in which 1 Bq decays at a rate of 1 disintegration/second. The rate of decay of a given isotope is constant over time and is not influenced by pressure, temperature, or chemical combination. It is expressed in terms of physical half-life, the length of time required for half of the original number of atoms in a given radioactive sample to decay.

Sources

Nuclides are obtained from reactors, generators, and cyclotrons. The most common sources for nuclear medicine nuclides are generators and cyclotrons. Isotopes from cyclotrons are usually expensive.

Measurement

The measurement of exposed radiation includes the roentgen (R), which is the amount of energy per kilogram of air. The rad (radiation absorbed dose) is more meaningful because it describes the amount of energy imparted to matter by ionizing radiation per unit mass of irradiated material at the place of interest. The rem (radiation equivalent, man) is a unit of human biologic dose as a result of exposure to different types of ionizing radiation. For γ and X-rays, 1 rem = 1 rad.

RADIONUCLIDES

The total number of radionuclides is uncertain because the number of very short lived radionuclides that have yet to be characterized is large. There are at least 3,000 radionuclides including those that are stable and known to decay, stable but not observed to decay, experimentally observed to decay, and artificially produced. The most widely used radionuclides for imaging or treatment of endocrine conditions include technetium-99m (Tc-99m) pertechnetate, iodine (I)-131, iodine (I)-123, sestamibi, metaiodobenzylguanidine (MIBG), I-131-Norcholesterol (NP-59), 18-fluorodeoxyglucose (FDG), and indium (In)-111. A list of the radionuclides used in endocrinology along with their uses and features is shown at the end of the chapter (Table 20-1).

Technetium-99m Pertechnetate

Tc-99m pertechnetate is used for thyroid scintigraphy because of the many features it offers compared with I-123. Tc-99m pertechnetate competes for the same transport symporter as iodine, causing active transport of the radionuclide into the thyroid gland. Because it gives off γ rays during its radioactive decay, Tc-99m pertechnetate allows the γ camera to visualize its location. Due to the nature of its energy, the γ ray (140 keV) offers better resolution and less radiation than I-131. Because Tc-99m pertechnetate is produced by a generator, it is cheap, readily available, and has a relatively short half-life of 6 hours as compared to the 13-hour half-life of I-123 (which is cyclotron-produced and expensive), making Tc-99m pertechnetate generally a more desirable radionuclide for everyday workload. However, TC-99m pertechnetate is not organified in the gland as are iodine isotopes, which may lead to faster washing out of the tissue. Rarely, a nodule that has maintained the trapping function and has lost organification may be photopenic (cold) in an I-123 scan and can be photon intense (hot) in a technetium scan, thus resulting in discordance. Common indications for the use of Tc-99m pertechnetate are evaluation of hyperthyroid nodules, goiter, and congenital hypothyroidism.

Iodine-131

I-131 is a radioactive isotope of elemental iodine, which has a half-life of roughly 8 days. It emits both γ and β radiation as it decays; however, the vast majority of the radiation given off by I-131 is in the form of β particles, which only travel several millimeters from the nucleus of the isotope. These β particles are very destructive to the surrounding tissues and will cause mutation and apoptosis in the cells. Therefore, it is this property of I-131 that is used primarily for therapeutic indications to radioactively ablate tissue. The thyroid follicular cells will actively absorb any isotope of iodine in the body, thereby concentrating most of the radioactive I-131 within the gland, thereby drastically limiting the destructive properties of the isotope to only the thyroid and spare surrounding tissues. I-131 is given orally for ablating residual thyroid tissue after thyroidectomy for thyroid cancer, functioning thyroid metastases, and ablation of hyperthyroid tissue. Radioiodine-induced thyroiditis is an adverse effect of tissue destruction. In this situation, the thyroid follicular cells may release much higher amounts of thyroid hormone in response to the tissue apoptosis and, in turn, cause transient hyperthyroidism. Often pretreatment with propylthiouracil or methimazole is necessary prior to I-131 ablation—particularly in patients with heart conditions and those who cannot tolerate a hyperthyroid exacerbation.

Because β particles only travel several millimeters from the site of fission, they cannot be visualized on external cameras. The γ radiation that I-131 emits in its decay is visible on a γ camera. I-131 is the imaging modality used for whole-body scans to detect metastases from thyroid cancer, which requires much smaller doses than does radioablation. Its advantage when used for imaging is that it is significantly cheaper to produce than I-123.

Iodine-123

I-123, a radioisotope of elemental iodine, is the most commonly used nuclide for imaging of the thyroid gland because it is trapped by the thyroid symporters and organified in the gland. Its half-life (13.2 hours) is much shorter than that of I-131. This allows visualization of not only anatomic but also physiologic characteristics of the gland. As the radionuclide undergoes decay, it emits γ rays, which are picked up by a γ camera. This radionuclide does not emit β particles during its decay, making it unsuitable for radioablative therapy unlike I-131. The most common indications for using I-123 include the evaluation of hyperthyroid nodules, suspected discordant nodules, and substernal goiter. It is also used to evaluate and quantify iodine uptake by the thyroid gland prior to undergoing I-131 ablation treatment.

Technetium-99m Sestamibi

Metoxyisobutyl-isonitrile (MIBI) is a molecule that nonspecifically concentrates in the mitochondria and cytoplasm of cells when there are elevated membrane potentials across phospholipid bilayers. This localization to mitochondria correlates to cells with elevated metabolic states. Consequently, MIBI was first developed as a myocardial perfusion–imaging agent but was later noted to have affinity for certain hypermetabolic adenomas and tumors, such as thyroid and parathyroid adenomas. Prior to the use of sestamibi in parathyroid imaging, thallium-201 was used. Sestamibi shows a greater affinity for parathyroid tissue and exhibits a differential in its association and washout with thyroid and parathyroid glands. These different kinetics of sestamibi between thyroid and parathyroid tissue are used to create an early and 2 hour–delayed image that allows for superior visualization of the parathyroid tissue. The sestamibi portion of the compound molecule acts as the biologic tissue localizer, whereas the Tc-99m undergoes radioactive decay to emit γ rays, which are picked up by the γ camera.

Iodine-123 and Iodine-131 Metaiodobenzlguanidine

Metaiodobenzylguanidine (MIBG), or *iobenguane*, is an analog of the neurotransmitter norepinephrine (NE). Various neural crest and neuroendocrine tissues take up the molecule in high concentration relative to that of surrounding tissue because it is similar to NE. This is due to the action of the NE transporter in sympathetically innervated tissue. MIBG is typically labeled with I-123 or I-131, depending on whether imaging or ablation of neuroendocrine tissue is desired. MIBG is the biologic agent in this combination because it will localize to the tissue. The iodine isotope is the radionuclide that allows visualization on the γ camera. MIBG has been used to localize various neuroendocrine tumors, particularly those in the adrenal medulla, such as pheochromocytomas and neuroblastomas. More recently, MIBG has been used for myocardial scintigraphy to diagnose heart failure and cardiomyopathies.

18-Fluorodeoxyglucose

18-Fluorodeoxyglucose (18-FDG) is a radiotracer that is a glucose analog (deoxyglucose) with a substituted fluorine atom that does not enter the full metabolic pathway of glucose. This inability of the FDG to be fully metabolized causes the molecule to build up in tissues that have high metabolic activity. This radiotracer is used in oncologic staging and follow-up to detect the presence of tumors that are metabolically active. 18-FDG is commonly used to evaluate poorly differentiated thyroid carcinoma, because it has poor iodine uptake due to its anaplastic quality. Iodine and 18-FDG uptake are reciprocals in thyroid carcinomas as well-differentiated indolent tumors will have high iodine uptake and low 18-FDG uptake. Poorly differentiated, rapidly growing tumors will show the opposite on imaging. 18-FDG PET scan can also be used to differentiate benign from malignant pheochromocytomas, insofar as malignant tumors are typically more highly metabolically active than benign adenomas and will more avidly uptake the fluorinated glucose molecules along with normal glucose.

Indium-111 OctreoScan

Indium-111 (In-111) decays by electron transfer and has a physical half-life of 68 hours. It emits γ rays at approximately 171 and 245 keV. This isotope is used to localize neuroendocrine tumors because In-111 is chelated to a somatostatin-like molecule (octreotide) that binds to somatostatin receptors on the cell surface of most neuroendocrine tumors.

Ga-68 is a generator-produced positron emitter that is labeled with a sandostatin analog. It is used in Europe for diagnosing and localizing neuroendocrine tumors and as an investigational new drug in the United States. Two other sandostatin-labeled analogs, Y-90 and Lu-177, have been used for the treatment of metastatic neuroendocrine tumors in both Europe and Asia.

CLINICAL APPLICATIONS

The applications of nuclear medicine to endocrinology include imaging and treatment of disorders involving thyroid, parathyroid, adrenal, and neuroendocrine glands.

Thyroid Gland

The thyroid gland is embryologically derived from the ventral wall of the pharynx, from where it migrates caudally from the base of the tongue down the neck to the level of the cricoid cartilage. The thyroglossal duct, a remnant of the migration of the thyroid, is usually obliterated *in utero*. The thyroid gland has two lobes, each approximately 5×2 cm, and each weighs 15 to 30 g. The two lobes are connected by a narrow isthmus across the ventral portion of the trachea. The main function of the thyroid gland is to produce thyroxine (T_4) and triiodothyronine (T_3). In the process, ionized iodide is actively transported into the thyroid gland by the sodium iodide symporter on the follicular cells and then organified. Radiotracers aimed at thyroid imaging take advantage of the gland's ability to concentrate iodine within the body.

Radioactive Iodine Uptake and Scintigraphy

Radioactive iodine uptake (RAIU) is a functional study of the thyroid gland and is used to quantify the amount of iodine the gland can trap and organify. The study is carried out as follows: The patient is given a known quantity of I-123 in the form of a pill, and measurements of the amount of uptake are taken 4 and 24 hours later. The amount of uptake by the thyroid is read by a γ probe, which detects levels of emission. The RAIU study is followed by imaging with a γ camera, which provides a visual representation of the gland's anatomy. The normal values range 5% to 15% at 4 hours and 15% to 30% at 24 hours. The anatomy of the thyroid gland and clarification of any disease process can be evaluated by determining the characteristic pattern of emission of the I-123 in the thyroid gland. The indications for thyroid scintigraphy include the evaluation of a patient with: 1) a single thyroid nodule or, diffuse enlargement of the thyroid gland and laboratory evidence of a suppressed serum thyroid-stimulating hormone (TSH), 2) a multinodular goiter (MNG) and laboratory evidence of a suppressed serum TSH, 3) a large MNG with extension into the mediastinum, 4) suspicion of ectopic thyroid tissue, and 5) subclinical hyperthyroidism.

Patient Preparation

Thyroid imaging with nuclides is dependent on radioactive iodine. Proper preparation of the patient's thyroid gland is essential for obtaining a quality study. Because the study utilizes radioactive material, the patient must not be pregnant; because iodine is excreted in the milk, the patient should not breastfeed for 3 days after the study. The patient should not ingest any iodine-containing medicine or food for at least 7 days prior to the study. If the patient is on antithyroid therapy, such as methimazole, it should be stopped 7 days prior to the study. Because iodinated contrast contains a significant amount of free iodine, the patient should not receive iodinated contrast at least 6 weeks prior to the study. In postoperative thyroid cancer patients, the TSH must be elevated prior to imaging. This is done so that the thyroid gland will avidly take up any radioactive iodine given during the study and will allow for a greater detection of any small remaining tumor. A serum TSH level ≥ 30 mIU/L is optimal. This level can be achieved in one of two ways. The patient can either stop thyroid-hormone replacement well in advance of the study, allowing the body to naturally upregulate TSH, or the patient can receive recombinant TSH (rhTSH) just prior to the study. The rhTSH is used when the patient cannot tolerate a hypothyroid state for a prolonged period of time. In addition to withdrawal of thyroid-hormone replacement, patients are advised to follow a low-iodine diet for several weeks prior to the study.

Thyroid Nodule

The first step in evaluating the patient with a thyroid nodule is to rule out an underlying hyperfunctioning disorder, which is done by measuring the serum TSH. If the TSH level is normal, the next step is to ultrasound the nodule to evaluate the size, structure, and diffuse changes in the surrounding thyroid gland. This will also enable the clinician to locate the best area for biopsy, if needed. Several sonographic features of the nodule suggest an increased risk for malignancy including microcalcifications, hypoechogenicity, irregular margins, predominant solid composition, intranodular vascularity, and the absence of a hypoechogenic "halo" around the nodule. Patients who have the known risk factors for malignancy and have these sonographic features should undergo a fine needle–aspiration (FNA) biopsy of the nodule.

If the serum TSH level is high, a serum free T_4 level and a thyroid peroxidase antibody (TPOAb) should be obtained to determine if hypothyroidism and/or lymphocytic thyroiditis are present. However, abnormal biochemical values cannot exclude a malignancy, and the patient should undergo an ultrasound evaluation.

If a hyperfunctioning state is discovered (low TSH and high free T_4), radioiodine scintigraphy can be performed to differentiate nodules with low uptake (cold nodules) from those with high uptake (hot nodules). Hot nodules are almost always benign, whereas cold nodules have a 5% to 15% risk for malignancy. The presence of a hot nodule on scintigraphy can rule out malignancy with a high degree of confidence and spare the patient further work-up. Some hot nodules show autonomous hyperfunctioning behavior. If there is an autonomous nodule, the pattern on Tc-99m pertechnetate or I-123 imaging will show a hot nodule, but all the surrounding extranodular thyroid tissue will be cold due to the autonomous nodule's increased synthetic activity, which will suppress the surrounding thyroid tissue and cause a discrepancy in iodine uptake. Such a pattern suggests that the autonomous nodule is a benign, hyperfunctioning adenoma.

If the nodule is malignant, and the patient undergoes surgical thyroidectomy, often a remnant of the gland is left behind that can be identified on thyroid scintigraphy. The thyroid remnant can be removed using I-131 radioablation treatment. Postoperative ablation has reduced recurrence rates and disease-specific mortality. Once all thyroid remnants are ablated, the patient can then be followed using the biochemical marker thyroglobulin.

Ectopic Thyroid Tissue

Radioactive emission outside the gland is referred to as an **extrathyroidal activity pattern**. Areas of extrathyroidal activity associated with true ectopic tissue are lingual thyroid, prominent pyramidal lobe of the thyroid, thyroglossal cyst, and mediastinal thyroid. Thyroglossal duct cysts are rarely visualized on scintigraphy due to the low density of functional follicles in the remnants. If they are identified, they are typically midline. Mediastinal thyroid tissue is typically better visualized with I-123 as opposed to Tc-99m due to better contrast with surrounding tissue. Occasionally, extrathyroidal activity may be due to an artifact. For example, due to iodine contained in saliva, the esophagus may incorrectly mimic an extrathyroidal activity pattern.

Thyroiditis

Tc-99m pertechnetate or radioiodine imaging can be used to narrow the differential diagnosis for subacute thyroiditis and thyrotoxicosis caused by Graves disease. The pattern of γ emission from the radionuclide can help identify the correct diagnosis. If the Tc-99m or I-123 pattern is cold (very little emission), then the diagnosis is likely to be silent or subacute thyroiditis. If the Tc-99m scan shows a multinodular localization, then the diagnosis is most likely a MNG or Plummer disease. If the gland shows both hot (increased emission) and diffuse emission on the Tc-99m scan, then the diagnosis is either Graves disease or early Hashimoto thyroiditis. Thyroid antibody testing will differentiate these two conditions. A TSH-receptor antibody is present in individuals with Graves disease whereas antithyroperoxidase and antithyroglobulin antibodies are present in individuals with Hashimoto thyroiditis.

Graves Disease

Graves disease, also referred to as *toxic diffuse goiter*, is caused by autoantibodies against TSH receptors in the follicular cells of the thyroid gland. The entire thyroid gland is uniformly affected by the thyroid-stimulating antibodies, thus accounting for the characteristic imaging findings on thyroid scintigraphy, which include a diffusely enlarged gland with uniformly distributed increase in uptake of radioiodine. In Graves disease, radioiodine is used not only for diagnostic imaging but also for calculating the dose of I-131 for therapy. Effective treatment with I-131 ablation should make the patient hypothyroid. With exogenous synthetic thyroid-hormone replacement, the patient should become clinically and biochemically euthyroid.

Multinodular Goiter

Multinodular goiter (MNG) presents clinically with an enlarged thyroid gland but will show a diffusely heterogenous localization pattern on either Tc-99m or I-123 scintigraphy (Figure 20-1). This pattern may or may not include discrete hot nodules. Typically, if hot nodules are present, the surrounding thyroid tissue becomes suppressed and shows a

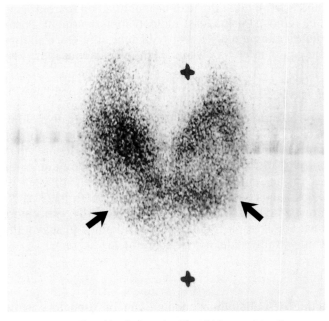

FIGURE 20-1. Thyroid scintigraphy. Thyroid image detecting presence of multiple nodules (*arrows*). (From Willis MC. Medical Terminology: A Programmed Learning Approach to the Language of Health Care. Baltimore, MD: Lippincott Williams & Wilkins; 2002.)

decreased uptake. By using quantitative RAIU, MNG can be differentiated from Graves disease. MNG patients have either normal or mildly elevated (20% to 40%) 24-hour uptake, whereas Graves patients have a 24-hour uptake ranging 50% to 80%. Radio-iodine I-131 can be used to treat toxic MNG just as with Graves disease. Only a single oral dose of I-131 is required, and many patients with toxic MNG will subsequently become euthyroid with the destruction of the hyperfunctioning tissue. However, 45% of patients do become permanently hypothyroid and require lifelong thyroid-hormone supplementation.

Parathyroid Glands

The parathyroid glands are derived from the dorsal endoderm of the third and fourth pharyngeal pouches. The fourth pouch forms the superior parathyroid, and the third pouch contributes to the inferior parathyroid, which often follows the recurrent laryngeal nerve to the arch of the aorta and results in an ectopic location. The normal glands are usually 5 to 7 mm by 3 to 4 mm, weighing approximately 40 to 60 mg. There are usually four parathyroid glands. The top two glands are usually midway along the posterior borders of the thyroid gland. The location of the lower two glands is variable, and they can be found anywhere from the carotid bifurcation to the mediastinum. These lower two glands are found near the lower poles of the thyroid gland in only about 40% of the population.

The parathyroid glands maintain homeostasis of calcium levels in the blood, triggering hormone secretion when levels fall below a concentration of 8.5 mg/dL. The chief cells of the parathyroid are responsible for secretion of parathyroid hormone (PTH), which opposes the effects of calcitonin. PTH stimulates osteoclast activity in the bones, causing bone resorption and an increase in serum calcium level. PTH also controls phosphate homeostasis by reducing reabsorption of phosphate in the nephron, thereby decreasing serum phosphate levels.

Parathyroid Scintigraphy

Tc-99m sestamibi (Figure 20-2A) is the gold standard for imaging patients with hyperparathyroidism, because the radiotracer has better imaging qualities than its two predecessors: selenium-75-methionine and thallium-201/Tc-99m. The MIBI portion of the ligand is the biologic tracer, which accumulates in the mitochondria of cells. Because adenomas are hypermetabolic, they have higher ratios of mitochondria-rich cells than the surrounding tissue, allowing for good contrast in the concentrations of tracer accumulation. The sensitivity of locating a solitary adenoma in a patient with primary hyperparathyroidism with this technique is 88%. Visualization of the tracer is by two-dimensional planar γ camera or a SPECT. Either modality provides a three-dimensional localization of the radiotracer, and, therefore, the adenoma. Many centers have hybrid imaging with both a CT scan and γ camera (Figure 20-2B). This allows both SPECT and CT scans to be performed in the same sitting, enabling exact localization of a parathyroid adenoma. Parathyroid scintigraphy is primarily used in the evaluation of primary and secondary hyperparathyroidism.

Hyperparathyroidism

A measurement of the serum PTH level is the initial diagnostic test in the evaluation for hyperparathyroidism. Scintigraphy is used to localize hyperfunctioning parathyroid tissue and guide surgical resection. Because parathyroid tissue is usually located along or within the thyroid gland, it is important to be able to determine the difference between the two types of tissues. In order to make a visual distinction between parathyroid and

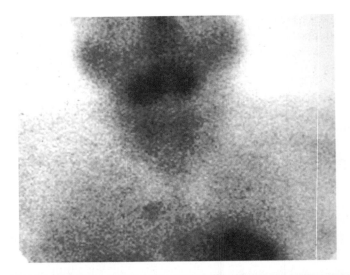

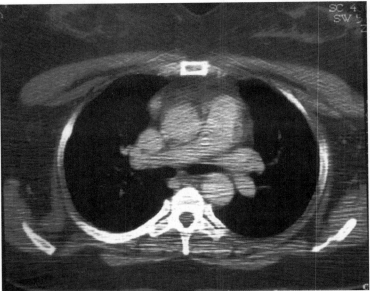

FIGURE 20-2. Ectopic parathyroid adenoma in a 43-year-old man.
(A) Tc-99m MIBI image shows focal uptake in the mediastinum.
(B) CT scan shows a soft tissue nodule in the anterior mediastinum.
(**A,B:** Courtesy of Raghuveer Halkar, MD, Department of Radiology,
Division of Nuclear Medicine, Emory University School of Medicine.)

thyroid tissue, two different methods of Tc-99m sestamibi scintigraphy can be used: dual phase and dual isotope with subtraction.

Dual-phase protocols are based on the principle that parathyroid tissue retains the MIBI radiotracer longer than the surrounding thyroid tissue. In order to maximize the difference between the thyroid and parathyroid glands, two sets of images are taken. One is taken 15 minutes postinjection and the other 1 to 3 hours postinjection. A parathyroid lesion will be seen on the latter imaging. All tumors are different, and some have long retention of radiotracer, whereas others have short retention. This method of imaging has significant limitations because the parathyroid lesion has a fast washout time of the radiotracer.

Parathyroid scintigraphy can also use the subtraction protocol. In this procedure, two radiotracers are used concurrently, Tc-99m-MIBI and I-123. The Tc-99m-MIBI labels both the thyroid and parathyroid glands, whereas the thyroid-specific I-123 only localizes in the thyroid gland. This method works on the principle that Tc-99m and I-123 emit γ rays of different energy levels. After both radiotracers are infused simultaneously, images are taken by the γ cameras. The thyroid images are digitally subtracted by the computer, thus visualizing only parathyroid tissue. This method has been found to have more sensitivity than the dual-phase protocol.

The cause of hyperparathyroidism is a solitary hyperfunctioning adenoma 80% of the time. It is seen as a single focal lesion of increased radiotracer uptake. Most of these adenomas occur posterior to the lower section of the thyroid gland; however, up to 20% of adenomas are ectopic. It should be noted that parathyroid carcinoma is indistinguishable from a functioning adenoma on scintigraphy.

Adrenal Glands

The paired adrenal glands lie in the retroperitoneum just superior to the kidneys. The glands contain two embryologically distinct regions: the adrenal cortex and the adrenal medulla. The function of the cortex, derived from mesodermal tissue, is to secrete steroid-derived hormones. The three areas within the adrenal cortex are each responsible for secretion of distinct steroid hormones. The most superior region, the zona glomerulosa, secretes mineralocorticoids such as aldosterone. The middle and largest region, the zona fasciculata, making up 80% of the cortex, secretes glucocorticoids such as cortisol. The innermost region, the zona reticularis, secretes weak androgens such as dehydroepiandrosterone and androstenedione. The adrenal medulla, derived from the neural crest cells, secretes NE and epinephrine. The indications for adrenal scintigraphy include the evaluation of: 1) an adrenocortical hyperfunctioning disorder, 2) an adrenal medullary disorder, and 3) a nonhyperfunctioning adrenal mass.

Adrenal Cortex

The disorders of the adrenal cortex that utilize nuclear medicine techniques include the evaluation for Cushing syndrome, primary hyperaldosteronism, and hyperandrogenism.

Cushing Syndrome

Cushing syndrome is characterized clinically and biochemically by excess cortisol production. This excess may be the result of direct stimulation from the adrenal glands or by secondary stimulation by adrenocorticotropic hormone (ACTH) from the pituitary gland. ACTH-dependent Cushing syndrome causes both of the adrenal glands to hypertrophy symmetrically. I-131-Norcholesterol (NP-59) scintigraphy is used to image and characterize this condition and will show a pattern of symmetric bilateral uptake of the radiotracer. However, this diagnosis is made from biochemical tests coupled with an MRI of the head to look for a pituitary adenoma. In up to 70% of cases, anatomic CT or MRI imaging shows diffuse enlargement of the adrenal glands.

Primary hypercortisolism or ACTH-independent Cushing syndrome may be due to an adrenal adenoma, an adrenal carcinoma, or bilateral nodular hyperplasia. An adrenal adenoma will show a discrete unilateral area in the affected gland when using NP-59. However, NP-59 is not readily available and is rarely used in the United States. If an adrenal carcinoma is present, no visualization of radiotracer will occur in either adrenal gland because carcinomas are more differentiated and do not uptake a sufficient quantity of radiotracer to be visible on scintigraphy. In the case of bilateral nodular hyperplasia, the pattern will show a heterogenous asymmetric bilateral visualization of the radiotracer in the adrenals.

Primary Hyperaldosteronism

The etiology of primary hyperaldosteronism is due to either an aldosterone-secreting adenoma or bilateral hyperplasia of the zona glomerulosa. Scintigraphy requires prepping the patient with a dexamethasone suppression test prior to imaging. This reduces the amount of ACTH-dependent uptake of NP-59 in other areas of the adrenal cortex. Daily injections of dexamethasone (a glucocorticoid) are given for at least 5 days. Visualization of the adrenal glands on NP-59 scintigraphy at 5 days postinjection is evidence of normal tissue. Aldosterone-secreting adenomas are diagnosed if visualization of a *unilateral* pattern is seen prior to 5 days, whereas adrenal hyperplasia is diagnosed if visualization of a *bilateral* pattern is seen prior to 5 days.

Adrenal Hyperandrogenism

In patients with suspected adrenal etiologies for hyperandrogenism, NP-59 scintigraphy can be used to more completely evaluate the disorder. Dexamethasone suppression is also used prior to imaging to decrease ACTH-dependent radiotracer uptake, thereby accentuating the uptake in the zona reticularis. The diagnosis is based on visualization of the radiotracer in relation to the timing postinjection of dexamethasone. If *unilateral* visualization of the adrenals is seen prior to 5 days postinjection, the diagnosis of an adrenal androgen-secreting adenoma is established. If *bilateral* visualization is seen prior to 5 days, adrenal hyperplasia is confirmed. In patients who have bilateral visualization after 5 days, the scan is reported as normal.

Adrenal Medulla

The disorders of the adrenal medulla that utilize nuclear medicine techniques include the evaluation for pheochromocytoma, neuroblastoma, and nonhyperfunctioning adrenal mass.

Pheochromocytoma

Pheochromocytomas are diagnosed by a combination of laboratory analysis (urine and/or plasma metanephrines) and MRI scans. MIBG scintigraphy is used for localizing extra adrenal lesions and metastases. The characteristic appearance of a pheochromocytoma on MIBG scintigraphy is intense unilateral uptake in an adrenal gland (Figure 20-3). MIBG scanning has particular utility in the imaging of suspected metastatic pheochromocytoma because it can localize small foci throughout the body, which would have been missed by MRI or CT. The sensitivity and specificity of MIBG scintigraphy for detection of

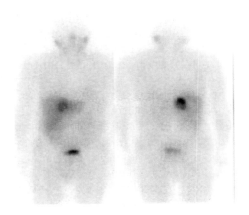

FIGURE 20-3. Pheochromocytoma in a 52-year-old man. I-123 MIBG image showing pheochromocytoma in the right adrenal with intense radiotracer uptake. (Courtesy of Raghuveer Halkar, MD, Department of Radiology, Division of Nuclear Medicine, Emory University School of Medicine.)

pheochromocytoma are 87% and 99%, respectively. Pheochromocytomas follow the **10% rule** in which 10% occur bilaterally, 10% are extra-adrenal, and 10% are malignant. Most pheochromocytomas are metabolically active and are good candidates for imaging with PET using 18-FDG, which is specific for a malignant pheochromocytoma.

Neuroblastoma

A neuroblastoma is usually detected initially by ultrasound when there is an abdominal mass detected on the physical examination. MIBG scintigraphy can be used to locate and characterize the lesion. It is successful in detection of the neuroblastoma in more than 90% of affected children. Images are taken at 24 and 48 hours and may show radiotracer concentration in the abdomen at the site of the tumor. Skeletal metastases are typically better seen on the 48-hour image. Depending on the avidity of MIBG uptake by the tumor, I-131 coupled with MIBG can be used as concomitant radio-ablative therapy along with chemotherapy.

Nonhyperfunctioning Adrenal Mass

Benign adrenal adenomas are fairly common in the general population, occurring at a prevalence of 2% to 9%. Recent advances and increasing use of tomographic imaging, such as CT and MRI, have led to incidental identification of masses in the adrenal glands. In the absence of a prior history of cancer, 95% of these lesions are benign. With a past history of cancer, the lesion may have a probability of malignancy approaching 50% (usually metastatic). Evaluation of an asymptomatic adrenal mass discovered on CT or MRI must be characterized as either functional or nonfunctional and either benign or malignant. The first step in the work-up of an adrenal mass is a biochemical assessment for subclinical Cushing syndrome, a pheochromocytoma, or hyperaldosteronism. The laboratory results coupled with the anatomic information from the CT or MRI imaging can provide the information needed to diagnose or characterize the mass. If the mass is still indeterminate, functional imaging using MIBG or 18-FDG PET can be done, which offers very high sensitivity and specificity.

Neuroendocrine Tumors

Peptide and hormone synthesis by neuroendocrine cells is inhibited by somatostatin, a 14-amino acid peptide that can be considered an "antigrowth" hormone because it inhibits the release of anterior pituitary hormones (ACTH, prolactin, TSH). Somatostatin inhibits the release of intestinal and pancreatic peptides including insulin, glucagon, gastrin, vasoactive intestinal peptide, gastric inhibitory polypeptide, secretin, motilin, and cholecystokinin. Theoretically, radionuclide-labeled somatostatin could bind to neuroendocrine tumors that contain somatostatin receptors, thereby facilitating the identification and imaging of the tumor and any metastases. Moreover, as an inhibitory substance, somatostatin can be given therapeutically to decrease the release of biologically active peptides and hormones overproduced by the neuroendocrine tumor, thereby helping to control or reduce tumor growth. The use of radiolabeled somatostatin is not practical. Because of its 14-amino acid chain, it consists of numerous covalent bonds that are readily disrupted by circulating plasma enzymes. Consequently, somatostatin has a very short biological half-life in circulation of only 2 to 4 minutes, which compromises its efficacy in diagnostic imaging. To circumvent this limitation, an 8-amino acid analog of somatostatin, octreotide, was developed, whose plasma half-life is nearly 2 hours. In-111, which decays by electron capture, is chelated to the octreotide molecule by diethyenetiaminepentacetic acid. The resulting molecule, 111-penetreotide binds to somatostatin receptors (subtypes 2 and 5). More than 80% of eneteropancreatic tumors express subtype 2 receptors, and therefore most neuroendocrine tumors can be localized with In-111 (Figure 20-4).

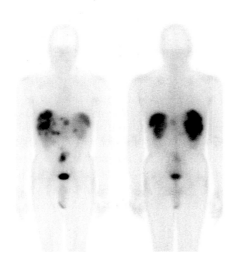

FIGURE 20-4. Primary carcinoid in a 54-year-old man. Indium-111 OctreoScan shows liver metastases and primary carcinoid in the terminal ileum. (Courtesy of Raghuveer Halkar, MD, Department of Radiology, Division of Nuclear Medicine, Emory University School of Medicine.)

TABLE 20-1.   Radionuclide Uses in Endocrinology

Radionuclide	Endocrine Uses	Features
Technetium-99m pertechnetate	Thyroid scintigraphy	Less radiation dose than I-131 and cheaper than I-123
		Not organified by thyroid
Iodine-131	Thyroid scintigraphy	Emits γ and β radiation
	Thyroid ablation	Concentrates in the thyroid
Iodine-123	Thyroid scintigraphy	Emits only γ radiation
		More expensive than I-131 and technetium pertechnetate
Technetium-99m sestamibi	Parathyroid scintigraphy	Affinity for parathyroid tissue
Iodine-123 or Iodine-131 MIBG	Pheochromocytoma Localization	Norepinephrine analog High uptake by neuroendocrine cell
	Neuroblastoma localization	
I-131-Norcholesterol (NP-59)	Adrenal cortical scintigraphy	Cholesterol analog
		Uptake regulated by ACTH and renin/angiotensin
18-FDG (fluorodeoxyglucose)	Oncologic staging and follow-up	Glucose analog
		Affinity for highly metabolically active cells
Indium-111 OctreoScan	Neuroendocrine tumor localization	Somatostatin analog
		High uptake by neuroendocrine cell

Notes: MIBG, metaiodobenzylguanidine; ACTH, adrenocorticotropic hormone.

CASE FOLLOW-UP

Our patient has symptoms of hyperthyroidism, an enlarged and firm thyroid gland, and a thyroid gland that is painful with palpation or swallowing. The most likely diagnosis is thyroiditis or, more specifically, De Quervein thyroiditis.

Initially our patient underwent RAIU using I-123 to image the thyroid gland. The scan showed an extremely low uptake.

Given the finding of a low uptake on the I-123 study along with symptoms of hyperthyroidism, viral thyroiditis, or De Quervain thyroiditis, was confirmed, and a biopsy was not necessary. However, if, she had low uptake and no signs of hyperthyroidism, an ultrasound-guided FNA biopsy of the thyroid nodule would have been performed.

REFERENCES and SUGGESTED READINGS

Avram AM, Fig LM, Gross MD. Adrenal gland scintigraphy. Semin Nucl Med. 2006;36(3):212–227.

Bahn RS Castro MR. Approach to the patient with nontoxic multinodular goiter. J Clin Endocrinol Metab. 2011;96(5):1202–1212.

Chien D, Jacene H. Imaging of parathyroid glands. Otolaryngol Clin North Am. 2010;43(2):399–415.

Cohen JI, Salter KD. Thyroid disorders: evaluation and management of thyroid nodules. Oral Maxillofac Surg Clin North Am. 2008;20(3):431–443.

Griggs WS, Divgi C. Radioiodine imaging and treatment in thyroid disorders. Neuroimaging Clin North Am. 2008;18(3):505–515, viii.

Ouyang T, et al. Imaging of the pituitary. Radiol Clin North Am. 2011;49(3):549–571, vii.

Palestro CJ, Tomas MB, Tronco GG. Radionuclide imaging of the parathyroid glands. Semin Nucl Med. 2005;35(4):266–276.

Sarkar SD. Benign thyroid disease: what is the role of nuclear medicine? Semin Nucl Med. 2006; 36(3):185–193.

Smith JR, Oates E. Radionuclide imaging of the thyroid gland: patterns, pearls, and pitfalls. Clin Nucl Med. 2004;29(3):181–193.

Soto GD, et al. Update in thyroid imaging. The expanding world of thyroid imaging and its translation to clinical practice. Hormones (Athens). 2010;9(4):287–298.

Taffel M, et al. Adrenal imaging: a comprehensive review. Radiol Clin North Am. 2012;50(2):219–243, v.

Taieb D, et al. Parathyroid scintigraphy: when, how, and why? A concise systematic review. Clin Nucl Med. 2012;37(6):568–574.

CHAPTER REVIEW QUESTIONS

1. In regards to I-131, all of the following are true except:

    A. It has a half-life of 8 days.
    B. It is ideally suited for imaging the thyroid gland.
    C. It emits both β and γ particles.
    D. It is useful for treating thyroid cancer.
    E. It is useful for treating Graves disease.

2. Thyroid scintigraphy is indicated in an individual presenting with any of the scenarios below except:

    A. Single thyroid nodule and laboratory evidence of a suppressed serum TSH
    B. Multinodular goiter and laboratory evidence of a suppressed serum TSH
    C. Large multinodular goiter with extension into the mediastinum

D. Elevated serum TSH level

E. Subclinical hyperthyroidism

3. A healthy 42-year-old female has no symptoms of thyroid disease, but is found to have a thyroid nodule on routine physical examination. Which of the following is the first step in evaluating the nodule?

A. Perform an ultrasound of the neck.

B. Perform a fine-needle aspirate (FNA) of the nodule.

C. Collect thyroid function studies.

D. Perform an I-131 uptake and scan.

E. Perform an I-123 uptake and scan.

4. All of the following neuroendocrine tumors can be localized using In-111 OctreoScan except:

A. Carcinoid

B. Gastrinoma

C. Parathyroid adenoma

D. Paraganglionoma

E. VIPoma

5. A 3-year-old child is suspected of having a neuroblastoma. In addition to chemotherapy, which of the following nuclides may be used to treat this child?

A. I-123

B. Technetium-99m pertechnetate

C. NP-59

D. 18-FDG

E. I-131 MIBG

CHAPTER REVIEW ANSWERS

1. The correct answer is B. I-131 is the radionuclide used for destroying thyroid tissue. The thyroid follicular cells will actively absorb any isotope of iodine in the body thereby concentrating the vast majority of the radioactive I-131 within the gland. The majority of the radiation given off by I-131 is in the form of β particles, which only travel several millimeters from the nucleus of the isotope. These β particles are very destructive to the surrounding tissues and can cause mutations and apoptosis in the cells. Although it is possible to image the thyroid gland with I-131, it does not produce as crisp an image as an image with I-123.

All of the other choices are true statements. I-131 has a half-life of about 8 days (**Choice A**), it emits both β particles and γ rays (**Choice C**) and is useful for treating both thyroid cancer (**Choice D**) and Graves disease (**Choice E**).

2. The correct answer is D. An individual with an elevated TSH level has primary hypothyroidism and usually does not require a nuclear imaging modality. All of the other choices are appropriate indications for thyroid scintigraphy.

3. The correct answer is C. The first step in evaluating an individual with a thyroid nodule is to determine if there is biochemical evidence of hypo- or hyperthyroidism. An individual with a suppressed serum TSH may have a hyperfunctioning nodule. Prior to determining the characteristics of the nodule, the clinician must know the TSH level.

4. The correct answer is C. A parathyroid adenoma can be evaluated using a technetium-99m (Tc-99m) sestamibi scan. Sestamibi exhibits a differential in its association and wash out with thyroid and parathyroid glands. The sestamibi portion of the compound molecule acts as the biologic tissue localizer, while the Tc-99m undergoes radioactive decay and emits γ rays which are visualized by the γ camera.

Indium-111 (In-111) is an isotope of indium that is chelated to an octreotide molecule (diethyenetiaminepentacetic acid). This molecule binds to somatostatin receptors (subtypes 2 and 5) on the cell surface. Neuroendocrine tumors including carcinoid (**Choice A**), gastrinoma (**Choice B**), paraganglionoma (**Choice D**), and VIPoma (**Choice E**) have somatostain receptors. Most neuroendocrine tumors express subtype 2 somatostatin receptors; therefore, In-111 is an ideal agent for scintigraphy.

5. The correct answer is E. Metaiodobenzylguanidine (MIBG) scintigraphy can be used to locate and characterize neuroblastomas. It is successful in detection of the neuroblastoma in more than 90% of affected children. Images are taken at 24 and 48 hours and may show radiotracer concentration in the abdomen at the site of the tumor. Skeletal metastases are typically better seen on the 48-hour image. Depending on the avidity of MIBG uptake by the tumor, I-131 coupled with MIBG can be used as concomitant radioablative therapy along with chemotherapy.

Surgical Approaches to Endocrine Disorders 21

Meredith Macnamara

Jyotirmay Sharma

CASE

A 6-year-old girl is brought to her pediatrician because her uncle recently had his thyroid gland removed due to thyroid cancer. She is healthy and denies recent illnesses, weight loss, or fever. She has no past medical or surgical history and is not taking any medications. Her family history is significant. Her paternal grandfather and both of her paternal uncles having had their thyroid glands removed for thyroid cancer. On examination, she appears healthy, in good spirits, and in no distress. Her thyroid gland appears normal, and she has no lymphadenopathy. Her vital signs are normal for age.

Laboratory serum studies are all within normal limits for age and reveal the following: thyroid-stimulating hormone (TSH) (2.3 mIU/L), free thyroxine (1.1 ng/dL), anti-thyroglobulin antibody (negative), antithyroperoxidase antibody (negative), total calcium (9.8 mg/dL), phosphate (3.1 mg/dL), and albumin (4.1 g/dL).

This chapter reviews the endocrine-related conditions that require surgical intervention to help the learner develop hypotheses that explore the etiology, evaluation, and treatment of our patient's condition. We review the work-up and provide a therapeutic plan at the end of the chapter so the learner will better understand the diagnosis. We recommend reviewing the pathophysiology of the endocrine disorders requiring surgical intervention in the earlier chapters in this book. There are many surgical procedures required for the treatment of endocrine disorders. This chapter is organized to best elucidate the endocrine conditions in which surgery is the first-line therapy.

(continues)

(continued)

OBJECTIVES

1. List the endocrine disorders that require surgery as first-line therapy.

2. Outline the indications for surgery in each endocrine disorder that requires surgery.

3. Discuss the surgical complications for each endocrine disorder that requires surgery.

PITUITARY GLAND

The pituitary gland is a small collection of tissue that has a dual origin (the pharynx for the adenohypophysis and brain for the neurohypophysis) attached to the hypothalamus by a stalk (Figure 21-1A). The pituitary gland hangs down from the brain and is located in a small cavity known as the *sella tursica*, which derives its name from the Turkish words describing its saddle shape. The gland is located in the center of the head at the juncture between the cranial cavity and nasal cavity.

Embryologically, the neurohypophysis and adenohypophysis are joined together during the developmental stage in a fetus. The cherry-shaped pituitary gland is attached by a pituitary stalk to the hypothalamus at the base of the brain. The posterior lobe, known as the *neurohypophysis*, is directly connected to the hypothalamus by the pituitary stalk. Just superior to the pituitary gland are the optic nerves, the optic chiasm, and the optic tracts; that conduct visual impulses to the brain. The hypothalamus lies superior to, and is connected to, the pituitary gland, via the pituitary stalk (Figure 21-1B).

A variety of tumors occur in the pituitary gland. Pituitary adenomas, which are benign, are the most common of these tumors. Metastatic cancer cells can also be found in the pituitary gland.

Benign pituitary adenomas can be divided into nonfunctioning and functioning tumors depending on the capability of tumor cells to produce hormones. Nonfunctioning pituitary adenomas do not produce active hormones by themselves, but mechanically can compress surrounding structures, such as normal pituitary gland and optic systems, that result in endocrine hypofunction due to either the compression itself, or as a consequence of subsequent surgery.

Functioning pituitary adenomas produce an overabundance of hormones including prolactinomas, adenomas that cause Cushing disease, adenomas that cause gigantism or acromegaly, and thyroid-stimulating hormone (TSH)–producing tumors.

Pituitary Gland Disorders

Pituitary gland disorders that require surgery are either those which are being secreted in excessive amounts or those that affect vision or secretion of other pituitary hormones.

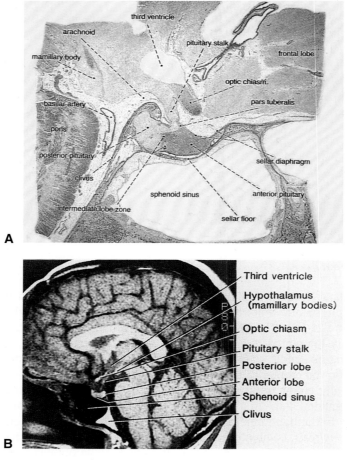

FIGURE 21-1. Pituitary gland. **(A)** Sagittal whole-mount section of normal pituitary gland and surrounding structures. The anterior (at right) and posterior (at left) lobes are clearly delineated. The pars tuberalis is the thin tongue-shaped portion of anterior lobe that extends for a short distance up the stalk. This diagram illustrates the proximity of the optic chiasm to the pituitary. Superior extension of a pituitary tumor may compress the optic chiasm with resultant visual field deficits, whereas downward extension may fill the sphenoid sinus (Luxol-Fast Blue–PAS). **(B)** Magnetic resonance imaging: sagittal view of the brain at the level of the pituitary stalk and gland. The clarity of the pituitary gland, stalk, hypothalamus, and optic chiasm is remarkable, making magnetic resonance imaging (MRI) an excellent imaging modality for the assessment of pituitary lesions. One advantage of MRI over computed tomography (CT) is the absence of bony artifact with MRI. (**A, B:** From Stacey E. Mills, Histology For Pathologists Third Edition, Philadelphia, PA: Lippincott Williams & Wilkins; 2007.)

Prolactinoma

Prolactinomas are the most common functioning pituitary adenomas. The excess production of prolactin results in amenorrhea, galactorrhea, infertility, and sexual dysfunction. Prolactinomas can also be treated with medications. In addition to the symptoms related to excess prolactin production, the mass effect created by the size, pressure, and swelling of the tumor may cause bitemporal hemianopsia due to pressure on the optic chiasm; vertigo, nausea, and vomiting. Treatment is indicated if mass effects from the tumor and/or significant effects of hyperprolactinemia are present. Most small tumors do not progress to macroadenomas. Therefore, patients with small tumors and minimal symptoms can be monitored closely with serial measurements of prolactin. Treatment with a dopamine agonist (i.e., bromocriptine or cabergoline) is the preferred treatment modality for patients with prolactinomas. Dopamine agonists potentiate the effect of dopamine on decreasing the synthesis and secretion of prolactin. It also decreases tumor cell division and growth, which can help alleviate symptoms of mass effect. When medication side effects or intolerance develops, a transsphenoidal pituitary adenomectomy is the preferred surgical treatment. Remission is defined as resolution of symptoms and normal prolactin levels. For microadenomas, remission is achieved in 85 % to 90 % of cases. For macroadenomas, surgical outcome is directly related to the size of the tumor and the preoperative prolactin level. Therefore, in patients with very large tumors, unless the patient is experiencing progressive visual loss or develops a pituitary infarction, dopamine agonists are the preferred treatment.

Acromegaly

Pituitary adenomas that produce growth hormone (GH) cause gigantism in children (due to their active growth plates) or acromegaly in adults. In acromegaly, the jaw, cheeks, fingers, and toes are thickened along with enlargement of soft tissues, such as the tongue, nose, and lips. Affected adult patients might find that their shoes or hats do not fit properly. GH-secreting pituitary adenomas are typically large tumors (macroadenomas, >10 mm in size) which may present with a mass effect and symptoms of excess GH or hypopituitarism due to destruction of adjacent pituitary tissue. Hypogonadism is the most common hormone deficiency experienced by a mass effect in patients with acromegaly. Patients often have symptoms of decreased libido, infertility or oligo/amenorrhea. As approximately 25 % of GH-secreting adenomas present with a prolactin-secreting component, the symptoms of hypogonadism may also be due to hyperprolactinemia.

Resection of the pituitary adenoma is the preferred treatment of patients with acromegaly. Goals of treatment include reduction of GH to normal levels and relief of the mass effect. Surgery offers rapid and effective resolution of symptoms. Transsphenoidal hypophysectomy involves removal of the tumor by tunneling through the sphenoid sinuses. These procedures normally relieve the pressure on surrounding brain regions and lead to lower GH levels. Complications of surgery include cerebrospinal fluid (CSF) leaks, meningitis, or damage to normal pituitary tissue. All of these surgically treated patients need lifelong hormone supplementation. In patients with large pituitary tumors or with residual tumors after surgery, the use of somastotastin analogs (e.g., octreotide or lanreotide) are effective in reducing GH secretion and reducing tumor size. Somatostatin is an endogenous peptide derived from the hypothalamus and gastrointestinal tract, and although somatostatin analogs are considered first-line pharmacotherapy for GH excess, GH and insulin-like growth factor (IGF)-1 levels are suppressed in less than 70 % of patients.

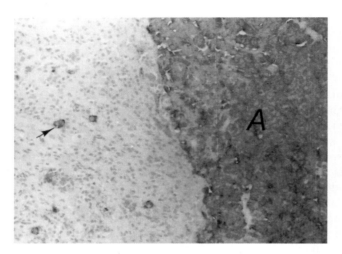

FIGURE 21-2. Immunohistochemical staining of an adrenocorticotropic hormone–producing adenoma from a patient with Cushing disease. The normal pituitary tissue on the left contains a few adrenocorticotropic hormone (ACTH)–positive cells (*arrow*). Magnification ×250. (From Mulholland MW, Lillemore KD, Doherty GM, et al. Greenfield's Surgery: Scientific Principles and Practice. 4th ed. Philadelphia, PA: Lippincott Williams & Wilkins; 2006.)

Cushing Disease

Cushing disease refers to those conditions caused by an adrenocorticotropic hormone (ACTH)–producing pituitary adenoma leading to hypercortisolism. Pituitary adenomas are responsible for 70% of endogenous Cushing syndrome. The presenting signs, symptoms, and diagnosis are discussed in detail in Chapter 10.

The diagnosis of Cushing disease is based on the clinical assessment and static and dynamic hormone testing. New diagnostic and imaging techniques have improved the sensitivity of microadenoma detection. Surgical resection is the preferred therapy for patients with Cushing disease. When the pituitary gland is completely removed, ACTH-producing adenomas contain excess corticotrophs as compared to unaffected, normal pituitary tissue (Figure 21-2). If surgical treatment fails to relieve symptoms, radiosurgery or medical treatments can be instituted. Transsphenoidal microsurgery remains the single best therapy when compared with drug or radiation treatment. The initial remission rate for microadenomas is 85% to 90% with an overall complication rate of only 3%. In those who fail the initial procedure, repeat surgery for a total hypophysectomy is beneficial, with remission rates of 50%. If this is unsuccessful, a bilateral adrenalectomy may be considered.

Thyroid-stimulating Hormone–secreting Adenoma

TSH-secreting pituitary adenomas account for <1% of all pituitary adenomas and cause secondary hyperthyroidism. Failure to recognize a TSH-secreting pituitary adenoma may lead to improper therapy and complications, including visual field defects due to compression of the optic chiasm or hypopituitarism.

TSH-secreting pituitary adenomas are a heterogeneous entity group with regards to their clinical presentation, hormonal profile, and therapeutic response. The endocrine effects include those related to hyperthyroidism, insofar as a primary elevation in TSH will result in overstimulation of thyroid hormone secretion from the thyroid gland. Hyperthyroidism is discussed in detail in Chapter 3. The primary treatment is surgical adenomectomy. If the patient is not a surgical candidate, medical therapy is used.

Pituitary Gland Surgery

For functional endocrine tumors, conventional transsphenoidal surgery has historically been performed under the operating microscope via a sublabial incision or intranasal incision (Figure 21-3). It requires 2 to 3 days of nasal packing and 3 to 5 days of hospital

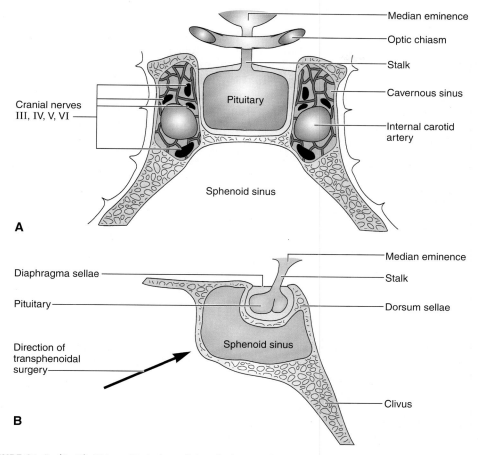

FIGURE 21-3. (A, B) Mid-sagittal view of the pituitary and surrounding bony structures. Note the approach for transsphenoidal surgery. Anterior is to the left. (From Mulholland MW, Lillemore KD, Doherty GM, et al. Greenfield's Surgery: Scientific Principles and Practice. 4th ed. Philadelphia, PA: Lippincott Williams & Wilkins; 2006.)

stay. Endoscopic pituitary tumor surgery is an alternative surgical approach and is performed through a nostril without conventional incisions. After surgery, nasal packing is not required. Postoperative discomfort is minimal, and hospital stay is frequently only overnight. This procedure does not require sublabial or nostril incisions and eliminates the need for occlusive postoperative packing used with the more conventional procedures. This method is minimally invasive because it directly approaches the tumor through the patient's nostril, thus eliminating facial swelling, decreasing postoperative pain, and resulting in faster recovery. This innovative procedure utilizes endoscopic technology to improve visualization of the pituitary gland, the tumor, and the other nearby anatomical structures.

Indications for Pituitary Surgery

Surgery is the first-line treatment for symptomatic pituitary adenomas, large nonfunctioning pituitary adenomas (macroadenomas), and pituitary apoplexy with compressive symptoms regardless of type. If medical treatment or radiotherapy is initially tried and fails, surgery is the next option particularly for prolactin- and GH-secreting tumors. Surgery provides prompt relief from excess hormone secretion and mass effect.

Complications of Pituitary Surgery

The overall mortality rate for transspheniodal surgery is <0.5%. Major morbidity occurs in <2% of patients and includes CSF leak, meningitis, stroke, intracranial hemorrhage, and visual loss. Less serious complications occur in <10% of patients and include nasal septal perforations and wound infections. Visual deficits in patients with nonfunctioning pituitary adenomas are almost always improved. Most patients with intact pituitary function preoperatively retain their normal function postoperatively. In those with preoperative pituitary deficiency approximately 25% regain function and the remainder are managed with hormone replacement therapy. Larger invasive tumors and giant adenomas are associated with a higher mortality.

THYROID GLAND

The thyroid gland is located posterior to the strap muscles of the neck (Figure 21-4). The lobes are near the thyroid cartilage and are connected in the midline by an isthmus just

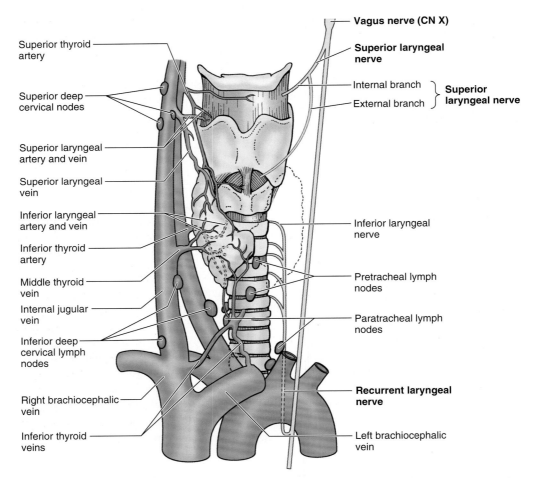

FIGURE 21-4. Nerves of the larynx. The laryngeal nerves are derived from the vagus (CN X) through the internal and external branches of the superior laryngeal nerve, and the inferior laryngeal nerve from the recurrent (inferior) laryngeal nerve. Notice the left recurrent laryngeal passing inferior to the arch of the aorta. (From Moore KL, Dalley AF. Clinically Oriented Anatomy. 4th ed. Baltimore, MD: Lippincott Williams & Wilkins; 1999.)

inferior to the cricoid cartilage. The thyroid gland is a small, flat, reddish tan, bilobed structure lying on either side of the larynx and trachea, with a flat band of similar tissue, the isthmus, that crosses the first three tracheal rings just below the cricoid cartilage. Projecting superiorly from the isthmus may be a slender strip of thyroid tissue, the pyramidal lobe, to either side of the midline.

The superior aspect of the thyroid gland is supplied by the superior thyroid artery. The inferior aspect is supplied by the inferior thyroid artery. The superior thyroid artery arises from the external carotid artery just above, at, or just below the bifurcation of the common carotid artery. The inferior thyroid artery arises from the thyrocervical trunk of the subclavian arteries. The inferior thyroid artery crosses the recurrent laryngeal nerve. Venous drainage occurs through the confluence of small surface veins into three main sets of veins: the superior, middle, and inferior thyroid veins. The superior and middle veins drain directly into the internal jugular veins, whereas the inferior veins drain into the brachiocephalic veins.

The recurrent laryngeal and superior laryngeal nerves surround the thyroid gland (Figure 21-4). The recurrent laryngeal nerves are susceptible to damage during a thyroidectomy because of their proximity to the gland and because they cross the inferior thyroid artery in a variable pattern. The right nerve branches from the vagus nerve as it crosses anteriorly to the right subclavian artery. The left nerve arises where the aorta crosses the vagus nerve. The recurrent laryngeal nerves cross the inferior thyroid artery at the middle third of the gland. It may cross anterior to, posterior to, or between the branches of the artery. Alternatively, it may exit directly from the carotid sheath and course from lateral to medial in a nonrecurrent manner from either above the inferior thyroid artery, or beneath it.

Thyroid Gland Disorders

The thyroid gland disorders that may require surgery include hyperthyroidism due to Graves disease and thyroid cancer.

Hyperthyroidism

Graves disease is the most common cause of hyperthyroidism. TSH-stimulating autoantibodies activate the TSH receptor, resulting in excess production of thyroid hormone. For individuals with Graves disease, treatment options include medical therapy (i.e., methimazole), I-131 ablation, and surgical removal. Radioablative and surgical procedures are definitive, and the majority of patients require lifetime thyroid replacement therapy.

The most common treatment of Graves disease for adults living in the United States is radioablative therapy. In children, the most common treatment is medical therapy. Although thyroidectomy is not the first-line treatment for most patients with hyperthyroidism, it is chosen if the patient develops an allergy, experiences side effects, or has a contraindication to medical or radioablative therapy. It is usually performed as initial therapy in patients with hyperthyroidism and severe exophthalmos, very large goiters, or pregnancy.

Other conditions causing hyperthyroidism include a hyperfunctioning thyroid nodule (i.e., Plummer disease) and viral thyroiditis. In those with only a nodule, a lobectomy could be performed. The pathophysiology and medical management of hyperthyroidism is discussed in detail in Chapter 3.

Thyroid Cancer

Thyroid cancer affects approximately 11 people per 100,000 each year and appears to be on the rise. Although the reason for the increase is not clear, it has been attributed to improved screening, obesity, radiation exposure, and diets low in fruits and vegetables.

The four types of thyroid carcinoma are papillary, follicular, medullary, and undifferentiated. The papillary form of thyroid cancer is the most common. Its histological appearance includes papillary projections into gland-like spaces. Tumor cells have "ground-glass" or "Orphan Annie" nuclei. Calcified spheres known as *psammoma bodies* may also be present. This cancer has a better prognosis than other forms of thyroid cancer, even when adjacent lymph nodes are involved. Total thyroidectomy is the treatment of choice. The overall 10-year survival is better than 95% in patients who undergo surgery with radioactive iodine ablation.

Follicular thyroid cancer is characterized histopathologically by relatively uniform follicles. It is more aggressive than the papillary form, but, similar to patients with papillary cancer with tumors <1.0 cm, the prognosis is very good.

Medullary thyroid carcinoma originates from the C cells of the thyroid that secrete calcitonin, which plays a role in calcium regulation. Histologically, the tumor resembles sheets of tumor cells in an amyloid-containing stroma. Medullary carcinoma can be associated with multiple endocrine neoplasia (MEN) syndromes 2A and 2B. The *RET* oncogene is implicated in those cases of medullary thyroid cancer associated with MEN and in familial medullary thyroid cancer (MTC).

Undifferentiated or anaplastic thyroid cancer tends to occur in older adults and has an extremely poor prognosis. Nonneoplastic thyroid nodules show no histological signs of malignancy and are generally the result of spontaneous glandular hyperplasia. The histological evaluation of the fine-needle aspirate (FNA) shows normal follicular cells with minimal nucleolar changes. Anaplastic thyroid cancer is highly unlikely to be curable by surgery or any other treatment modality and is in fact, usually unresectable due to its high propensity for invading surrounding tissues.

Thyroid Gland Surgery

Thyroid surgery is classified based on the amount of thyroid gland removed. The classification can be simplified to that of a thyroid lobectomy and a total thyroidectomy. A thyroid lobectomy is the total extracapsular removal of one lobe and the isthmus, leaving behind viable parathyroid glands and intact recurrent and superior laryngeal nerves. The surgeon and the endocrinologist commonly work together to determine the best surgery for the patient's thyroid disease.

Indications for Thyroid Gland Surgery

There are six major indications for thyroid surgery:

1. Thyroid cancer
2. Hyperthyroidism refractory to medical or radioablative therapy
3. Graves diseases with severe exophthalmos
4. Thyroid nodules with atypia or with suspicious or nondiagnostic FNA biopsy
5. Goiter with airway compressive symptoms
6. Cosmetic purposes in patients with a large goiter.

Complications of Thyroid Gland Surgery

The main complications of thyroidectomy are postsurgical hypothyroidism, local hematoma formation, recurrent laryngeal nerve injury, hypoparathyroidism, and thyroid storm.

A hematoma, although extremely rare, may develop in the area of resection and cause airway obstruction early in the postoperative period. Most hematomas (80%) occur within 6 hours of surgery. If it causes airway compromise, the surgeon must immediately remove the skin and strap muscle sutures and evacuate the hematoma. After the hematoma is evacuated, the patient is returned to the operating room for irrigation, control of hemorrhage, and repeat closure of the wound.

The recurrent laryngeal nerve should be identified during thyroidectomy. Great care must be taken to avoid traction or cautery injuries to the nerve. A unilateral recurrent laryngeal nerve injury causes paralysis of one vocal cord that results in hoarseness and difficulty clearing secretions but rarely in airway compromise. Most patients have improvement in symptoms with time and those with permanent unilateral vocal cord dysfunction rarely have a change in their voice. A bilateral recurrent nerve injury, on the other hand, can result in severe airway compromise that may require a tracheostomy. Any suspicion for recurrent laryngeal nerve dysfunction should be evaluated by direct laryngoscopy. In cases of bilateral nerve injury, the patient should be monitored in the intensive care unit, and the surgeon should have a low threshold for performing a tracheostomy.

Transient hypoparathyroidism occurs in up to 25% of patients undergoing a thyroidectomy. Permanent hypoparathyroidism occurs in less than 1% of patients. If it occurs, symptomatic hypocalcemia usually develops 16 to 24 hours after surgery. Administration of oral calcium and vitamin D replacement results in normalization of serum calcium level for most patients in <1 week.

Thyroid storm is a rare complication of a thyroidectomy because most patients with hyperthyroidism do not undergo the operation until their thyroid function and hemodynamic status is stable. This complication almost never occurs after thyroidectomy in adequately prepared patients but can occur in patients with untreated thyrotoxicosis who are undergoing nonthyroid operations. Treatment for individuals developing thyroid storm is discussed in detail in Chapter 3.

PARATHYROID GLAND

The parathyroid glands are pea-sized glands located at the top and bottom posterior borders of the lateral lobes of the thyroid gland (Figure 21-5). The glands are richly vascularized and consist primarily of chief cells and fat within a thin capsule of connective tissue.

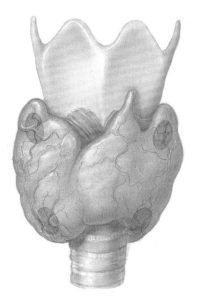

FIGURE 21-5. Parathyroid glands. (Asset provided by Anatomical Chart Co.)

The chief cells synthesize and secrete parathyroid hormone (PTH), which plays a major role in calcium homeostasis. The function of PTH and its relation to calcium homeostasis is discussed in detail in Chapters 4 and 5.

The superior thyroid glands are derived from the fourth branchial pouch, which also gives rise to the thyroid gland. The third branchial pouch gives rise to the inferior parathyroid glands and the thymus. Most patients have four parathyroid glands. Although not common, some patients (5%) have ectopic parathyroid tissue, the most common location of which, is in the thymus. This is important to consider in patients who have hyperparathyroidism and are being evaluated for surgery.

Parathyroid Gland Disorders

The most common cause of hypercalcemia that requires parathyroid surgery is hyperparathyroidism. Most other conditions that cause hypercalcemia do not require parathyroid gland surgery.

Hyperparathyroidism

Primary hyperparathyroidism is the result of overactive parathyroid glands that result in excessive production of PTH. The excess production of PTH directly increases calcium resorption from bone and reabsorption from the kidneys and indirectly increases calcium absorption from the small intestine by upregulating the 1α-hydroxylase enzyme and promoting increased production of calcitriol. The most common cause is a parathyroid adenoma that overproduces PTH, causing hypercalcemia. Secondary hyperparathyroidism is the result of elevated PTH levels in response to hypocalcemia. Tertiary hyperparathyroidism is seen in patients on dialysis or after renal transplant who develop hypercalcemia from elevated PTH levels. In over 80% of patients, a single adenoma is the cause of primary hyperparathyroidism, whereas in 20% of patients, hyperplasia or multiple adenomas are the cause. This distinction is important when determining the underlying cause and the therapeutic approach to be used. Parathyroid adenomas or parathyroid hyperplasia can exist as a single entity or as part of a MEN syndrome. MEN syndromes are discussed in detail in Chapter 17. Parathyroid carcinoma is a rare cause of primary hyperparathyroidism and is only present in about 1% of cases. Hyperparathyroidism and hypercalcemia is discussed in detail in Chapter 5.

Parathyroid Gland Surgery

Prior to surgery, all patients should undergo a localization study, such as cervical ultrasonography, computed tomography (CT) scan with intravenous (IV) contrast, or radionuclide scanning after an IV injection of Tc-99m-sestamibi, in order to reduce operative timing by limiting incision size. A curative parathyroidectomy not only results in improvement in the serum calcium level but also improves the bone density, neuropsychiatric symptoms, calciphylaxis, nephrocalcinosis, nephrolithiasis, and risk for cardiovascular complications. A parathyroidectomy is most commonly performed in patients with primary or tertiary hyperparathyroidism. There are several different approaches to parathyroid surgery including a conventional exploration through a low collar incision and a minimally invasive one. Regardless of the parathyroid surgery approach, imaging with I-123 and collection of intraoperative PTH (IOPTH) levels are essential for determining if the correct gland or glands have been removed.

A parathyroidectomy is usually performed under general anesthesia through a low collar incision, although local anesthesia is appropriate for elderly and high-risk patients as well as those undergoing minimally invasive radioguided parathyroidectomy (MIRP) or image-guided focal exploration. It is accompanied by measurement of IOPTH levels. If the PTH level is in the normal range within 5 minutes of excision of a suspected adenoma, it should be assumed that all hypersecreting tissue has been removed.

Limited or minimally invasive parathyroid exploration followed by measurement of IOPTH levels is appropriate when a preoperative sestamibi scan accurately localizes the enlarged adenoma. With the use of IOPTH and parathyroid localization, a less-extensive dissection can be performed with acceptable results in about 65% of patients. In the other 35% of patients, the preoperative localization studies are inconclusive or, IOPTH levels are consistent with multigland pathology. With the addition of IOPTH levels, the criteria for classification of abnormal parathyroid glands not only includes size, histology, and morphology, but also function. Patients who have persistently elevated IOPTH levels after a limited neck exploration should be converted to a bilateral neck exploration to determine if another PTH-secreting adenoma exists.

MIRP involves the injection of IV Tc-99m-sestamibi 1.5 to 2.5 hours prior to the operation. Guided by a gamma probe, the enlarged gland is removed, and absence of multigland disease is confirmed with IOPTH measurements. Failure of this limited approach, as documented by the IOPTH level, then requires a conventional cervical exploration. Finally, use of minimal access techniques, such as robotic or video-assisted parathyroidectomy that involves the insertion of an endoscope, or a trocar for insufflation of CO_2 and several small-sized operating ports for 2-mm instruments may be necessary.

A solitary parathyroid adenoma is present in approximately 80% of patients and should be excised. Double adenomas are present in <5% of patients, and excision is appropriate along with biopsy of the normal gland. Sporadic primary hyperplasia is best treated with subtotal parathyroidectomy (excision of three and a half glands), leaving a small, vascularized remnant. IOPTH levels can help guide the extent of surgery in patients with hyperplasia. An extremely low IOPTH (<5 pg/dL) at the conclusion of the surgery will determine the need for a parathyroid autograft and avoid permanent hypoparathyroidism. Patients with secondary or tertiary hyperparathyroidism, who are unlikely to be candidates for renal transplantation, should undergo either total parathyroidectomy with an autograft, or a near-total parathyroidectomy with a small, vascularized remnant.

Indications for Parathyroid Gland Surgery

There are eight major indications for parathyroidectomy:

1. Markedly elevated serum calcium (>1 mg/dL above upper limits of normal)
2. History of life-threatening hypercalcemia
3. Creatinine clearance reduced by 30% compared with age-matched normal subjects
4. Markedly elevated 24-hour urine calcium (>400 mg/day)
5. Nephrolithiasis
6. Osteitis fibrosa cystica
7. Substantially reduced bone mass as determined by direct measurement (e.g., >2 standard deviations below controls matched for age, gender, and ethnicity)
8. Neuromuscular symptoms of proximal weakness, atrophy, hyperreflexia, and gait disturbance.

Most patients with primary hyperparathyroidism are asymptomatic, and the disease is discovered by routine blood chemistry analysis. Most patients with asymptomatic hyperparathyroidism follow a benign clinical course with <20% developing complications, such as severe hypercalcemia or osteoporosis after 10 years of follow-up. For that reason, the National Institute of Health and the Endocrine Society recommend surgery in asymptomatic patients if age <50 years, progressive renal impairment, osteoporosis by low bone mineral density, or by a history of bone fracture.

Complications of Parathyroid Gland Surgery

The surgical stress of a parathyroidectomy is low, and blood transfusions are rarely needed. Postsurgical complications are similar to those after a thyroidectomy and include hypocalcemia due to postsurgical hypoparathyroidism, hematoma, and recurrent laryngeal nerve injury. Failure to normalize serum calcium levels occurs in less than 5% of patients and is usually due to multigland hyperplasia or recurrence of the disease.

PANCREAS

The pancreas is a retroperitoneal organ located at the level of the second lumbar vertebrae. Anatomically it is divided into a head, uncinate process, neck, body, and tail (Figure 21-6). Histologically, pancreatic tissue can be divided into pancreatic acini and islets of Langerhans. Pancreatic acini are the functional units of the exocrine pancreas and produce various polypeptides and enzymes involved in digestion. Islets of Langerhans are the functional units of the endocrine pancreas. They are composed of five cell types: α (alpha) cells that produce glucagon, β (beta) cells that produce insulin, δ (delta) cells that produce somatostatin, F cells that secrete pancreatic proteins, and ε (epsilon) cells that produce ghrelin. Islet cell tumors produce excess hormone commonly associated with MEN 1. MEN syndromes are discussed in detail in Chapter 17. The most common functional islet cell tumors are insulinomas and gastrinomas.

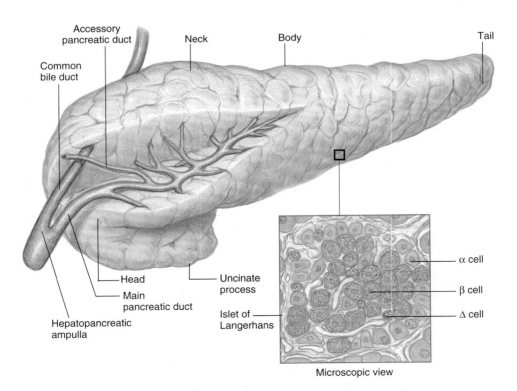

FIGURE 21-6. The areas of the pancreas. (Asset provided by Anatomical Chart Co.)

Pancreatic Disorders

The most common functional pancreatic tumor that requires surgery is the insulinoma. An insulinoma may be acquired or congenital. Neonates with gain-of-function gene mutations causing persistent hyperinsulinism hypoglycemia of infancy (PHHI) may benefit from surgery.

Insulinoma

The most common tumor of the endocrine pancreas is an insulinoma. This is a β cell–derived neoplasm that causes hyperinsulinism, characterized by the Whipple triad (symptoms of hypoglycemia, plasma glucose level <50 mg/dL, and relief of symptoms when glucose is raised to normal levels). Secretion of insulin by an insulinoma is not properly regulated by glucose, and the tumor will continue to secrete insulin resulting in hypoglycemia. Insulinomas cause hyperinsulinemic nonketotic hypoglycemia. The body's first defense system fails insofar as insulin levels do not drop in response to low plasma glucose concentrations. Elevated insulin levels inhibit lipolysis, gluconeogenesis, and glycogenolysis. In addition, insulin secretion inhibits glucagon secretion, the second defense mechanism in individuals with hypoglycemia. Insulinomas occur more commonly in women and at a mean age of 50 years. They are usually small (<2 cm), and >90% are benign. Hypoglycemia due to hyperinsulinism is discussed in detail in Chapter 6.

Once the diagnosis of hyperinsulinism is established biochemically, the location of the tumor must be accurately established. Since most insulinomas are small and difficult to detect by CT or magnetic resonance imaging (MRI), the intra-arterial calcium gluconate infusion test is used to assess insulin levels at different areas of the pancreas. In adults with insulinomas and children with PHHI, intra-arterial calcium infusion increases insulin secretion. This test is performed as follows: calcium gluconate is infused into the splenic, superior mesenteric, gastroduodenal, and celiac axis arteries. After each injection, blood is collected from the right hepatic vein. Because each artery supplies a different region of the pancreas (Figure 21-7), insulin and glucose levels collected after each injection may accurately locate the insulinoma. This information will limit the surgery to a small area of the pancreas (e.g., elevated insulin level after infusion in only one of the arteries) rather than remove the majority of the pancreas if the hyperinsulinism is diffuse.

In neonates with PHHI, a positron-emission tomography (PET) scan using 18-fluorodopamine can localize the area of hyperinsulinism insofar as the tracer has high uptake in areas with high insulin concentration.

Pancreatic Surgery

The majority (90%) of pancreatic tumors are benign and solitary. The surgical options include enucleation, distal pancreatectomy, or pancreaticoduodenectomy (Whipple operation). The laparoscopic approach provides easy visualization of the pancreas. The postoperative course is much easier and the recovery significantly shorter than in cases of standard laparotomy. The optimal surgical choice is enucleation of the tumor because the normal pancreas is spared, and postoperative hyperglycemia is prevented. Some tumors, however, are large, and a more formal resection such as a distal pancreatectomy is necessary.

Children with PHHI usually have diffuse rather than focal hyperinsulinism and require a 95% to 98% pancreatectomy to eliminate hypoglycemia. Unfortunately, >50% of children undergoing this large of a pancreatectomy develop hyperglycemia that requires insulin therapy within 10 years after surgery.

Medical treatment is necessary for those tumors that are surgically nonresectable, metastatic, or in individuals who are at a poor surgical risk. The most commonly used

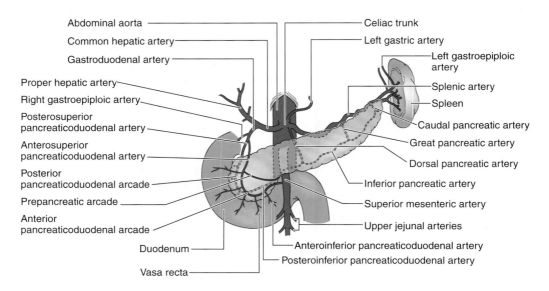

FIGURE 21-7. Arterial supply to the pancreas. (From Woodburne RT. Essentials of Human Anatomy. New York, NY: Oxford University Press; 1973.)

drugs to control hyperinsulinism are diazoxide and octreotide. Diazoxide is a potassium-channel activator that decreases insulin release from the insulin-secreting cells. Octreotide is a somatostatin analog that has diffuse and global effects on the inhibition of many hormones but also has a wide range of side effects. Diazoxide, because of its target at the islet cell, is the preferred medical therapy for insulinomas in nonoperative candidates.

Indications for Pancreatic Surgery

Surgery for insulinoma is indicated for treatment of hypoglycemia despite dietary and medical therapy. Individuals with small gastrinomas (<2.5 cm) should be managed medically because less than 20% of individuals undergoing surgical resection for a gastrinoma are disease free a year later. Due to the increased risk of malignancy, large gastrinomas (>2.5 cm) should be removed surgically.

Complications of Pancreatic Surgery

Complications may occur in up to 50% of patients, but most are minor. Most complications occur in patients undergoing the large operations (i.e., pancreatectomy or pancreaticoduodenectomy). After removal of a portion of the pancreas, the pancreatic duct or its small tributaries may not seal effectively and result in a leakage of pancreatic enzymes. Other complications include bleeding, abscess formation, pancreatitis, or development of a fistula.

ADRENAL GLAND

The adrenal glands are paired structures located superior to each of the kidneys (Figure 21-8). The adrenal gland is divided into an outer cortex and an inner medulla. The cortex originates from mesodermal tissue near the gonads on the adrenogenital ridge at the fifth week of gestation. Adrenocortical tissue is located in the ovaries, spermatic cord, and testes. The adrenal cortex is composed of three zones based on structure and

Anterior view

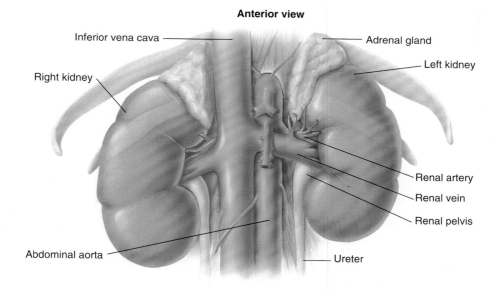

FIGURE 21-8. Adrenal glands. (Asset provided by Anatomical Chart Co.)

function: 1) zona glomerulosa, 2) zona fasciculata, and 3) zona reticularis. The outermost zona glomerulosa is responsible for production of the mineralocorticoids that maintain sodium, potassium, and fluid balance. The middle zona fasciculata is the largest zone and makes up 80% of the cortex. It produces glucocorticoids that affect metabolism of glucose and proteins. The innermost zona reticularis secretes androgens.

The adrenal medulla originates from the neural crest; it is ectodermal in origin. The adrenal medulla produces the catecholamines epinephrine, norepinephrine, and dopamine. These hormones activate the sympathetic nervous system (SNS) during periods of stress. The adrenal medulla secretes catecholamines under control of the SNS. Basal secretion of catecholamines is very low; however, under periods of stress, sympathetic activity results in release of catecholamines into the bloodstream in preparation for a "fight-or-flight" response. Epinephrine and norepinephrine act on multiple α- and β-adrenergic receptors to cause several different effects in target tissues. Vasoconstrictive and vasodilatory effects are prominent in different tissues, as are positive chronotropic and inotropic effects on the heart. Epinephrine and norepinephrine increase the metabolic rate, stimulate glycogenolysis, and raise blood glucose, free-fatty acid, and lactate levels. Epinephrine and norepinephrine also increase alertness.

Each adrenal gland is supplied by three sets of arteries: the superior adrenal (from the inferior phrenic artery), the middle adrenal (from the aorta), and the inferior adrenal (from the renal artery). These vessels branch into as many as 50 arterioles. The left adrenal vein empties into the ipsilateral renal vein, whereas the right adrenal vein drains directly into the inferior vena cava (Figure 21-9).

Adrenal Gland Disorders

The adrenal gland disorders that require surgery include adrenal adenomas, carcinomas, and pheochromocytomas. Because the symptoms adrenal masses produce are commonly subtle, individuals may not present to the clinician until significant morbidity has occurred. The individual with an adrenal adenoma and carcinoma may present with signs and symptoms of glucocorticoid (Cushing syndrome), mineralocorticoid (hyperaldosteronism), or androgen excess. Individuals with pheochromocytomas may be hypertensive and have

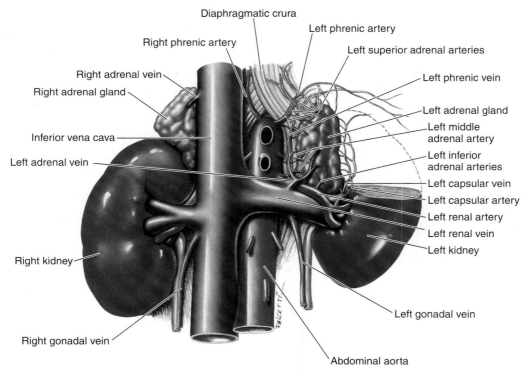

FIGURE 21-9. Blood supply to the adrenal glands. Schematic drawing showing the inferior vena cava, the aorta, the renal veins and arteries, and the relationship of these structures with the adrenal glands. Note the arterial and venous supply of the left adrenal gland. Only the vein of the right adrenal gland is shown. (From Uflacker R. Atlas of Vascular Anatomy: An Angiographic Approach. 2nd ed. Philadelphia, PA: Lippincott Williams & Wilkins; 2006.)

symptoms of headaches and sweating. Insofar as each of the adrenal conditions that require surgery present as an adrenal mass, they are presented and discussed as an adrenal mass, rather than each individually. Adrenal gland disorders are discussed in detail in Chapter 10 and pheochromocytomas are discussed in detail in Chapter 11.

Adrenal Mass

An adrenal mass is a preliminary term that has not yet been thoroughly delineated. It could be functional or nonfunctional, benign or malignant, and affect the cortex or the medulla. Masses that appear to have no correlation to a particular layer of the adrenal gland include metastatic lesions, cysts, ganglioneuromas, and hematomas. The widespread use of ultrasound, CT, and MRI scans over the past two decades has led to a significant increase in the number of these lesions identified. It is found in up to 4% of patients undergoing abdominal imaging.

The etiology of an adrenal mass depends on the layer of adrenal tissue involved.

Adrenal Cortex Mass

A cortical mass may be a functional or a nonfunctional adenoma or an adrenocortical cancer. Individuals with an adenoma of the adrenal cortical fasciculata that secretes excess glucocorticoid have Cushing syndrome and exhibit signs and symptoms of hypercortisolism; those with an adenoma of the adrenal cortical glomerulosa have hyperaldosteronism; and in those with an adenoma of the adrenal cortical reticularis have signs and symptoms of androgen excess. Not uncommonly, an adrenal adenoma or carcinoma can extend beyond just one layer of the adrenal cortex. These individuals, as might be expected, have clinical findings with excess secretion of multiple hormones.

Adrenal Medulla Mass

A medullary mass may be a benign or a malignant pheochromocytoma. A pheochromocytoma is a neuroendocrine tumor that usually arises in the adrenal medulla from chromaffin cells or is extra-adrenal from chromaffin tissue that failed to involute after birth. These tumors secrete excessive amounts of catecholamines (epinephrine, norepinephrine, and their metabolites). Most occur sporadically, but at least 25% are due to genetic mutations. A number of gene mutations are associated with familial pheochromocytoma. The pheochromocytoma is also a tumor of the MEN syndrome (type 2A or 2B). The MEN syndromes are discussed in detail in Chapter 17. The effects of catecholamine excess produce the clinical findings. The principal catecholamines produced by a pheochromocytoma are epinephrine, norepinephrine, homovanillic acid, and vanillylmandelic acid. These catecholamines activate $\alpha 1$, $\alpha 2$, $\beta 1$, and $\beta 2$ receptors. Norepinephrine, the catecholamine principally produced by extra-adrenal pheochromocytomas, has $\alpha 1$, $\alpha 2$, and $\beta 1$ effects. The most accurate case-finding method for identifying catecholamine-secreting tumors is measuring fractionated metanephrines and catecholamines in a 24-hour urine collection (sensitivity 98%, specificity 98%).

Adrenal Gland Surgery

A laparoscopic approach (with or without hand-assist) under general anesthesia is used when nonmalignant adrenal lesions <12 cm are to be excised. An open anterior transabdominal, flank extraperitoneal, or posterior retroperitoneal approach with resection of the 12th rib is used when an adrenal adenocarcinoma is large (>12 cm) or has extensive adhesions or when portal hypertension is present. Intermittent compression stockings are applied to the lower extremities before the operation begins. For patients with large vasoactive tumors, arterial blood pressure monitoring and central venous catheterization is often necessary.

Unilateral laparoscopic adrenalectomy is the treatment of choice for adrenal adenomas. Open adrenalectomies are required for carcinomas to prevent accidental release of cancerous cells. Surgical excision of an adrenocortical carcinoma is the only curative therapy. Transabdominal adrenalectomy, with excision of any involved structures such as liver, kidney, spleen, or pancreas is recommended. Postoperative chemotherapy with mitotane, the best anti-neoplastic agent available, may be necessary.

Laparoscopic adrenalectomy is associated with minimal blood loss, conversion to an open procedure <5% of the time, a short operating time, and only modest stress and morbidity. An open adrenalectomy, on the other hand, may be associated with moderate blood loss, longer operating times, and moderate stress.

Indications for Adrenal Gland Surgery

The indications for an adrenalectomy are: 1) benign adrenal tumor associated with hyperaldosteronism (Conn syndrome), Cushing syndrome, or pheochromocytoma; 2) large (>6 cm) nonfunctioning adrenal tumors; and 3) primary adrenal carcinoma.

Complications of Adrenal Gland Surgery

Complications from adrenalectomy are due to either the surgery or are specific to the type of tumor involved. Surgical complications include damage to the surrounding bowel, hemorrhage, infection, adhesions, and poor wound healing. For the surgical removal of a pheochromocytoma, an intraoperative hypertensive crisis due to massive release of catecholamines, or postoperative hypotension following catecholamine reduction, may cause an Addisonian crisis because removal of the glucocorticoid-secreting tumor may suppress the nonaffected adrenal gland by negative feedback from the obligatory excess steroid production preoperatively. A patient experiencing an Addisonian crisis during or shortly after an adrenalectomy should be treated with fluids and small, intermittent doses of IV pressor agents as needed. Postoperative hypotension is less frequent in patients who have had adequate preoperative α-adrenergic blockade and volume expansion.

Individuals with Cushing disease who have an inoperable pituitary adenoma may require a bilateral adrenalectomy to prevent hypercortisolism. If appropriate exogenous glucocorticoid is not administered, these patients may develop Nelson syndrome, in which corticotropin-releasing hormone stimulates adenomatous corticotropes to secrete ACTH. The ACTH secretory burst in patients with Nelson syndrome is more marked than in patients with untreated Cushing disease. The differences are likely due to unique tumoral secretory properties or hypothalamic injury related to the actual adenoma, or treatment of it, prior to bilateral adrenalectomy. Patients with Nelson syndrome develop significant hyperpigmentation because of the action of ACTH on melanocytes.

CASE FOLLOW-UP

Our patient's strong family history of thyroid cancer along with her clinical presentation makes thyroid cancer a leading diagnosis. Medullary carcinoma of the thyroid gland is the most likely inherited thyroid cancer. Many patients present late and only after developing signs and symptoms of thyroid cancer. Therefore, it is imperative that once there is a family history of thyroid cancer, all family members should undergo genetic testing for the presence of the *RET* proto-oncogene mutation.

Due to our patient's family history of medullary carcinoma of the thyroid gland, a serum calcitonin level is measured, and ultrasonography of her thyroid gland is obtained.

The ultrasound of her thyroid gland is normal, but her serum calcitonin level (21 pg/mL; normal range = 0 to 12) is elevated. Based on these findings and together with her family history, she most likely has medullary carcinoma of the thyroid. Because she does not have any of the classic symptoms, the cancer is likely in its early stages, and she would benefit from a thyroidectomy.

Medullary carcinoma of the thyroid originates from the parafollicular cells (C cells) that produce the hormone calcitonin. Approximately 25% of the causes are genetic due to a mutation in the *RET* proto-oncogene. When it is isolated, it is known as *familial medullary carcinoma of the thyroid*. When it coexists with tumors of the parathyroid gland and the adrenal gland (pheochromocytoma), it is referred to as *MEN 2*.

Mutations in the *RET* proto-oncogene lead to the expression of a mutated receptor tyrosine kinase protein that is involved in the regulation of cell growth and development. Hereditary medullary carcinoma of the thyroid is inherited as an autosomal dominant trait. DNA analysis makes it possible to identify children

(continues)

CASE FOLLOW-UP (*continued*)

who carry the mutant gene. If the entire thyroid gland is surgically removed at any early age (i.e., before the tumor metastasizes), a cure is usually achieved.

Because our patient is symptom free, there is enough time to collect a DNA analysis and determine if she has a mutation of the *RET* proto-oncogene.

Within a few weeks, genetic analysis reveals that she does have a mutation of the *RET* proto-oncogene that is characteristic of familial medullary carcinoma of the thyroid gland.

She undergoes a total thyroidectomy 2 months after presenting to her pediatrician. The surgery is uneventful but does include the reimplantation of her parathyroid glands into her sternocleidomastoid muscle. The following day she is started on replacement levothyroxine therapy.

There are no complications from her surgery, and her calcium and phosphate levels remain in the normal range postoperatively. She has routine follow-up visits to her pediatric endocrinologist every 6 months for height, weight, and thyroid-function monitoring. Serum calcitonin, calcium, and phosphate levels are performed yearly as long as they remain in the normal range and she is symptom free.

REFERENCES and SUGGESTED READINGS

Adelman DT, Liebert KJ, Nachtigall LB, Lamerson M, Bakker B. Acromegaly: the disease, its impact on patients, and managing the burden of long-term treatment. Int J Gen Med. 2013;6:31–38.

Ahmad R, Hammond JM. Primary, secondary, and tertiary hyperparathyroidism. Otolaryngol Clin North Am. 2004;37(4):701–713.

Bliss RD, Gauger PG, Delbridge LW. Surgical approach to the thyroid gland: surgical anatomy and the importance of technique. World J Surg. 2000;24:891–897.

Bokhari AR, Davies MA, Diamond T. Endoscopic transphenoidal pituitary surgery: a single surgeon experience and the learning curve. Br J Neurosurg. 2013;27(1):44–49.

Colao A, Savastano S. Medical treatment of prolactinomas. Nat Rev Endocrinol. 2011;7:267–278.

Eigelberger MS, Cheah WK, Ituarte PHG, Streja L, Duh QY, Clark OH. The NIH criteria for parathyroidectomy in asymptomatic primary hyperparathyroidism. Are they too limited? Ann Surg. 2004;239(4):528–535.

Ellison TA, Edil BH. The current management of pancreatic neuroendocrine tumors. Adv Surg. 2012; 46:283–296.

Ezzat S. Acromegaly. Endocrinol Metab Clin North Am. 1997;26(4):703–723.

Fraker DL, Harsono H, Lewis R. Minimally invasive parathyroidectomy: benefits and requirements of localization, diagnosis, and intraoperative PTH monitoring. Long-term results. World J Surg. 2009;33(11):2256–2265.

Jho HD, Carrau RL. Endoscopic pituitary surgery: an early experience. Surg Neurol. 1997;47:213–223.

Kamran SC, Marqusee E, Kim MI, et al. Thyroid nodule size and prediction of cancer. J Clin Endocrinol Metab. 2013;98(2):564–570.

Kienitz T, Quinkler M, Strasburger CJ, Ventz M. Long term management in five cases of TSH-secreting pituitary adenomas: a single center study and review of the literature. Euro J Endocrinol. 2007; 157:39–46.

Klibanski, A. Clinical practice. Prolactinoma. N Engl J Med. 2010;362:1219–1225.

Lucas JW, Zada G. Endoscopic surgery for pituitary tumors. Neurosurg Clin North Am. 2012;23(4): 555–569.

Martins RG, Agrawal R, Berney DM, et al. Differential diagnosis of adrenocorticotropic hormone-independent Cushing syndrome: role of adrenal venous sampling. Endocr Pract. 2012;18(6):e153–e157.

Mazzaferri EL. An overview of the management of papillary and follicular thyroid carcinoma. Thyroid 1999;9(5):421–427.

Nayak B, Burman K. Thyrotoxicosis and thyroid storm. Endocrinol Metab Clin North Am. 2006;35(4):663–686.

Patel SK, Christiano LD, Eloy JA, Liu JK. Delayed postoperative pituitary apoplexy after endoscopic transsphenoidal resection of a giant pituitary macroadenoma. J Clin Neurosci. 2012;19(9):1296–1298.

Patterson ME, Mao CS, Yeh MW, et al. Hyperinsulinism presenting in childhood and treatment by conservative pancreatectomy. Endocr Pract. 2012; 18(3):e52–e56.

Pradeep PV, Agarwal A, Baxi M, Agarwal G, Gupta SK, Mishra SK. Safety and efficacy of surgical management of hyperthyroidism: 15-year experience from a tertiary care center in a developing country. World J Surg. 2007;31(2):306–312.

Prejbisz A, Lenders JW, Eisenhofer G, Januszewicz A. Mortality associated with phaeochromocytoma. Horm Metab Res. 2013;45(2):154–158.

Raff H, Findling JW. A physiologic approach to diagnosis of the Cushing syndrome. Ann Intern Med. 2003;138(12):980–991.

Young WF. Clinical practice. The incidentally discovered adrenal mass. N Engl J Med. 2007;356(6):601–610.

CHAPTER REVIEW QUESTIONS

1. A 32-year-old man is concerned about his risk for developing thyroid cancer. His past medical history is insignificant. He does not smoke or consume alcohol. His family history reveals that his father, paternal uncle, and paternal grandmother had thyroidectomies for thyroid cancer. Which of the following tests is most effective in predicting his risk for developing thyroid cancer?

   A. Annual physical exam
   B. Frequent self-exam of the neck
   C. Annual head and neck CT
   D. Periodic calcitonin measurement
   E. DNA testing for a mutation of the *RET* proto-oncogene

2. A 38-year-old woman presents with a 6-month history of headaches and difficulty with vision. She also states that it is difficult for her to see vehicles on the sides of her car while she is driving. Her past medical history is unremarkable, and she has not been taking any medications. She smokes a pack of cigarettes per day and has done so for the past 10 years. On visual field exam, she has a defect in her peripheral vision. The patient undergoes transsphenoidal surgery, and an adenoma is removed. Which of the following would not be a complication of this type of surgery?

   A. Leakage of CSF
   B. Hypothyroidism
   C. Meningitis
   D. Cushing syndrome
   E. GH deficiency

3. A 60-year-old man is admitted to the hospital with pneumonia. His medical history is significant for hypertension, diabetes mellitus, and kidney stones. He also has severe degenerative disk disease of the lumbar spine and complains of constant lower back pain. During his hospitalization, the laboratory report shows an elevated serum calcium level (12.8 mg/dL; normal = 8.5 to 10.5) and low phosphate level (1.9 mg/dL; normal = 3.0 to 4.5). A serum PTH level is then ordered; the result is elevated (185 pg/mL; normal = 10 to 60). Of the following, which is the best method for managing this patient?

   A. Treatment with oral phosphate therapy and repeat labs in 1 month
   B. Thyroidectomy
   C. Minimally invasive parathyroidectomy regardless of the preoperative sestamibi scan
   D. Hemodialysis and repeat labs in 1 week
   E. Conventional parathyroidectomy with collection of intraoperative parathyroid hormone (IOPTH) levels after parathyroid removal

4. Within 10 minutes after undergoing an adrenalectomy, a 27-year-old man develops hypotension that responds to fluid therapy. Prior to the procedure he was normotensive, but during initial manipulation of the adrenal gland, he became hypertensive. His serum sodium and potassium levels were normal prior to, during, and after surgery. What was the most likely preoperative diagnosis?

A. Hyperaldosteronism
B. Cushing syndrome
C. Pheochromocytoma
D. Adrenal cortical carcinoma
E. Ganglioneuroma

5. A 45-year-old woman is evaluated in the office for a 7-kg (14.4 lb) weight gain over the past 2 years. She complains that she usually awakens in the middle of the night trembling, weak, and sweating, a condition that is relieved after she eats crackers and drinks a cola. Initial laboratory findings reveal a serum glucose level of 30 mg/dL. Laboratory studies repeated the next day reveal a serum glucose of 34 mg/dL with a simultaneous cortisol of 19 µg/dL and an insulin level of 13 mIU/L. All of the following would be appropriate steps in managing this patient *except*:

A. Calcium gluconate infusion to assess insulin levels
B. Measurement of serum ACTH
C. CT scan of the abdomen
D. MRI of the abdomen
E. Treatment with octreotide

CHAPTER REVIEW ANSWERS

1. The correct answer is E. DNA testing for a mutation of the *RET* proto-oncogene should be performed in those patients with a family history of medullary carcinoma of the thyroid or MEN 2. A genetic test can be performed from a peripheral blood sample at any age. If the DNA test is positive, a total thyroidectomy is indicated, because the risk of developing medullary thyroid carcinoma is near 100%.

An annual physical exam (**Choice A**) should be performed in all patients with or without a medical history. However, in patients with a family history of medullary carcinoma of the thyroid, the tumor has metastasized by the time findings are discovered on physical exam. Frequent self-examination of the neck (**Choice B**) is not very helpful because by the time a patient recognizes an abnormality on the neck the cancer may have metastasized. Annual head and neck CT scans (**Choice C**) are expensive and may not show a significant change until the cancer has metastasized. Periodic calcitonin measurements (**Choice D**) are useful after total thyroidectomy for a medullary carcinoma of the thyroid to determine if residual tumor is present but are less sensitive than a DNA analysis.

2. The correct answer is D. Cushing syndrome, or excess production of cortisol, is not a complication of transsphenoidal surgery for removal of a GH-secreting adenoma. Based on the clinical description, this woman has a GH-secreting mass in her pituitary gland that requires transsphenoidal removal. All of the other choices are potential complications from this type of surgery.

A leakage of CSF (**Choice A**) and meningitis (**Choice C**) are nonendocrine complications of transsphenoidal surgery. Hormone deficiencies due to removal of a pituitary tumor such as hypothyroidism (**Choice B**), adrenal insufficiency, and GH deficiency (**Choice E**) are endocrine-related complications to transsphenoidal surgery.

---

3. The correct answer is E. A conventional parathyroidectomy with collection of intra-operative parathyroid hormone (IOPTH) levels after gland removal is the best option for this man who has primary hyperparathyroidism and likely has experienced symptoms for a long time.

Treatment with oral phosphate therapy and repeat labs in 1 month (**Choice A**) is not an appropriate treatment for primary hyperparathyroidism. This man is symptomatic and needs relief now. Oral phosphate may slightly reduce his serum calcium; however, it would likely not reduce it to normal and would most likely promote kidney stones. A thyroidectomy (**Choice B**) would be inappropriate as his thyroid function is normal. He needs to have the parathyroid adenoma(s) removed. A minimally invasive parathyroidectomy, regardless of the preoperative sestamibi scan (**Choice C**), is not the best option because it is not diagnostic. Although the minimally invasive approach is the recommended surgical treatment, it is best when the sestamibi scan is diagnostic to accurately localize the adenoma(s). Hemodialysis and repeat labs in 1 week (**Choice D**) is not appropriate because there is no evidence or history of renal failure, hyperkalemia, or metabolic acidosis.

---

4. The correct answer is C. This patient developed hypertension during surgery because the surgeon was manipulating the adrenal mass. He then developed hypotension soon after the mass was removed. This sequence is characteristic of a pheochromocytoma.

If the patient had hyperaldosteronism (**Choice A**) he most likely would have been hypertensive prior to the surgery. He would not have been normotensive initially then hypertensive during surgery, and hypotensive after surgery and still maintain normal electrolytes. If the patient had Cushing syndrome (**Choice B**), he may have been hypertensive before surgery but would be unlikely to develop hypertension during the surgery and hypotensive postoperatively. For an adrenal cortical carcinoma (**Choice D**), these blood pressure findings would likely only occur if the electrolytes were abnormal. Removal of a ganglioneuroma (**Choice E**) should have no effect on blood pressure.

---

5. The correct answer is B. This woman has an insulinoma, and there is no need to measure serum ACTH levels. All of the other choices are appropriate for evaluation or treatment of a patient with an insulinoma. With hypoglycemia, the woman's cortisol level is the appropriate counterregulatory response, indicating that it is unnecessary to pursue adrenal insufficiency as a cause for her hypoglycemia.

For a patient suspected of having an insulinoma, performing an arterial calcium gluconate infusion (**Choice A**) to assess insulin levels around the pancreas is appropriate. An imaging study, such as a CT scan (**Choice C**) or MRI of the abdomen (**Choice D**), is appropriate to accurately locate a pancreatic mass. In patients who are not good surgical candidates or who need medical therapy while awaiting surgery, treatment with octreotide (**Choice E**), a somatostatin analog, is an appropriate choice because it inhibits insulin secretion.

Index

Page numbers followed by *f* indicate figures; those followed by *t* indicate tables.